Advances in Human Services and Public Health (AHSPH) Book Series

Jennifer Martin
RMIT University, Australia

ISSN:2475-6571
EISSN:2475-658X

Mission

The well-being of the general public should be a primary concern for any modern civilization. Ongoing research in the field of human services and public healthcare is necessary to evaluate, manage, and respond to the health and social needs of the global population.

The **Advances in Human Services and Public Health (AHSPH)** bc high-quality reference publications focused on the latest methodologies, too managing the health and social welfare of the public. The AHSPH book s evant for healthcare professionals, policy makers, government officials, and research in this field.

Coverage

- Public Welfare
- Domestic Violence
- Health Policy
- Access to Healthcare Services
- Youth Development
- Public Funding
- Social Welfare Policy
- Medicare and Medicaid
- Healthcare Reform
- Poverty

IGI Global is currently accepting manuscripts for publication within this series. To submit a proposal for a volume in this series, please contact our Acquisition Editors at Acquisitions@igi-global.com or visit: http://www.igi-global.com/publish/.

The Advances in Human Services and Public Health (AHSPH) Book Series (ISSN 2475-6571) is published by IGI Global, 701 E. Chocolate Avenue, Hershey, PA 17033-1240, USA, www.igi-global.com. This series is composed of titles available for purchase individually; each title is edited to be contextually exclusive from any other title within the series. For pricing and ordering information please visit http://www.igi-global.com/book-series/advances-human-services-public-health/102256. Postmaster: Send all address changes to above address.

Titles in this Series

For a list of additional titles in this series, please visit: www.igi-global.com/book-series/advances-human-services-public-health/102256

Ecological and Evolutionary Perspectives on Infections and Morbidity
P.A. Azeez (Salim Ali Centre for Ornithology and Natural History, Coimbatore, India) P.P. Nikhil Raj (Amrita Vishwa Vidyapeetham University, India) and R. Mohanraj (Bharathidasan University, ndia)
Medical Information Science Reference • © 2022 • 315pp • H/C (ISBN: 9781799894148) • US $295.00

Modern Challenges and Approaches to Humanitarian Engineering
Yiannis Koumpouros (University of West Attica, Greece) Angelos Georgoulas (University of West Attica, Greece) and Georgia Kremmyda (University of Warwick, UK)
Engineering Science Reference • © 2022 • 321pp • H/C (ISBN: 9781799891901) • US $215.00

Societal Resilience and Response to Contagious Diseases and Pandemics
Amal Adel Abdrabo (Faculty of Education, Alexandria University, Egypt) and Aly Abdel Razek Galaby (Faculty of Arts, Alexandria University, Egypt)
Information Science Reference • © 2022 • 344pp • H/C (ISBN: 9781799889731) • US $215.00

Tactical Sciences for Biosecurity in Animal and Plant Systems
Kitty F. Cardwell (Oklahoma State University, USA) and Keith L. Bailey (Charles River Laboratories, Inc., USA)
Information Science Reference • © 2022 • 454pp • H/C (ISBN: 9781799879350) • US $195.00

Handbook of Research on Interdisciplinary Perspectives on the Threats and Impacts of Pandemics
Şahver Omeraki Çekirdekci (Haliç University, Turkey) Özlem İngün Karkış (Doğuş University, Turkey) and Suna Gönültaş (Doğuş University, Turkey)
Information Science Reference • © 2022 • 556pp • H/C (ISBN: 9781799886747) • US $245.00

Smart Cities and Machine Learning in Urban Health
J. Joshua Thomas (UOW Malaysia KDU Penang University College, Malaysia) Vasiliki Geropanta (Technical University of Crete, Greece) Anna Karagianni (Technical Chamber of Greece, Greece) Vladimir Panchenko (Russian University of Transport, Russia) and Pandian Vasant (MERLIN Research Center, TDTU, Vietnam)
Information Science Reference • © 2022 • 269pp • H/C (ISBN: 9781799871767) • US $195.00

Handbook of Research on Digital Citizenship and Management During Crises
Erdem Öngün (Trakya University, Turkey) Nilüfer Pembecioğlu (Istanbul University, Turkey) and Uğur Gündüz (Istanbul University, Turkey)
Information Science Reference • © 2022 • 440pp • H/C (ISBN: 9781799884217) • US $275.00

IGI Global
PUBLISHER of TIMELY KNOWLEDGE

701 East Chocolate Avenue, Hershey, PA 17033, USA
Tel: 717-533-8845 x100 • Fax: 717-533-8661
E-Mail: cust@igi-global.com • www.igi-global.com

Assessing the Effects of Emerging Plastics on the Environment and Public Health

Sung Hee Joo
University of Seoul, South Korea

IGI Global
PUBLISHER of TIMELY KNOWLEDGE

A volume in the Advances in Human Services and Public Health (AHSPH) Book Series

Published in the United States of America by
IGI Global
Engineering Science Reference (an imprint of IGI Global)
701 E. Chocolate Avenue
Hershey PA, USA 17033
Tel: 717-533-8845
Fax: 717-533-8661
E-mail: cust@igi-global.com
Web site: http://www.igi-global.com

Library of Congress Cataloging-in-Publication Data

Names: Joo, Sung Hee, editor.
Title: Assessing the effects of emerging plastics on the environment and public health / Sung Hee Joo, editor.
Description: Hershey, PA : Engineering Science Reference, [2022] | Includes bibliographical references and index. | Summary: "With plastic pollution concerns growing globally, especially the production, consumption, and disposal of face masks, medical gloves, personal protective equipment and plastic dishes, this book is about assessing harmful effects of plastics on the environment and public health"-- Provided by publisher.
Identifiers: LCCN 2022970008 (print) | LCCN 2022970009 (ebook) | ISBN 9781799897231 (hardcover) | ISBN 9781799897248 (paperback) | ISBN 9781799897255 (ebook)
Subjects: LCSH: Plastics--Environmental aspects. | Plastics--Health aspects.
Classification: LCC TD798 .A85 2022 (print) | LCC TD798 (ebook) | DDC 620.1/923--dc23/eng/20220301
LC record available at https://lccn.loc.gov/2022970008
LC ebook record available at https://lccn.loc.gov/2022970009

This book is published in the IGI Global book series Advances in Human Services and Public Health (AHSPH) (ISSN: 2475-6571; eISSN: 2475-658X)

British Cataloguing in Publication Data
A Cataloguing in Publication record for this book is available from the British Library.

Table of Contents

Detailed Table of Contents

Plastic pollution is a global transboundary threat to the planet's marine resources. Tracking pollution is crucial to implement effective marine management strategies on coastal and island regions, where mismanaged plastics are most at risk of entering the ocean. However, the uncertainty of sources and pathways of marine litter poses a major challenge to the assessment of marine pollution. This chapter reviews the principal sectors and human activities contributing to plastic pollution, the mechanisms by which plastic enters the ocean, and some possible drivers of marine litter, including the growing role of coastal tourism on small developing islands. It also outlines future directions for meaningfully integrating research, material accounting, and prevention actions to mitigate the infiltration of plastic pollution in the marine environment, via proper monitoring, assessment, and reporting on plastic material flows from source to sink.

Microplastics are the newly identified pollutant of this century, yet they are already detected everywhere worldwide. Microplastic pollution in global marine environments has been intensively reported. Evidence of microplastic pollution is emerging in other environments, including land, freshwater, atmosphere, and organisms. Public concerns were also raised about microplastic pollution around them. From terrestrial environments, through freshwater environments, finally to marine environments, is a major transportation route of microplastic pollution. Human activities are the fundamental source of microplastic pollution. Cities, with the highest population density on this planet, are important sources of microplastic pollutants.

It is unavoidable that microplastics (MPs; <5 mm in diameter) are becoming widespread in agroecosystem. However, these changes act upon the agroecosystem with far-reaching but poorly understood consequences on ecosystem functions and subsequent plant-soil health. MPs could change a broad of essential soil biogeochemical processes by effecting soil properties, forming specific microbial hotspots, inducing diversed influences on microbial functions. The physical damage or chemical toxicity on soil organisms and plants caused by MPs may influence plant health. Due to the C contained in MPs, it contributes to the accumulation of soil organic matter as well dissolved organic matter. This further stimulates microbial activity and consequently CO2 and N2O emissions. Enhanced soluble C released from the decomposition of bioplastics increases microbial nutrient immobilizatization and thus causes competition between plants and microbes. Although MPs may confer some benefits in agroecosystems, it is thought that these will be far outweighed by the potential disbenefits.

Chapter 6
Preventive Measures for Plastic Pollution 111
Bupe Getrude Mwanza, University of Zambia, Zambia

The production of plastics has rapidly overwhelmed the world's ability to manage it, hence the demanding environmental issues on plastics pollution. The negative effects of plastics have become omnipresent and prompted many studies to be conducted leading to a global treaty. This study focused on reviewing measures for preventing plastic pollution in the environment. Based on the literature review approach, seven key measures are identified: recycling prioritization, utilization of bio-based and biodegradable plastics, improvement of waste collection systems, awareness and education in communities, extended producer responsibility (EPR) enforcement, strengthen stakeholder engagement, and technology and innovations. The study concludes by providing practical recommendations that should be implemented contextually.

Chapter 7
Study of the Potential Impact of Microplastics and Additives on Human Health 128
Ranjit Barua, Omdayal Group of Institutions, India
Debasish Banerjee, Omdayal Group of Institutions, India
Sumit Bhowmik, Omdayal Group of Institutions, India

The spreading and abundance of micro and nano plastics into the world are so wide that many researchers used them as main pointers of the modern and contemporary period defining a new historical era. However, the inferences of microplastics are not yet systematically understood. There is the significant difficulty involved to know their impact due to dissimilar physical-chemical characteristics that make micro-plastics complex stressors. Micro-plastics carry toxic chemicals in the ecosystems, therefore serving as vectors of transport, and, on the other hand, a combination of dangerous chemicals that are further voluntarily during their manufacture as additives to increase polymer properties and extend their life. In this chapter, the authors prominently discuss the different kinds of literature on micro and nano-plastic exposure pathways and their probable risk to human health to encapsulate present information with the target of enhanced attention, upcoming study in this area, and information gaps.

In the contemporary world, the menace of plastic pollution dovetailed with the current pandemic scenario is a globally rising concern which is affecting every life form on Earth. Plastics hold several properties like ductility that permit the material to be casted and given numerous shapes and forms for various commercial uses. When summed up, it has benefited mankind by becoming an indispensable part of our lives. But the negative impacts associated with it lurks behind silently. Most of the plastic polymers manufactured today are highly resistant to degradation, and the accumulation of these complex and persistent materials are not only causing serious damage to the environment, but also to human health. Additives are added during the manufacturing process to improve the life of these synthetic polymers. The excessive usage of plastic products has resulted in accumulation of the hazardous chemicals, associated with plastic polymers in human body about which this chapter discusses further.

Plastic contamination in the ocean has recently received a lot of attention. Plastic production has been growing and its use spread to many sectors. More than 80% of plastic enters the ocean from land-based sources, with the remaining having ocean-based sources. Once in the ocean, plastic undergoes fragmentation and degradation that lead to the formation of microplastics (MPs) and nanoplastics (NPs), and their dimensions are becoming an environmental concern. Thus, this chapter provides an overview of the effects of MPs and NPs on marine organisms, from bacteria to fish. Plastic affects marine organisms from molecular to population levels but some knowledge gaps exist regarding the biogeochemical cycle of plastic, how it behaves and is distributed in the aquatic-sediment compartment and in deep-sea. Moreover, more attention is necessary concerning NPs ecotoxicological effects already detected and because not all polymer types and size effects have been investigated. In addition, risk assessment of plastic particles is needed to characterize their risks and for data to be comparable.

Pollution by microplastics is a recent global problem owing to their preponderance in various matrices like air, water, biota, sediment, or soil and has become a global concern for the future generation sustainability. The mushrooming concerns about the detrimental effects of microplastics (MPs) on biota in response to its crescive detection and quantification in the aqueous ecosystems is looming large since last few decades, and it's a need of the hour for a thorough ecological risk assessment. The chapter highlights the MP production, release, and transport pathways along with its detrimental impacts on the aquatic biota at different levels of biological organization with available degradation approaches.

Plastics are one of the essential materials due to their low cost and properties. Plastics are used almost everywhere including food packaging, home appliance, agriculture, automobile, electrical insulators, medical instruments, etc. However, due to the low biodegradability of conventional plastics, they remain in the environment for a very long time and thus pose a serious threat to our environment. Getting rid of these plastics is very difficult. The burning of plastics produces harmful chemicals that negatively impact the environment (e.g., global warming) and human health. Plastic management via recycling is an incomplete measure to address the environmental impacts of plastic. Therefore, there is a demand for developing alternative plastic materials that will be more environmentally friendly. Bioplastics have attracted much attention as a potential replacement for conventional plastics. This chapter will focus on the development, properties, and applications of various bioplastics. The biodegradability of the bioplastics will also be discussed.

The ever-growing demand and consumption of plastic has created irrevocable havoc on earth. The exponential increase in the production of plastic is expected to create 2,134 million tons of waste by 2050, which surpasses the fish mass in the oceans. With no proper reuse or recycling policies and gruesome exploitation of this persistent pollutant, plastic has started accumulating and overflowing beyond control. The prevalence and the undefined harm from micro and nano plastic pollution calls for a vigilant screening and periodic upgradation of analytical methodology for efficient and standard reporting. This chapter aims to provide a summary of currently available extraction protocols and instrumental methodologies for microplastics analysis in various environmental samples to fully understand the implications it possesses.

Identification and quantification of microplastics (MPs) pollution levels in all the environmental compartments including water, sediments, and biota are an hourly need. MPs analytical techniques in water, sediments, and biota consist of several laborious steps including sampling, sample handling, and analytical techniques for identification and quantification. Studies have employed a wide variety of techniques resulting in variation in MPs abundance and characteristics. MPs reporting techniques also vary between different studies. The sampling techniques, digestion reagents, the temperature applied, density separation reagents, and the techniques utilized cause significant impacts on the recovery rate of the MPs particles from samples. 20-10 µm has become the lower reliable, practical limit for MPs due to the limitations in identification methods. Since there is many more MPs research to be done, there is an urgency of establishing reliable and efficient standard methodologies for MPs monitoring enabling comparison of studies from different parts of the world.

The aim of this chapter is to investigate the environmental effect of plastics (macroplastic and microplastic)

Preface

The term "plastic" has been well known to the public for many years. Yet serious issues related to plastic pollution have just recently been recognized—in particular, the escalated negative impacts of plastic pollution on the environment and public health. Plastic pollution has been a growing concern globally, especially under the current COVID-19 pandemic, including but not limited to the production, consumption, and disposal of face masks, medical gloves, personal protective equipment and plastic dishes. Thus, there is a significant need for assessing harmful effects of plastics on the environment and public health. Still, the manufacturing of plastic goods and products is expected to continuously grow over the next decade.

This book covers plastic pollution in the environment, including (1) background information, as well as the sources and pathways of plastics; (2) characterization and analysis; (3) environmental risks; (4) public health risk; (5) microplastics and nanoplastics in the aquatic environment, particularly challenges and threats to aquatic organisms; (6) preventive measures; (7) current status and future challenges of microplastics in the agroecosystems; and (8) development of bioplastics and biodegradable plastics. More specifically, the content of this book focuses on assessing the risks of plastics (including nano- and micro-plastics) released into the environment, and it is designed to educate fundamental aspects of plastic materials, including potential risks to the public health and environment, approaches to assessing their harmful effects, prevention of plastic pollution, and environmentally sound technologies for recycling plastics and/or converting them into renewable energy sources. Risk assessment of plastics is required to evaluate currently available treatment technologies and identify the significance of plastic pollution.

A brief summary of each chapter in the book is presented here.

CHAPTER 1: SOURCES AND PATHWAYS OF MARINE LITTER – A GLOBAL ASSESSMENT OF PLASTIC POLLUTION IN COASTAL AND ISLAND REGIONS

Plastic pollution is a global transboundary threat to the planet's marine resources. Tracking pollution is crucial to implement effective marine management strategies on coastal and island regions, where mismanaged plastics are most at risk of entering the ocean. However, the uncertainty of sources and pathways of marine litter poses a major challenge to the assessment of marine pollution. This chapter reviews the principal sectors and human activities contributing to plastic pollution, the mechanisms by which plastic enters the ocean, and some possible drivers of marine litter, including the growing role of coastal tourism on small developing islands. It also outlines future directions for meaningfully integrating research, material accounting, and prevention actions to mitigate the infiltration of plastic pollution in the marine environment, via proper monitoring, assessment, and reporting on plastic material flows from source to sink.

CHAPTER 2: A REVIEW OF MICROPLASTIC POLLUTION CHARACTERISTICS IN GLOBAL URBAN FRESHWATER CATCHMENTS

Microplastics are the newly identified pollutant of this century, yet they are already detected everywhere worldwide. Microplastic pollution in global marine environments has been intensively reported. Evidence of microplastic pollution is emerging in other environments, including land, freshwater, atmosphere and organisms. Public concerns were also raised about microplastic pollution around them. From terrestrial environments, through freshwater environments, finally to marine environments, is a major transportation route of microplastic pollution. Human activities are the fundamental source of microplastic pollution. Cities, with the highest population density on this planet, are important sources of microplastic pollutants. This chapter focuses on urban freshwater environments, the first receptor and major transporter of urban microplastics. By reviewing microplastic pollution in global urban freshwater catchments, urban microplastic pollution characteristics were clarified, and the key information to prevent urban microplastic discharge was sought.

CHAPTER 3: MICROPLASTICS IN THE ENVIRONMENT – SOURCES, PATHWAYS, AND ABUNDANCE

Microplastics in the environment pose a significant threat to the entire ecosystem. Household activity, industrial activity, tyre wear and tear, construction, incineration, plastic litters, landfill, and agricultural activities are the major sources of microplastics in the environment. Microplastics can freely float and adapt between different environmental mediums in the ecosystem due to their lightweight and low-density characteristics. Eventually, microplastics entering the ocean from different pathways result in accumulation and widespread distribution in the marine environment. The frequent interaction between microplastic and aquatic environments accumulates the microplastics in live organisms. The microplastic accumulation and exposure to animals and humans will also affect the ecosystem. This chapter seeks to understand the sources, pathways, and abundance of microplastics in a different environment. The study also highlighted the future research prospects for mitigation of plastic towards environment protection.

CHAPTER 4: MICROPLASTICS AND NANOPLASTICS IN AQUATIC ENVIRONMENTS – CHALLENGES AND THREATS TO AQUATIC ORGANISMS

Marine trash can be found all around the oceans. Debris enters oceans through a variety of sources, including but not limited to sources onshore, vessels, and other marine infrastructure. Plastics are often the most significant component of marine debris, contributing up to 100% of floating trash. Microplastics (MPs) or nanoplastics (NPs), which are fragmented or otherwise minute plastic materials, have remained a source of environmental concern. This chapter traces the different avenues of NPs and MPs in an aquatic setting along with their origin. The toxic impacts of NPs and MPs on the marine ecosystem have been discussed in detail. This chapter also highlights the toxicity comparison of MPs/NPs and the brief analytical techniques for their mitigation. The available data suggests that the prolonged presence of NPs and MPs in the aquatic systems could have long-term repercussions. The more empirical and doctrinal study is pertinent for a better understanding of systemic toxicity caused by MPs/NPs, as well as the underlying mechanism.

CHAPTER 5: THE FATE, CONSEQUENCES, AND FUTURE CHALLENGES OF MICROPLASTICS IN AGROECOSYSTEMS

It is unavoidable that the accumulation of microplastics (MPs) with diameter less than 5 mm will influence environment, due to the increasing production but the slow degradation rates of MPs. Here, our objective is to assess whether MPs represent an emerging threat to soil quality and plant health in agroecosystems. We conclude the physical damage or chemical toxicity on soil organisms and plants caused by MPs may influence plant health. Due to the C contained in the MPs, it contributes to the accumulation of soil organic matter (SOM) as well dissolved organic matter (DOM). This further stimulates microbial activity and consequently enhances the production of CO2 and N2O. Due to the various nature of MPs found in soils, e.g., polymer type, shape, size, and concentration, we also find differing impacts on SOM, nutrients, as well as greenhouse gases emissions. Although MPs may confer some benefits in agroecosystems (e.g., enhanced soil structure, aeration), it is thought that these will be far outweighed by the potential disbenefits.

CHAPTER 6: PREVENTIVE MEASURES OF PLASTIC POLLUTION

The production of plastics has rapidly overwhelmed the world's ability to manage it and hence the demanding environmental issues on plastics pollution. The negative effects of plastics have become so omnipresent and prompted many studies to be conducted leading to a global treaty. This study focused on reviewing measures for preventing plastic pollution in the environment. Based on the literature review approach, seven key measures are identified; recycling prioritization, utilization of bio-based and biodegradable plastics, improvement of waste collection systems, awareness and education in communities, extended producer responsibility (EPR) enforcement, strengthen stakeholder engagement and technology and innovations. The study concludes by providing practical recommendations that should be implemented contextually.

CHAPTER 7: STUDY OF THE POTENTIAL IMPACT OF MICROPLASTICS AND ADDITIVES ON HUMAN HEALTH

The spreading and abundance of micro and nano plastics into the world are so wide that many researchers used them as main pointers of the modern and contemporary period defining a new historical era. Though, the inferences of microplastics are not yet systematically understood. There is the significant difficulty involved to know their impact due to dissimilar physical-chemical characteristics that make micro-plastics complex stressors. Micro-plastics carry toxic chemicals in the ecosystems, therefore serving as vectors of transport, and, on the other hand, a combination of dangerous chemicals that are further voluntarily during their manufacture as additives to increase polymer properties and extend their life. In this chapter, we prominently discuss the different kinds of literature on micro and nano-plastic exposure pathways and their probable risk to human health to encapsulate present information with the target of enhanced attention upcoming study in this area and fill information gaps.

CHAPTER 8: THE EFFECTS OF (MICRO AND NANO) PLASTICS ON THE HUMAN BODY – NERVOUS SYSTEM, RESPIRATORY SYSTEM, DIGESTIVE SYSTEM, PLACENTAL BARRIER, SKIN, AND EXCRETORY SYSTEM

In the present contemporary world, the menace of plastic pollution clubbed with the current pandemic scenario, is a globally rising concern which is affecting every life form on Earth. Plastics hold several properties like ductility that permits the material to be casted and given numerous shapes and forms for various commercial uses. When summed up, it has benefited mankind by becoming an indispensable part of our lives. But the negative impacts associated with it lurks behind silently. Most of the plastic polymers manufactured today are highly resistant to degradation, and the accumulation of these complex and persistent materials are not only causing serious damage to the environment, but also to human health. Additives are added during the manufacturing process to improve the life of these synthetic polymers. The excessive usage of plastic products has resulted in accumulation of the hazardous chemicals, associated with plastic polymers in human body about which this chapter discusses further

CHAPTER 9: IMPACTS OF MICRO- AND NANOPLASTIC IN THE MARINE ENVIRONMENT

Plastic contamination in the ocean has recently received a lot of attention. Plastic production has been growing and its use spread to many sectors. More than 80% of plastic enters the ocean from land-based sources, with the remaining having ocean-based sources. Once in the ocean, plastic undergoes fragmentation and degradation that lead to the formation of microplastics (MPs) and nanoplastics (NPs) and their dimensions are becoming an environmental concern. Thus, this chapter provides an overview of the effects of MPs and NPs on marine organisms, from bacteria to fish. Plastic affect marine organisms from molecular to population levels but some knowledge gaps exist regarding the biogeochemical cycle of plastic, how it behaves and is distributed in the aquatic-sediment compartment and in deep-sea. Moreover, more attention is necessary concerning NPs ecotoxicological effects already detected and because not all polymer types and sizes effects have been investigating, In addition, risk assessment of plastic particles is needed, to characterize their risks, and for data to be comparable

CHAPTER 10: IMPACTS OF MICROPLASTICS ON THE HYDROSPHERE (AQUATIC ENVIRONMENT)

The comforts and uses of plastics have undeniably impacted the mankind in a way such that the help has become a reason of worry for the future generations. The mushrooming concerns about the detrimental effects of microplastics (MPs) on biota in response to its crescive detection and quantification in the marine and freshwater ecosystems, is looming large since last few decades. The infiltration of MPs and its smaller versions into the hydrosphere has been documented as the problem with the anthropogenic angle as the major contributor till date. The present chapter highlights the MPs production, release, and transport pathway along with its impacts on the aquatic biota in terms of a cocktail of adverse effects. It is hence a pressing need to develop methods for the degradation and removal of MPs which have collected over the years of its unregulated use playing havoc since recent times with a lot more yet to come.

CHAPTER 11: DEVELOPMENT OF BIOPLASTICS AND BIODEGRADABLE PLASTICS

Plastics are one of the essential materials due to their low cost and properties. Plastics are used almost everywhere including, food packaging, home appliance, agriculture, automobile, electrical insulators, medical instruments, etc. However, due to the low biodegradability of conventional plastics, they remain in the environment for a very long time and thus, pose a serious threat to our environment. Getting rid of these plastics is very difficult. The burning of plastics produces harmful chemicals that negatively impact the environment (e.g., global warming) and human health. Plastic management via recycling is an incomplete measure to address the environmental impacts of plastic. Therefore, there is a demand for developing alternative plastic materials that will be more environmentally friendly. Bioplastic has attracted much attention as a potential replacement for conventional plastics. This chapter will focus on the development, properties, and applications of various bioplastics. The biodegradability of the bioplastics will also be discussed.

CHAPTER 12: ANALYSIS OF PLASTICS

The ever-growing demand and consumption of plastic has created an irrevocable havoc on earth from last several decades. The exponential increase in the production of plastic from 2.3 million tons worldwide in 1950 to 448 million tons in 2015 is expected to double by 2050. With no proper reuse or recycling policies and gruesome exploitation of this persistent pollutant, plastic has started accumulating and overflowing beyond control. The prevalence and the undefined harm from micro and nano plastic pollution calls for a vigilant screening and periodic upgradation of analytical methodology for efficient and standard reporting. This chapter provides a mere attempt to provide a summary of suitable methodology for analysis of various environment samples and fully understand the implications it possesses.

CHAPTER 13: MICROPLASTICS ANALYTICAL TECHNIQUES IN WATER, SEDIMENTS, AND BIOTA

Identification and quantification of microplastics (MPs) pollution levels in all the environmental compartments including water, sediments, and biota are an hourly need. MPs analytical techniques in water, sediments, and biota consist of several laborious steps including sampling, sample handling, and analytical techniques for identification and quantification. Studies have employed a wide variety of techniques resulting in variation in MPs abundance and characteristics. MPs reporting techniques also vary between different studies. The sampling techniques, digestion reagents, the temperature applied, density separation reagents and the techniques utilized, cause significant impacts on the recovery rate of the MPs particles from samples. 20-10 μm has become the lower reliable, practical limit for MPs due to the limitations in identification methods. Since there are many more MPs research to be done, there is an urgency of establishing reliable and efficient standard methodologies for MPs monitoring enabling comparison of studies from different parts of the world.

CHAPTER 14: ENVIRONMENTAL EFFECT OF PLASTICS DURING THE ANTHROPOCENE AND THE GREAT ACCELERATION

The aim of this chapter is to investigate the environmental effect of plastics (macroplastic and microplastic) during the Anthropocene and the Great Acceleration. Plastic production has worldwide increased since 1950. For instance, many Tunisian regions such as Bizerte, Kerkennah and Gabes witness a proliferation of plastic and microplastic, the manifestation of the plastic invasion is obviously noticed dispersed within continental and marine environments. The detection of microplastic needs an extraction protocol and the use of the infrared spectroscopy. Added to their esthetic pollution, effect of plastics on environment and human health remains controversial. On the other hand, microplastic fragments obtained after the partial destruction of plastic represent more serious danger. These fragments are integrated within the pedosphere, hydrosphere and biosphere. They may be eaten by animals, including humans. Plastics are also good and safe niches for pathogenic viruses. They are considered as motivators of the Anthropocene virology.

The book allows readers to critically think of ways of avoiding or at least minimizing plastic contamination and advocating/educating risk assessment of plastics with contaminants in the environment. The significance of plastic pollution is illustrated through case studies, along with tracking of the ultimate fate of plastics in heterogeneous environmental conditions. Compared to other existing books in the area, this book evaluates potential risks of micro- and nano-plastics, especially in the aquatic environment, and reviews applications of modeling tools and prevention approaches, using technologies to minimize plastic pollution through the development of biodegradable plastics or recycling and reusing plastics in environmentally friendly ways. The book stands out from the competition in terms of addressing recent hot topics on plastic pollution in the environment, especially in the COVID-19 pandemic situation.

In addition to discussing the future outlook based on case studies, this book contributes to the field of micro/nanoplastics research in that it offers new knowledge and recent updates on (1) the risk assessment of plastics in the environment, (2) preventive measures and modeling tools for assessing plastic pollution, (3) characterization and analysis of plastics, and (4) the current status and future challenges of microplastics in agroecosystems.

Readers, particularly those in the field of toxicology, materials, environmental policy, public health, and water treatment, will benefit from this book's content and educational features, in perspectives of providing knowledge in the environmental field, namely the current status and technology developments for avoiding or minimizing plastic contamination, case studies used to assess environmental and public health risks of micro- and nano-plastics, and educational recommendations in resolving issues with global plastic pollution. The target audience includes research scientists and engineers, industry consultants, practitioners, students (both undergraduate and graduate), and also entry-level professionals including those with non-major educational backgrounds. For this audience, the book will be an essential reference, providing fundamental information for practice and research. The book is also recommended for students whose major is in the field of environmental science, materials and environmental engineering, public health, or chemistry.

Sung Hee Joo
University of Seoul, South Korea

Acknowledgment

The editor greatly acknowledges all those who contributed to the success of this book. This book was not possible without all the contributors who served as the authors. Production of a book often requires a significant investment of time to ensure both the quality and quantity of contents of the particular theme. As such, the editor greatly appreciates the reviewers who have contributed constructive comments and suggestions to enhance the quality of all chapters for the book. All the feedback, suggestions, and recommendations were valuable and strengthened the content of the new fields in micro/nanoplastics research. The editor acknowledges all the authors in the book and particular acknowledgements go to the following fellows. Dr. Gabriela Fernandez, Ms. Carol Maione, Dr. Huadong Zang, Dr. Soumen Basu, Dr. Tejraj Aminabhavi, Dr. Bupe Getrude Mwanza, Mr. Yuyao Xu, Dr. Kaustubha Mohanty, Dr. Md Saquib Hasnain, Dr. Judy Lee, Dr. Marie Enfrin, Dr. Filippo Giustozzi, Dr. Sandhya Babel, Dr. Gilberto Dias de Alkimin, Dr. Sadasivam Anbumani, Dr. Sanchari Biswas, Dr. Nitai Giri, Dr. Devarati Bagchi, Dr. Jie Zhou. The editorial assistant, Rowan Rumbaugh, is also grateful for the assistance of all the contributors. Finally, the editor acknowledges the funding provided by Korea Environment Industry & Technology Institute (KEITI) through Post Plastic, a specialized program of the Graduate School funded by Korea Ministry of Environment (MOE).

Chapter 1
Sources and Pathways of Marine Litter:
A Global Assessment of Plastic Pollution in Coastal and Island Regions

Carol Maione
Politecnico di Milano, Italy

Gabriela Fernandez
San Diego State University, USA

ABSTRACT

Plastic pollution is a global transboundary threat to the planet's marine resources. Tracking pollution is crucial to implement effective marine management strategies on coastal and island regions, where mismanaged plastics are most at risk of entering the ocean. However, the uncertainty of sources and pathways of marine litter poses a major challenge to the assessment of marine pollution. This chapter reviews the principal sectors and human activities contributing to plastic pollution, the mechanisms by which plastic enters the ocean, and some possible drivers of marine litter, including the growing role of coastal tourism on small developing islands. It also outlines future directions for meaningfully integrating research, material accounting, and prevention actions to mitigate the infiltration of plastic pollution in the marine environment, via proper monitoring, assessment, and reporting on plastic material flows from source to sink.

INTRODUCTION

In just over a century, plastic has gone from being hailed as a "*scientific wonder*" to becoming an "*environmental scourge*" (Plummer, 2018). In fact, the social and economic benefits associated with plastic materials made them so popular that they have been documented in the most remote corners of the planet (Andrady & Neal, 2009; Thompson et al., 2009). Plastic pollution is defined as the totality of plastic accumulation in the environment, as well as the ecological impacts associated with its production,

DOI: 10.4018/978-1-7998-9723-1.ch001

consumption, mismanagement, and emissions related to end-of-life practices (Nielsen et al., 2020). The scale of plastic pollution is striking, causing US$75 billion social and environmental costs every year (UNEP, 2014a). It has been estimated that over 8 million metric tons of plastics enter our oceans every year (Jambeck et al., 2015), and this flow is expected to nearly triple by 2040 (The Pew Charitable Trust & SYSTEMIQ, 2020), with tremendous consequences for the subsistence of marine life (Derraik, 2002).

A growing body of research has reported that plastic litter is one of the most serious threats to the underwater world, making the study of marine plastic pollution a key priority (Li et al., 2016). However, our knowledge of the magnitude and distribution of plastic pollution in the planet's oceans is relatively new and there is still much uncertainty about the sources and pathways of marine pollution (Thompson et al., 2004; Cózar et al. 2014). This is due to the difficulties in assessing provenience (the geographic origin of the debris and the sector that is primary responsible for its release), means of release (the mechanisms by which the debris enters the marine environment), and entry points (where the release occurred) of plastic debris (Veiga et al., 2016). To bridge these gaps, existing assessment frameworks consider the annual amount of mismanaged plastic waste produced by coastal populations. In fact, it has been estimated that plastics consumed within a 50 km distance from the coast are at "*high risk of entering the ocean*" via direct littering, inland waterways, wastewaters, or transported by wind and tides (Jambeck et al., 2015).

This chapter explores the most common sources and pathways of plastic pollution in coastal and island regions, where mismanaged plastic waste is at the highest risk of becoming marine pollution, and it provides tangible implications and solutions to detect plastics in these areas. Coastal environments suffer particularly from plastic pollution, as they host hotspots for the production, accumulation, and release of plastic debris (Li et al., 2016). Second, coastal sites are exposed to the negative effects of plastic pollution, ranging from environmental degradation to jeopardy of marine ecosystems (Cózar et al., 2014; Lamb et al., 2018). A third element of concern is that marine pollution can impoverish local economies via reduced investments in coastal development (McIlgorm et al., 2011; Jang et al., 2014) and decline of coastal- and marine-dependent activities (e.g., fishing, mariculture, and tourism) (Mohammed, 2002; Staehr et al., 2018). In addition to the challenges experienced by coasts, islands face several barriers related to environmental management such as the limited physical space for storing and treating waste, a lack of resources to implement efficient waste infrastructure, higher waste management costs, and difficulty of implementing plastics circularity locally (Eckelman et al., 2014). Ultimately, understanding the distribution patterns of marine litter in coastal and island regions is crucial to unfold the impacts on the marine environment and root causes of marine pollution.

The chapter is organized as follows: the next section presents background information on plastic waste and its management. The main focus of the chapter is on the sources and pathways of marine litter and plastic pollution, including a case study on the role of coastal tourism in marine pollution. Next, a number of priority solutions and recommendations on monitoring and reporting on plastic pollution are presented. The chapter suggests some future research directions to integrate existing monitoring approaches. Finally, concluding remarks are provided.

Figure 1. Present plastic end-of-life management routes
Source: ISWA (2017).

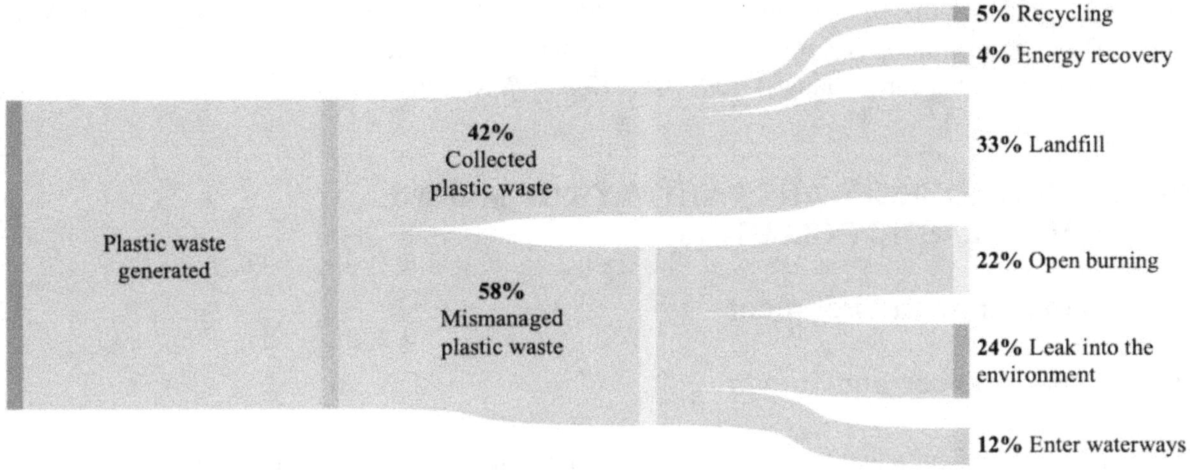

BACKGROUND

Managing Plastic Waste and Pollution

Consumption of plastics has spread rapidly due to their great versatility and mechanical properties, that made them affordable, durable, and good quality materials (Andrady & Neal, 2009; Thompson et al., 2009). The convenience that plastics offer, however, has led to a throwaway culture that reveals the material's dark side of single-use plastic (Everaert et al., 2018). Plastics can in fact become problematic when waste materials are not handled properly after disposal and end up in unregulated landfills, are illegally burnt, or enter the environment, from where they can eventually reach the ocean (Barnes et al., 2009; Jambeck et al., 2015) (Figure 1). It has been estimated that nearly 60% of all plastics ever produced have accumulated in the environment, where they are still present in the form of waste and pollution (Geyer et al., 2017). Global plastic leakage is estimated in the order of 10 million tonnes per year (mt/year), with yearly values ranging from 4.8 mt/year to 12.7 mt/year (Jambeck et al., 2015), to 8.28 mt/year (UNEP, 2018c), 12.2 mt/year (EUNOMIA, 2016), or 10 mt/year (Boucher & Friot, 2017).

Plastic pollution in the planet's oceans has long been recognized as a pressing environmental issue (Haward, 2018). Nonetheless, land-based plastic pollution, which roughly accounts for 80% of all marine litter (Jambeck et al., 2015), remained unregulated for decades. In 2014, world leaders jointly committed to "*prevent[ing] and significantly reduc[ing] marine pollution of all kinds, in particular from land-based activities, including marine debris*" making the issue of plastic pollution a top global priority (SDG 14: Life Below Water) (UN, 2015). In the following years, the United Nations advanced several resolutions and targets with the aim of protecting and restoring ocean health via urgent actions such as the retention of land-based and sea-based anthropogenic pollution (e.g., UNEP, 2014b, 2016b, 2017, 2019a; UNGC, 2020).

These global actions were further bolstered by the enforcement of local-based environmental policies in an effort to reduce land-based plastic pollution. Examples of local-based policies are the ban on the manufacture, retail, distribution, and import of plastic shopping bags in African countries (Greenpeace,

2020), the ban of tourism-related plastic import into tropical islands (e.g., Government Communication Unit, 2019), the phaseout of single-use plastic items (cotton bud sticks, tableware, balloons, food containers, cigarette butts, bags, wrappers, and sanitary items) in European countries (EC, 2019; WWF et al., 2020), and restrictions on microplastics from land-based sources (e.g. microbeads contained in cosmetics and personal care products) (EC, 2018; Kentin & Kaarto, 2018).

IDENTIFYING SOURCES AND PATHWAYS OF MARINE LITTER AND PLASTIC POLLUTION

Plastics in Marine Environment

Marine Litter Sources and Trends

Marine litter sources are widely distributed in the marine environment. Coastal and island regions can be subject to marine pollution from local, regional, or even distant, as litter can be transported by ocean currents and wind drift (Boucher & Friot, 2017). Identifying the origin and transport mechanisms of marine litter is a difficult and uncertain task, as debris can be generated from a number of sea-based or land-based, and originate from near or distant sources. At present, different assessment methods are employed to determine primary sources and drivers of marine pollution, as well as potential deficiencies in the production, consumption, and waste management systems that can result in marine litter. Assessing marine litter is necessary to identify hotspots of plastic pollution, establish appropriate targets, and design and implement pollution management strategies. Ultimately, the results from marine litter assessments can support key considerations to prevent macro- and microplastics waste from entering the ocean.

Primary Polluting Sectors in Coastal and Island Regions

Based on culture, habits, and waste disposal practices, key contributing sectors in coastal and island regions include but are not limited to: households, the retail sector, tourism, shipping, fisheries, building and construction, and the plastic industry. Table 1 lists the most popular plastics by sector and related entry points to the marine environment. The volume of plastic entering the ocean depends largely on the extent and effectiveness of wastewater and solid waste collection and management.

Household waste is considered one of the most consistent contributors of plastic pollution along coastal and island regions globally. Individuals contribute to marine litter in different ways, for example by visiting marine or coastal regions, but also in everyday life through littering on land or direct disposal into coastal waters. Domestic activities can also contribute to pollution at local beaches through excessive irrigation and washing activities. These activities can carry a wide range of pollutants from domestic solid waste and dust to fertilizer, pesticide, herbicide, automobile fluid, paint, animal waste, and other chemicals into the storm drain system and, from there, they can flow untreated into channels, harbors, and the ocean endangering marine life. The most commonly used plastics by households are associated with food handling and preparation (e.g., containers and wrapping), single-use tableware (e.g., cups, cutlery, and plates), cleaning supplies, clothing, sporting, and cosmetics (UNEP, 2016a). Moreover, microfiber clothing and cosmetics are primary sources of microplastic that can be released into the environment via laundry and washing (Fendall & Sewell, 2009; Free et al., 2014). Managing domestic

Table 1. Most common plastic types by sector

ID	Sectors	Plastic items	Entry points
1	Household (public litter)	Plastic shopping bags, beverage bottles, food wrapping, containers, tableware, cleaning supplies, clothing, sport equipment, and cosmetics.	Rivers, coastal
2	Retail	Containers, food wrapping, and plastic shopping bags.	Rivers, coastal
3	Tourism	Beverage bottles, food wrapping, tableware, sportswear, fishing equipment, sport equipment, and beauty care products.	Rivers, coastal, marine
4	Shipping	Food wrapping, tableware, beverage bottles, and containers.	Coastal, marine
5	Fisheries	Fishing equipment, including abandoned, lost or otherwise discarded fishing gear (ghost gear).	Coastal, marine
6	Building and construction	Window profiles, pipes, insulation layers, packaging, utensils, and plastic components (e.g., screws, bolt covers, silicones).	Rivers, coastal
7	Plastic industry	Plastic components and wrapping.	Rivers, coastal

refuse at home can allow consumers to avoid large volumes of waste, particularly of recyclables, to be sent to landfills, or be illegally dumped or abandoned in the environment, thereby losing potential for material recovery (UNEP, 2018c).

One of the fastest growing marine polluters are retailers in the business of fast-moving consumer goods, such as food, beverages, toiletries, and retail products including clothing (fast fashion) and accessories. These products often come in plastic packaging: polyethylene terephthalate (PET) bottles and high-density polyethylene (HDPE) containers which account for the biggest share of plastic packaging, followed by low-density polyethylene (LDPE) wrappings and plastic shopping bags, and polystyrene (PS), polypropylene (PP), and polyvinyl chloride (PVC) containers (Europen, 2009). Retailers have high annual turnovers and therefore contribute to the input of large amounts of plastic packaging into the market. To address this packaging inflow, roadmaps for the integration of circular economy principles within the retail sector have been advanced (e.g., Gong et al., 2020), including zero-waste strategies, commitment to partnerships with recycling companies and global pacts, lighter packaging, and maximization of resource efficiency (UNEP, 2016a; James, 2019). In addition, to facilitate consumer response, retailers and producers need to provide clearly visible substitutes or upstream solutions. For example, companies like Patagonia have also launched merchandise from recyclable plastic materials. In 2021, 89% of their polyester line used recycled polyester fabrics from beverage bottles, thereby saving 3.3 million pounds of CO2 associated with the extraction and processing of fossil fuels, while educating customers to be environmentally conscious (Patagonia, 2021).

Coastal and ship-based tourism represent a primary source of litter in many regions, with major hotspots distributed across the Mediterranean Sea, Caribbean, Southeast Asia, and small developing islands (GESAMP, 2016). The problem is exacerbated by poor management of solid waste (training, technology, funding, infrastructure, education, and political support), a lack of resources, a disconnect between those benefiting from the activity (tourists, restaurant owners, tour operators) and those dealing with the consequences of increased waste generation (local communities), and very often by direct, deliberate, or accidental littering of shorelines (ARCADIS, 2012). In addition, tourism services in small developing islands can lead to the importation of very large quantities of food and other consumer goods with the accompanying packaging, creating a huge challenge for effective waste management (Jang et al., 2014).

Although regulated by international laws and regulations based on the International Convention for the Prevention of Pollution from Ships (MARPOL), the shipping sector still represents an alarming and continuing source of marine litter, both due to accidental release (such as collisions or storm damage) and illegal disposal of plastics at sea (UNEP, 2016a). Through the years, there has been a great expansion of trade in manufactured goods from Asia to Europe to North America, of which a significant fraction was composed of plastics (e.g., pellets and nurdles) transported in container vessels. Unfortunately, shipping accidents result in major losses of macro and microplastics at sea each year. In the winter months between 2020 and 2021 alone, over 3,000 shipping containers fell into the Pacific Ocean causing alarming numbers of marine pollution, which posed serious risks to the health of ocean, marine life, and marine activities (Lydon, 2021). Moreover, despite this great danger, no actions and policy measures are taken to track the containers lost at sea and manage their contents, resulting in high environmental costs (Lydon, 2021).

Fishing-related debris is one of the most frequent types of beach and marine litter, and has been increasingly associated with risks of entanglement, ingestion, and contamination of wandering bird colonies along the coast (UNEP, 2016a). It has been estimated that approximately 70% by weight of floating macroplastic debris in the ocean is fishing-related (Eriksen et al., 2014). This can be due to several regional factors such as the type of gear, the educational level of the fishing workers, inefficient fishing methods, gear conflicts with other fishers and maritime users, or the value of the catch compared with the cost of the net and the event of fishing (Gilman, 2015). Not only do fisheries largely contribute to marine pollution, but it has been observed that marine plastic debris may cause a reduction in fishing income as a result of reduced fishing days due to the presence of litter (FAO, 2017).

The building and construction sector is considered the second largest utilizer of plastic materials, accounting for 19% of the total share of plastic in use (PlasticsEurope, 2019). Plastics used by the building and construction industry include PP (pipes), HDPE (pipes), PVC (window frames, profiles, floor and wall covering, cable insulation, finishing materials), PS (insulation and foams), and other plastic resins (roofing sheets and protective coatings) (PlasticsEurope, 2019). In addition, many building materials, including both plastic and non-plastic sources, arrive at the construction site wrapped in plastic packaging. Furthermore, constructions can cause severe environmental impacts not only directly, but also indirectly through the activities associated with use, maintenance, and demolition of buildings and structures. Finally, surface runoff and urban runoff from the construction of roads, buildings, ports, channels, and harbours, can carry plastic debris, soil, materials, minerals, and other materials into the sea, with major harm for wildlife habitats.

Finally, plastic waste can originate at all stages of the plastic supply chain, making the plastic industry one the fastest growing plastic polluters worldwide. The plastic industry encompasses all industrial actors along the plastic supply chain: from producers located at the first stage of the supply chain; converters, manufacturers, and brand owners covering core functions such as processing semi-finished and finished products; distributors supplying such products to the market; and finally waste management companies and recyclers (James, 2019). To comprehensively understand the plastic footprint of the plastic industry, it is important to understand plastic production trends, distribution of plastic products from producers to end consumers, and their end-of-life management. In recent years, the plastic industry has worked actively to reduce its plastic footprint, including developing better infrastructure to manage plastic waste, promoting environmental education campaigns, building capacity to improve resource use, and scaling up plastic recycling (The Pew Charitable Trusts & SYSTEMIQ, 2020). Moreover, industries are now looking for alternative products made of sustainably sourced or recycled materials, and innovative industrial processes to make plastic recycling more economically viable.

Figure 2. Coastal and island sources of macroplastics and related means of release
Adapted from UNEP (2016a)

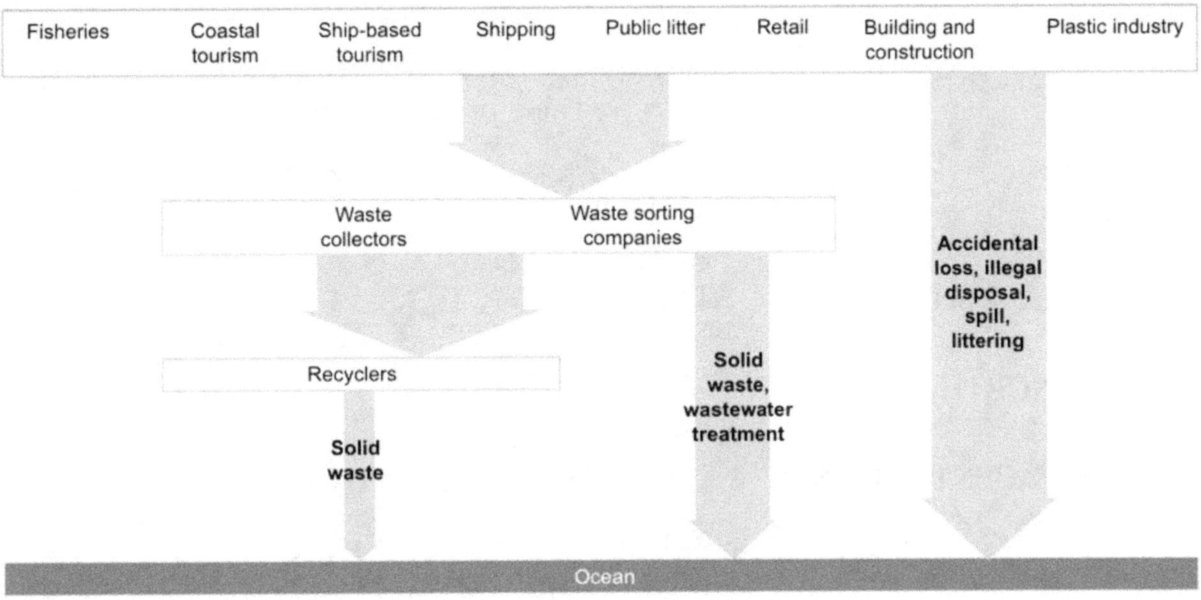

Release of Macroplastics in Coastal and Island Regions

Higher abundance of macroplastics has been found in coastal waters, particularly in regions with denser coastal populations, inadequate waste collection and management, intensive fisheries, and high levels of coastal tourism. The problem is enlarged by inadequate waste management infrastructure and practices, as well as by intentional or unintentional material loss, especially in areas with least adapted waste management facilities (Boucher & Friot, 2017). Scholars from around the world have assessed a number of plastic items in our oceans. Such items include large plastic pieces such as abandoned fishing nets, traps, rope, and plastic bags that wash up on beaches or accumulate in ocean currents (Boucher & Friot, 2017). This litter arises from various economic sectors and activities, either directly or indirectly. Figure 2 summarizes the main sources of marine pollution found in coastal and island regions, including land-based sources such as urban runoff, littering, inadequate waste disposal and management, industrial activities, and construction, and sea-based sources, such as fishing, nautical activities, and tourism.

Release of Microplastics in Coastal and Island Regions

Land-based sources of microplastics include cosmetics and personal care products, textiles and clothing (synthetic fibres), terrestrial transport (dust from tyres) and plastic producers and fabricators (plastic resin pellets used in plastics manufacture), while sea-based sources appear to be dominated by the maritime sector (UNEP, 2016a). In addition, under the influence of weather conditions such as photolysis, weathering, disintegration, and other physical transformations, larger plastic particles break down into smaller fragments, adding up to the amounts of microplastics from sea-based sources (Cózar et al. 2014; Sharma et al., 2021). Figure 3 shows regional differences in microplastics release and composition. These differences are the result of varied patterns and pathways that depend on local characteristics,

Figure 3. Global release of microplastics to the world oceans by geographical area and primary sources (%)
Source: Boucher & Friot (2017)

	Synthetic textiles	Tyres	Road markings	Marine coatings	Personal care products	Plastic pellets
INDIA & SOUTH ASIA	15,9	1,1	0,3	0,1	0,8	0
NORTH AMERICA	2,6	11,5	1,9	1	0,1	0,1
EUROPE & CENTRAL ASIA	4	8,6	2,4	0,6	0,2	0,1
CHINA	10,3	2,5	1,3	1,2	0,5	0
EAST ASIA & OCEANIA	6,3	5,3	1,6	1,5	0,3	0
SOUTH AMERICA	2,9	5,1	0,9	0	0,2	0
AFRICA & MIDDLE EAST	4	3,2	0,6	0,4	0,5	0

such as population density, gross domestic product (GDP), cultural habits, and the effectiveness of local infrastructure to retain waste.

Marine Litter Pathways

It has been estimated that 80% of plastic debris floating in the oceans originate from land-based sources and reach the marine environment via rivers, waterways, or transported by wind and tide (Jambeck et al., 2015). In 2010, between 4.8 and 12.7 million tonnes of plastic waste were released into the ocean from coastal regions (Jambeck et al., 2015), and an additional 1.2 to 2.4 million tonnes of plastic reached the ocean through inland riverways (Lebreton et al., 2017). Once plastics enter the ocean, they can be transported for long distances before being deposited and can transform (e.g., macro-debris can break down into smaller fragments) (Born & Brüll, 2021). However, these circulation mechanisms are still poorly understood and can depend on a number of contextual factors, including geographical location, meteorological conditions, hydrodynamics, and the characteristics of the local ecosystems (ISWA, 2017).

River Systems

About 90% of the world's population lives within a close distance from freshwater bodies (10 km or less) (Kummu et al., 2011), and especially in urban areas, rivers collect urban waste, sewage and wastewaters, industrial discharges, and various pollutants (EEA, 2016). It is not surprising then that a key input of marine plastic pollution is through rivers. Inland rivers are considered responsible for nearly 48% of marine litter from land-based sources and, in particular, rivers within 50 km from the coast account for 20% of marine pollution (Lebreton et al., 2017). Rivers are also primary carriers of microplastics from domestic and industrial sources (Thompson et al., 2009).

Estimates show that 20 rivers account for approximately 67% of the global river input annually, most of which are located in Asia (86%). River Yangtze, in southern China, is considered the world's top polluting river, with an annual inflow of 333,000 tons, equivalent to over 4% of ocean plastic pollution (Lebreton et al., 2017). Smaller volumes of river plastic originate from Africa (7.8%), South America (4.8%), North and Central America (0.9%), Europe (0.3%), and lastly Australia and the Pacific region (0.02%) (Lebreton et al., 2017). The composition of river plastics can vary greatly in these regions as it depends on the land uses (e.g., residential, industrial, commercial), the social practices of local populations, and the nature of commercial and industrial activities in the catchment area (UNEP, 2016a; ISWA, 2017). Moreover, the effectiveness of solid waste management systems has a great influence on the inputs to river systems and substantial regional differences can be expected (UNEP, 2016a).

Drainage and Sewage Systems

Wastewater is another primary carrier of plastic debris. Like rivers, drainage and sewage systems can become convenient dumping sites collecting municipal solid waste, street litter, and waste overflowing from littering, dumpsites, and waste storage facilities (ISWA, 2017; UNEP, 2018b). Waste transport is especially problematic during rain events (and wet seasons where present), when rain can mobilize large volumes of waste from sidewalks and waste collection stations (ISWA, 2017). This situation is further exacerbated in areas with poor and malfunctioning infrastructure, where waste can clog drains causing serious flooding.

During heavy rain events, untreated wastewater can also find its way to rivers or directly into the ocean, in particular in absence of wastewater treatment plants (ISWA, 2017). This is especially critical in regions with low rates of wastewater treatment. Lower middle-income and low-income countries present percentages of untreated wastewater of 72% and 92% respectively, with higher risk of contaminating water bodies (WWAP, 2017).

Transport by Wind

Most plastics, and especially packaging plastics, are lightweight and therefore are more at risk of being transported by wind (Kukulka et al., 2012). Wind can in fact blow plastic waste out of trash cans, dumpsites, or other waste management facilities and carry them into water bodies (ISWA, 2017). Transport by wind is influenced by several factors. First, the nature of plastic debris, including weight, density, size, and polymer type, can make plastics more susceptible to being transported by wind (Browne et al., 2010). Not surprisingly, studies assessing plastic debris carried along estuarine shorelines observed a greater abundance of microplastics, and in particular denser microplastic particles, compared to macroplastic debris (e.g., Kukulka et al., 2012). Another factor is related to the site conditions, such as meteorological conditions (e.g., wind speed, direction, and turbulence) and depositional environments (Browne et al., 2010; Thiel et al., 2011; Kukulka et al., 2012).

Wind can also determine microplastics distribution and circulation in the atmosphere. Microplastics are literally falling from the sky through rainwater and the air we breathe (e.g., Simon, 2021; Fleming, 2020; Johnson, 2019; Imster, 2020), flushed from land into the sea and aquatic environments (UNEP, 2021). Scientists have found that over 90% of rainwater samples contain microplastics (Fleming, 2020; Simon, 2020; Johnson, 2019). These plastic particles can originate from cities, industrial activities, agricultural fields, roads, or dust, and transported by wind, can saturate the surrounding environment (Simon, 2021). Therefore, it is nearly impossible to determine their exact pathways from source to sea.

Littering

No unified data on the total contributions of littering to marine plastic pollution exist. It was estimated that approximately 2% of the total mass of waste generated is littered, and 25% of this amount is not captured into existing waste management systems (Jambeck et al., 2015), for a total loss of 0.8 million tons of plastic to the environment (Jambeck et al., 2015; UNEP, 2018c; Ryberg et al., 2019). Direct deposit and discharge of plastic into the world's seas remain a primary input of marine litter.

Littering can be linked to a wide range of coastal and marine activities: (i) coastal tourism, during all beach-based and land-based activities, and from tourism-related commercial activities in proximity of the shoreline (ECORYS, 2013, 2016); (ii) commercial and recreational fishing, via abandonment and loss of of fishing gears, ancillary items, and release of galley waste (UNEP, 2016a); (iii) ship-based tourism, when cruise ships are not equipped with proper systems to manage on-board wastes and solid waste is discarded ashore at ports and on small islands (UNEP, 2016a); and (iv) maritime transport, including unregulated disposal of plastic waste from ships and spillage of pellets from cargos (UNEP, 2016a).

Losses from Plastic Value Chain

Although rare, losses of microplastics may occur during production, handling, and processing of plastics (UNEP, 2018c). Loss of plastic pellets mainly results from accidental spills at the plant level; however, given their limited and punctual scope, limited data exist on these quantities. A general value used for estimations of plastic spills from industrial plants is that of 0.4 g/kg of plastic material, resulting from a study conducted on plastic losses at a polystyrene plant (Sundt et al., 2014). These quantities are likely to end up in the drainage system of industrial facilities, from where they are treated in wastewater treatment plants for microbeads removal (Magnusson et al., 2016). As a result, the total loss of microplastics from industrial production to the environment is estimated to be between 0.01 million tons (Magnusson et al., 2016; UNEP, 2018c) and 0.02 million tons (Ryberg et al., 2019). Microplastics losses from transport and handling of plastic pellets are estimated to vary between 0.0005% and 0.01%, with an average value of 0.005%, of the total losses to the environment, for an amount of 0.02 million tons (Magnusson et al., 2016).

More consistent losses occur downstream in the plastic value chain. Plastic use and consumption accounts for nearly 3.3 million tons of plastic leakage annually, from packaging and consumer products, transportation (e.g., tyre abrasion, road markings), and other applications (e.g., textile, building and construction, fishing), and end-of-life management for an estimated 5.1 million tons (Ryberg et al., 2019; UNEP, 2016a). However, different sources may report different numbers and regional differences are to be accounted for when calculating plastic losses to the environment, as many contextual factors can come into play, such as the presence of initiatives to reduce material losses from industrial sources and increase material efficiency, the effectiveness of local waste management systems, and economic and industrial practises among others.

Tides, Ocean Currents, and Debris Circulation

Once plastic enters the ocean, it can translocate for a long time, becoming a transboundary pollution issue (UNEP & GRID-Arendal, 2016). Circulation and geographical distribution of marine plastic debris are influenced by entry points and transport mechanisms, and are subject to prevailing winds, waves, and ocean currents (Rech et al., 2014). It is also not surprising that, during these movements, larger particles can break down into smaller fragments (micro- or nanoplastics) that, due to their morphological characteristics, are even more susceptible to being transported by tides and ocean currents (ISWA, 2017).

Surface circulation is dominated by five major ocean currents or gyres, namely North Atlantic, South Atlantic, North Pacific, South Pacific, and Indian Ocean gyres. These five gyres are well-known spots for debris accumulation at the sea surface (Law et al., 2010, 2014; Cózar et al., 2014; Eriksen et al., 2014; Van Sebille et al., 2020), registering debris concentrations as high as 10 kg/square km (Cózar et al., 2015; Van Sebille et al., 2015). In addition to the five major plastic patches, recent studies have observed floating plastic regions of new formation in the Arctic region (Bergmann et al., 2015; Van Sebille et al., 2012), Southern Ocean and Antarctic islands (Eriksson et al., 2013), Mediterranean, Southeast Asian, and Bengal seas (Cózar et al., 2015; UNEP, 2016a).

The vertical movement of ocean currents, or sedimentation, is also affected by environmental factors. For example, in oceans, a lower ocean temperature and higher salinity result in an increase of high-density polymers in the water column (Kowalski et al., 2016). Therefore, composition of plastics in the established compartment is strongly affected by polymer type, where variation in the composition within the same compartment is likely explained by variations in environmental factors such as salinity and temperature.

Plastic particles do not float at the sea surface forever. When it starts to sink, plastic debris moves along the so-called ocean conveyor belt, a moving system of deep-ocean current circulation caused by cold, dense water sinking and drifting plastics towards deeper waters (UNEP & GRID-Arendal, 2016). Once plastic reaches deeper parts of the ocean, and eventually deposits on the seabed becoming benthic litter, its pathways are even less understood, suggesting that further research is needed.

Difficulty in Determining Marine Litter Sources and Pathways

Forecasting plastic pollution is a challenging endeavor. At the global level, much uncertainty remains, which explains the discrepancies in plastic pollution estimates. These uncertainties can either be structural, when they are related to the understanding of the mechanisms and pathways of the leakage, or data-related, when they pertain to the availability of reliable datasets (EUNOMIA, 2016). The latter is especially of concern in certain countries where lack of resources, limited education, and technological challenges among others can limit transparency and traceability of plastic pollution flows.

Moreover, there are a number of problems with existing material flow accounting approaches, that can make pollution management a hard-to-reach perspective. Firstly, the lack of a standardized computations or datasets to calculate mismanaged waste and leakages; thus, different approaches yield different results. Secondly, littering estimations are by nature complex to produce: litter may be identified from municipality cleaning operators' statistics, but not for the fraction that falls through the cracks (e.g., leakage). This fraction is by definition not measured and very difficult to calculate (e.g., for the calculation of municipal plastic waste, governments create proxies based on hypothetical situations) (Jambeck et al., 2015). Lastly, release rates from mismanaged waste are rarely based on evidence and rather hypothetical. This is because the release pathways are poorly understood and release rates, therefore, provide indicative estimates describing somewhere between 10% and 40% of their global variability (Jambeck et al, 2015; UNEP, 2018a). As a result, these rates fail to capture regional and local variations, with possible implications for the management of plastic pollution flows. In addition, contextual factors such as socio-cultural behaviors (e.g., littering habits), climatic conditions (e.g., effect of rain or wind on dispersal of waste from dumpsites), and geographic characteristics (e.g., distance to shore and waterways) are expected to have a significant influence on the extent, distribution, and spatiotemporal variability of plastic pollution (Kukulka et al, 2012).

As a consequence, measuring and forecasting plastic pollution and its impacts on coastal and island regions is a complex and challenging task. Nonetheless, developing a more specific and actionable methodology to quantify plastic pollution flows requires overcoming some of these uncertainties. Possible solutions encompass the use of material circularity models to map and monitor leakage pathways, coordinated efforts to collect data on plastic and pollution, or priority actions to monitor plastic pollution locally (e.g., citizen science, geospatial analysis, environmental campaigns).

Identifying Sources of Marine Litter on Small Islands: The Case of Zanzibar, Tanzania, Africa

The Zanzibar archipelago offers a rich case for studying marine pollution within a naturally bounded environment. Located some 30 km off the eastern coast of Tanzania in the Western Indian Ocean, the archipelago underwent an exceptional coastal development over the past decades (Sharpley & Ussi, 2014). Coastal tourism became one of the largest income-generating sectors in Zanzibar; but, on the flip side, it was responsible for an enormous increase in waste generation (Ally et al., 2014; Lange, 2015; Staehr et al., 2018). At present, the volume of plastic waste produced by the tourism sector remains unknown. However, the hotels' location and direct access to the beach suggest that plastic waste can find an easy route into the ocean (Mohammed, 2002). Furthermore, the many tourism activities taking place on the beach or in the water, such as boat tours, snorkeling, and recreational fishing, are associated with increased marine littering (Interviews, Tourism worker; Maione, 2019).

This section presents a study of the main drivers of plastic pollution on Zanzibar's tourism beaches, sources, and pathways of marine plastic pollution to depict a comprehensive analysis of the role of coastal tourism in plastic pollution on small islands. Data were collected during a scientific expedition conducted in 2018, during the high tourism season, at four tourism locations on the Unguja island (Figure 4). For data collection, 57 key stakeholders from the tourism sector (hotel staff, human resources coordinators, hotel managers, and restaurant owners), local operators (tour guides, drivers, and vendors) and waste workers (waste pickers, street sweepers, municipal officers, and private waste management companies) were interviewed to explore (i) the perception of tourism and its role in plastic pollution, (ii) the state of waste facilities on tourism beaches, and (iii) tourists' littering practices (for a detailed description of the interview process see Maione (2019)). In addition, the authors conducted observations and macro-debris surveys at all sites to assess the amounts, composition, and primary sources of beach litter (for a detailed description of the survey process see Maione (2021)).

Figure 4. Map of the sampling locations on Unguja island, Zanzibar (Tanzania): (1) Stone Town, (2) Nungwi, (3) Uroa, and (4) Fumba

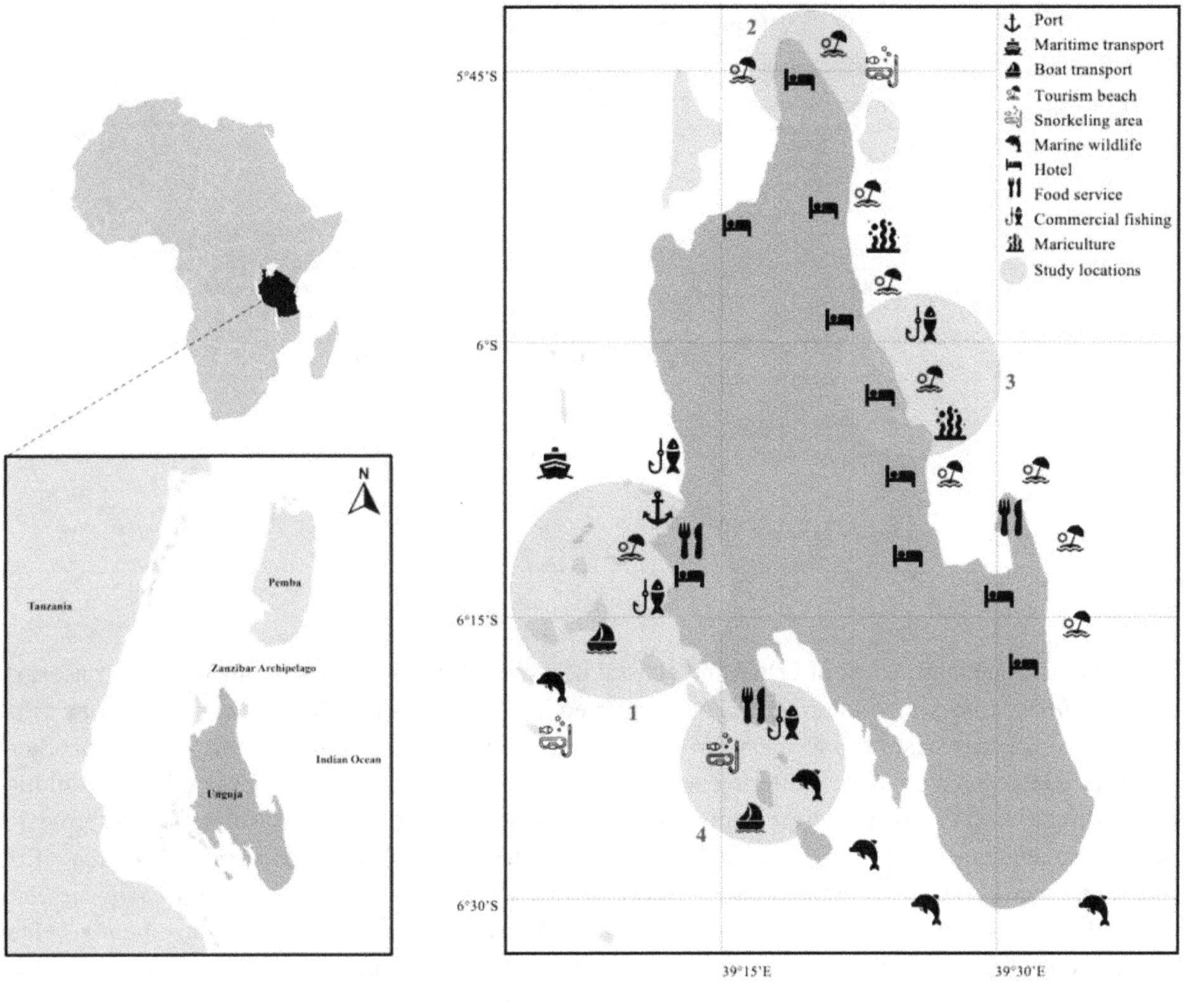

Drivers of Plastic Pollution on Tourism Beaches

In general, the majority of the study's participants reported that waste generation was greater during high tourism season, suggesting that tourism is a primary waste-generating sector on the island. Some waste pickers indicated that, during the high tourism season, the amount of solid waste doubled in their areas of operation. In particular, they observed a greater amount of plastic beverage bottles, which are usually associated with tourism consumption since "*people here [Zanzibaris] don't drink bottled water because it's expensive*" (Interviews, Hotel manager; Maione, 2019). However, because of the exclusion of many tourism activities from the municipal waste management services, it is likely that this amount was largely underestimated.

Interview respondents indicated that the persistence of plastic litter on Zanzibar's tourism beaches was primarily driven by five factors, as shown in Figure 5. First, marine littering was mentioned by all

Figure 5. Overview of the interview findings on the five major drivers of beach plastic pollution and related sub-drivers

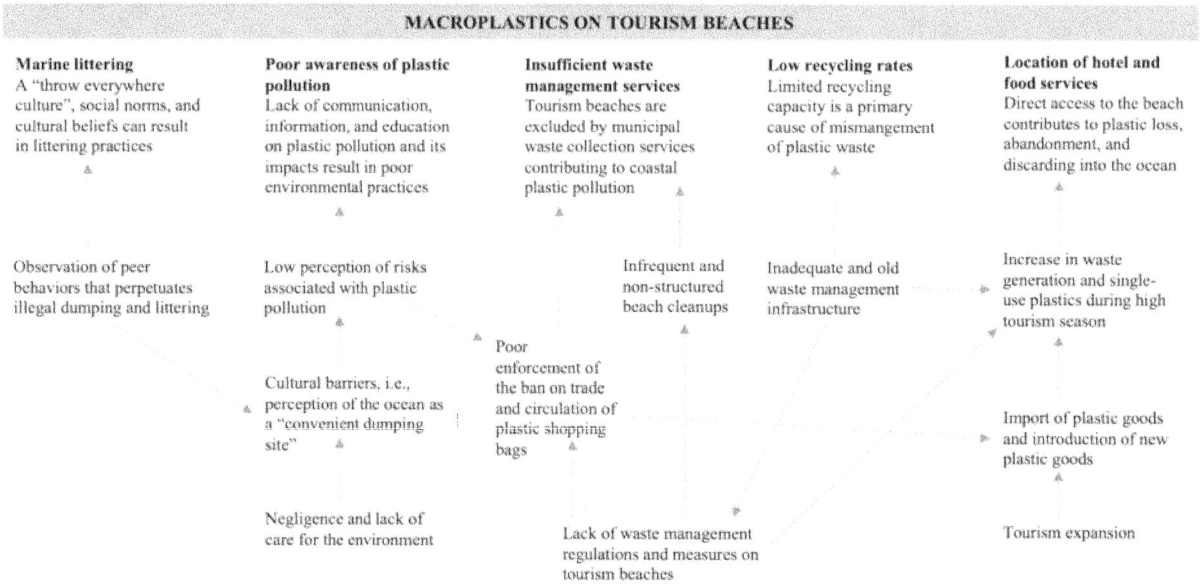

respondents as a major driver of beach and coastal pollution. Interviewees used the term "*throw everywhere culture*" to describe littering practices adopted by Zanzibaris that "*don't care where they throw trash*", and tourists who "*throw everything in the sea from the boats*" (Interviews, Tourism workers; Maione, 2019). Second, marine littering was often associated with poor awareness of plastic pollution and its impacts on the local environment. A third driver of marine pollution was insufficient provision of waste management services, especially on coastal tourism sites. This is due to the inability of the municipal waste sector to provide regulations for all stakeholders (e.g., waste-generating activities such as hotels and food services, private companies supplying waste collection and management services, waste and recycling associations) on one hand, and the absence of waste collection activities in coastal areas, where most of the tourism facilities are located, resulting in the mismanagement of tourism-related waste (Blomstrand & Silander Hagström, 2014). Finally, the proximity of hotels and food services to the beach was another main driver of beach pollution. Waste workers reported that the majority of plastic litter found on the main tourism beach in Stone Town came from Forodhani Gardens, an open-air food market located along the beach. Dominant plastic litter items included single-use plastic food containers, shopping bags, tableware, straws, and beverage bottles.

Sources of Marine Plastic Pollution

Observations conducted in the coastal city of Stone Town showed the greatest heterogeneity of marine plastics. Sampled plastic litter was linked to four primary sources: (i) residential households, (ii) tourism, (iii) building and construction sector, (iv) small businesses and commercial services, as shown in Table 2. Tourism was also found to be a primary source of marine plastic pollution in the sites of Nungwi, Uroa, and Fumba. In these areas, hotels, resorts, and tourism coastal attractions (e.g., beach visits, beach sports, recreational fishing, boat tours, and diving centers) were associated with input beach accumulations, in the form of plastic beverage bottles, followed by plastic shopping bags and other single-use plastics. Littering during boat tours and other tourism activities was a major pathway of marine plastic pollution, confirming the interview findings that marine littering and poor awareness of plastic pollution were major drivers of beach litter. In addition, the lack of waste facilities in the area significantly contributed to the mismanagement of plastic waste. Plastics from fishing constituted another major source of marine pollution. Secondary sources of plastic pollution were tourism-related commercial activities and residential households.

Implications for Small Developing Islands

The Zanzibar archipelago presents several challenges related to the management of waste and pollution on small developing islands with underdeveloped waste management infrastructure. As other small islands, Zanzibar is bounded by limited physical space for collecting, storing, and processing solid waste. This is coupled with the absence of an adequate waste management infrastructure and results in large amounts of waste and recyclables being lost or dispersed in the natural environment (Mohee et al., 2015). In particular, the volumes of plastic waste generated on the island vary greatly between high and low tourism season, with implications on the management of different solid waste flows (Maione, 2021).

Another challenge pertains to the high costs of collecting and managing waste, especially in areas that are not formally included in the waste management services provided by the Zanzibar Municipal Council. Other economic barriers encompass the cost of collection vehicles and equipment, costs associated with the recycling process (e.g., purchase of recycling machineries, fixed and maintenance costs to operate recycling facilities), and low revenues from the recycling sector (Bhadra et al., 2017). Furthermore, small developing islands generally present underdeveloped end-markets for recycled plastics and difficulty of developing local circular economy models (Eckelman et al., 2014). This is also due to the fact that most plastics are produced elsewhere (on the mainland Tanzania, in other African or international countries), and subsequently imported in Zanzibar in the form of semi-finished or finished plastic goods, mostly used for tourism consumption.

Furthermore, studying tourism-related plastics is of massive importance to understand the numerous effects of plastic pollution on small islands like Zanzibar, that heavily rely on marine resources and tourism incomes. These effects can range from well-documented risks for marine organisms, such as ingestion, entanglement, or chemical contamination (Cózar et al., 2014), to degradation of reef areas (Lamb et al., 2018), to less-known economic damages associated with the degradation of ecotourism environments and attractions. In these areas, plastic pollution can cause a decrease in the number of tourists and beach activities, and consequent loss of tourism revenues (Jang et al., 2014; McIlgorm et al., 2011). If no action is taken to stop plastic from entering the ocean, coastal-dependent activities such as commercial and recreational fishing, daily beach visits, snorkeling, diving, boat tours, and mariculture, are predicted to see a rapid decline (Staehr et al., 2018).

Table 2. Summary of observations conducted in Stone Town. Adapted from Maione (2019, 2021)

Sampling site	Data collected	Description	Photos
Forodhani Gardens food market	Littering practices	Food wrapping, packaging, and tableware abandoned in the environment.	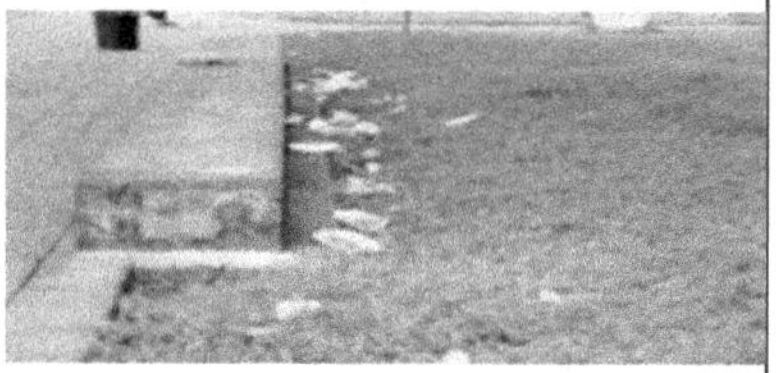
Forodhani Gardens food market	Source, amount, and type of plastic litter	0.2 kg of domestic plastics including cleaning supplies containers. 47.2 kg of plastics from the building and construction sector including wrapping, containers, and small plastic components. 20.7 kg of plastics from the commercial sectors including plastic shopping bags, containers, and small plastic components. 47.9 kg of tourism plastics including beverage bottles, tableware, food wrapping, takeaway containers, and plastic shopping bags.	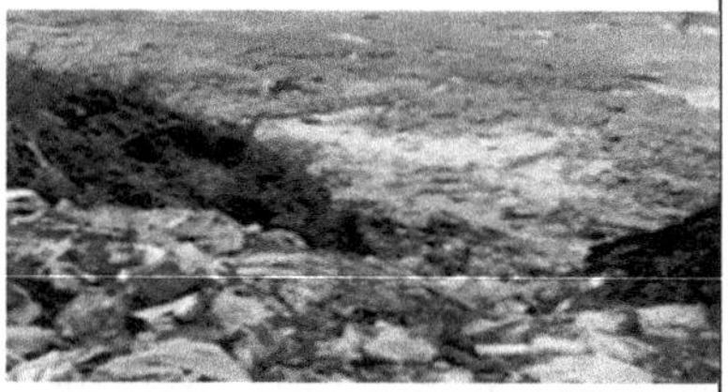
Shoreline walkway	Number, location, type, and conditions of waste facilities	Counted 30 trash cans, squared stone containers with a metal grid skeleton, sized 0.5 m x 0.5 m. Distanced 10 m and aligned with urban furniture. Emptied on a daily basis between 10:00 am and 12:00 pm.	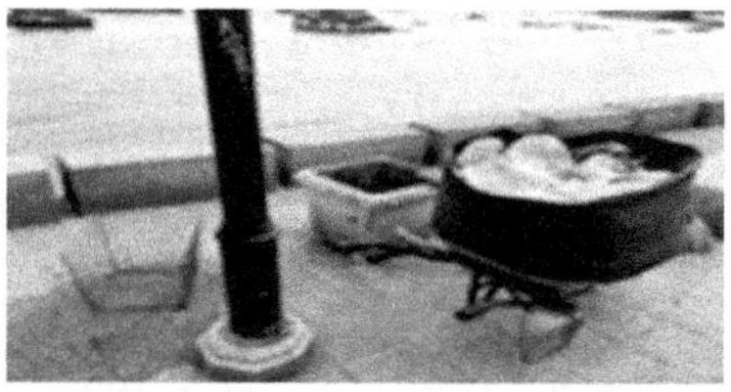
Open sea	Littering practices	Discarding beverage bottles from boat tours in the sea.	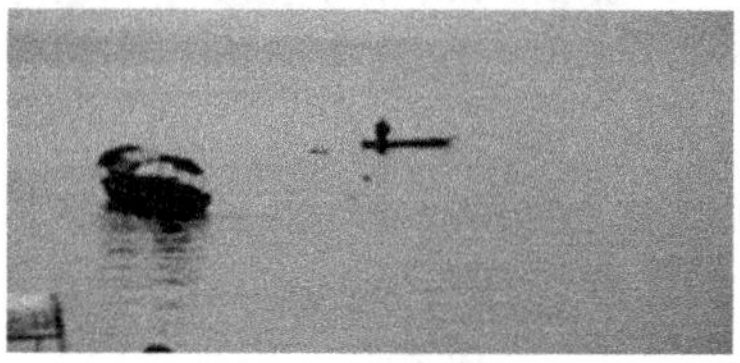
Port	Source, amount, and type of plastic litter	26.8 kg of domestic plastics including plastic shopping bags, flip flops, rubbers, cleaning supplies containers, tyres, and fishing equipment. 9.3 kg of plastics from the building and construction sector including wrapping, containers, and small plastic components. 1.4 kg of plastics from the commercial sector including plastic shopping bags, food wrapping, and supplies containers. 4.8 kg of tourism plastics including beverage bottles and plastic shopping bags.	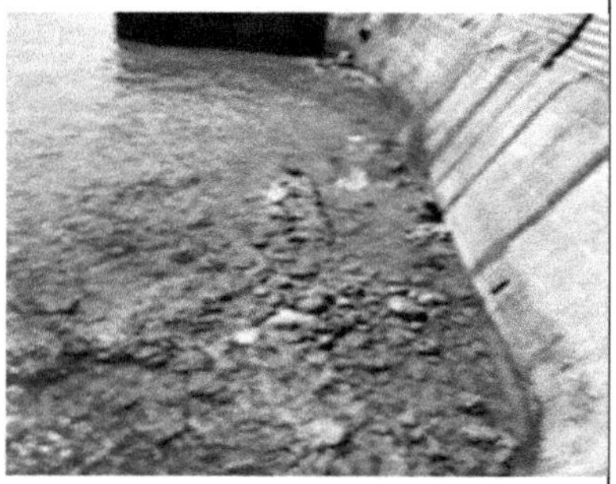

continued on following page

Table 2. Continued

Sampling site	Data collected	Description	Photos
Shangani beach	Source, amount, and type of plastic litter	20.8 kg of domestic plastics including plastic shopping bags, food wrapping, houseware, flip flops, rubbers, cleaning supplies containers, tyres, fishing equipment, and clothing. 18.3 kg of plastics from the building and construction sector including wrapping containers and small plastic components. 10.9 kg of plastics from the commercial sector including plastic shopping bags, containers, and small plastic components. 17.6 kg of tourism plastics including beverage bottles, tableware, food wrapping, containers, plastic shopping bags, flip flops, recreational fishing equipment, and sporting equipment.	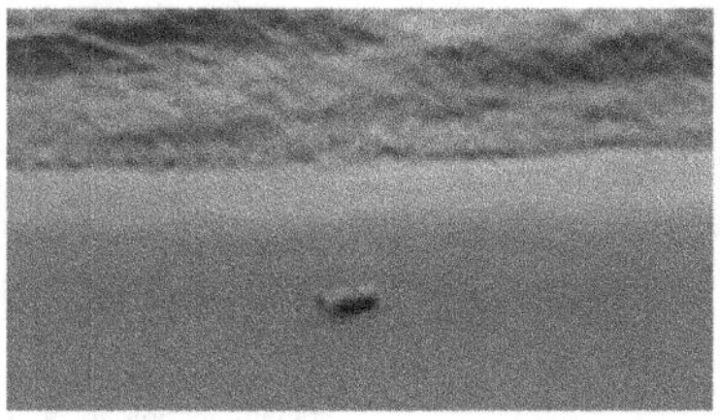

SOLUTIONS AND RECOMMENDATIONS

Monitoring and Reporting on Marine Litter

Our present understanding of marine pollution is not sufficient to calculate trends and volumes of plastic debris in the marine environment and the totality of their ecological impacts (JRC, 2013). Current assessments provide in fact patchy information on the original sources and pathways of plastic pollution, and the types of marine debris; hence, much uncertainty remains in the calculation of marine litter amounts. These difficulties can partially be attributed to the degree of maturity of commonly used assessment protocols, their testing, and their effectiveness in capturing local and global dynamics. Moreover, methods to analyze and quantify marine litter are not standardized, both in terms of methodologies and outputs, which can make a comparison of results difficult, if not impossible.

Monitoring has been defined as "*the repeated measurement of a characteristic of the environment, or of a process, in order to detect a trend in space or time*" (Jambeck et al., 2015). In particular, marine litter monitoring consists of the repeated collection, quantification (by item count or weight), and characterization (into waste material categories) over a specific period of time (Barnardo & Ribbink, 2020). As such, monitoring and reporting on plastic flows is of massive importance, especially with regard to materials' fate at the end of their useful life (Jambeck et al., 2015; Geyer et al., 2017). The results of marine litter monitoring should answer four main questions pertaining to: (i) the type and distribution of land-based and sea-based sources of plastic pollution; (ii) the pathways and transport mechanisms of marine pollution from source to sea; (iii) the amounts and types of debris concentrations; and (iv) the spatio-temporal variability of these concentrations (Barnardo & Ribbink, 2020).

Monitoring can be conducted at different scales (macro, meso, micro) depending on the specific characteristics of the sampling site and the assessment's objectives. Table 3 presents three levels of analysis that can be employed as separate assessments or combined and integrated to provide a deeper analysis of macro- and microplastics altogether.

Table 3. Toolkit of monitoring methodologies at the macro-, meso-, and micro-level

Scale	Open issues	Survey questions	Methodology	Objectives	Collected data	References
Macro-level (e.g., coastal regions across international borders, river basins, transboundary waters)	•Limited traceability associated with different systems for material/pollution monitoring and accounting. •Different policies and measures to allocate resources, and keep material flows accountable. •Lack of information exchange across borders. •Uneven use and communication of data analytics.	•What are the magnitude, location, and temporal variability of plastic accumulations? •What are the composition, spatio-temporal distribution, and abundance of plastic accumulations? •What are the main physical and anthropogenic processes influencing the transport and accumulation of plastics?	•Space-based observation of magnitude, spatio-temporal distribution, and accumulation of marine plastic pollution. •Spectrometric analysis of observed pollution. •Proximity sensing (e.g., sensors, drones) data acquisition on pollution.	•Provide real-time or nearly real-time data acquisition, wide area coverage, and high spatial resolution. •Provide a consistent global, harmonized system for assessing plastic particles swirling in transboundary waters.	•Satellite imagery of plastic pollution. •Aerial photos of pollution.	Maione & Fernandez, 2021; Topouzeli et al., 2019; Biermann et al., 2020
Meso-level (e.g., beach, tourism site, coastal waters)	•Paucity of data on sources and amounts of marine plastic pollution. •Uncertainty about sources and pathways of marine pollution.	•Where are the areas where litter is most prevalent? •How much litter occurs in the selected study site? •What is the litter composition (wet, recyclable, non-recyclable)? •What are the principal types of material (e.g., plastic, paper, metal, etc.)? •What are the principal litter items? •Does the amount of litter vary across different transects? •What are possible variables that affect the input of litter at sea?	•In-situ assessment and quantification of plastic litter via litter counting (visual inspection of debris). •Litter separation by material type and debris classification.	•Capture spatio-temporal variability of beach and coastal plastic pollution over time (e.g., measurements can be repeated over several consecutive days and across time). •Provide a more accessible litter assessment using basic, cost-effective tools (e.g., logbook, pencils, measuring tape, litter bags, and buckets).	•Marine litter amounts (count and weight). •Marine litter density (kg/ transect). •Photographic evidence. •Information on sampling conditions (e.g., location, GPS coordinates, time, procedure).	NOWPAP, 2007; JRC, 2013; Lippiatt et al., 2013; Barnardo & Ribbink, 2020
Micro-level (e.g., water samples, shore sediments, biota)	•Limited data on ecological and biological impacts of plastic on native species. •Uncertainty about the translocation of microplastics across trophic levels.	•What are the abundance, distribution, and variability of microplastics? •What is the incidence of encounter between microplastics and native species (e.g., resulting in ingestion)? •How does plastic pollution affect the subsistence (e.g., feeding behavior) of native species?	•Sampling of water. •Sampling of shore sediments containing plastic particles. •Sampling of fish, birds, bivalves, or crustaceans.	•Quantify smaller fragments like microplastics and nanoplastics. •Assess specific impacts of plastic pollution, such as the incidence of encounters between plastic particles and marine organisms, as well as related effects (e.g., biological effects, ecological effects, changes in fish feeding behavior, or debris translocation across trophic levels).	•Number and type (beads, fibers, fragments, films, or foams) of plastic particles. •Particle size (length and area). •Dominant particle color (e.g., blue, black, red, or orange).	GESAMP, 2015; Free et al., 2014; Ory et al., 2017; Kundu et al., 2021

CONCLUSION

Marine litter and plastic pollution present a serious threat to the planet's oceans. Assessing sources and pathways of marine plastics is of utmost importance; however, knowledge gaps and uncertainty in numbers, entry points, and transport mechanisms persist. This chapter presents a global assessment of plastic pollution in coastal and island regions, emphasizing the role and contributions of different sea-based and land-based pollution sources, their origins, means of release, and physical means by which plastic debris enters the sea. Among the numerous sources of plastic pollution, the contributions of coastal tourism to plastic pollution are emphasized, especially in areas that heavily rely on tourism resources for their development. The chapter discusses some priority solutions for assessing the magnitude and extent of plastic swirling in water bodies using a combination of monitoring approaches. Proposed solutions aim to provide harmonized information on the fate of plastics to deepen the understanding of their ecological impacts on the marine environment, and to provide stakeholders with implications on plastic's end-of-life management and ways to retain plastics within the economic system. Finally, future research could address the role of emergent sectors in plastic pollution, including the impacts of marine litter sources on ocean industries and livelihoods, as well as projections and estimations of the global ocean plastic burden following ongoing system changes.

REFERENCES

Ally, B., Ismail, S. N. S., & Rasdi, I. (2014). Municipal solid waste management of Zanzibar: Current practice, the challenges and the future. *International Journal of Current Research and Academic Review, 1*, 5-19. http://www.ijcrar.com/special/1/Biubwa%20Ally,%20et%20al.pdf

Andrady, A. L., & Neal, M. A. (2009). Applications and societal benefits of plastics. *Philosophical Transactions of the Royal Society of London. Series B, Biological Sciences, 364*(1526), 1977–1984. doi:10.1098/rstb.2008.0304 PMID:19528050

ARCADIS. (2012). *Case study on the plastic cycle and its loopholes in the four European regional seas areas*. European Commission DG Environment Framework contract. ENV.D.2./ETU/2011/0041

Barnardo, T., & Ribbink, A. J. (2020). *African Marine Litter Monitoring Manual*. African Marine Waste Network. Sustainable Seas Trust, Port Elizabeth. https://sst.org.za/wp-content/uploads/2020/07/Barnardo-Ribbink-2020_African-Marine-Litter-Monitoring-Manual.pdf

Barnes, D. K., Galgani, F., Thompson, R. C., & Barlaz, M. (2009). Accumulation and fragmentation of plastic debris in global environments. *Philosophical Transactions of the Royal Society of London. Series B, Biological Sciences, 364*(1526), 1985–1998. doi:10.1098/rstb.2008.0205 PMID:19528051

Bergmann, M., Sandhop, N., Schewe, I., & D'Hert, D. (2016). Observations of floating anthropogenic litter in the Barents Sea and Fram Strait, Arctic. *Polar Biology, 39*(3), 553–560. doi:10.100700300-015-1795-8

Bhadra, J., Al-Thani, N., & Abdulkareem, A. (2017). Recycling of polymer-polymer composites. In *Micro and nano fibrillar composites (MFCs and NFCs) from polymer blends* (pp. 263–277). Woodhead Publishing. doi:10.1016/B978-0-08-101991-7.00011-X

Biermann, L., Clewley, D., Martinez-Vicente, V., & Topouzelis, K. (2020). Finding plastic patches in coastal waters using optical satellite data. *Scientific Reports, 10*(1), 1–10. doi:10.103841598-020-62298-z PMID:31913322

Blomstrand, E., & Silander Hagström, T. (2014). *Waste management and production systems; The case of Zanzibar*. https://www.diva-portal.org/smash/get/diva2:853136/FULLTEXT01.pdf

Born, M. P., & Brüll, C. (2021). From model to nature— A review on the transferability of marine (micro-) plastic fragmentation studies. *The Science of the Total Environment*. Advance online publication. doi:10.1016/j.scitotenv.2021.151389 PMID:34808157

Boucher, J., & Friot, D. (2017). *Primary microplastics in the oceans: A global evaluation of sources* (Vol. 10). Gland, Switzerland: IUCN. https://holdnorgerent.no/wp-content/uploads/2020/03/IUCN-report-Primary-microplastics-in-the-oceans.pdf

Browne, M. A., Galloway, T. S., & Thompson, R. C. (2010). Spatial patterns of plastic debris along estuarine shorelines. *Environmental Science & Technology, 44*(9), 3404–3409. doi:10.1021/es903784e PMID:20377170

Cózar, A., Echevarría, F., González-Gordillo, J. I., Irigoien, X., Úbeda, B., Hernández-León, S., Palma, A. T., Navarro, S., García-de-Lomas, J., Ruiz, A., Fernandez-de-Puelles, M. L., & Duarte, C. M. (2014). Plastic debris in the open ocean. *Proceedings of the National Academy of Sciences of the United States of America, 111*(28), 10239–10244. doi:10.1073/pnas.1314705111 PMID:24982135

Cózar, A., Sanz-Martín, M., Martí, E., González-Gordillo, J. I., Ubeda, B., Gálvez, J. Á., Irigoien, X., & Duarte, C. M. (2015). Plastic accumulation in the Mediterranean Sea. *PLoS One, 10*(4), e0121762. doi:10.1371/journal.pone.0121762 PMID:25831129

Derraik, J. G. (2002). The pollution of the marine environment by plastic debris: A review. *Marine Pollution Bulletin, 44*(9), 842–852. doi:10.1016/S0025-326X(02)00220-5 PMID:12405208

EC (European Commission). (2018). *A European Strategy for Plastics in a Circular Economy*. https://ec.europa.eu/environment/strategy/plastics-strategy_en

EC (European Commission). (2019). *Directive on single-use plastics*. https://eur-lex.europa.eu/legal-content/EN/TXT/PDF/?uri=CELEX:32019L0904&from=EN

Eckelman, M. J., Ashton, W., Arakaki, Y., Hanaki, K., Nagashima, S., & Malone-Lee, L. C. (2014). Island waste management systems: Statistics, challenges, and opportunities for applied industrial ecology. *Journal of Industrial Ecology, 18*(2), 306–317. doi:10.1111/jiec.12113

ECORYS. (2013). *Study in Support of Policy Measures for Maritime and Coastal Tourism at EU Level*. ECORYS.

ECORYS (2016). *Study on Specific Challenges for a Sustainable Development of Coastal and Maritime Tourism in Europe*. doi:10.2826/94993

EEA (European Environmental Agency). (2016). *Restoring European rivers and lakes in cities improves quality of life*. https://www.eea.europa.eu/highlights/restoring-european-rivers-and-lakes

Eriksen, M., Lebreton, L. C., Carson, H. S., Thiel, M., Moore, C. J., Borerro, J. C., Galgani, F., Ryan, P. G., & Reisser, J. (2014). Plastic pollution in the world's oceans: More than 5 trillion plastic pieces weighing over 250,000 tons afloat at sea. *PLoS One*, *9*(12), e111913. doi:10.1371/journal.pone.0111913 PMID:25494041

Eriksson, C., Burton, H., Fitch, S., Schulz, M., & van den Hoff, J. (2013). Daily accumulation rates of marine debris on sub-Antarctic island beaches. *Marine Pollution Bulletin*, *66*(1-2), 199–208. doi:10.1016/j.marpolbul.2012.08.026 PMID:23219394

EUNOMIA. (2016). *Plastics in the Marine Environment*. https://www.eunomia.co.uk/reports-tools/plastics-in-the-marine-environment/

Europen. (2009). *The European Shopping Baskets – Packaging trends for Fast Moving Consumer Goods in Selected European Countries*. Europen, The European Organization for packaging and the environment. https://www.leanbusinessireland.ie/includes/documents/Public%2520Phase%2520I%2520ESB%2520Report%5B1%5D.pdf

Everaert, G., Van Cauwenberghe, L., De Rijcke, M., Koelmans, A. A., Mees, J., Vandegehuchte, M., & Janssen, C. R. (2018). Risk assessment of microplastics in the ocean: Modelling approach and first conclusions. *Environmental Pollution*, *242*, 1930–1938. doi:10.1016/j.envpol.2018.07.069 PMID:30061084

FAO (Food and Agriculture Organization of the United Nations). (2017). *Microplastics in fisheries and aquaculture. Status of knowledge on their occurrence and implications for aquatic organisms and food safety*. FAO. https://www.fao.org/3/I7677E/I7677E.pdf

Fendall, L. S., & Sewell, M. A. (2009). Contributing to marine pollution by washing your face: Microplastics in facial cleansers. *Marine Pollution Bulletin*, *58*(8), 1225–1228. doi:10.1016/j.marpolbul.2009.04.025 PMID:19481226

Fleming, S. (2020). *Scientists find plastic pollution in the rain and in the air we breathe*. https://www.weforum.org/agenda/2020/07/scientists-find-plastic-pollution-in-the-rain-and-in-the-air-we-breathe/

Free, C. M., Jensen, O. P., Mason, S. A., Eriksen, M., Williamson, N. J., & Boldgiv, B. (2014). High-levels of microplastic pollution in a large, remote, mountain lake. *Marine Pollution Bulletin*, *85*(1), 156–163. doi:10.1016/j.marpolbul.2014.06.001 PMID:24973278

GESAMP. (2015). *Sources, fate and effects of microplastics in the marine environment: A global assessment*. GESAMP. https://ec.europa.eu/environment/marine/good-environmental-status/descriptor-10/pdf/GESAMP_microplastics%20full%20study.pdf

GESAMP. (2016). *Sources, fate and effects of microplastics in the marine environment: Part 2 of a global assessment*. GESAMP. http://www.gesamp.org/publications/microplastics-in-the-marine-environment-part-2

Geyer, R., Jambeck, J. R., & Law, K. L. (2017). Production, use, and fate of all plastics ever made. *Science Advances*, *3*(7), e1700782. doi:10.1126ciadv.1700782 PMID:28776036

Gilman, E. (2015). Status of international monitoring and management of abandoned, lost and discarded fishing gear and ghost fishing. *Marine Policy*, *60*, 225–239. doi:10.1016/j.marpol.2015.06.016

Gong, Y., Putnam, E., You, W., & Zhao, C. (2020). Investigation into circular economy of plastics: The case of the UK fast moving consumer goods industry. *Journal of Cleaner Production*, *244*, 118941. doi:10.1016/j.jclepro.2019.118941

Government Communication Unit. (2019). *Notice to travellers planning to visit Tanzania*. The United Republic of Tanzania Vice President's Office.

Greenpeace. (2020). *34 Plastic Bans in Africa. A Reality Check*. https://www.greenpeace.org/africa/

Haward, M. (2018). Plastic pollution of the world's seas and oceans as a contemporary challenge in ocean governance. *Nature Communications*, *9*(1), 1–3. doi:10.103841467-018-03104-3 PMID:29445166

ISWA (International Solid Waste Association). (2017). *Prevent marine plastic litter - now!* ISWA Marine Task Force. https://marinelitter.iswa.org/fileadmin/user_upload/Marine_Task_Force_Report_2017/ISWA_report170927_interactive_lowres.pdf

Jambeck, J. R., Geyer, R., Wilcox, C., Siegler, T. R., Perryman, M., Andrady, A., Narayan, R., & Law, K. L. (2015). Plastic waste inputs from land into the ocean. *Science*, *347*(6223), 768–771. doi:10.1126cience.1260352 PMID:25678662

James, G. (2019). *The Plastics Landscape: Risk and opportunities along the value chain*. Principles for Responsible Investment. https://www.unpri.org/plastics/risks-and-opportunities-along-the-plastics-value-chain/4774.article

Jang, Y. C., Hong, S., Lee, J., Lee, M. J., & Shim, W. J. (2014). Estimation of lost tourism revenue in Geoje Island from the 2011 marine debris pollution event in South Korea. *Marine Pollution Bulletin*, *81*(1), 49–54. doi:10.1016/j.marpolbul.2014.02.021 PMID:24635983

Johnson, S. (2019). *'It is raining plastic': Microplastics found in U.S. rainwater*. https://bigthink.com/the-present/microplastics-rainwater/

JRC. (2013). *Guidance on Monitoring of Marine Litter in European Seas*. Joint Research Centre of the European Commission, Ispra, EUR 26113 EN. https://mcc.jrc.ec.europa.eu/documents/201702074014.pdf

Kentin, E., & Kaarto, H. (2018). An EU ban on microplastics in cosmetic products and the right to regulate. *Review of European, Comparative & International Environmental Law*, *27*(3), 254–266. doi:10.1111/reel.12269

Kowalski, N., Reichardt, A. M., & Waniek, J. J. (2016). Sinking rates of microplastics and potential implications of their alteration by physical, biological, and chemical factors. *Marine Pollution Bulletin*, *109*(1), 310–319. doi:10.1016/j.marpolbul.2016.05.064 PMID:27297594

Kukulka, T., Proskurowski, G., Morét-Ferguson, S., Meyer, D. W., & Law, K. L. (2012). The effect of wind mixing on the vertical distribution of buoyant plastic debris. *Geophysical Research Letters*, *39*(7), n/a. Advance online publication. doi:10.1029/2012GL051116

Kummu, M., De Moel, H., Ward, P. J., & Varis, O. (2011). How close do we live to water? A global analysis of population distance to freshwater bodies. *PLoS One*, *6*(6), e20578. doi:10.1371/journal.pone.0020578 PMID:21687675

Kundu, A., Shetti, N. P., Basu, S., Reddy, K. R., Nadagouda, M. N., & Aminabhavi, T. M. (2021). Identification and removal of micro-and nano-plastics: Efficient and cost-effective methods. *Chemical Engineering Journal, 421*, 129816. doi:10.1016/j.cej.2021.129816 PMID:34504393

Lamb, J. B., Willis, B. L., Fiorenza, E. A., Couch, C. S., Howard, R., Rader, D. N., True, J. D., Kelly, L. A., Ahamd, A., Jompa, J., & Harvell, C. D. (2018). Plastic waste associated with disease on coral reefs. *Science, 359*(6374), 460–462. doi:10.1126cience.aar3320 PMID:29371469

Lamprecht, A. (2013). *The abundance, distribution and accumulation of plastic debris in Table Bay, Cape Town, South Africa* [Master's dissertation]. University of Cape Town. http://hdl.handle.net/11427/6633

Lange, G. M. (2015). Tourism in Zanzibar: Incentives for sustainable management of the coastal environment. *Ecosystem Services, 11*, 5–11. doi:10.1016/j.ecoser.2014.11.009

Law, K. L., Morét-Ferguson, S., Maximenko, N. A., Proskurowski, G., Peacock, E. E., Hafner, J., & Reddy, C. M. (2010). Plastic accumulation in the North Atlantic subtropical gyre. *Science, 329*(5996), 1185–1188. doi:10.1126cience.1192321 PMID:20724586

Law, K. L., Morét-Ferguson, S. E., Goodwin, D. S., Zettler, E. R., DeForce, E., Kukulka, T., & Proskurowski, G. (2014). Distribution of surface plastic debris in the eastern Pacific Ocean from an 11-year data set. *Environmental Science & Technology, 48*(9), 4732–4738. doi:10.1021/es4053076 PMID:24708264

Lebreton, L. C., Van Der Zwet, J., Damsteeg, J. W., Slat, B., Andrady, A., & Reisser, J. (2017). River plastic emissions to the world's oceans. *Nature Communications, 8*(1), 1–10. doi:10.1038/ncomms15611 PMID:28589961

Li, W. C., Tse, H. F., & Fok, L. (2016). Plastic waste in the marine environment: A review of sources, occurrence and effects. *The Science of the Total Environment, 566*, 333–349. doi:10.1016/j.scitotenv.2016.05.084 PMID:27232963

Lippiatt, S., Opfer, S., & Arthur, C. (2013). *Marine debris monitoring and assessment: recommendations for monitoring debris trends in the marine environment.* NOAA. https://repository.library.noaa.gov/view/noaa/2681

Lydon, T. (2021). *3,000 Shipping Containers Fell Into the Pacific Ocean Last Winter.* https://therevelator.org/container-ship-accidents/

Magnusson, K., Eliaeson, K., Fråne, A., Haikonen, K., Olshammar, M., Stadmark, J., & Hultén, J. (2016). *Swedish sources and pathways for microplastics to the marine environment.* https://www.diva-portal.org/smash/record.jsf?pid=diva2%3A1549783&dswid=4554

Maione, C. (2019). *Emergence of plastic pollution on tourism beaches in Zanzibar, Tanzania* [Master's Thesis]. University of Michigan. http://hdl.handle.net/2027.42/148801

Maione, C. (2021). Quantifying plastics waste accumulations on coastal tourism sites in Zanzibar, Tanzania. *Marine Pollution Bulletin, 168*, 112418. doi:10.1016/j.marpolbul.2021.112418 PMID:33930645

Maione, C., & Fernandez, G. (2021). Plastic Detection Using a Multi-method Approach: Comparative Case Studies from Coastal Tourism Sites. In *Abstracts of 1st International Symposium on Plastic Pollution: Removal, Analysis, and Risk Assessment of Microplastics* (pp. 23-27). AIJR. 10.21467/abstracts.119

McIlgorm, A., Campbell, H. F., & Rule, M. J. (2011). The economic cost and control of marine debris damage in the Asia-Pacific region. *Ocean and Coastal Management*, *54*(9), 643–651. doi:10.1016/j.ocecoaman.2011.05.007

Mohammed, S. M. (2002). Pollution management in Zanzibar: The need for a new approach. *Ocean and Coastal Management*, *45*(4-5), 301–311. doi:10.1016/S0964-5691(02)00060-1

Mohee, R., Mauthoor, S., Bundhoo, Z. M., Somaroo, G., Soobhany, N., & Gunasee, S. (2015). Current status of solid waste management in small island developing states: A review. *Waste Management (New York, N.Y.)*, *43*, 539–549. doi:10.1016/j.wasman.2015.06.012 PMID:26116009

Ng, Y. T., Lu, W. F., & Song, B. (2014). Quantification of end-of-life product condition to support product recovery decision. *Procedia CIRP*, *15*, 257–262. doi:10.1016/j.procir.2014.06.086

Nielsen, T. D., Hasselbalch, J., Holmberg, K., & Stripple, J. (2020). Politics and the plastic crisis: A review throughout the plastic life cycle. *Wiley Interdisciplinary Reviews. Energy and Environment*, *9*(1), e360. doi:10.1002/wene.360

NOWPAP. (2007). *Guidelines for Monitoring Litter on the Beaches and Shorelines of the Northwest Pacific Region*. NOWPAP CEARAC. http://hdl.handle.net/20.500.11822/27232

Ocean Conservancy. (2015). *Stemming the Tide: Land-based strategies for a plastic-free ocean*. McKinsey & Company and Ocean Conservancy. https://oceanconservancy.org/wp-content/uploads/2017/04/full-report-stemming-the.pdf

Ory, N. C., Sobral, P., Ferreira, J. L., & Thiel, M. (2017). Amberstripe scad Decapterus muroadsi (Carangidae) fish ingest blue microplastics resembling their copepod prey along the coast of Rapa Nui (Easter Island) in the South Pacific subtropical gyre. *The Science of the Total Environment*, *586*, 430–437. doi:10.1016/j.scitotenv.2017.01.175 PMID:28196756

Patagonia. (2021). *Recycled Polyester*. https://eu.patagonia.com/it/en/our-footprint/recycled-polyester.html

PlasticsEurope. (2019). *Plastics - the Facts 2019. An analysis of European plastic production, demand and waste data*. https://plasticseurope.org/wp-content/uploads/2021/10/2019-Plastics-the-facts.pdf

Plummer, R. (2018). *Plastic fantastic: How it changed the world*. https://www.bbc.com/news/business-42646025

Rech, S., Macaya-Caquilpán, V., Pantoja, J. F., Rivadeneira, M. M., Madariaga, D. J., & Thiel, M. (2014). Rivers as a source of marine litter–a study from the SE Pacific. *Marine Pollution Bulletin*, *82*(1-2), 66–75. doi:10.1016/j.marpolbul.2014.03.019 PMID:24726186

Ryberg, M. W., Hauschild, M. Z., Wang, F., Averous-Monnery, S., & Laurent, A. (2019). Global environmental losses of plastics across their value chains. *Resources, Conservation and Recycling*, *151*, 104459. doi:10.1016/j.resconrec.2019.104459

Sharma, S., Basu, S., Shetti, N. P., Nadagouda, M. N., & Aminabhavi, T. M. (2021). Microplastics in the environment: Occurrence, perils, and eradication. *Chemical Engineering Journal*, *408*, 127317. doi:10.1016/j.cej.2020.127317 PMID:34017217

Sharpley, R., & Ussi, M. (2014). Tourism and governance in small island developing states (SIDS): The case of Zanzibar. *International Journal of Tourism Research, 16*(1), 87–96. doi:10.1002/jtr.1904

Simon, M. (2020). *Plastic Rain Is the New Acid Rain.* https://www.wired.com/story/plastic-rain-is-the-new-acid-rain/

Simon, M. (2021). *Plastic Is Falling From the Sky. But Where's It Coming From?* https://www.wired.com/story/plastic-is-falling-from-the-sky/

Staehr, P. A., Sheikh, M., Rashid, R., Ussi, A., Suleiman, M., Kloiber, U., Dahl, K., Tairova, Z., Strand, J., Kuguru, B., & Muhando, C. (2018). Managing human pressures to restore ecosystem health of zanzibar coastal waters. *J. Aquac. Mar. Biol, 7*(2), 59–70. doi:10.15406/jamb.2018.07.00185

Sundt, P., Schulze, P.-E., & Syversen, F. 2014. *Sources of microplastic- pollution to the marine environment.* Miljødirektoaret/Norwegian Environment Agency. https://d3n8a8pro7vhmx.cloudfront.net/boomerangalliance/pages/507/attachments/original/1481155578/Norway_Sources_of_Microplastic_Pollution.pdf?1481155578

The Pew Charitable Trusts & SYSTEMIQ. (2020). *Breaking the Plastic Wave: A Comprehensive Assessment of Pathways Towards Stopping Ocean Plastic Pollution.* https://www.pewtrusts.org/-/media/assets/2020/10/breakingtheplasticwave_mainreport.pdf

Thiel, M., Hinojosa, I. A., Joschko, T., & Gutow, L. (2011). Spatio-temporal distribution of floating objects in the German Bight (North Sea). *Journal of Sea Research, 65*(3), 368–379. doi:10.1016/j.seares.2011.03.002

Thompson, R. C., Olsen, Y., Mitchell, R. P., Davis, A., Rowland, S. J., John, A. W., McGonigle, D., & Russell, A. E. (2004). Lost at sea: Where is all the plastic? *Science, 304*(5672), 838–838. doi:10.1126cience.1094559 PMID:15131299

Thompson, R.C., Swan, S.H., Moore, C.J., & Vom Saal, F.S. (2009). *Our plastic age.* doi:10.1098/rstb.2009.0054

Topouzelis, K., Papakonstantinou, A., & Garaba, S. P. (2019). Detection of floating plastics from satellite and unmanned aerial systems (Plastic Litter Project 2018). *International Journal of Applied Earth Observation and Geoinformation, 79*, 175–183. doi:10.1016/j.jag.2019.03.011

UN. (2015). *The 17 Goals.* https://sdgs.un.org/goals

UNEP. (2014a). *Valuing Plastic: The Business Case for Measuring, Managing and Disclosing Plastic Use in the Consumer Goods Industry.* UN Environment Programme. http://hdl.handle.net/20.500.11822/9238

UNEP. (2014b). *Annex I. UNEA Resolution 1/6 Marine plastic debris and microplastics.* https://wedocs.unep.org/bitstream/handle/20.500.11822/17562/Marine%20Plastic%20Debris%20and%20Microplastic%20Technical%20Report%20Advance%20Copy%20Ann.pdf?%20sequence=2&isAllowed=y

UNEP. (2016a). *Marine Plastic Debris and Microplastics – Global Lessons and Research to Inspire Action and Guide Policy Change.* UN Environment Programme. https://wedocs.unep.org/handle/20.500.11822/7720

UNEP. (2016b). *2/11. Marine plastic litter and microplastics.* https://wedocs.unep.org/bitstream/handle/20.500.11822/11186/K1607228_UNEPEA2_RES11E.pdf?sequence=1&isAllowed=y

UNEP. (2017). *3/7. Marine litter and microplastics.* https://wedocs.unep.org/bitstream/handle/20.500.11822/22773/K1800210%20-%20UNEP-EA-3-RES-7%20-%20Advance.pdf?sequence=15&isAllowed=y

UNEP. (2018a). *Report of the first meeting of the ad hoc open-ended expert group on marine litter and microplastics.* UN Environment Programme. https://papersmart.unon.org/resolution/uploads/k1801471.pdf

UNEP. (2018b). *Africa Waste Management Outlook.* UN Environment Programme. https://wedocs.unep.org/20.500.11822/25514

UNEP. (2018c). *Mapping of global plastics value chain and plastics losses to the environment (with a particular focus on marine environment).* UN Environment Programme. http://hdl.handle.net/20.500.11822/26745

UNEP. (2019a). *4/6. Marine plastic litter and microplastics.* https://wedocs.unep.org/bitstream/handle/20.500.11822/28471/English.pdf?sequence=3&isAllowed=y

UNEP. (2021). *Drowning In Plastics - Marine Litter and Plastic Waste Vital Graphics.* UN Environment Programme and GRID-Arendal, Nairobi and Arendal. https://wedocs.unep.org/xmlui/bitstream/handle/20.500.11822/36964/VITGRAPH.pdf

UNEP & GRID-Arendal. (2016). *Marine Litter Vital Graphics.* UN Environment Programme and GRID-Arendal, Nairobi and Arendal. https://www.unep.org/resources/report/marine-litter-vital-graphics

UNGC. (2020). *Ocean Stewardship 2030. Ten ambitions and recommendations for growing sustainable ocean business.* New York: UN Global Compact. https://ungc-communications-assets.s3.amazonaws.com/docs/publications/Ocean-Stewardship-2030-Report.pdf

Van Sebille, E., Aliani, S., Law, K. L., Maximenko, N., Alsina, J. M., Bagaev, A., Bergmann, M., Chapron, B., Chubarenko, I., Cózar, A., Delandmeter, P., Egger, M., Fox-Kemper, B., Garaba, S. P., Goddijn-Murphy, L., Hardesty, B. D., Hoffman, M. J., Isobe, A., Jongedijk, C. E., ... Wichmann, D. (2020). The physical oceanography of the transport of floating marine debris. *Environmental Research Letters, 15*(2), 023003. doi:10.1088/1748-9326/ab6d7d

Van Sebille, E., England, M. H., & Froyland, G. (2012). Origin, dynamics and evolution of ocean garbage patches from observed surface drifters. *Environmental Research Letters, 7*(4), 044040. doi:10.1088/1748-9326/7/4/044040

Van Sebille, E., Wilcox, C., Lebreton, L., Maximenko, N., Hardesty, B. D., Van Franeker, J. A., Eriksen, M., Siegel, D., Galgani, F., & Law, K. L. (2015). A global inventory of small floating plastic debris. *Environmental Research Letters, 10*(12), 124006. doi:10.1088/1748-9326/10/12/124006

Veiga, J. M., Fleet, D., Kinsey, S., Nilsson, P., Vlachogianni, T., Werner, S., Galgani, F., Thompson, R. C., Dagevos, J., Gago, J., Sobral, P., & Cronin, R. (2016). *Identifying sources of marine litter.* MSFD GES TG Marine Litter Thematic Report. *JRC Technical Report, EUR, 28309.* Advance online publication. doi:10.2788/018068

WWAP (United Nations World Water Assessment Programme). (2017). T*he United Nations World Water Development Report 2017. Wastewater: The Untapped Resource.* UNESCO. https://wedocs.unep.org/20.500.11822/20448

WWF, EMF, & BCG. (2020). *The business case for a UN treaty on plastic pollution.* WWF. https://www.plasticpollutiontreaty.org/UN_treaty_plastic_poll_report.pdf

KEY TERMS AND DEFINITIONS

End-of-Life: A product reaches its end-of-life when it no longer satisfies users. End-of-life conditions may include a change in the product's dimension from the original ones, lower cleanliness level which can negatively affect the product's use, and reduced performance due to extensive use of the product over time (Ng et al., 2014).

Litter Pathway: Physical and/or technical means by which pollution enters the marine environment and transport mechanisms (Veiga et al., 2016)

Litter Source: Refers to the means of release of marine litter, including the primary sectors and human activities generating plastic pollution, their geographic origin and location (Veiga et al., 2016).

Microplastics: Plastic particles, 5 mm in size or smaller. Microplastics can generate in-water from the breakdown of larger plastic debris or on-land, where they are generally found in personal care products (e.g., dental hygiene products and cosmetics) or clothing (Fendall & Sewell, 2009; Free et al., 2014).

Monitoring: Refers to an array of approaches, technologies, and instruments used to detect, map, and monitor a specific phenomenon (e.g., plastic pollution) via communication of real-time or nearly real-time data.

Plastic Pollution: Is the totality of plastic accumulation in the environment. It is associated with ecological impacts and emissions from plastic production, consumption, leakages from littering practices and inefficiencies in waste management infrastructure, and impacts related to recycling and other waste treatment processes (Nielsen et al., 2020).

Plastic-Waste Leakage: Refers to the spillage of unmanaged plastic waste that originates on land and reaches the ocean (Ocean Conservancy, 2015).

Chapter 2
A Review of Microplastic Pollution Characteristics in Global Urban Freshwater Catchments

Yuyao Xu
University of Nottingham, Ningbo, China

Jun He
University of Nottingham, Ningbo, China

Faith Ka Shun Chan
University of Nottingham, Ningbo, China

Thomas Stanton
Loughborough University, UK

Matthew F. Johnson
University of Nottingham, UK

ABSTRACT

Microplastics are the newly identified pollutant of this century, yet they are already detected everywhere worldwide. Microplastic pollution in global marine environments has been intensively reported. Evidence of microplastic pollution is emerging in other environments, including land, freshwater, atmosphere, and organisms. Public concerns were also raised about microplastic pollution around them. From terrestrial environments, through freshwater environments, finally to marine environments, is a major transportation route of microplastic pollution. Human activities are the fundamental source of microplastic pollution. Cities, with the highest population density on this planet, are important sources of microplastic pollutants. This chapter focuses on urban freshwater environments, the first receptor, and major transporter of urban microplastics. By reviewing microplastic pollution in global urban freshwater catchments, urban microplastic pollution characteristics were clarified, and the key information to prevent urban microplastic discharge was sought.

DOI: 10.4018/978-1-7998-9723-1.ch002

INTRODUCTION

Background

Microplastics are plastic material ranging in size from 1 μm to 5 mm and are listed as an emerging marine pollutant (Hitchcock, 2020; Horton, Walton, et al., 2017). Marine microplastic pollution is ubiquitous, even recorded in deep oceans and polar seas that are inaccessible to humans (Alice et al., n.d.; Angiolillo et al., 2021; Mason et al., 2016; Van Cauwenberghe et al., 2013). Previously documented sources of marine microplastics include the degradation and fragmentation of larger plastic litter in the ocean (Andrady, 2011; Cole et al., 2011). However, the findings of several recent studies demonstrate that riverine transport of microplastics is also a noteworthy source of microplastic pollution in the marine environment (Bondelind et al., 2020; Mai et al., 2019; van Wijnen et al., 2019). It has also been suggested that current estimates of microplastic concentrations in the marine environment are underestimates because they do not fully account for the role of freshwater systems in transporting microplastics to the oceans (R. Hurley et al., 2018).

Microplastics are found across the terrestrial land surface, in the atmosphere, and in human food, beverages and even infant milk products (Ferraz et al., 2020). Evidence of microplastic pollution has been reported in river systems, globally, including the Thames River in the UK (Horton, Svendsen, et al., 2017; Rowley et al., 2020), the Great Lakes in the US (Baldwin et al., 2016; Mason et al., 2016), the Yangtze River in China (J. Fan et al., 2021; Li et al., 2019), the Sinos River in Brazil (Ferraz et al., 2020) and the Nakdong River in South Korea (Eo et al., 2019). These microplastics are distributed in various environmental matrices in freshwater systems, including surface water, water columns, sediments, and aquatic organisms.

The ingestion of microplastics by aquatic organisms has been widely reported and is believed to cause physical damage. Some microplastics have sharp edges that can injure the organs and tissues of organisms. Microplastics can also accumulate in organisms and clog their digestive systems (Carreras-Colom et al., 2018; R. R. Hurley et al., 2017; Maaghloud et al., 2021; Peters & Bratton, 2016). In addition to the physical damage, ingestion of microplastics may also pose toxicological risks, as plastic materials may contain or adsorb organic or inorganic chemical contaminants. Moreover, the monomers released from polymers also have toxicological effects (He et al., 2020). However, the exact hazards of microplastics to organisms remains contentious because many studies are performed in laboratory settings with concentrations of microplastics far in excess of those found in the environment (Boucher et al., 2016; C. Y. Chen et al., 2021; Rochman et al., 2013).

The term 'microplastics' was first defined in the marine environment in 2004 (Thompson, 2004), yet plastic materials have been widely used globally for over half a century. Hou et al. (2021) investigated historical samples of urban freshwater fish held in the Chicago Museum in the USA and found no microplastic particles in samples from before the 1950s. In contrast, there was a significant increasing trend in the number of microplastics in the fish samples from the middle of the last century to 2018. Similar historical data on microplastic pollution can be obtained by investigating microplastic contamination in soil or sediment cores with similar results (Fan et al., 2019; Matsuguma et al., 2017; Van Cauwenberghe et al., 2013). This suggests that human society is facing a serious challenge of a pollutant that has been spreading and accumulating in the environment for more than half a century.

Microplastics in Freshwater Environment

Despite large unknowns in the impact of microplastics on ecosystems, there is no doubt that there microplastic pollution occurs in freshwater environments and that fluvial (riverine) systems continue to transport large quantities of microplastics to the marine environment (Wang et al., 2021). Microplastic contamination can be divided into primary and secondary microplastics. Primary microplastics refer to the plastic particles that are manufactured in the micro-scale size, such as raw plastic pellets and microbeads added to the Personal Care Products (PCPs). Secondary microplastics refer to the micro-scale plastic particles released from larger plastic items that degrade and/or break down when exposed to the environment due to physical, chemical and other factors (Fan et al., 2019). Both primary and secondary microplastics are derived from emissions associated with human activities. Urban settlements are the most densely populated areas and contain diverse plastic industries and channels of plastic consumption. Therefore, urban areas are an important source of microplastics (Xu et al., 2020). It also follows that urban freshwater environments are the first waterbodies to be contaminated by the emission of microplastics, and a key source of microplastic downstream.

Haberstroh et al. (2021) claim that plastic pollution in freshwater systems is not as well understood by the academic community as it is in marine systems. This view is equally appropriate in the field of microplastics. Andrady (2011) and Cole et al. (2011) reviewed microplastic pollution in the ocean and Eerkes-Medrano et al. (2015) and Horton et al. (2017) reviewed microplastics in freshwater environments. These reviews invariably point to the fact that there are large research gaps, particularly in freshwater environments, including the role played by urban freshwater systems. Few reviews have been conducted on microplastics in urban freshwater environments; for example, Xu et al. (2020) reviewed microplastic pollution in Chinese urban freshwater catchments and related policy management.

As described above, human activities in cities are the major source of various emerging plastic and microplastic pollutants, yet the processes and mechanisms of how such pollutants are emitted from cities and spread to the rest of environment are not well understood. Urban emissions of these pollutants are in turn closely linked to the economic development of human societies. Microplastic pollution are not only accumulating in the global environment but are also being ingested and inhaled by humans. The current knowledge of microplastics determines the trade-off between current economic development and the control of these pollutants, especially when microplastic pollution has implication for biological and human health. Understanding the patterns of microplastic pollution in urban water is an important part of the study of urban microplastic emissions through the water environment. This chapter aims to critically review the current research on microplastics in urban freshwater environments, discussing the spatial and temporal distribution patterns of microplastics in global urban inland waterbodies, and to discuss the characteristics of microplastic pollution in urban freshwater environments. This chapter fills a gap in the current literature by extending the perspective to a review of microplastic pollution in global urban freshwater environments. This chapter collected relevant publications included on the Web of Science (search term: *"microplastic* AND (urban OR city OR cities)"*) up to November 2021, accumulating over 300 available publications. Following sections presented a summary of several representative research among those publications.

The accounts of microplastic concentrations reviewed next are in the units used in the original publications. These units expressed in those different ways are usually interchangeable. Readers can directly feel it is also clear that not only different methods are being used in microplastics research, but there is also no uniform form of reporting on the findings of microplastic pollution.

THE ROLE OF URBAN FRESHWATER IN MICROPLASTIC POLLUTION

A Receiver of Microplastic Pollution

Urban freshwater catchments play two roles in microplastic pollution; they are a receiver and transporter of plastics. As receivers, microplastic abundances have been documented in different environmental matrices in urban freshwater catchments. Xu et al. (2021) reported average microplastic concentrations of 1620.16 ± 878.22 n/m^3 and 1696.08 ± 983.52 n/m^3 during the wet season and dry season respectively, along surface water of the Fenghua River in Ningbo City, China. In the water column of the Santa Cruz River, USA, an average of 195 ± 2.2 (standard error) no./L of microplastics were measured (Eppehimer et al., 2021). A mean microplastic concentration of 914 ± 844 particles/kg (dry weight) or 1793 ± 1275 particles/m^2 was found in the sediments of the Salford Quays basin, Manchester city centre, UK by Hurley et al. (2017). These concentrations in urban freshwaters are typically higher than in less populated areas. For example, Di and Wang (2018) recorded the average microplastic concentrations in rural, suburban and urban areas as 3208 ± 1540 n/m^3, 4366 ± 2855 n/m^3 and 6201 ± 3034 n/m^3 respectively, across the surface water of the Three Gorges Reservoir in China. The research conducted in the surface water of northern Lake Victoria in Africa also found that sampling sites located in urban or semi-urban areas had the highest microplastic concentration (0.69 – 2.19 particles/m^3), compared to other sampling sites set in a rural community (0.199 - 1.0 particles/m^3) and set in the vicinity of river inflows (0.02 - 0.14 particles/m^3) (Egessa et al., 2020).

The high concentrations of microplastics in urban areas, is often accompanied by a higher diversity in microplastic shape, size, colour and polymer type. Hayes et al. (2021) compared the microplastic abundance of two rivers and beaches in South Australia between urban areas and non-urban areas and found that low urbanized areas have fewer types of polymers. Similarly high concentrations and diversities of microplastics have been widely documented in global urban freshwater environments (Dahms et al., 2020; Gopinath et al., 2020; Xu et al., 2020).

Relatively stable freshwater environments, such as lakes and sediments, may act as sinks for microplastic particles, holding microplastic pollution for a long time than in the flowing water. The impact of the longer-term storage of microplastics on local water bodies and aquatic life is still widely debated. However, the storage of microplastics in these matrices is not permanent. Natural (e.g. flooding, extreme weather) and artificial modification of channel and/or catchment hydromorphology can lead to these microplastics entering the active aquatic environment again. For example, Ji et al. (2021) found that dredged freshwater sediment storage was placed on the land whilst awaiting permanent disposal, with sediments able to disperse and contaminate the surrounding soil and surface waters. In addition, high flows can also entrain microplastics from sediments into the flow (Xu et al., 2020). Regulation of water levels in reservoirs can also moves microplastics from stable waterbodies (i.e. reservoirs) to the more active, downstream river environment (Di & Wang, 2018).

A Transporter of Microplastic Pollution

The fluvial freshwater system acts as a transporter of microplastics from urban environments towards other locations. Annually, 15963 ± 11268 tons of microplastics are estimated to be discharged from the Pearl River (China) to the South China Sea, with multiple megacities located in the Pearl River basin contributing to that discharge (Fan et al., 2019). 152 – 291 billion pieces of microplastics were predicted to be discharged from the Warnow estuary (an urbanized shipping channel in Mecklenburg-Western Pomerania, Germany) into the Baltic Sea every year (Piehl et al., 2021). Nihei et al. (2020) calculated that the entirety of Japan discharges 210 – 4776 t/yr microplastics and macroplastics towards the ocean, with the highly urbanized cities, especially Tokyo, Nagaya and Osaka, predicted to dominate that discharge. 95% of the plastic collected from the rivers in Florida, the United States were microplastics, where urban catchments released a much larger microplastic load than sparsely populated upstream areas (Haberstroh, Arias, Yin, & Wang, 2021).

High microplastic loads are not the only reason that may make urban microplastic discharges particularly important. The water quality of urban environments have been influenced by industrial and human activities over extended time periods and, thus, urban water bodies may contain complex pollutant mixtures. Given the lipophilicity and irregular surface texture of microplastics, they tend to adsorb and carry organic contaminants, metal pollutants, and even pathogenic colonies and viruses already found in the environment (Caruso, 2019; Rochman et al., 2013; Su et al., 2021). Microplastics may spread these environmental risks across a larger area by improving their mobility. However, this may be counterbalanced during transportation if microplastics become retained, and accumulate, in low-flow areas that induce deposition (Haberstroh, Arias, Yin, Sok, et al., 2021).

The mechanisms of microplastic movement in the aquatic environment are complex and have not been determined yet. It is also clear that the density of microplastics is an important control on their distribution in freshwater environments. Microplastics can be formed from a diverse array of polymers, which can have different densities. The density of microplastics may also be altered by contaminants or biofilms on their surface. It is highly likely that less dense microplastics will remain suspended in the flow and be relatively rapidly expelled into estuarine and marine environments, whereas denser microplastics are likely to interact with riverbed sediments, being temporally stored and moved towards marine environments over a longer timescale.

Chen et al. (2021) reported a mean microplastic concentration of 4.39 ± 5.11 p/L in the surface water of the Langat River Basin (Malaysia), but a mean concentration of 45.86 ± 24.76 p/L in the downstream estuary, which was over 10 fold higher than the upstream river section. Estuaries thus may be potential reservoirs of microplastics (Defontaine et al., 2020), likely relating to their depositional nature and the mixing of freshwater and seawater. The dynamics of microplastics in estuaries remains a research gap, especially urban estuaries.

MICROPLASTICS IN URBAN FRESHWATER ENVIRONMENT

The Spatial Characteristics of Microplastic Pollution

Several studies have identified a negative linear correlation between microplastic concentrations and the distance from urban centres. The surface water of twenty urban waterbodies was investigated in Wuhan City, China, where microplastic concentrations ranged from 1660.0 ± 639.1 to 8925 ± 1591 n/m^3 (Wang et al., 2017), with a negative linear relationship that microplastic concentration increased with the distance from the city centre decreased ($p < 0.001$; $r = -0.895$), which means high concentrations of microplastics were easy to detect at the sampling sites closed to city centre. A similar significant negative linear relationship was also recorded in the study of city creeks, rivers, and small waterbodies in Shanghai City, China ($p < 0.05$) (Luo et al., 2019). However, many previous studies have failed to detect a similar statistical trend with Wang et al. (2017) and Luo et al. (2019), such as on the Vistula River in Poland (Sekudewicz et al., 2021) and the Fenghua River in China (Xu, Chan, Johnson et al., 2021) where no obvious statistical linear relationship was found between microplastic concentrations and the distance from city centre. The distance from city centres is a spatial indicator of the degree of urbanization of a sampling point. Due to the differences in urban planning, urbanism, and urban dynamics among cities, spatial location will not always be indicative of the level of urbanization, nor microplastic discharge.

Ghaffari et al. (2019) concluded that urbanization level and population density are the main factors affecting the distribution of macro-, meso- and micro-plastic pollution, followed by natural factors. Therefore, some research groups have used population density and local economic status as indicators of urbanization to observe the trend of microplastic abundance. For example, Fan et al. (2019) documented a positive linear correlation between microplastic concentration and both the population density ($R^2 = 0.772$; $p < 0.01$) and gross domestic product ($R^2 = 0.746$; $p < 0.01$), in the sediment of the Pearl River catchment, China. However, Zhao et al. (2015) suggested that microplastic abundance does not always linearly relate to the population density and economic status as they only indicate local plastic pollution conditions. Ferraz et al. (2020) did not find that microplastic pollution in river surface water showed any change with urbanization level, but found high concentrations in the location of a city, hypothesized to be due to urban sewage treatment plants, and also upstream in some localized rural areas, hypothesized to be due to the direct discharge of sewage.

The variability in microplastic sources and complexity of their transport, means that spatial linear relationships between microplastic concentrations and urban factors are unlikely to hold true in many situations. Microplastics have both point source (e.g. wastewater outflows) and diffuse sources (e.g. run-off, litter, plastic degradation). A linear distribution of microplastic concentration is more likely where several major point sources are varying or being arranged in a certain pattern in urban centers but the reality is often more complex. For example, Huang et al. (2021) documented concentrations of micro-plastics ranging from high to low in commercial/public/entertainment areas, residential areas, industrial areas and natural areas, respectively. Di and Wang (2018) reported a microplastic concentration peak in the sediment of a rural area rather than of urban areas, even though microplastic concentrations generally increased from rural to urban areas. A possible reason was local factories and wastewater emissions in rural areas (Di & Wang, 2018). It has also been documented that the discharges from wastewater treatment plants may alter the distribution patterns of microplastics in non-urban areas (Hurley et al., 2018). Therefore, how to effectively evaluate the role of urbanization in microplastic freshwater pollution is still an important topic.

The Temporal Characteristics of Microplastic Pollution

Wang et al. (2017) summarized the factors influencing microplastic abundance patterns into four points, which are: 1. the properties of microplastics, 2. the hydrological conditions, 3. surroundings and 4. meteorological conditions. The properties of microplastics (e.g. microplastic density) and surrounding conditions (e.g. local population density) often influence spatial patterns of microplastics, while the hydrological conditions and meteorological conditions may contribute to the temporal patterns of freshwater microplastic abundances.

Fan et al. (2019) discovered the microplastic concentration in surface water was significantly higher in autumn (1.19 ± 1.01 items/L) than in spring (0.29 ± 0.10 items/L) and summer (0.27 ± 0.11 items/L) in the Pearl River catchment in China, due to the dilution effect of more frequent rainfall during wet seasons.

Haberstroh et al. (2021) suggested low water flows during the dry season may allow microplastics to accumulate in water bodies, while frequent storm events during the wet season can release large quantities of plastic particles. Hurley et al. (2018) found that after a summer flood, the urban catchment area of Manchester, UK had a significant reduction in riverbed microplastics, with an average reduction of 64%, and urban microplastic hot spots disappeared, consistent with the conclusion by Haberstroh et al. (2021). Therefore, rainfall can be significant in washing microplastics into waterways and re-entraining those stored in sediments back into the water column.

Studies that conduct comparative sampling before and after rainfall or storm events, both high-frequency sampling (Hitchcock, 2020) and low-frequency sampling (Eppehimer et al., 2021) found a significant increase in microplastic concentration. For example, a significant increment in microplastic concentration was observed after a storm event in the surface water samples from Cooks River estuary, Australia, from 400 particles/m^3 before the storm to 17383 particles/m^3 (over 40 fold) 12 hours after the storm began (Hitchcock, 2020). Microplastic concentration continued to increase for two days after the storm and quickly decreased during the following five days (Hitchcock, 2020). In contrast, there was no significant variation in microplastic concentrations before (1170.8 $\pm$ 953.1 n/m^3) and after (1245.8 $\pm$ 531.5 n/m^3) typhoons in the water column (subsurface water) in three urban estuaries in China (Zhao et al., 2015). Additionally, the accumulation effects during the dry season mentioned by Haberstroh et al. (2021) are not consistent with the findings of Ji et al. (2021), where 29031 $\pm$ 5869 n/kg dw (17780 – 37780 n/kg dw) of microplastics were collected from the sediment of an urban river of Wenzhou, China during the wet season while a smaller concentration (24784 $\pm$ 6953 n/kg dw (13710 – 37610 n/kg dw)) was found during the dry season. Moreover, some past research has not even identified seasonal differences in microplastic pollution in freshwaters (Xu, Chan, Johnson, et al., 2021). As such, urbanized areas may impact expected temporal trends driven by natural events, modulating their impact on the entrainment and continued transport of plastics in freshwaters.

Two key points for future research are whether urban microplastic pollution patterns are impacted by seasonality. The factors affecting the seasonality of microplastic pollution are complex, including atmospheric deposition, precipitation, river flow, tidal processes and the seasonal activities of the population (e.g., agricultural, aquacultural and industrial productions). The dilution, wash and microplastic input effects from increased rainfall-runoff may lead to high concentration in the wet season, high concentration in the dry season, or no significant seasonal difference at all according to the literature. This is likely due to location specific characteristics affecting the relative significance of dilution and increased inputs of microplastics. It is also possible that sample strategies may account for discrepancies in findings. For example, Eo et al. (2019) found that microplastic concentrations in surface water were three times higher than at intermediate depths. Zhao et al. (2015) postulate that density differences in microplastic particles and sampling locations could also be a reason for non-significant seasonal results in some studies.

Despite some contention, precipitation remains important to the input of microplastics in urban freshwater environments. Hitchcock (2020) regarded storm events as the "hot moment" of microplastic pollution, during which microplastics on land and in water are briefly connected. According to records in a Mexican city, rainwater runoff was estimated to contribute 8 x 10^5 to 3 x 10^6 particles/ha of microplastics to adjacent water bodies per year (de Jesus Pinon-Colin et al., 2020). Eo et al. (2019) estimated that 70 – 80% of annual microplastics were emitted during the wet season in the Nakong River, South Korea, and the estimates of annual emissions using the surface water data during the rainy season were 13 times higher than estimates using yearly average data. A unique fact in urban areas is the rapid and significant runoff generated by impermeable surfaces can carry street dust from vehicle exhaust and tires; both important sources of microplastic pollution (Abbasi et al., 2017). The specific effects of rainfall events are also influenced by geographical and anthropogenic factors in and around the freshwater basin (Haberstroh, Arias, Yin, & Wang, 2021). Thus, it is also crucial to avoid the direct input of rainwater runoff towards the urban freshwater environment, to control the global microplastic discharge (Hitchcock, 2020).

MICROPLASTIC MORPHOLOGICAL CHARACTERISTICS

The previous subsections reviewed the role of urban freshwater environments in microplastic pollution and the spatial and temporal characteristics of microplastics in urban freshwater systems, in terms of microplastic concentrations. However, concentrations are not all that distinguishes microplastic pollution. For a better understanding of the originating sources of microplastics collected from the environment, the microplastic research community usually classify the microplastic particles by their shape, size, colour and polymer type.

Microplastic Shape

Microplastics are typically categorized by their shape into fragments (hard microplastics with an irregular shape), films (membrane-like microplastics), pellets (spherical microplastics) and fibres (wirelike microplastics). However, the naming and classification methods of those shapes are not unified. For example, some studies name microplastic fragments and those that sit between fragment and film, as a microplastic sheet (Fan et al., 2019; Lee et al., 2018; Zhang et al., 2019). Since microplastic foams, plastic microbeads, and raw plastic pellets can all be spherical but of different sources, some literature may classify these types of microplastics separately, or name them as microplastic granules (Battulga et al., 2020; Chen et al., 2020b; Hurley et al., 2018). Some research may name microplastic fibres as lines or filaments (Dahms et al., 2020).

The dominance of microplastic fibres in microplastic samples has been widely documented in global urban freshwater environments (Ferraz et al., 2020; Xu, Chan, Stanton, et al., 2021). 96% of total microplastics collected from the surface water of the Langat River Basin in Malaysia were microplastic fibres (Chen et al., 2021). Microplastic fibres represented 93.5% - 93.8% of the total microplastic particles collected from the sediment of Suzhou Creek, Shanghai City, China (Chen et al., 2020a) and represented 95.0% of the microplastics ingested by *Chironomus* sp. larvae in the Braamfontein Spruit in South Arica (Dahms et al., 2020).

The prevalence of microplastic fibres in urban freshwaters has been related to incomplete treated sewage discharged by WWTPs and non-treated laundry sewage discharged by residential areas. Urban WWTPs receive a huge amount of laundry sewage from urban residents, which usually contains a high proportion of synthetic fibres (Xu, Chan, Stanton, et al., 2021). A WWTP of Sari City in Iran had a microplastic removal rate of 96.70% with a microplastic concentration in effluent as 423 ± 44.9 MP/m^3, where microplastic fibres were 77.5% of the total (Petroody et al., 2020). We collected all the publications from the Web of Science on wastewater/sewage treatment plants in global urban freshwater environments. By November 2021, a total of 51 publications were published, five of which did not mention the shape of microplastics in the water samples. Of the remaining 46 articles, 35 publications reported that fibres were the dominant microplastic shape in water samples. The microplastic removal rate was recorded between 44.55% (Tadsuwan & Babel, 2021) and 100% (Wei et al., 2020) across all 51 publications, most being between 80% and 99%. Although these WWTPs appeared to have a relatively high microplastic removal rate, they remain one of the major sources of microplastic and microfibre pollution in urban freshwater receptors. For example, 131.35 ± 95.36 MP/L of microplastics was found in the effluent of an industrial WWTP in the city of Cádiz, Spain (Franco et al., 2021) and 276-1030 items/L of microplastics were found in the effluent of WWTPs in the cities of Tianjin and Beijing, Xi'an in China (Wang et al., 2020). More seriously, not all of the wastewaters will be treated by WWTPs. For instance, there was only one municipal sewage treatment plant in the entire Sinos River Basin, which could only treat 10% of the total urban daily wastewater (Ferraz et al., 2020). The remaining sewage water is likely to end up in rainwater drains and waterways. In urban storm runoff water in Tijuana, Mexico, microplastic fibres represented 68% - 87% of total samples (de Jesus Pinon-Colin et al., 2020). WWTPs may also return contaminated sludge to nearby catchments for fertilizers, providing another potential route via runoff, for microplastics to reach waterways (Ferraz et al., 2020).

In addition to municipal sewage, aquacultural and fishing activities are one of the main sources of microplastic fibres in the environment. For example, a high proportion of microplastic fibres were observed in the Lake Victoria, Africa, where fishing activities were frequent (Egessa et al., 2020).

Microplastic fragments come from the fragmentation of plastic wastes in the environment while films and foams may come from the fragmentation of widely used packaging materials or containers (Di & Wang, 2018; Xu et al., 2020). Such shapes can dominated microplastic populations; for example, fragments represented 56.1% and 83.1% of microplastic samples in both the surface water (2074 ± 3651 MPs/m^3) and sediment (3726 ± 9030 MPs/m^2) of Ravi River, Lahore, Pakistan (Irfan et al., 2020). In general, large proportions of fragments occur more frequently in sediment samples than in surface waters, presumably because many fragments are larger than microfibres and may be higher density. An example is microplastic films being dominant in the surface water of Adour Estuary, France, while in the subsurface water samples and bottom water samples, fragments were the largest proportion (Defontaine et al., 2020).

Plastic microbeads were widely used in PCPs and cosmetics (Bayo et al., 2017), which have recently been prohibited in many countries including the US, UK, South Korea and China (Xu et al., 2020). Perhaps because of the positive influences of microbead legislation in recent years, microbeads often make up a relatively small proportion of total microplastic particles in urban freshwater environments (Xu, Chan, Johnson, et al., 2021). The main pathway of microbeads entering water bodies is sewage water (Boucher et al., 2016). Compared to microbeads, microplastic foams (i.e. particles eroded from polystyrene) were more common in urban freshwater samples, with Hurley et al. (2017) identifying that 87% of spheric microplastics were foams in sediment samples from Manchester, UK. It is also worth noting that macro-, meso- and micro-plastic foams can absorb other microplastics. For example, along the shore of the Tuul River in Mongolia, 5 – 141 microplastics were observed to adhere to each plastic foam particle (Battulga et al., 2020).

Microplastic Size

Currently, the microplastic research community groups microplastics according to different size ranges to evaluate the size distribution pattern of microplastics. However, the size categories vary substantially between publications, which pose a challenge to comparison across research studies and sites. Despite this, in most studies it is the smallest size groups that account for the largest proportion. For example, particles between 0.355 – 0.500 mm accounted for 57.63% of total surface water microplastics (7.428 ± 3.678 SE pieces/m^3) in the Lam Tsuen River in Hongkong China (Cheung et al., 2019). Similarly, the smallest microplastics (0.050 – 0.332 mm) accounted for 89% of total surface water microplastics in Cooks River estuary, Australia (Hitchcock, 2020). In the sediments of an urban river of Wenzhou, Zhejiang Province, China, 75.4% - 91.1% of microplastics belonged to the smallest size group (< 0.3 mm) (Ji et al., 2021). The same is broadly true in organism tissues. For example, in the fish *Leuciscus cephalus, Capoeta trutta, Alburnus chalcoides, Capoeta damascina, Barbus capito, Cyprinion macrostomum* and *Luciobarbus caspius* collected from Kermanshah city, Iran, the smallest microplastics were also the most common (Heshmati et al., 2021).

Smaller microplastic sizes, especially those associated with secondary microplastics, may imply a longer retention history in the environment. With depth in the sediment of the Pearl River Catchment, the proportion of microplastics smaller than 0.45 mm also increased, indicating the fragmentation of microplastics increased with time (Fan et al., 2019). Smaller microplastics may also have higher bioavailability as they can be readily ingested by small aquatic organisms and microorganisms (Angiolillo et al., 2021; Piarulli et al., 2020). Although small-sized microplastics are usually most abundant, larger-sized microplastics usually dominate the mass of samples. For example, Fan et al. (2019) found that the smallest microplastic group accounted for an average of 60.6% ± 10.6% (water sample) / 45.0% ± 4.3% (sediment sample) of the total number of microplastics, but it was the largest microplastic class that accounted for 56.4% ± 9.4% (water sample) / 64.5% ± 7.0% (sediment sample) of the total microplastic mass. This could be important information for modelling the load and transport of microplastics in the riverine system in the future.

Microplastic Colour

Several publications document the colours of collected microplastics. The most common colours mentioned in previous research include transparent, white, blue and black. There are no clear standards for recording microplastic colours, thus, the results can be subjective.

In reviewed literature, white and transparent were the most common microplastic colours in waterbodies. Transparent microplastics accounted for 56% of total microplastics in the surface water of the Ofanto River, Italy (Campanale et al., 2020). The average proportions of white and transparent microplastics in the Pearl River Catchment (China) were 62.6% ± 13.5% in the surface water and 51.0% ± 7.0% in sediment, respectively (Fan et al., 2019). Transparent microplastics accounted for 21.4% - 75.0% of total microplastics in the sediment of the Lagoon of Bizerte (Abidli et al., 2017). In the environment, microplastic exposed to sunlight may fade and increase the proportion of colourless microplastics (Fan et al., 2021). In addition, in the laboratory extraction of microplastics from environmental media, strong oxidizing chemicals including hydrogen peroxide, concentrated sulfuric acid and/or concentrated hydrochloric acid are often used to digest the organic matter. This process can also discolour some microplastic samples (Xu, Chan, Johnson, et al., 2021).

In organisms, the dominance of colourless microplastics decreases, with blue and black microplastics more commonly found. Black microplastics dominated in the Duck mussel (*Anodonta anatina*) from the River Höjeå: Genarp and Värpinge in southern Sweden (Berglund et al., 2019). Blue microplastics were dominant in the *Chironomus* sp. larvae from the Braamfontein Spruit, Johannesburg, in South Africa (Dahms et al., 2020). This phenomenon may involve the selective ingestion of microplastics by organisms. The selective ingestion of microplastics by organisms may also be related to biofilms and bacterial communities coating the surface of microplastics, as this is a potential source of nutrients for aquatic organisms (Hurley et al., 2017). However, it is still unclear whether aquatic organisms are preferentially choosing microplastics that are black and blue in colour, or whether microbial communities prefer to adhere to microplastics with dark colours.

Polymer Types

The microplastic research community uses a diverse range of spectrometers to identify the polymer types of collected microplastics. Polyethylene (PE) and polypropylene (PP) tend to dominate in surface water environments due to their low density and wide use. For example, accounted for 43.8% - 50.8% and 39.0% - 41.4% of the identified microplastics from the surface water of five major cities in Japan (Abeynayaka et al., 2020). 58.33% and 56.99% of identified microplastics were PE in the surface water and sediment of the Netravathi River, India (Amrutha & Warrier, 2020). PP was the dominant polymer (38% of identified microplastics) in the sediment of West River, Pearl River system, China (Huang et al., 2021). PP and PE may dominate samples in sediments because of biofouling on the surface, changing their density and causing them to sink (Di & Wang, 2018). PP and PE are also very common, being used widely as food packaging, pipes, textile fibres, agricultural mulching, fishery equipment, and containers (Gopinath et al., 2020). In comparison to PE and PP, Polyethylene terephthalate (PET) is more widely distributed in sediments, such as in the Suzhou Creek in China (Chen et al., 2020a) and the Thames river basin in the UK (Horton, Svendsen, et al., 2017). PET has relatively high density and is used as textile fabrics, building materials, and other fibrous products (Fan et al., 2019). Most products of PP, PE and PET are recyclable. Therefore, the large quantities of these polymers in the environment implies a lack of recycling and reuse of relevant plastic products (Hayes et al., 2021).

He et al. (2020) found that in the sediment of Brisbane River (Australia), sampling sites with high microplastic abundance were not found to have high hazard scores, while the two sites with the highest hazard scores had microplastic concentration less than 10 mg/kg in the sediment. This was because two polymer types; polyvinylidene chloride and polyacrylonitrile, were detected in the sample which are more hazardous than other, more commonly found polymers such as PP, PE and PET. The calculation of a hazard score takes into account the mass of microplastics and the toxicity index of the monomer released by each type of microplastic. There polymer type can have a significant impact on the potential hazard risk of microplastics found in the environment, and using a hazard score can help identify risks, not obvious when only looking at concentrations and/or mass of plastics.

DEVELOPMENT STATUS AND MICROPLASTIC POLLUTION

Due to the current lack of unified methods for sampling, extracting, identifying and reporting microplastics, comparison of results between studies is challenging. However, the general trends identified above suggest different concentrations of microplastics found in different nations can be related to development status. It is clear that microplastics occur in substantially different concentrations between different regions, and through time. For example, in Chinese surface water, microplastics have been reported as 2990 – 9870 n/m^3 in West River (Huang et al., 2021), 1597 – 12611 n/m^3 of microplastics in the Three Gorges Reservoir (Di & Wang, 2018), 14400 (± 5100 n/m^3) in Suzhou Creek, 26200 (± 9600 n/m^3) in Huangpu River (Chen et al., 2020a). However, in other countries, especially developed countries, the surface microplastic concentrations tend to be much lower; for example, 1.6 ± 2.3 n/m^3 in major cities in Japan (Abeynayaka et al., 2020), 0.05 – 32 n/m^3 in 29 Great Lakes tributaries in the USA (Baldwin et al., 2016), 0 - 3.88 n/m^3 in the Adour Estuary in France (Defontaine et al., 2020) and 0.87 ± 1.24 n/m^3 in Garonne River in France (Garcia et al., 2021). This may also be in part due to the export of waste from developed countries to developing countries.

The surface water microplastic concentrations in other developing countries include 56 – 2328 n/m^3 in the Netravathi River in India (Amrutha & Warrier, 2020), 4.39 ± 5.11 to 45.86 ± 24.76 p/L (4390 ± 5110 to 45860 ± 24760 n/m^3) in the Langat River basin in Malaysia (Chen et al., 2021) and 2074 ± 3651 Mps/m^3 in Ravi River, Pakistan (Irfan et al., 2020). Developed countries have significantly lower microplastic concentrations in the surface water than developing countries, and the situation is similar for sediment matrices. This may be related to the high population density, active industrial production and immature waste management in developing countries.

SOLUTIONS AND RECOMMONDATIONS

The chemical stability and low degradation rate of plastic materials mean that most microplastic particles can persist in the environment for a long time. Although the recycling of plastic materials and the promotion of degradable plastics can reduce future microplastic emissions, it is still difficult to address the microplastic pollution that has been already left in the environment. Padervand et al. (2020) summarized several promising methods available for removing microplastics from the environment, which includes adsorbing microplastics using microalgae, using dynamic membranes or membrane bioreactors removing microplastics from waterbodies, trapping microplastics by using activated sludge, electrocoagulation, photocatalytic degradation, biological degradation, and advanced techniques used by WWTPs (filtration, settling and coagulation). However, these technologies usually have one or several of the following drawbacks, including the inability to treat the collected microplastics, high-energy consumption, low removal rates, and selective removal of microplastics. Meanwhile, available microplastic removal techniques do not sufficiently deal with current microplastic emissions, resulting in a large number of microplastics entering the freshwater environment through municipal wastewater.

This chapter makes seven recommendations to slow down the continued accumulation of microplastic particles in the environment, based on the current state of microplastic pollution in urban freshwaters. First, the production and consumption of plastic products that present a clear environmental hazard and for which alternatives are available (such as microbeads and ultra-thin plastic bags) should be limited. Secondly, the recycling of plastic wastes should be promoted. Third, the techniques used by urban WWTPs should be upgraded, particularly in developing areas. Fourth, the popularization and dissemination of knowledge of microplastic pollution should be strengthened among the global public. Fifth, research into the mechanisms of microplastic movement and dynamism in the environment should be promoted. Sixth, research on microplastic removal and elimination technologies should be encouraged. Last, the methods to collect the macro-plastic litter in the urban environment should be developed. The first four recommendations aim to reduce the intensity of microplastic emissions, while the last three recommendations aim to find ways to reduce the total amount of microplastics in the environment.

In addition, there is currently a lack of uniform methods and reporting standards for microplastics research in the academic community. This makes cross-study comparisons difficult and seriously hampers progress in reaching regional or even global conclusions on microplastic pollution. This is not conducive to advancing the implementation of the above recommendations. A unified approach to research is worth advocating and should be promoted in a step-by-step manner. Until then, the academic community should first improve the standards for reporting the findings of microplastics studies (Cowger et al., 2020; Provencher et al., 2020), including the requirement to provide all key sampling parameters and microplastics identification approaches, so that studies using the same sampling or identification methods can be quickly compared between regions.

CONCLUSION

This chapter reviews the current state of microplastic pollution in urban freshwater basins, globally. Microplastic pollution in the urban freshwater environment is characterized by high concentrations, high diversity, and high correlation with local human activities. Microplastic pollution in the global urban freshwater environment may have a similar pattern of microplastic types, such as the prevalence of microplastic fibres, but there are also differences, particularly between developed and developing countries. Given that microplastic emissions are increasing year by year, there is a need for interventions to control the freshwater microplastic discharge from cities. However, there are still large research gaps relating to the mechanisms of microplastic pollution in urban freshwater environments. There are currently significant discrepancies in the methodologies and data reported in studies worldwide, making cross-study comparisons difficult. This adds to the many challenges in reviewing publications in this chapter. Future studies should attempt to harmonize the methods and standardize data reporting.

ACKNOWLEDGMENT

This research was supported by the National Natural Science Foundation of China (NSFC) (Grant number: 41850410497); the National Key R&D Program of China (Grant number: 2019YFC1510400) and the Faculty of Science and Engineering (FoSE) Postgraduate Research Scholarship of the University of Nottingham Ningbo China.

REFERENCES

Abbasi, S., Keshavarzi, B., Moore, F., Delshab, H., Soltani, N., & Sorooshian, A. (2017). Investigation of microrubbers, microplastics and heavy metals in street dust: A study in Bushehr city, Iran. In Environmental Earth Sciences (Vol. 76, Issue 23). Springer. doi:10.100712665-017-7137-0

Abeynayaka, A., Kojima, F., Miwa, Y., Ito, N., Nihei, Y., Fukunaga, Y., Yashima, Y., & Itsubo, N. (2020). Rapid Sampling of Suspended and Floating Microplastics in Challenging Riverine and Coastal Water Environments in Japan. In Water (Vol. 12, Issue 7). MDPI. doi:10.3390/w12071903

Abidli, S., Toumi, H., Lahbib, Y., & El Menif, N. T. (2017). The First Evaluation of Microplastics in Sediments from the Complex Lagoon-Channel of Bizerte (Northern Tunisia). In Water Air and Soil Pollution (Vol. 228, Issue 7). Springer International Publishing AG. doi:10.100711270-017-3439-9

Alice, P., Maud, G., Dominique, B., & Julien, G. (n.d.). Micro- and nanoplastic transfer in freezing saltwater: Implications for their fate in polar waters. In *Environmental Science-Processes & Impacts*. Royal Soc Chemistry. doi:10.1039/D1EM00280E

Amrutha, K., & Warrier, A. K. (2020). The first report on the source-to-sink characterization of microplastic pollution from a riverine environment in tropical India. In *Science of the Total Environment* (Vol. 739). Elsevier. doi:10.1016/j.scitotenv.2020.140377

Andrady, A. L. (2011). Microplastics in the marine environment. *Marine Pollution Bulletin*, *62*(8), 1596–1605. doi:10.1016/j.marpolbul.2011.05.030 PMID:21742351

Angiolillo, M., Gerigny, O., Valente, T., Fabri, M.-C., Tambute, E., Rouanet, E., Claro, F., Tunesi, L., Vissio, A., Daniel, B., & Galgani, F. (2021). Distribution of seafloor litter and its interaction with benthic organisms in deep waters of the Ligurian Sea (Northwestern Mediterranean). In Science of the Total Environment (Vol. 788). Elsevier. doi:10.1016/j.scitotenv.2021.147745

Baldwin, A. K., Corsi, S. R., & Mason, S. A. (2016). Plastic Debris in 29 Great Lakes Tributaries: Relations to Watershed Attributes and Hydrology. In Environmental Science & Technology (Vol. 50, Issue 19, pp. 10377–10385). Amer Chemical Soc. doi:10.1021/acs.est.6b02917

Battulga, B., Kawahigashi, M., & Oyuntsetseg, B. (2020). Behavior and distribution of polystyrene foams on the shore of Tuul River in Mongolia. In *Environmental Pollution* (Vol. 260). ELSEVIER SCI LTD., doi:10.1016/j.envpol.2020.113979

Bayo, J., Martinez, A., Guillen, M., Olmos, S., Roca, M.-J., & Alcolea, A. (2017). Microbeads in Commercial Facial Cleansers: Threatening the Environment. In Clean-Soil Air Water (Vol. 45, Issue 7). Wiley. doi:10.1002/clen.201600683

Berglund, E., Fogelberg, V., Nilsson, P. A., & Hollander, J. (2019). Microplastics in a freshwater mussel (Anodonta anatina. In N. Europe (Ed.), *Science of the Total Environment* (Vol. 697). Elsevier. doi:10.1016/j.scitotenv.2019.134192

Bondelind, M., Sokolova, E., Nguyen, A., Karlsson, D., Karlsson, A., & Bjorklund, K. (2020). Hydrodynamic modelling of traffic-related microplastics discharged with stormwater into the Gota River in Sweden. In Environmental Science and Pollution Research (Vol. 27, Issues 19, SI, pp. 24218–24230). Springer Heidelberg. doi:10.100711356-020-08637-z

Boucher, C., Morin, M., & Bendell, L. I. (2016). The influence of cosmetic microbeads on the sorptive behavior of cadmium and lead within intertidal sediments: A laboratory study. In *Regional Studies in Marine Science* (Vol. 3, pp. 1–7). Elsevier Science BV. doi:10.1016/j.rsma.2015.11.009

Campanale, C., Stock, F., Massarelli, C., Kochleus, C., Bagnuolo, G., Reifferscheid, G., & Uricchio, V. F. (2020). Microplastics and their possible sources: The example of Ofanto river in southeast Italy. In *Environmental Pollution* (Vol. 258). Elsevier Sci Ltd. doi:10.1016/j.envpol.2019.113284

Carreras-Colom, E., Constenla, M., Soler-Membrives, A., Cartes, J. E., Baeza, M., Padros, F., & Carrasson, M. (2018). Spatial occurrence and effects of microplastic ingestion on the deep-water shrimp Aristeus antennatus. In *Marine Pollution Bulletin* (Vol. 133, pp. 44–52). Pergamon-Elsevier Science Ltd. doi:10.1016/j.marpolbul.2018.05.012

Caruso, G. (2019). Microplastics as vectors of contaminants. *Marine Pollution Bulletin*, *146*, 921–924. doi:10.1016/j.marpolbul.2019.07.052 PMID:31426238

Chen, C.-Y., Lu, T.-H., Yang, Y.-F., & Liao, C.-M. (2021). Toxicokinetic/toxicodynamic-based risk assessment of freshwater fish health posed by microplastics at environmentally relevant concentrations. In *Science of the Total Environment* (Vol. 756). Elsevier. doi:10.1016/j.scitotenv.2020.144013

Chen, H., Jia, Q., Zhao, X., Li, L., Nie, Y., Liu, H., & Ye, J. (2020a). The occurrence of microplastics in water bodies in urban agglomerations: Impacts of drainage system overflow in wet weather, catchment land-uses, and environmental management practices. *Water Research*, *183*, 116073. doi:10.1016/j.watres.2020.116073 PMID:32599427

Chen, H., Jia, Q., Zhao, X., Li, L., Nie, Y., Liu, H., & Ye, J. (2020b). The occurrence of microplastics in water bodies in urban agglomerations: Impacts of drainage system overflow in wet weather, catchment land-uses, and environmental management practices. In *Water Research* (Vol. 183). Pergamon-Elsevier Science Ltd. doi:10.1016/j.watres.2020.116073

Chen, H. L., Gibbins, C. N., Selvam, S. B., & Ting, K. N. (2021). Spatio-temporal variation of microplastic along a rural to urban transition in a tropical river. In *Environmental Pollution* (Vol. 289). Elsevier Sci Ltd. doi:10.1016/j.envpol.2021.117895

Cheung, P. K., Hung, P. L., & Fok, L. (2019). River Microplastic Contamination and Dynamics upon a Rainfall Event in Hong Kong, China. In Environmental Processes-An International Journal (Vol. 6, Issue 1, pp. 253–264). Springer International Publishing AG. doi:10.100740710-018-0345-0

Cole, M., Lindeque, P., Halsband, C., & Galloway, T. S. (2011). Microplastics as contaminants in the marine environment: A review. *Marine Pollution Bulletin*, *62*(12), 2588–2597. doi:10.1016/j.marpolbul.2011.09.025 PMID:22001295

Cowger, W., Booth, A. M., Hamilton, B. M., Thaysen, C., Primpke, S., Munno, K., Lusher, A. L., Dehaut, A., Vaz, V. P., Liboiron, M., Devriese, L. I., Hermabessiere, L., Rochman, C., Athey, S. N., Lynch, J. M., Lynch, J. M., Frond, H. D., Gray, A., Jones, O. A. H., ... Nel, H. (2020). Reporting Guidelines to Increase the Reproducibility and Comparability of Research on Microplastics. *Applied Spectroscopy*, *74*(9), 1066–1077. doi:10.1177/0003702820930292 PMID:32394727

Dahms, H. T. J., van Rensburg, G. J., & Greenfield, R. (2020). The microplastic profile of an urban African stream. In *Science of the Total Environment* (Vol. 731). Elsevier. doi:10.1016/j.scitotenv.2020.138893

de Jesus Pinon-Colin, T., Rodriguez-Jimenez, R., Rogel-Hernandez, E., Alvarez-Andrade, A., & Wakida, F. T. (2020). Microplastics in stormwater runoff in a semiarid region, Tijuana, Mexico. In *Science of the Total Environment* (Vol. 704). Elsevier. doi:10.1016/j.scitotenv.2019.135411

Defontaine, S., Sous, D., Tesan, J., Monperrus, M., Lenoble, V., & Lanceleur, L. (2020). Microplastics in a salt-wedge estuary: Vertical structure and tidal dynamics. In *Marine Pollution Bulletin* (Vol. 160). Pergamon-Elsevier Science Ltd. doi:10.1016/j.marpolbul.2020.111688

Di, M., & Wang, J. (2018). Microplastics in surface waters and sediments of the Three Gorges Reservoir, China. *The Science of the Total Environment*, *616–617*, 1620–1627. doi:10.1016/j.scitotenv.2017.10.150 PMID:29050832

Eerkes-Medrano, D., Thompson, R. C., & Aldridge, D. C. (2015). Microplastics in freshwater systems: A review of the emerging threats, identification of knowledge gaps and prioritisation of research needs. *Water Research, 75*, 63–82. doi:10.1016/j.watres.2015.02.012 PMID:25746963

Egessa, R., Nankabirwa, A., Ocaya, H., & Pabire, W. G. (2020). Microplastic pollution in surface water of Lake Victoria. In *Science of the Total Environment* (Vol. 741). Elsevier. doi:10.1016/j.scitotenv.2020.140201

Eo, S., Hong, S. H., Song, Y. K., Han, G. M., & Shim, W. J. (2019). Spatiotemporal distribution and annual load of microplastics in the Nakdong River, South Korea. In *Water Research* (Vol. 160, pp. 228–237). Pergamon-Elsevier Science Ltd. doi:10.1016/j.watres.2019.05.053

Eppehimer, D. E., Hamdhani, H., Hollien, K. D., Nemec, Z. C., Lee, L. N., Quanrud, D. M., & Bogan, M. T. (2021). Impacts of baseflow and flooding on microplastic pollution in an effluent-dependent arid land river in the USA. In Environmental Science and Pollution Research (Vol. 28, Issue 33, pp. 45375–45389). Springer Heidelberg. doi:10.100711356-021-13724-w

Fan, J., Zou, L., & Zhao, G. (2021). Microplastic abundance, distribution, and composition in the surface water and sediments of the Yangtze River along Chongqing City, China. In Journal of Soils and Sediments (Vol. 21, Issue 4, pp. 1840–1851). Springer heidelberg. doi:10.100711368-021-02902-5

Fan, Y., Zheng, K., Zhu, Z., Chen, G., & Peng, X. (2019). Distribution, sedimentary record, and persistence of microplastics in the Pearl River catchment, China. In *Environmental Pollution* (Vol. 251, pp. 862–870). Elsevier Sci Ltd. doi:10.1016/j.envpol.2019.05.056

Ferraz, M., Bauer, A. L., Valiati, V. H., & Schulz, U. H. (2020). Microplastic Concentrations in Raw and Drinking Water in the Sinos River, Southern Brazil. In Water (Vol. 12, Issue 11). MDPI. doi:10.3390/w12113115

Franco, A. A., Arellano, J. M., Albendin, G., Rodriguez-Barroso, R., Quiroga, J. M., & Coello, M. D. (2021). Microplastic pollution in wastewater treatment plants in the city of C?diz: Abundance, removal efficiency and presence in receiving water body. In *Science of the Total Environment* (Vol. 776). Elsevier. doi:10.1016/j.scitotenv.2021.145795

Garcia, A. G., Suarez, D. C., Li, J., & Rotchell, J. M. (2021). A comparison of microplastic contamination in freshwater fish from natural and farmed sources. In Environmental Science and Pollution Research (Vol. 28, Issue 12, pp. 14488–14497). Springer Heidelberg. doi:10.100711356-020-11605-2

Ghaffari, S., Bakhtiari, A. R., Ghasempouri, S. M., & Nasrolahi, A. (2019). The influence of human activity and morphological characteristics of beaches on plastic debris distribution along the Caspian Sea as a closed water body. In Environmental Science and Pollution Research (Vol. 26, Issue 25, pp. 25712–25724). Springer Heidelberg. doi:10.100711356-019-05790-y

Gopinath, K., Seshachalam, S., Neelavannan, K., Anburaj, V., Rachel, M., Ravi, S., Bharath, M., & Achyuthan, H. (2020). Quantification of microplastic in Red Hills Lake of Chennai city, Tamil Nadu, India. In Environmental Science and Pollution Research (Vol. 27, Issues 26, SI, pp. 33297–33306). Springer Heidelberg. doi:10.100711356-020-09622-2

Haberstroh, C. J., Arias, M. E., Yin, Z., Sok, T., & Wang, M. C. (2021). Plastic transport in a complex confluence of the Mekong River in Cambodia. In Environmental Research Letters (Vol. 16, Issue 9). IOP Publishing Ltd. doi:10.1088/1748-9326/ac2198

Haberstroh, C. J., Arias, M. E., Yin, Z., & Wang, M. C. (2021). Effects of Urban Hydrology on Plastic Transport in a Subtropical River. In ACS ES&T WATER (Vol. 1, Issue 8, pp. 1714–1727). Amer Chemical Soc. doi:10.1021/acsestwater.1c00072

Hayes, A., Kirkbride, K. P., & Leterme, S. C. (2021). Variation in polymer types and abundance of microplastics from two rivers and beaches in Adelaide, South Australia. In *Marine Pollution Bulletin* (Vol. 172). Pergamon-Elsevier Science Ltd. doi:10.1016/j.marpolbul.2021.112842

He, B., Duodu, G. O., Rintoul, L., Ayoko, G. A., & Goonetilleke, A. (2020). Influence of microplastics on nutrients and metal concentrations in river sediments. In Environmental Pollution (Vol. 263, Issue A). Elsevier Sci Ltd. doi:10.1016/j.envpol.2020.114490

Heshmati, S., Makhdoumi, P., Pirsaheb, M., Hossini, H., Ahmadi, S., & Fattahi, H. (2021). Occurrence and characterization of microplastic content in the digestive system of riverine fishes. In *Journal of Environmental Management* (Vol. 299). Academic Press Ltd- Elsevier Science Ltd. doi:10.1016/j.jenvman.2021.113620

Hitchcock, J. N. (2020). Storm events as key moments of microplastic contamination in aquatic ecosystems. In *Science of the Total Environment* (Vol. 734). Elsevier. doi:10.1016/j.scitotenv.2020.139436

Horton, A. A., Svendsen, C., Williams, R. J., Spurgeon, D. J., & Lahive, E. (2017). Large microplastic particles in sediments of tributaries of the River Thames, UK - Abundance, sources and methods for effective quantification. In Marine Pollution Bulletin (Vol. 114, Issue 1, pp. 218–226). Pergamon-Elsevier Science Ltd. doi:10.1016/j.marpolbul.2016.09.004

Horton, A. A., Walton, A., Spurgeon, D. J., Lahive, E., & Svendsen, C. (2017). Microplastics in freshwater and terrestrial environments: Evaluating the current understanding to identify the knowledge gaps and future research priorities. *The Science of the Total Environment*, *586*, 127–141. doi:10.1016/j.scitotenv.2017.01.190 PMID:28169032

Hou, L., McMahan, C. D., McNeish, R. E., Munno, K., Rochman, C. M., & Hoellein, T. J. (2021). A fish tale: A century of museum specimens reveal increasing microplastic concentrations in freshwater fish. In Ecological Applications (Vol. 31, Issue 5). Wiley. doi:10.1002/eap.2320

Huang, S., Peng, C., Wang, Z., Xiong, X., Bi, Y., Liu, Y., & Li, D. (2021). Spatiotemporal distribution of microplastics in surface water, biofilms, and sediments in the world's largest drinking water diversion project. In *Science of the Total Environment* (Vol. 789). Elsevier. doi:10.1016/j.scitotenv.2021.148001

Hurley, R., Woodward, J., & Rothwell, J. J. (2018). Microplastic contamination of river beds significantly reduced by catchment-wide flooding. In Nature Geoscience (Vol. 11, Issue 4, p. 251+). Nature Publishing Group. doi:10.103841561-018-0080-1

Hurley, R. R., Woodward, J. C., & Rothwell, J. J. (2017). Ingestion of Microplastics by Freshwater Tubifex Worms. In Environmental Science & Technology (Vol. 51, Issue 21, pp. 12844–12851). Amer Chemical Soc. doi:10.1021/acs.est.7b03567

Irfan, M., Qadir, A., Mumtaz, M., & Ahmad, S. R. (2020). An unintended challenge of microplastic pollution in the urban surface water system of Lahore, Pakistan. In Environmental Science And Pollution Research (Vol. 27, Issue 14, pp. 16718–16730). Springer heidelberg. doi:10.100711356-020-08114-7

Ji, X., Ma, Y., Zeng, G., Xu, X., Mei, K., Wang, Z., Chen, Z., Dahlgren, R., Zhang, M., & Shang, X. (2021). Transport and fate of microplastics from riverine sediment dredge piles: Implications for disposal. In Journal of Hazardous Materials (Vol. 404, Issue A). Elsevier. doi:10.1016/j.jhazmat.2020.124132

Lee, H., Byun, D.-E., Kim, J. M., & Kwon, J.-H. (2018). Desorption of Hydrophobic Organic Chemicals from Fragment-Type Microplastics. *Ocean Science Journal*, *53*(4), 631–639. doi:10.100712601-018-0051-x

Li, L., Geng, S., Wu, C., Song, K., Sun, F., Visvanathan, C., Xie, F., & Wang, Q. (2019). Microplastics contamination in different trophic state lakes along the middle and lower reaches of Yangtze River Basin. *Environmental Pollution*, *254*, 112951. doi:10.1016/j.envpol.2019.07.119 PMID:31374488

Luo, W., Su, L., Craig, N. J., Du, F., Wu, C., & Shi, H. (2019). Comparison of microplastic pollution in different water bodies from urban creeks to coastal waters. In *Environmental Pollution* (Vol. 246, pp. 174–182). Elsevier Sci Ltd. doi:10.1016/j.envpol.2018.11.081

Maaghloud, H., Houssa, R., Bellali, F., El Bouqdaoui, K., Ouansafi, S., Loulad, S., & Fahde, A. (2021). Microplastic ingestion by Atlantic horse mackerel (Trachurus trachurus) in the North and central Moroccan Atlantic coast between Larache (35 degrees 30 ` N) and Boujdour (26 degrees 30 ` N). In *Environmental Pollution* (Vol. 288). Elsevier Sci Ltd. doi:10.1016/j.envpol.2021.117781

Mai, L., You, S.-N., He, H., Bao, L.-J., Liu, L.-Y., & Zeng, E. Y. (2019). Riverine Microplastic Pollution in the Pearl River Delta, China: Are Modeled Estimates Accurate? In Environmental Science & Technology (Vol. 53, Issue 20, pp. 11810–11817). Amer Chemical Soc. doi:10.1021/acs.est.9b04838

Mason, S. A., Kammin, L., Eriksen, M., Aleid, G., Wilson, S., Box, C., Williamson, N., & Riley, A. (2016). Pelagic plastic pollution within the surface waters of Lake Michigan, USA. In Journal of Great Lakes Research (Vol. 42, Issue 4, pp. 753–759). Elsevier Sci Ltd. doi:10.1016/j.jglr.2016.05.009

Matsuguma, Y., Takada, H., Kumata, H., Kanke, H., Sakurai, S., Suzuki, T., Itoh, M., Okazaki, Y., Boonyatumanond, R., Zakaria, M. P., Weerts, S., & Newman, B. (2017). Microplastics in Sediment Cores from Asia and Africa as Indicators of Temporal Trends in Plastic Pollution. In Archives of Environmental Contamination and Toxicology (Vol. 73, Issues 2, SI, pp. 230–239). Springer. doi:10.100700244-017-0414-9

Nihei, Y., Yoshida, T., Kataoka, T., & Ogata, R. (2020). High-Resolution Mapping of Japanese Microplastic and Macroplastic Emissions from the Land into the Sea. In Water (Vol. 12, Issue 4). MDPI. doi:10.3390/w12040951

Padervand, M., Lichtfouse, E., Robert, D., & Wang, C. (2020). Removal of microplastics from the environment. A review. *Environmental Chemistry Letters*, *18*(3), 807–828. doi:10.100710311-020-00983-1

Peters, C. A., & Bratton, S. P. (2016). Urbanization is a major influence on microplastic ingestion by sunfish in the Brazos River Basin, Central Texas, USA. In *Environmental Pollution* (Vol. 210, pp. 380–387). Elsevier Sci Ltd. doi:10.1016/j.envpol.2016.01.018

Petroody, S. S. A., Hashemi, S. H., & van Gestel, C. A. M. (2020). Factors affecting microplastic retention and emission by a wastewater treatment plant on the southern coast of Caspian Sea. In *Chemosphere* (Vol. 261). Pergamon-Elsevier Science Ltd. doi:10.1016/j.chemosphere.2020.128179

Piarulli, S., Vanhove, B., Comandini, P., Scapinello, S., Moens, T., Vrielinck, H., Sciutto, G., Prati, S., Mazzeo, R., Booth, A. M., Van Colen, C., & Airoldi, L. (2020). Do different habits affect microplastics contents in organisms? A trait-based analysis on salt marsh species. In *Marine Pollution Bulletin* (Vol. 153). Pergamon-Elsevier Science Ltd. doi:10.1016/j.marpolbul.2020.110983

Piehl, S., Hauk, R., Robbe, E., Richter, B., Kachholz, F., Schilling, J., Lenz, R., Fischer, D., Fischer, F., Labrenz, M., & Schernewski, G. (2021). Combined Approaches to Predict Microplastic Emissions Within an Urbanized Estuary (Warnow, Southwestern Baltic Sea). In Frontiers in Environmental Science (Vol. 9). Frontiers Media SA. doi:10.3389/fenvs.2021.616765

Provencher, J. F., Covernton, G. A., Moore, R. C., Horn, D. A., Conkle, J. L., & Lusher, A. L. (2020). Proceed with caution: The need to raise the publication bar for microplastics research. *The Science of the Total Environment*, *748*, 141426. doi:10.1016/j.scitotenv.2020.141426 PMID:32814297

Rochman, C. M., Hoh, E., Kurobe, T., & Teh, S. J. (2013). Ingested plastic transfers hazardous chemicals to fish and induces hepatic stress. *Scientific Reports*, *3*(1), 3263. doi:10.1038rep03263 PMID:24263561

Rowley, K. H., Cucknell, A.-C., Smith, B. D., Clark, P. F., & Morritt, D. (2020). London's river of plastic: High levels of microplastics in the Thames water column. In *Science of the Total Environment* (Vol. 740). Elsevier. doi:10.1016/j.scitotenv.2020.140018

Sekudewicz, I., Dabrowska, A. M., & Syczewski, M. D. (2021). Microplastic pollution in surface water and sediments in the urban section of the Vistula River (Poland). In *Science of the Total Environment* (Vol. 762). Elsevier, doi:10.1016/j.scitotenv.2020.143111

Su, Y., Zhang, Z., Zhu, J., Shi, J., Wei, H., Xie, B., & Shi, H. (2021). Microplastics act as vectors for antibiotic resistance genes in landfill leachate: The enhanced roles of the long-term aging process. In *Environmental Pollution* (Vol. 270). Elsevier Sci Ltd. doi:10.1016/j.envpol.2020.116278

Tadsuwan, K., & Babel, S. (2021). Microplastic contamination in a conventional wastewater treatment plant in Thailand. In Waste Management & Research (Vol. 39, Issues 5, SI, pp. 754–761). Sage Publications Ltd. doi:10.1177/0734242X20982055

Thompson, R. C., Olsen, Y., Mitchell, R. P., Davis, A., Rowland, S. J., John, A. W. G., McGonigle, D., & Russell, A. E. (2004). Lost at Sea: Where Is All the Plastic? *Science*, *304*(5672), 838–838. doi:10.1126cience.1094559 PMID:15131299

Van Cauwenberghe, L., Vanreusel, A., Mees, J., & Janssen, C. R. (2013). Microplastic pollution in deep-sea sediments. *Environmental Pollution*, *182*, 495–499. doi:10.1016/j.envpol.2013.08.013 PMID:24035457

van Wijnen, J., Ragas, A. M. J., & Kroeze, C. (2019). Modelling global river export of microplastics to the marine environment: Sources and future trends. *The Science of the Total Environment*, *673*, 392–401. doi:10.1016/j.scitotenv.2019.04.078 PMID:30991329

Wang, R., Ji, M., Zhai, H., & Liu, Y. (2020). Occurrence of phthalate esters and microplastics in urban secondary effluents, receiving water bodies and reclaimed water treatment processes. *The Science of the Total Environment*, *737*, 140219. doi:10.1016/j.scitotenv.2020.140219 PMID:32783843

Wang, W., Ndungu, A. W., Li, Z., & Wang, J. (2017). Microplastics pollution in inland freshwaters of China: A case study in urban surface waters of Wuhan, China. *The Science of the Total Environment*, *575*, 1369–1374. doi:10.1016/j.scitotenv.2016.09.213 PMID:27693147

Wang, Z., Zhang, Y., Kang, S., Yang, L., Shi, H., Tripathee, L., & Gao, T. (2021). Research progresses of microplastic pollution in freshwater systems. *The Science of the Total Environment*, *795*, 148888. doi:10.1016/j.scitotenv.2021.148888 PMID:34328911

Wei, S., Luo, H., Zou, J., Chen, J., Pan, X., Rousseau, D. P. L., & Li, J. (2020). Characteristics and removal of microplastics in rural domestic wastewater treatment facilities of China. *The Science of the Total Environment*, *739*, 139935. doi:10.1016/j.scitotenv.2020.139935 PMID:32540663

Xu, Y., Chan, F. K. S., He, J., Johnson, M., Gibbins, C., Kay, P., Stanton, T., Xu, Y., Li, G., Feng, M., Paramor, O., Yu, X., & Zhu, Y.-G. (2020). A critical review of microplastic pollution in urban freshwater environments and legislative progress in China: Recommendations and insights. *Critical Reviews in Environmental Science and Technology*, •••, 1–44. doi:10.1080/10643389.2020.1801308

Xu, Y., Chan, F. K. S., Johnson, M., Stanton, T., He, J., Jia, T., Wang, J., Wang, Z., Yao, Y., Yang, J., Liu, D., Xu, Y., & Yu, X. (2021). Microplastic pollution in Chinese urban rivers: The influence of urban factors. *Resources, Conservation and Recycling*, *173*, 105686. doi:10.1016/j.resconrec.2021.105686

Xu, Y., Chan, F. K. S., Stanton, T., Johnson, M. F., Kay, P., He, J., Wang, J., Kong, C., Wang, Z., Liu, D., & Xu, Y. (2021). Synthesis of dominant plastic microfibre prevalence and pollution control feasibility in Chinese freshwater environments. *The Science of the Total Environment*, *783*, 146863. doi:10.1016/j.scitotenv.2021.146863 PMID:33872912

Zhang, J., Zhang, C., Deng, Y., Wang, R., Ma, E., Wang, J., Bai, J., Wu, J., & Zhou, Y. (2019). Microplastics in the surface water of small-scale estuaries in Shanghai. *Marine Pollution Bulletin*, *149*, 110569. doi:10.1016/j.marpolbul.2019.110569 PMID:31546109

Zhao, S., Zhu, L., & Li, D. (2015). Microplastic in three urban estuaries, China. *Environmental Pollution*, *206*, 597–604. doi:10.1016/j.envpol.2015.08.027 PMID:26312741

ADDITIONAL READING

Stanton, T., Kay, P., Johnson, M., Chan, F. K. S., Gomes, R. L., Hughes, J., Meredith, W., Orr, H. G., Snape, C. E., Taylor, M., Weeks, J., Wood, H., & Xu, Y. (2021). It's the product not the polymer: Rethinking plastic pollution. *WIREs. Water*, *8*(1). Advance online publication. doi:10.1002/wat2.1490

Xu, Y., Chan, F. K. S., He, J., Johnson, M., Gibbins, C., Kay, P., Stanton, T., Xu, Y., Li, G., Feng, M., Paramor, O., Yu, X., & Zhu, Y.-G. (2020). A critical review of microplastic pollution in urban freshwater environments and legislative progress in China: Recommendations and insights. *Critical Reviews in Environmental Science and Technology*, 1–44. doi:10.1080/10643389.2020.1801308

KEY TERMS AND DEFINITIONS

Biofilm: The same as 'Biofouling' in this chapter.

Biofouling: In this chapter, it means the accumulation or the colonization of microorganism adhering on the surface of microplastics.

Macroplastic: Plastic in size larger than 2.5 cm in the environment.

Mesoplastic: Plastic debris in size between 5 mm and 2.5 cm.

Microplastic: Plastic debris in size between 0.001 mm and 5 mm in the environment.

Surface Water: Usually refers to the water layer 0 – 25 cm deep in a waterbody. The exact depth range is defined differently in publications.

Water Column: Generally, refers to the water layer other than the surface water.

Chapter 3
Microplastics in the Environment:
Sources, Pathways, and Abundance

Naveenkumar Ashok Yaranal
Indian Institute of Technology, Guwahati, India

Senthilmurugan Subbiah
Indian Institute of Technology, Guwahati, India

Kaustubha Mohanty
Indian Institute of Technology, Guwahati, India

ABSTRACT

Microplastics in the environment pose a significant threat to the entire ecosystem. Household activity, industrial activity, tyre wear and tear, construction, incineration, plastic litter, landfill, and agricultural activities are the major sources of microplastics in the environment. Microplastics can freely float and adapt between different environmental mediums in the ecosystem due to their lightweight and low-density characteristics. Eventually, microplastics entering the ocean from different pathways result in accumulation and widespread distribution in the marine environment. The frequent interaction between microplastic and aquatic environments accumulates the microplastics in live organisms. The microplastic accumulation and exposure to animals and humans will also affect the ecosystem. This chapter seeks to understand the sources, pathways, and abundance of microplastics in a different environment. The study also highlights the future research prospects for mitigation of plastic towards environment protection.

INTRODUCTION

The widespread use of plastic may be attributed to their numerous attractive properties. Plastics are affordable, flexible, durable, lightweight, waterproof, easy to clean and sterilize, and act as insulators, among other things (Bergmann et al., 2015; Lebreton & Andrady, 2019). Plastics are commonly used

DOI: 10.4018/978-1-7998-9723-1.ch003

in packaging, automotive, household leisure, electrical and electronic parts, building and construction materials, sports products, and the agricultural sector (Elizalde-Velázquez & Gómez-Oliván, 2021). Plastic production has grown exponentially, with large-scale production starting in the 1950s around 1.5 million tons per year to 348 million tons in the 2017s (Plastics Europe, 2018; WHO, 2019). Historically the global production of plastic materials has increased by around 8 - 10% each year (Crawford & Quinn, 2016; Peixoto et al., 2019). Plastic production is expected to double by 2025 and more than triple by 2050, based on the projected global population growth rate and existing consumption and waste patterns (FAO, 2017). Due to improper plastic waste disposal, a significant number of plastics eventually end up in the marine ecosystem via household materials, industrial discharge, wastewater treatment plants (WWTPs), incineration, landfills, and rivers. This has resulted in increasing quantities of plastic pollution in oceans worldwide. (Aslam et al., 2020; Crawford & Quinn, 2016; Henry et al., 2019). The occurrence and distribution of large plastic litter in the marine environment have been extensively documented (Ajith et al., 2020; Du et al., 2020). However, with prolonged physical, chemical, and biological weathering, these larger plastic materials eventually fragment, resulting in macro, meso, micro, and nanoplastics (Golwala et al., 2021).

Microplastic enters the environment as primary and secondary sources. These microplastics are ubiquitous in the atmospheric, terrestrial, and aquatic environment, mainly due to inappropriate plastic disposal and insufficient waste management (Ajith et al., 2020). Landfills, the most prominent technique of solid waste management, are the main repository and disseminator of microplastics, including both primary and secondary microplastics (Golwala et al., 2021). Different environmental conditions (such as rain and wind) facilitate the transport of landfilled microplastics to the surrounding ecosystem. Furthermore, due to inadequate separation, microplastics from different consumer commodities and microfibers from synthetic clothes are potential sources of microplastics in WWTPs (Z. Zhang & Chen, 2020). The majority of microplastics enter aquatic streams after passing through WWTPs (De Falco et al., 2018; Talvitie et al., 2017). The retained microplastics accumulates in sludge or biosolids applied for agricultural activities may result in microplastic contamination in agricultural soil (Q. Li et al., 2019; Y. Zhou et al., 2020). The majority of plastic waste created in industrial operations and small workshops are discharged immediately into the environment without treatment (Du et al., 2020). Finally, microplastics reach into the sea from diverse sources and are dispersed by ocean currents. Widespread deposition and distribution of microplastics raise a concern about their interaction and potential consequences on marine ecosystems. The gradual increase of microplastic in the sea will lead to significant accumulation in coastal and marine environments (Bergmann et al., 2015).

A schematic diagram of sources, pathways, and toxic effects of microplastic is shown in **Fig. 1**. Animal and humans are directly or indirectly exposed to microplastics. Direct exposure of pollutions to organisms occurs through different mediums, including water and air. Indirect exposure, on the other hand, occurs through the food chain or in conjunction with other chemicals (additives, heavy metals, and POPs). In general, direct exposure causes significant toxicity in the near term, whereas indirect exposure can cause long-term organ damage (Du et al., 2020). Microplastics are harmful to a variety of fish and invertebrates because they can cause digestive tract blockage, inflammation, reproductive disorders, growth rate inhibition, oxidative and pathological stress (Rist et al., 2019; Sana et al., 2020). According to Rist et al. (2018), more than 700 aquatic species were adversely affected, including birds, turtles, whales, blue mussel, sand hopper, crab, pacific oyster (Carr et al., 2016; Chapman, 2007; Leslie et al., 2017; Rios Mendoza et al., 2018a; Rist et al., 2018).

Figure 1. Schematic diagram of sources, pathways, and toxic effects of microplastics

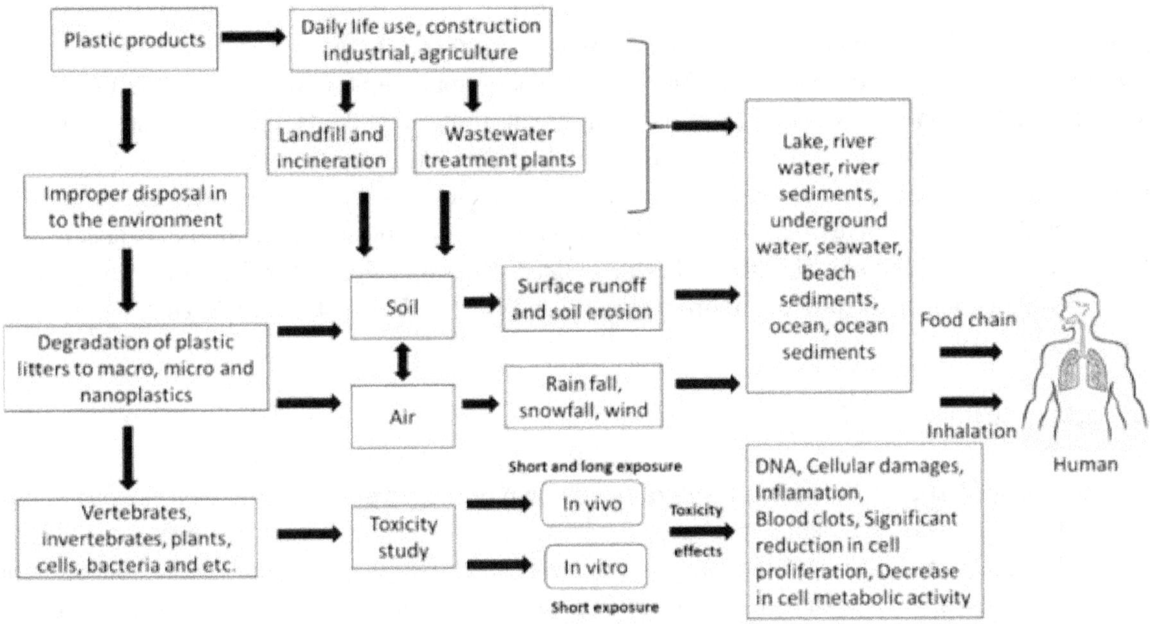

Microplastics have been found in air, potable water, and table salt, indicating that they can enter the human body in various ways (Kankanige & Babel, 2020; Yaranal et al., 2021a). Recent investigations show microplastics have been observed in human lungs, digestive tract, placenta, and feces (Pauly et al., 1998; Ragusa et al., 2021; Schwabl et al., 2019; Toussaint et al., 2019). Since microplastics can harm various organisms, the possibility of humans being harmed by microplastics must be considered. Since humans are the final consumers of microplastic-affected seafood, there is a substantial risk of microplastic transfer to humans (Cox et al., 2019; Wright & Kelly, 2017). The effects of microplastics on both the environment and human health are not completely understood. Knowing all microplastic sources, pathways, and abundance in atmospheric, terrestrial, and aquatic environments is essential to understand better and control microplastic pollution. The current chapter reviewed the possible sources, pathways, and abundance of microplastics in air, soil, freshwater, and sea environments. Based on the review, the future prospects are discussed.

SOURCES AND PATHWAYS OF MICROPLASTICS

The plastic industry has outgrown exponentially, and the use of plastics has increased in recent years. It has been predicted that the usage will double in the next 20 years (Perren et al., 2018). On the other side, the unregulated disposal practices of plastics have resulted in aquatic, terrestrial, and now atmospheric environments. All three environments are interconnected through diverse pathways and sources that can affect the microplastic accumulation and flux in these matrices. Microplastics, based on their origin, are classified into primary and secondary categories (Blair et al., 2019; Boucher & Friot, 2017; Herbort et al., 2018).

Primary Microplastics

Primary microplastics are manufactured to serve exclusive purposes in many domestics or industrial applications. The cosmetic and cleaning products such as soaps, make-up foundation, body scrubs, lotions, toothpaste, peeling, baby products, nail polish, sunscreen, insect repellents, and synthetics clothes are the major sources (Carr et al., 2016; Veerasingam et al., 2020). The industry originated feedstocks used in plastic manufacturing, plastic resin powder/pellet spillage during air-blasting, 3D printer ink (Rios Mendoza et al., 2018b), and textile fibers also lead to a high level of plastics and microplastic generation in the environment (Talvitie et al., 2017). Textiles release microplastics in the form of synthetic fibers to the atmosphere during the process of production to end use (De Falco et al., 2018; Henry et al., 2019; Stanton et al., 2019).

Secondary Microplastics

Secondary microplastics, formed as a result of breakdown of bigger plastic items such as bottles, bags, toys, construction materials, paints, packaging materials, electronics items, and vehicle tyre (Carr et al., 2016; Da Costa et al., 2016). Secondary microplastics are also generated during the collection and disposal of municipal solid waste and as the result of anthropogenic actions such as littering (Du et al., 2020; Horton, Walton, et al., 2017). Considering the enormous volume of macroplastics entering the environment, secondary microplastics are seen as a major contributor to microplastic contamination in the environment. Plastic items are weathered as they travel through the environment, creating microplastics as a result of mechanical fragmentation, chemical, and biological degradation. These factors lead to continuous temporal changes in the physical and chemical characteristics of plastics (Cai et al., 2018; Oliveira et al., 2020; Singh & Sharma, 2008; Zbyszewski et al., 2014). Photodegradation of the polymer matrix causes bond breakage and brittleness in plastics, leading them to disintegrate. Among others, Cai et al. (2018) studied the impact of UV exposure for three polymers types of polystyrene (PS), polypropylene (PP), and polyethylene (PE). Their exposure studies have revealed that the pellet surface homogenous texture changed drastically over months of exposure, where cracks and flakes were common patterns of this degradation process.

Pathways and Accumulation of Microplastics into Various Environment

Microplastics exist in the atmospheric, terrestrial, and aquatic environments. The physical processes influenced by climatic forces play a key role in the specific distribution of microplastic among diverse environments (K. Zhang et al., 2017). The significant factors in the conveyance of microplastic are wind, river, surface runoff, flooding, tides, etc. Recent investigations have found that considerable quantities of fibers have been transferred by atmospheric fallout, particularly in densely populated areas. Wind can transfer these particles in the atmosphere to terrestrial and aquatic environments. The microplastic sources, transport pathways, and accumulation among different environments are depicted in Fig. 2.

Atmospheric environment: The climatic and seasonal conditions play an essential role in the deposition and concentration of the microplastic in the atmosphere. The density and buoyancy affect the vertical distribution of microplastic in the atmosphere. The highest concentration is generally found near to terrestrial region. Very few researches have been conducted on microplastic contamination in the atmosphere. The first study on microplastic in the urban environment was conducted by Dris et al.

Figure 2. Sources, pathways and accumulation of microplastic in atmospheric, terrestrial, and aquatic environments

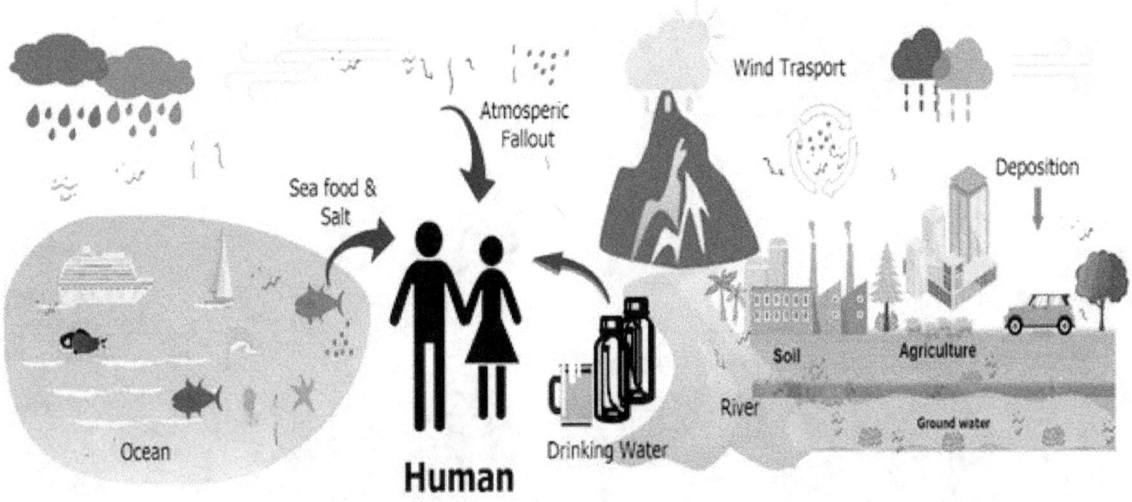

(2015). The microplastics in the urban environment are often associated with extensive human activity. Like synthetic fabrics, urban dust, construction materials, industrial pollutants, landfills, agricultural practices and plastic materials are all potential microplastic sources in the atmosphere (G. Chen et al., 2020; Qiu et al., 2020; Y. Zhang et al., 2020). Microplastics were easily dispersed by wind and might stay for a long period in the atmosphere, transferring it to remote places (Trainic et al., 2020). The climatic parameters, including wind, precipitation, temperature, are dependent factors for microplastic distribution in atmospheric environment (Prata, 2018). After being discharged into the air, microplastics are conveyed and settle in terrestrial and marine environments.

Terrestrial environment: The presence of a wide range of microplastic debris in the terrestrial environment is primarily due to excessive use and their improper disposal (J. Li et al., 2020). Due to non-degradability and various other properties, microplastics may remain in the environment for a longer period, affecting biodiversity and the environment, including the growth and reproduction of plants and organisms (Kumar et al., 2020; W. Li et al., 2020). Arable soils can be polluted with microplastics via various pathways. On the one hand, microplastics enters the agricultural soil through sewage sludge, digested residues, irrigation with polluted waters, polymer-based fertilizer and pesticides, atmospheric deposition, littering, plastics items from landfills, and surface runoff (Da Costa et al., 2016; Sujathan et al., 2017; Talvitie et al., 2017). Microplastics in agricultural soils, on the other hand, are created by the degradation of plastic materials utilized in agricultural practices (M. Liu et al., 2018; Rehm et al., 2021). Due to its remarkable benefits, PE and polyvinyl chloride (PVC) composed mulch films have become extensively used in global agricultural production. Plastic mulch is widely used in agriculture practices and covers around 20 million hectares of farmlands worldwide, where China alone accounts for nearly 90% of it (Yang et al., 2021; Y. Zhou et al., 2020). In 2016, globally, 4 million tons of plastic film was used in agriculture and predicted to rise to 5.6 million tons per year by 2030. The removal of the mulching film from the agriculture field is a time-consuming and labor-intensive task; as a result, certain parts of it are left on farms, either purposely or inadvertently. Different organisms, including

Figure 3. Sources, accumulation and transport of microplastics in soils

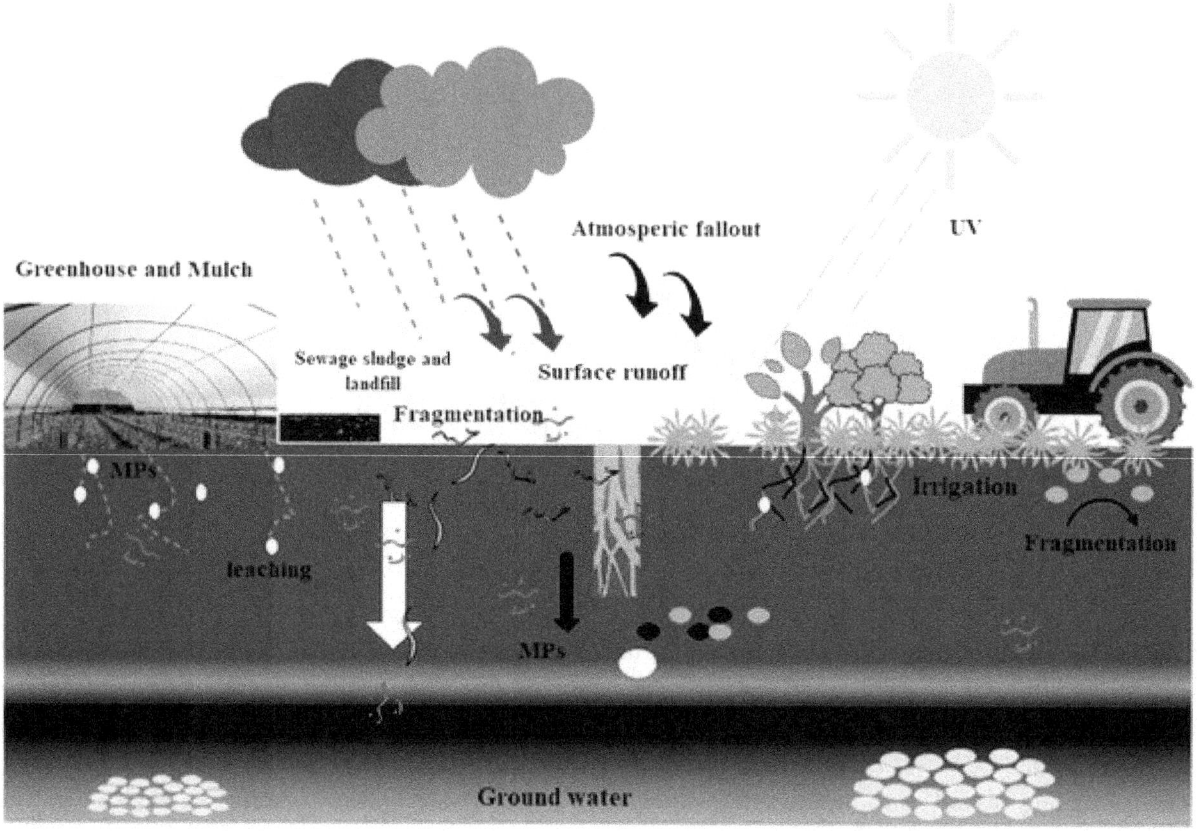

earthworms, can aid in the production of microplastics and nanoplastics from larger plastic fragments (Kumar et al., 2020; Piehl et al., 2018). Considering current overall understanding of possible microplastic sources in agricultural soils, in-situ soil contamination data is limited, owing to the difficulty of detecting microplastics in the soil (Möller et al., 2020). According to J. Li et al. (2020), agricultural soil is highly porous media; thus, particles (0.1–6.0 µm) can easily move vertically along with the soil. Based on the different studies on estimates of microplastics in the soil, the agriculture soil is considered as a major microplastic sink. It is sometimes debated whether the accumulation of microplastics in the soil leads to a permanent or whether it is lost again through leaching into groundwater or surface runoff and erosion. Because agricultural soils are particularly prone to erosion, the possibility of microplastics being transported by surface runoff is of major importance (Y. Chen et al., 2020; Rehm et al., 2021). The highest plastic transport was recorded in the Rhône River a few days after rainfall events, demonstrating that surface runoff may have a significant impact on microplastics intake to water bodies when compared to other processes (Castro-Jiménez et al., 2019). The studies of Piehl et al. (2018) and B. Zhou et al. (2020) found that frequent uses of plastic material in the farmland are major contributors to plastic pollution in the agricultural fields. In addition, careless disposal and displacement of plastics by wind were the primary routes for input to croplands.

Aquatic environment: Microplastic enters the freshwater via different pathways, significantly from the discharge of urban drainage systems, road runoff, WWTPs effluent, agriculture, wind, and fisheries and aquaculture (C. Wang et al., 2021; WHO, 2019). The microplastics present in cosmetics, cleaning products, and microfibers from cloth can enter the aquatic environment through industrial or domestic drainage systems. According to De Falco et al. (2018), the primary microplastics infiltrate the aquatic environment through WWTPs in urban areas. Surface runoff from agricultural fields and urban areas is another significant source of microplastics in surface water (WHO, 2019). Additionally, data suggests that tyres and road markings may contribute to microplastic contamination, with storm-water runoff as a major pathway for plastic particles to reach surface waterways. Wind dispersal may transport larger plastic objects and their degradation products into aquatic ecosystems (Horton, Svendsen, et al., 2017; Horton, Walton, et al., 2017; Xu et al., 2021).

Microplastics reach the marine environment mainly through rivers, airborne, plastic litters degradation, loss of fishing gears, aquaculture, shipping, tourism activities, urban and industrial (onshore and offshore) effluents (Yaranal et al., 2021b). According to research calculations, every year, approximately 4.8 to 12.7 million metric tons of plastics waste ends up in the marine ecosystem (Veerasingam et al., 2020) in that nearly 1.15 to 2.41 million metric tons of plastics reaches through rivers (Kim et al., 2018; Lebreton & Andrady, 2019). Land-based plastic debris contributes to 80% of all plastic garbage in the ocean (Issac & Kandasubramanian, 2021; Y. Li et al., 2020). Estuaries and coastal lagoons are where the bulk of aquaculture species are cultivated. The significant use of plastic materials in the fishing and aquaculture sectors is the primary cause of microplastic pollution in the ocean (Du et al., 2020; Thiele et al., 2021). There are no global estimates on the amount of plastic garbage produced by the fisheries and aquaculture industries. The Republic of Korea has produced the first national estimate of fisheries and aquaculture debris input to marine environments, with an annual input of approximately 51,000 tons of plastics (Jang et al., 2014; Lusher et al., 2017). According to Eriksen et al. (2014), the oceans already contain more than five trillion particles of plastic weighing more than 2,50,000 tones. These microplastics are a hundred times lower on the sea surface than predicted, lending credence to the notion that most microplastics sink and collect in the core region of the ocean. Some have been found frozen in the Arctic ocean ice, which has become a global sink for microplastics (Kanhai et al., 2020). Microplastics with densities lower than seawater float at the surface layer or are suspended in the water column with neutral density, whereas microplastics with densities higher than seawater are concentrated in marine benthic regions (Ajith et al., 2020; Y. Li et al., 2020). Some of the factors, such as turbulence and biofouling, increase the density of microplastics.

MICROPLASTICS ABUNDANCE

Atmospheric Environment

The most vital element for survival is air. However, breathing polluted air is hazardous to health. Researchers have found airborne microplastics among the various contaminants in the atmosphere. Dris et al. (2017), Cai et al. (2017), and Liu et al. (2019) observed the presence of microplastic fibers in indoor, outdoor, and working places. The presence of microplastics in the atmosphere are summarized in **Table 1**. From **Table 1**, it can be seen that various researchers have identified the presence of varied microplastics in terms of shape, size, and composition in different cities of the world, viz. 118 particles m^{-2} day^{-1} in Greater Paris, France (Dris et al., 2015); 175 - 313 particles m^{-2} day^{-1} in Dongguan City (Cai et al., 2017); 365 $\pm$ 69 particles m^{-2} day^{-1} in French Pyrenees (Allen et al., 2019) and 136.5 and 512.0

particles m^{-2} day^{-1} in Hamburg, Germany (Klein & Fischer, 2019). According to Dris et al. (2017), the amount of microplastics in indoor air (1 – 60 fibres m^{-3}) was substantially greater than in outside air (0.3 - 1.5 fibres m^{-3}). This is because microplastics are typically formed by mechanical wear or degradation of textile apparel and bedding such as pillows, blankets, and curtains due to closed or semi-closed compartments, as explained by (Prata, 2018). In Denmark, Vianello et al. (2019) observed the presence of airborne microplastics in three-flats and found that PE, polyester, polyamide (PA), and PP were the most prevalent types. Catarino et al. (2018), in Edinburg, collected the household fibers fallout during a meal with concentrations and deposition rate of 5 ± 3.3 - 10 ± 4.2 particle m-3 and 1666.8 - 1671.84 particles m-2 day-1, respectively. The study of Kaya et al. (2018), Abbasi et al. (2019), Patchaiyappan et al. (2021), and Su et al. (2020) and Yukioka et al. (2020) confirmed the microplastics pollution in roadside dust from urban and rural areas. According to studies related to multiple correlation and principal component analysis, urbanization, rainfall and snow have significant role on roadside microplastic deposition (Su et al., 2020). The airborne microplastics were identified in the West Pacific Ocean and North Atlantic Ocean atmosphere by Liu et al. (2019) and Trainic et al. (2020). The deposition of the microfibers on snow and mosses from the atmosphere was also confirmed by Bergmann et al. (2019) and Roblin and Aherne (2020). These findings, therefore, confirm the ubiquitous existence of microplastics in the global ecosystem.

Atmospheric microplastics have vertical distribution features due to density and buoyancy, with higher concentrations towards the ground. The low density and small size make the microplastic distributed easily by wind. The deposition rate varied with location, depending on the climate conditions and seasonality. Across various altitudes of atmospheres, the highest concentration of microplastics was reported at 1.7 m above the ground (Qiu et al., 2020). Dris et al. (2015) and Dris et al. (2016), in their study using the rain sampling method, observed a greater number of microplastics in urban areas compared to suburban areas with less population density. Similarly, Liu et al. (2019a, 2019b, 2019c) observed the higher concertation of microplastics in land-based sampling to sea air due to the dilution effect of sea air and human activity. Rain and snow play an important role in microplastics deposition (Allen et al., 2019; Gasperi et al., 2018). The above studies confirmed that the climate conditions, seasonality, population density, and sampling methodology may also influence the deposition and concentration of microplastics. However, knowledge about microplastics in atmospheric is limited. Therefore, more research is required to focus on the origin and fate of microplastics in different regions.

Terrestrial Environment

Microplastics presence and dispersion in soils have not been well investigated; however, the current data (Table 1) demonstrated that microplastic contamination exists in soil matrices globally. The presence of microplastics in soil affects the growth, reproduction, and immune system of organisms (W. Li et al., 2020). According to Liu et al. 2018, microplastics can occur in topsoil as well as subsurface soils; however, research on microplastic pollution in the soil is minimal. Some of the researchers, such as Fuller and Gautam (2016), conducted the first survey of the concentration and distribution of microplastics in industrial soil. Furthermore, microplastics have been identified in parks, gardens, wetlands (Yang et al., 2021), industrial farmlands (Fuller & Gautam, 2016), and floodplain soils (Scheurer & Bigalke, 2018). The average microplastics found in industrial soils of Sydney were 300 - 67,500 mg kg^{-1} and 5.5 mg kg^{-1} or 593 items kg^{-1} of microplastics in floodplain soil of Switzerland (Fuller & Gautam, 2016; Scheurer & Bigalke, 2018). Many researchers have identified the presence of microplastics in farmland soils of

Table 1. Worldwide abundance and characteristics of atmospheric microplastics

Study area and air type	Identification	Sample preparation method	Shape	Size (μm)	Composition	Microplastics abundance	Reference
Paris, France (urban outdoor)	Stereomicroscope	Filtration	Fibres, fragments	100- 1,000	N/A	29 - 280 particles m^{-2} day^{-1}; Average:118 particles m^{-2} day^{-1}	(Dris et al., 2015)
Paris, France (urban and sub-urban outdoor)	Stereomicroscope, μ-FTIR	Filtration (1.6 μm, GF)	Fibers	50 – 5,000	RY, PET, PU, PA	Urban average:110 ± 96 particles m^{-2} day^{-1}; Sub-urban average: 53 ± 38 particles m^{-2} day^{-1}	(Dris et al., 2016)
Paris, France (indoor and outdoor)	Stereomicroscope, μ-FTIR	Vacuum pump + density separation ($ZnCl_2$) + filtration (1.6 GF)	Fibres	50 – 4,850	RY, PE, PA, PP, PET	Indoor: 1 - 60 fibers m^{-3} (1586-11,130 fibers m^{-2} day^{-1}); Outdoor: 0.3 - 1.5 fibers m^{-3}	(Dris et al., 2017)
Edinburgh, UK (indoor home)	Fluorescence microscope, μ-FTIR	Density separation (NaCl) + filtration	Fibres	≥ 500	PET, PUR	5±3.3 - 10±4.2 particles m^{-3}	(Catarino et al., 2018)
Aarhus, Denmark (indoor)	μ-FTIR	Filtration	Fibres	4 - 400	PES, PE, nylon	1.7 – 16.2 particles m^{-3}	(Vianello et al., 2019)
Dongguan, China (urban outdoor)	Stereomicroscope, μ-FTIR, SEM	Filtration (1 μm, GF)	Fibres, fragments, foams, films	200 – 4,200	PE (14%), PP (9%), PS (4%)	175 - 313 particles m^{-2} day^{-1}	(Cai et al., 2017)
Shanghai, China (urban - outdoor)	Stereomicroscope, μ-FTIR	Filtration (1.6 μm, GF)	Fibres, fragment, granule	23 - 9,555	PE, PET, PES, PAN, RY	0 - 4.18 particles m^{-3}	(K. Liu, Wang, Fang, et al., 2019)
Shanghai, China	Microscope, μ-FTIR	Filtration	Fibres, fragments, and microbeads	< 5,000	PET, PE, PP, PA and PS	0.05 to 0.07 particles m^{-3}	(K. Liu, Wang, Wei, et al., 2019)
Hamburg, Germany (metropolitan area)	Fluorescence microscope, μ-Raman spectroscopy	Digestion (NaClO) + filtration	Fragments and fibres	< 63 – 5,000	PE, PVA, and PET	136.5 and 512 particles m^{-2} day^{-1}	(Klein & Fischer, 2019)
Pyrenees mountains, France (remote mountain area)	Stereomicroscope, μ-FTIR	Filtration	Fragments, films, fibers	25 - 2,600	PS, PE, PP, PVC, PET	365 ± 69 particles m^{-2} day^{-1}	(Allen et al., 2019)
Snow from Europe and artic (Alps, N. Germany, Artic)	Stereomicroscope, μ-FTIR	Filtration (0.2 μm, aluminum oxide)	Fibers	11 - 5000	PE, rubber, PA, PS and polyester	0 - 154 × 103 N $liter^{-1}$	(Bergmann et al., 2019)
Asaluyeh County, Iran (suspended dust, urban dust-outdoor)	Fluorescence microscope, SEM-EDS	Digestion (30% H_2O_2) + density separation (NaI) + filtration	Spherules, films, fragments, fibers	2 - 1,000	N/A	900 MPs and 250 micro rubbers in 15 gm dust sample. Average: 0.3 - 1.1 particles m^{-3}	(Abbasi et al., 2019)
Victoria, Australia (roadside dust from rural and urban area)	Stereomicroscope, μ-FTIR	Dust collected (sweeping) + screening + digestion (30% H_2O_2) + density separation (NaCl) + filtration	Fiber, fragment, film and pellet	20 – 4,700	Polyester and PP	20.6 to 529.3 items kg^{-1}	(Su et al., 2020)
Kusatsu, Japan, Da Nang, Vietnam, and Kathmandu, Nepal (road dust)	Stereomicroscope, ATR-FTIR	Digestion (30% H_2O_2) + density separation (NaI) + filtration	Fragments, film, fibers, and granules	100 - 5000	Rubbers, PE, PP, PS and PET	Kusatsu: 2.0 ± 1.6 pieces m^{-2}; Da Nang: 19.7 ± 13.7; Kathmandu: 12.5 ± 10.1 pieces m^{-2}	(Yukioka et al., 2020)
Chennai, India (suspended dust - outdoor)	Fluorescence microscope, μ-Raman, SEM-EDS	Digestion (0.05 M Fe + 30% H_2O_2) + density separation (NaI) + filtration	Fragments	> 50 - < 5000	PVC, PE, PTFE	227.94 ± 91.37 particles/100g dust sample	(Patchaiyappan et al., 2021)
Ireland (mosses from lakes catchment)	Stereomicroscope, Raman spectroscopy	Digestion (0.05 M Fe + 30% H_2O_2) + filtration	Fibers	< 4,310		24 g^{-1} dry weight of mosses	(Roblin & Aherne, 2020)
West Pacific Ocean (sea air)	Stereomicroscope, μ-FTIR	Filtration (GF)	Fibers, fragment, granule, microbeads	20 - 500	PET, PE-PP, PS, EP, others	0-1.37 particles m^{-3}	(K. Liu, Wu, et al., 2019)
North Atlantic Ocean (sea air)	Stereomicroscope, μ-Raman	Filtration	N/A	1-100	PP, PE, PP, poly-silicone	N/A	(Trainic et al., 2020)

China and reported a high concentration ranging from 50 - 12,560 MPs kg^{-1} (Y. Chen et al., 2020; M. Liu et al., 2018; J. Wang et al., 2017; B. Zhou et al., 2020; Q. Zhou et al., 2016) as show in **Table 2**. Low and high numbers of microplastics were found in the agricultural soil of Germany (0.34 - 0.36 MPs kg^{-1}) and Spain (190 – 5,190 MPs kg^{-1}), respectively (Piehl et al., 2018; Van den Berg et al., 2020). Microplastic accumulation in the soil with sewage sludge and mulching applications was confirmed by Piehl et al. (2018) and B. Zhou et al. (2020). The study of Van den Berg et al. (2020) also showed that farmlands without sludge applications had an average of 2,030 microplastics kg^{-1} while farmland with sludge application had an average of 5,190 microplastics kg^{-1}. B. Zhou et al. (2020) observed higher amount of microplastics in mulching soil than non-mulching soil, with an average of 571 pieces kg^{-1}

and 263 pieces kg^{-1}, respectively. The above studies revealed that microplastic content increased with mulching and sewage sludge applications in the farmland. The mesoplastics are likely to break down further and degrade into the finer particle, and thus increasing microplastic pollution. The variation in abundance of microplastics mainly depends on the continuing damage and degradation of the film mulch over time due to biotic and abiotic factors. Many factors, such as cultivation, fertilization, and sampling sites, are the main reason for the diversified abundance of microplastics in different regions. Based on review data, it is evident that microplastics in the terrestrial environment is rapidly increasing. Eco friendly materials, techniques and fertilizers in agricultural practices can reduce the microplastic presence. Easy standard sampling procedure should be developed and adopted for identification and quantification of microplastics in terrestrial environment.

Aquatic Environment

Microplastics were identified in variable concentrations in freshwater and sediment depending on the region. Microplastics that are not trapped in sewage sludge throughout the treatment process end up in aquatic streams (Horton et al., 2017). Freshwater bodies are the primary sources of drinking water for people and are suspected of becoming possible sources of microplastics exposure to humans. The microplastics detected around the world, including lakes, rivers, sediments, beaches, and seawater, are presented in table 3. The microplastics concentration in surface water viz. 379 - 12,611 MPs m^{-3} in fresh water of China (Di & Wang, 2018; Lin et al., 2018), 58 – 1,265 items m^{-3} in Antuã River of Portugal (Rodrigues et al., 2018), 2.68 - 3.36 particles m^{-3} in lake of Italy (Fischer et al., 2016), 67 - 11,532 MPs m^{-3} in Meuse and Dommel rivers of Netherland (Mintenig et al., 2020), and 3.52 to 32.05 particles m^{-3} in Carpathian basin of Europe (Bordós et al., 2019) was reported. While the concentration of microplastic in the sediment of the same water system was observed in the range of 25 - 7924 items m^{-3} in China (Di & Wang, 2018; Lin et al., 2018), 18 - 629 items m^{-3} in Portugal (Rodrigues et al., 2018), 234 particles m^{-3} in Italy (Fischer et al., 2016), and 0.46 to 1.62 particles m^{-3} in Europe (Bordós et al., 2019). Recent researchers in India Selvan et al. (2021) identified the presence of microplastics in groundwater. Moreover, J. Wang et al. (2017) reported that the microplastic concentrations in sediment are much higher than that in freshwater. Microplastics abundance in freshwater and sediment is generally higher in China when compared to other countries (Table 3); the rise in concentration is attributed to the rapid economic development of the country. Studies in China, Kores, Netherland, Italy, Turkey, and Tunisia reported the highest microplastics pollution in seawater and sediments (Yaranal et al., 2021b). Coastal areas recorded the maximum concentrations of microplastics (Kang et al., 2015; Lots et al., 2017; Nel & Froneman, 2015). Deep-sea sediments act as a major sink for microplastics (Kanhai et al., 2019, 2020); however, different factors influence the distribution of microplastics in marine water such as topography, ocean currents, wind, and human activities (Pan et al., 2019; Yaranal et al., 2021b).The concentration of microplastics in the ocean varied with different regions. For instance, the average abundance of seawater was around 1.15 particles m^{-3} in the Atlantic Ocean (Kanhai et al., 2017); 1.0×10^4 MPs km^{-2} in the North-western Pacific Ocean (Pan et al., 2019); 2 - 17 MPs/L in sea ice from Arctic Central Basin and 0 - 18 MPs m^{-3} in seawater beneath ice floes of Arctic Ocean (Kanhai et al., 2020).

The microplastics ingestion by aquatic organisms can cause several negative health impacts. Therefore, the role of researchers in future works is important in 1) identifying the sources of microplastics to aquatic environment; 2) development of new technologies to prevent microplastics dispersion in aquatic system; 3) preparation of alternative eco-friendly polymeric materials.

Table 2. Worldwide abundance and characteristics of terrestrial microplastics

Study area	Identification	Shape	Size (μm)	Sample preparation	Microplastics abundance	Composition	Reference
Sydney, Australia (soil from industrial area)	ATR-FT-IR	N/A	< 1mm	Sieve	300 – 67, 500 mg kg^{-1}	PVC, and PE	(Fuller & Gautam, 2016)
Shandong, China (coastal soil)	Stereomicroscope, SEM-EDS	Granules, fragment fibers, films	< 4.7 mm	Density separation (NaI) + filtration	634 MPs kg^{-1}	N/A	(Q. Zhou et al., 2016)
Switzerland (floodplain)	Microscope, FT-IR	N/A	< 1 mm	Digestion (HNO_3) + density separation (NaCl, $ZnCl_2$) + filtration (0.45 μm)	55.5 mg kg^{-1} or 593 particles kg^{-1}	PE, PS, and PP	(Scheurer & Bigalke, 2018)
Southeast Germany (farmland soil)	Stereomicroscope, ATR-FT-IR	Films and fragments	< 5mm	Digestion (H_2O_2) + filtration	0.34 ± 0.36 MPs kg^{-1}	PE, PS, and PP	(Piehl et al., 2018)
Shanghai, China (farmland soil)	μ-FT-IR	Fibers, fragments, films, and pellets	< 5 mm	Digestion (H_2O_2) + density separation (NaCl) + filtration (20 μm)	Top soil: 78 ± 12.91; Deep soil: 62.50±12.97 items kg^{-1}	PP and PE	(M. Liu et al., 2018)
Nanjing and Wuxi, China (farmland soil)	μ-FT-IR	Fibers, fragments	< 5 mm	Digestion (H_2O_2 + H_2SO_4) + density separation (NaCl, ZnCl2) + filtration (2 μm)	420–1,290 MP items kg^{-1}	PE and PP	(Q. Li et al., 2019)
Wuhan, China (vegetable farmland soil)	Stereomicroscope, μ-Raman spectroscopy	Fibers and microbeads	< 5 mm	Density separation ($ZnCl_2$) + filtration (0.45 μm)	320 to 12,560 items kg^{-1}	PA, and PP	(Y. Chen et al., 2020)
Shihezi City, Xinjiang, China (farmland soil)	Microscope, SEM ATR-FT-IR	Film	< 5 mm	Flotation + filtration	40.35 mg kg^{-1}	PE and others	(W. Li et al., 2020)
Hangzhou Bay, China (farmland soil)	Stereomicroscope, μ- FT-IR	Fragments, films, fibers	< 5 mm	Density separation (NaCl) + filtration	Mulching soils: 571 pieces kg^{-1}; Non-mulching soils: 263 pieces kg^{-1}; Irrigation water: 3.9 – 17 pieces/L	PE, PP, PA polyester, rayon, and acrylic	(B. Zhou et al., 2020)
USA (wetland)	Microscope, ATR-FT-IR	Fibers and fragments	< 5 mm	Digestion (H_2O_2) + filtration	1,270 ± 150 MPs kg^{-1} Or 23200 ± 2500 MPs m^{-2}	PS, PE, and synthetic rubber	(Helcoski et al., 2020)
Valencia, Spain (sewage sludge and soil)	Microscope, μ-FT-IR	Fragment, fibers, film and foam	< 5 mm	Density separation (NaI) + filtration	Sewage sludge: 18,000 ± 15,940 and 32,070 ± 19,080 MPs kg^{-1}; Soil without sludge: 930 ± 740 and 1,100 ± 570 MPs kg^{-1}; Soil with sludge: 2,130 ± 950 and 3,060 ± 1,680 MPs kg^{-1}	PP, and PVC	(Van den Berg et al., 2020)
Mellipilla, Chile (crop lands and pastures)	Microscope, μ-FT-IR	Film, fibers and fragments	< 5 mm	Density separation (NaCl, $ZnCl_2$) + filtration	Crop land: 306 ± 360 particles kg^{-1}; Pastures: 184 ± 266 particles kg^{-1}	Acrylates, PU, PE, PP and PA	(Corradini et al., 2021)

CONCLUSION

The frequent utility of plastic in daily life, inadequate disposal, and improper waste management leads to the wide distribution of microplastics in atmospheric, terrestrial, and aquatic environments. The various household, industrial and construction activities are the major sources for the microplastic depository. The increasing application of plastic in daily life is a major concern for the environment. The microplastic accumulation and exposure to animals and humans will also affect the ecosystem health. Eventually, microplastics entering the ocean from different pathways result in accumulation and widespread distribution in the marine environment. The present study showed that the microplastic sources are diverse and can migrate from one environment to another environment in the ecosystem through different pathways.

WAY FORWARD

Microplastics are ubiquitous in the environment, however, knowledge of sampling methodology and concentration of microplastics in atmospheric, terrestrial, and aquatic regions is minimal. Therefore, the inclusion of alternative standard sampling methodology and more studies may facilitate the comparison

Table 3. Worldwide abundance and characteristics of aquatic microplastics

Study area and sample type	Identification methods	Sample preparation method	Size (μm)	Composition	Microplastics abundance	Reference
China, Three Gorges Reservoir	Microscope, μ-Raman spectroscopy	Digestion (30% H_2O_2) + filtration (0.45 μm, GF)	< 5000	PC, PE, PP, PS, PVC	Surface water: 1,597– 12,611 MPs m^{-3}; Sediment: 25 – 300 MPs kg^{-1}	(Di & Wang, 2018)
China, Pearl River	Stereo light microscope, μ-FTIR	Digestion (30% H_2O_2) + filtration	20 - 5000	PP, PE, PET	Surface water: 379–7,924 items m^{-3}; Sediment: 80 – 9,597 MPs kg^{-1}	(Lin et al., 2018)
Portugal, Antuã River	Stereomicroscope, ATR-FTIR	Digestion (Fe + 30% H_2O_2) + density separation ($ZnCl_2$), filtration (0.45 μm)	55 - 5000	PP, PE, PS, PET	Surface water: 58 - 1,265 items m^{-3}; Sediment: 18–629 items kg^{-1}	(Rodrigues et al., 2018)
Italy, Lake Chiusi,	UV- microscope, SEM	Digestion (HCl) + density separation (NaCl), filtration (0.45 μm)	< 5000	N/A	Surface water: 2.68–3.36 particles m^{-3}; Sediment: 234 particles kg^{-1}	(Fischer et al., 2016)
Europe, Carpathian basin	Microscope, ATR-FTIR	Density separation (NaCl), filtration	200-5000	PE, PP, PTFE, PS	Surface water: 3.52 – 32.05 particles m^{-3}; Sediment: 0.46 – 1.62 particles kg^{-1}	(Bordós et al., 2019)
Netherland, Meuse and Dommel river	Stereomicroscope, μ-FTIR, ATR-FTIR	Digestion (H_2O_2), density separation ($ZnCl_2$), vacuum filtration	<25 - 1000	PE, PP, and EPDM	Surface water: 67 – 11,532 MPs m^{-3}	(Mintenig et al., 2020)
India, Ground, surface water	Stereomicroscope, ATR-FTIR, AFM, ICP-OES	Digestion (Fe + 30% H_2O_2) + filtration	300 - 5000	PP, PA, PE, and PVC	Ground water: 10.1 particles/L Surface water: 19.9 particles /L	(Selvam et al., 2021)
Germany, Drinking water treatment plants	Microscope, μ-Raman spectroscopy	Vacuum filtration	5 - 1000	PE, PET, PP, PA	197 MPs m^{-3} (raw water), 1–102 MPs m^{-3} (DWTP), 6 - 74 MPs m^{-3} (Tap water)	(Pittroff et al., 2021)
Korea, Geoje island, Seawater	Microscope, FTIR	N/A	<5000, and >5000	PE, PP, PES, ALK, PS	0.62– 15,560 particles m^{-3}	(Kang et al., 2015)
European, beach sediments (13 different countries)	Microscope, Raman spectroscopy	Density separation + filtration	< 5000	PES, PE, PP	72±24 -1,512 ±187 MPs kg^{-1}	(Lots et al., 2017)
South Africa, South-eastern coastline seawater and beach sediments	Microscope	Vacuum filtration	< 5000	N/A	Seawater: 275.9–1,215 particles m^{-3}; beach Sediment: 688.9–3,308 particles m^{-2}	(Nel & Froneman, 2015)
China, Maowei Seawater	Microscope, μ-FTIR	Vacuum filtration	< 5000	PP, PE, PES, PA, PS	1,200–10,100 particles m^{-3}	(Zhu et al., 2019)
North-western Pacific	Microscope, μ-Raman spectroscopy, SEM-EDX	Digestion (Fe + H_2O_2), density separation (NaCl) + filtration (0.2 μm)	< 5000	PE, PP, PA	1.0 x 10^4 items km^{-2}	(Pan et al., 2019)
India, beach sediment	Microscope, μ-Raman spectroscopy, FESEM-EDX	Digestion (H_2O_2) + density separation (NaCl) + filtration (0.2 μm)	< 5000	PE and PP	664 ± 114 MPs kg^{-1}	(Yaranal et al., 2021b)
Atlantic Ocean	Microscope, FTIR	Filtration (GF)	250 - 5000	PES, PA, acrylic	Seawater: 1.15 ± 1.45 particles m^{-3}	(Kanhai et al., 2017)
Arctic Ocean, sea ice and seawater beneath ice floes	Microscope, FTIR	Filtration (GF)	100-5000	PVC, PA, polyester	Sea ice: 2 – 17 particles /L; Ice floes: 0 - 18 particles m^{-3}	(Kanhai et al., 2020)

of microplastics distribution in various environments. These studies will provide detailed data on microplastic in different environments, which may be helpful in the futuristic plan for sustainable management and protection of environment and ecosystem health. Therefore, the development of new technologies and resources for the alternative materials to replace and mitigate plastic items is necessary. Further, the implementation of effective plans and technologies for solid and sludge waste management towards microplastics fate, degradation, and utilization is equally essential.

REFERENCES

Abbasi, S., Keshavarzi, B., Moore, F., Turner, A., Kelly, F. J., Dominguez, A. O., & Jaafarzadeh, N. (2019). Distribution and potential health impacts of microplastics and microrubbers in air and street dusts from Asaluyeh County, Iran. *Environmental Pollution, 244*, 153–164. doi:10.1016/j.envpol.2018.10.039 PMID:30326387

Ajith, N., Arumugam, S., Parthasarathy, S., Manupoori, S., & Janakiraman, S. (2020). Global distribution of microplastics and its impact on marine environment—a review. In Environmental Science and Pollution Research (Vol. 27, Issue 21, pp. 25970–25986). doi:10.100711356-020-09015-5

Allen, S., Allen, D., Phoenix, V. R., Le Roux, G., Durántez Jiménez, P., Simonneau, A., Binet, S., & Galop, D. (2019). Atmospheric transport and deposition of microplastics in a remote mountain catchment. *Nature Geoscience, 12*(5), 339–344. doi:10.103841561-019-0335-5

Aslam, H., Ali, T., Mortula, M. M., & Attaelmanan, A. G. (2020). Evaluation of microplastics in beach sediments along the coast of Dubai, UAE. *Marine Pollution Bulletin, 150*(November), 110739. doi:10.1016/j.marpolbul.2019.110739

Bergmann, M., Gutow, L., & Klages, M. (2015). Marine anthropogenic litter. In M. B. L. Gutow & M. Klages (Eds.), *Marine Anthropogenic Litter*. Springer., doi:10.1007/978-3-319-16510-3

Bergmann, M., Mützel, S., Primpke, S., Tekman, M. B., Trachsel, J., & Gerdts, G. (2019). White and wonderful? Microplastics prevail in snow from the Alps to the Arctic. *Science Advances, 5*(8), eaax1157. Advance online publication. doi:10.1126ciadv.aax1157 PMID:31453336

Blair, R. M., Waldron, S., Phoenix, V. R., & Gauchotte-Lindsay, C. (2019). Microscopy and elemental analysis characterisation of microplastics in sediment of a freshwater urban river in Scotland, UK. *Environmental Science and Pollution Research International, 26*(12), 12491–12504. doi:10.100711356-019-04678-1 PMID:30848429

Bordós, G., Urbányi, B., Micsinai, A., Kriszt, B., Palotai, Z., Szabó, I., Hantosi, Z., & Szoboszlay, S. (2019). Identification of microplastics in fish ponds and natural freshwater environments of the Carpathian basin, Europe. *Chemosphere, 216*, 110–116. doi:10.1016/j.chemosphere.2018.10.110 PMID:30359912

Boucher, J., & Friot, D. (2017). Primary microplastics in the oceans: A global evaluation of sources. In Primary microplastics in the oceans: A global evaluation of sources. doi:10.2305/IUCN.CH.2017.01.en

Cai, L., Wang, J., Peng, J., Tan, Z., Zhan, Z., Tan, X., & Chen, Q. (2017). Characteristic of microplastics in the atmospheric fallout from Dongguan city, China: Preliminary research and first evidence. *Environmental Science and Pollution Research International, 24*(32), 24928–24935. doi:10.100711356-017-0116-x PMID:28918553

Cai, L., Wang, J., Peng, J., Wu, Z., & Tan, X. (2018). Observation of the degradation of three types of plastic pellets exposed to UV irradiation in three different environments. *The Science of the Total Environment, 628–629*, 740–747. doi:10.1016/j.scitotenv.2018.02.079 PMID:29454214

Carr, S. A., Liu, J., & Tesoro, A. G. (2016). Transport and fate of microplastic particles in wastewater treatment plants. *Water Research, 91*, 174–182. doi:10.1016/j.watres.2016.01.002 PMID:26795302

Castro-Jiménez, J., González-Fernández, D., Fornier, M., Schmidt, N., & Sempéré, R. (2019). Macro-litter in surface waters from the Rhone River: Plastic pollution and loading to the NW Mediterranean Sea. *Marine Pollution Bulletin, 146*, 60–66. doi:10.1016/j.marpolbul.2019.05.067 PMID:31426199

Catarino, A. I., Macchia, V., Sanderson, W. G., Thompson, R. C., & Henry, T. B. (2018). Low levels of microplastics (MP) in wild mussels indicate that MP ingestion by humans is minimal compared to exposure via household fibres fallout during a meal. *Environmental Pollution, 237*, 675–684. doi:10.1016/j.envpol.2018.02.069 PMID:29604577

Chapman, P. M. (2007). Microplastic an emerging contaminant of potential concern. *Integrated Environmental Assessment and Management, 3*(2008), 1. doi:10.1897/IEAM_2008-022.1

Chen, G., Feng, Q., & Wang, J. (2020). Mini-review of microplastics in the atmosphere and their risks to humans. In Science of the Total Environment (Vol. 703). doi:10.1016/j.scitotenv.2019.135504

Chen, Y., Leng, Y., Liu, X., & Wang, J. (2020). Microplastic pollution in vegetable farmlands of suburb Wuhan, central China. *Environmental Pollution, 257*, 113449. doi:10.1016/j.envpol.2019.113449 PMID:31706776

Corradini, F., Casado, F., Leiva, V., Huerta-Lwanga, E., & Geissen, V. (2021). Microplastics occurrence and frequency in soils under different land uses on a regional scale. *The Science of the Total Environment, 752*, 141917. doi:10.1016/j.scitotenv.2020.141917 PMID:32892050

Cox, K. D., Covernton, G. A., Davies, H. L., Dower, J. F., Juanes, F., & Dudas, S. E. (2019). Human Consumption of Microplastics. *Environmental Science & Technology, 53*(12), 7068–7074. doi:10.1021/acs.est.9b01517 PMID:31184127

Crawford, C. B., & Quinn, B. (2016). Microplastic Pollutants. In Microplastic Pollutants. doi:10.1016/C2015-0-04315-5

Da Costa, J. P., Santos, P. S. M., Duarte, A. C., & Rocha-Santos, T. (2016). (Nano)plastics in the environment - Sources, fates and effects. *The Science of the Total Environment, 566–567*, 15–26. doi:10.1016/j.scitotenv.2016.05.041 PMID:27213666

De Falco, F., Gullo, M. P., Gentile, G., Di Pace, E., Cocca, M., Gelabert, L., Brouta-Agnésa, M., Rovira, A., Escudero, R., Villalba, R., Mossotti, R., Montarsolo, A., Gavignano, S., Tonin, C., & Avella, M. (2018). Evaluation of microplastic release caused by textile washing processes of synthetic fabrics. *Environmental Pollution, 236*, 916–925. doi:10.1016/j.envpol.2017.10.057 PMID:29107418

Di, M., & Wang, J. (2018). Microplastics in surface waters and sediments of the Three Gorges Reservoir, China. *The Science of the Total Environment, 616–617*, 1620–1627. doi:10.1016/j.scitotenv.2017.10.150 PMID:29050832

Dris, R., Gasperi, J., Mirande, C., Mandin, C., Guerrouache, M., Langlois, V., & Tassin, B. (2017). A first overview of textile fibers, including microplastics, in indoor and outdoor environments. *Environmental Pollution, 221*, 453–458. doi:10.1016/j.envpol.2016.12.013 PMID:27989388

Dris, R., Gasperi, J., Rocher, V., Saad, M., Renault, N., & Tassin, B. (2015). Microplastic contamination in an urban area: A case study in Greater Paris. *Environmental Chemistry, 12*(5), 592–599. doi:10.1071/EN14167

Dris, R., Gasperi, J., Saad, M., Mirande, C., & Tassin, B. (2016). Synthetic fibers in atmospheric fallout: A source of microplastics in the environment? *Marine Pollution Bulletin, 104*(1–2), 290–293. doi:10.1016/j.marpolbul.2016.01.006 PMID:26787549

Du, J., Xu, S., Zhou, Q., Li, H., Fu, L., Tang, J., Wang, Y., Peng, X., Xu, Y., & Du, X. (2020). A review of microplastics in the aquatic environmental: Distribution, transport, ecotoxicology, and toxicological mechanisms. *Environmental Science and Pollution Research International, 27*(11), 11494–11505. doi:10.100711356-020-08104-9 PMID:32088821

Elizalde-Velázquez, G. A., & Gómez-Oliván, L. M. (2021). Microplastics in aquatic environments: A review on occurrence, distribution, toxic effects, and implications for human health. *The Science of the Total Environment, 780*, 146551. doi:10.1016/j.scitotenv.2021.146551 PMID:33773347

Fischer, E. K., Paglialonga, L., Czech, E., & Tamminga, M. (2016). Microplastic pollution in lakes and lake shoreline sediments - A case study on Lake Bolsena and Lake Chiusi (central Italy). *Environmental Pollution, 213*, 648–657. doi:10.1016/j.envpol.2016.03.012 PMID:27104923

Fuller, S., & Gautam, A. (2016). A Procedure for Measuring Microplastics using Pressurized Fluid Extraction. *Environmental Science & Technology, 50*(11), 5774–5780. doi:10.1021/acs.est.6b00816 PMID:27172172

Gasperi, J., Wright, S. L., Dris, R., Collard, F., Mandin, C., Guerrouache, M., Langlois, V., Kelly, F. J., & Tassin, B. (2018). Microplastics in air: Are we breathing it in? *Current Opinion in Environmental Science & Health, 1*, 1–5. doi:10.1016/j.coesh.2017.10.002

Golwala, H., Zhang, X., Iskander, S. M., & Smith, A. L. (2021). Solid waste: An overlooked source of microplastics to the environment. *The Science of the Total Environment, 769*, 144581. doi:10.1016/j.scitotenv.2020.144581 PMID:33482549

Helcoski, R., Yonkos, L. T., Sanchez, A., & Baldwin, A. H. (2020). Wetland soil microplastics are negatively related to vegetation cover and stem density. *Environmental Pollution, 256*, 113391. doi:10.1016/j.envpol.2019.113391 PMID:31662247

Henry, B., Laitala, K., & Klepp, I. G. (2019). Microfibres from apparel and home textiles: Prospects for including microplastics in environmental sustainability assessment. *The Science of the Total Environment, 652*, 483–494. doi:10.1016/j.scitotenv.2018.10.166 PMID:30368178

Herbort, A. F., Sturm, M. T., Fiedler, S., Abkai, G., & Schuhen, K. (2018). Alkoxy-silyl Induced Agglomeration: A New Approach for the Sustainable Removal of Microplastic from Aquatic Systems. *Journal of Polymers and the Environment, 26*(11), 4258–4270. doi:10.100710924-018-1287-3

Horton, A. A., Svendsen, C., Williams, R. J., Spurgeon, D. J., & Lahive, E. (2017). Large microplastic particles in sediments of tributaries of the River Thames, UK – Abundance, sources and methods for effective quantification. *Marine Pollution Bulletin, 114*(1), 218–226. doi:10.1016/j.marpolbul.2016.09.004 PMID:27692488

Horton, A. A., Walton, A., Spurgeon, D. J., Lahive, E., & Svendsen, C. (2017). Microplastics in freshwater and terrestrial environments: Evaluating the current understanding to identify the knowledge gaps and future research priorities. *The Science of the Total Environment, 586*, 127–141. doi:10.1016/j.scitotenv.2017.01.190 PMID:28169032

Issac, M. N., & Kandasubramanian, B. (2021). Effect of microplastics in water and aquatic systems. *Environmental Science and Pollution Research, 28*(16), 19544–19562. doi:10.1007/s11356-021-13184-2

Jang, Y. C., Lee, J., Hong, S., Lee, J. S., Shim, W. J., & Song, Y. K. (2014). Sources of plastic marine debris on beaches of Korea: More from the ocean than the land. *Ocean Science Journal, 49*(2), 151–162. doi:10.1007/s12601-014-0015-8

Kang, J. H., Kwon, O. Y., Lee, K. W., Song, Y. K., & Shim, W. J. (2015). Marine neustonic microplastics around the southeastern coast of Korea. *Marine Pollution Bulletin, 96*(1–2), 304–312. doi:10.1016/j.marpolbul.2015.04.054 PMID:25979811

Kanhai, L. D. K., Gardfeldt, K., Krumpen, T., Thompson, R. C., & O'Connor, I. (2020). Microplastics in sea ice and seawater beneath ice floes from the Arctic Ocean. *Scientific Reports, 10*(1), 1–11. doi:10.103841598-020-61948-6 PMID:32193433

Kanhai, L. D. K., Johansson, C., Frias, J. P. G. L., Gardfeldt, K., Thompson, R. C., & O'Connor, I. (2019). Deep sea sediments of the Arctic Central Basin: A potential sink for microplastics. *Deep-sea Research. Part I, Oceanographic Research Papers, 145*, 137–142. doi:10.1016/j.dsr.2019.03.003

Kanhai, L. D. K., Officer, R., Lyashevska, O., Thompson, R. C., & O'Connor, I. (2017). Microplastic abundance, distribution and composition along a latitudinal gradient in the Atlantic Ocean. *Marine Pollution Bulletin, 115*(1–2), 307–314. doi:10.1016/j.marpolbul.2016.12.025 PMID:28007381

Kankanige, D., & Babel, S. (2020). Smaller-sized micro-plastics (MPs) contamination in single-use PET-bottled water in Thailand. *The Science of the Total Environment, 717*, 137232. doi:10.1016/j.scitotenv.2020.137232 PMID:32062244

Kim, J. S., Lee, H. J., Kim, S. K., & Kim, H. J. (2018). Global Pattern of Microplastics (MPs) in Commercial Food-Grade Salts: Sea Salt as an Indicator of Seawater MP Pollution. *Environmental Science & Technology, 52*(21), 12819–12828. doi:10.1021/acs.est.8b04180 PMID:30285421

Klein, M., & Fischer, E. K. (2019). Microplastic abundance in atmospheric deposition within the Metropolitan area of Hamburg, Germany. *The Science of the Total Environment*, *685*, 96–103. doi:10.1016/j.scitotenv.2019.05.405 PMID:31174127

Kumar, M., Xiong, X., He, M., Tsang, D. C. W., Gupta, J., Khan, E., Harrad, S., Hou, D., Ok, Y. S., & Bolan, N. S. (2020). Microplastics as pollutants in agricultural soils. *Environmental Pollution*, *265*, 114980. doi:10.1016/j.envpol.2020.114980 PMID:32544663

Lebreton, L., & Andrady, A. (2019). Future scenarios of global plastic waste generation and disposal. *Palgrave Communications*, *5*(1), 6. Advance online publication. doi:10.105741599-018-0212-7

Leslie, H. A., Brandsma, S. H., van Velzen, M. J. M., & Vethaak, A. D. (2017). Microplastics en route: Field measurements in the Dutch river delta and Amsterdam canals, wastewater treatment plants, North Sea sediments and biota. *Environment International*, *101*, 133–142. doi:10.1016/j.envint.2017.01.018 PMID:28143645

Li, J., Song, Y., & Cai, Y. (2020). Focus topics on microplastics in soil: Analytical methods, occurrence, transport, and ecological risks. *Environmental Pollution*, *257*, 113570. doi:10.1016/j.envpol.2019.113570 PMID:31767234

Li, Q., Wu, J., Zhao, X., Gu, X., & Ji, R. (2019). Separation and identification of microplastics from soil and sewage sludge. *Environmental Pollution*, *254*, 113076. doi:10.1016/j.envpol.2019.113076 PMID:31472456

Li, W., Wufuer, R., Duo, J., Wang, S., Luo, Y., Zhang, D., & Pan, X. (2020). Microplastics in agricultural soils: Extraction and characterization after different periods of polythene film mulching in an arid region. *The Science of the Total Environment*, *749*, 141420. doi:10.1016/j.scitotenv.2020.141420 PMID:32836118

Li, Y., Zhang, H., & Tang, C. (2020). *A review of possible pathways of marine microplastics transport in the ocean.* Anthropocene Coasts. doi:10.1139/anc-2018-0030

Lin, L., Zuo, L. Z., Peng, J. P., Cai, L. Q., Fok, L., Yan, Y., Li, H. X., & Xu, X. R. (2018). Occurrence and distribution of microplastics in an urban river: A case study in the Pearl River along Guangzhou City, China. *The Science of the Total Environment*, *644*, 375–381. doi:10.1016/j.scitotenv.2018.06.327 PMID:29981986

Liu, K., Wang, X., Fang, T., Xu, P., Zhu, L., & Li, D. (2019). Source and potential risk assessment of suspended atmospheric microplastics in Shanghai. *The Science of the Total Environment*, *675*, 462–471. doi:10.1016/j.scitotenv.2019.04.110 PMID:31030152

Liu, K., Wang, X., Wei, N., Song, Z., & Li, D. (2019). Accurate quantification and transport estimation of suspended atmospheric microplastics in megacities: Implications for human health. *Environment International*, *132*, 105127. doi:10.1016/j.envint.2019.105127 PMID:31487610

Liu, K., Wu, T., Wang, X., Song, Z., Zong, C., Wei, N., & Li, D. (2019). Consistent Transport of Terrestrial Microplastics to the Ocean through Atmosphere. *Environmental Science & Technology*, *53*(18), 10612–10619. doi:10.1021/acs.est.9b03427 PMID:31408609

Liu, M., Lu, S., Song, Y., Lei, L., Hu, J., Lv, W., Zhou, W., Cao, C., Shi, H., Yang, X., & He, D. (2018). Microplastic and mesoplastic pollution in farmland soils in suburbs of Shanghai, China. *Environmental Pollution*, *242*, 855–862. doi:10.1016/j.envpol.2018.07.051 PMID:30036839

Lots, F. A. E., Behrens, P., Vijver, M. G., Horton, A. A., & Bosker, T. (2017). A large-scale investigation of microplastic contamination: Abundance and characteristics of microplastics in European beach sediment. *Marine Pollution Bulletin*, *123*(1–2), 219–226. doi:10.1016/j.marpolbul.2017.08.057 PMID:28893402

Lusher, A., Hollman, P., & Mendozal, J. (2017). Microplastics in fisheries and aquaculture: Status of knowledge on their occurrence and implications for aquatic organisms and food safety. *FAO Fisheries and Aquaculture Technical Paper*, *615*, 147.

Mintenig, S. M., Kooi, M., Erich, M. W., Primpke, S., Redondo- Hasselerharm, P. E., Dekker, S. C., Koelmans, A. A., & van Wezel, A. P. (2020). A systems approach to understand microplastic occurrence and variability in Dutch riverine surface waters. *Water Research*, *176*, 115723. doi:10.1016/j.watres.2020.115723 PMID:32220661

Möller, J. N., Löder, M. G. J., & Laforsch, C. (2020). Finding Microplastics in Soils: A Review of Analytical Methods. *Environmental Science & Technology*, *54*(4), 2078–2090. doi:10.1021/acs.est.9b04618 PMID:31999440

Nel, H. A., & Froneman, P. W. (2015). A quantitative analysis of microplastic pollution along the south-eastern coastline of South Africa. *Marine Pollution Bulletin*, *101*(1), 274–279. doi:10.1016/j.marpolbul.2015.09.043 PMID:26433774

Oliveira, J., Belchior, A., da Silva, V. D., Rotter, A., Petrovski, Ž., Almeida, P. L., Lourenço, N. D., & Gaudêncio, S. P. (2020). Marine Environmental Plastic Pollution: Mitigation by Microorganism Degradation and Recycling Valorization. *Frontiers in Marine Science*, *7*, 1007. doi:10.3389/fmars.2020.567126

Pan, Z., Guo, H., Chen, H., Wang, S., Sun, X., Zou, Q., Zhang, Y., Lin, H., Cai, S., & Huang, J. (2019). Microplastics in the Northwestern Pacific: Abundance, distribution, and characteristics. *The Science of the Total Environment*, *650*, 1913–1922. doi:10.1016/j.scitotenv.2018.09.244 PMID:30286357

Patchaiyappan, A., Dowarah, K., Zaki Ahmed, S., Prabakaran, M., Jayakumar, S., Thirunavukkarasu, C., & Devipriya, S. P. (2021). Prevalence and characteristics of microplastics present in the street dust collected from Chennai metropolitan city, India. *Chemosphere*, *269*, 128757. doi:10.1016/j.chemosphere.2020.128757 PMID:33183789

Pauly, J. L., Stegmeier, S. J., Allaart, H. A., Cheney, R. T., Zhang, P. J., Mayer, A. G., & Streck, R. J. (1998). Inhaled cellulosic and plastic fibers found in human lung tissue. *Cancer Epidemiology, Biomarkers & Prevention*, *7*(5), 419–428. PMID:9610792

Peixoto, D., Pinheiro, C., Amorim, J., Oliva-Teles, L., Guilhermino, L., & Vieira, M. N. (2019). Microplastic pollution in commercial salt for human consumption: A review. In *Estuarine* (Vol. 219, pp. 161–168). Coastal and Shelf Science., doi:10.1016/j.ecss.2019.02.018

Perren, W., Wojtasik, A., & Cai, Q. (2018). Removal of Microbeads from Wastewater Using Electrocoagulation. *ACS Omega*, *3*(3), 3357–3364. doi:10.1021/acsomega.7b02037 PMID:31458591

Piehl, S., Leibner, A., Löder, M. G. J., Dris, R., Bogner, C., & Laforsch, C. (2018). Identification and quantification of macro- and microplastics on an agricultural farmland. *Scientific Reports, 8*(1), 1–9. doi:10.1038/s41598-018-36172-y

Pittroff, M., Müller, Y. K., Witzig, C. S., Scheurer, M., Storck, F. R., & Zumbülte, N. (2021). Microplastic analysis in drinking water based on fractionated filtration sampling and Raman microspectroscopy. *Environmental Science and Pollution Research International, 28*(42), 59439–59451. Advance online publication. doi:10.100711356-021-12467-y PMID:33511538

Prata, J. C. (2018). Airborne microplastics: Consequences to human health? *Environmental Pollution, 234*, 115–126. doi:10.1016/j.envpol.2017.11.043 PMID:29172041

Qiu, R., Song, Y., Zhang, X., Xie, B., & He, D. (2020). Microplastics in Urban Environments: Sources, Pathways, and Distribution. Handbook of Environmental Chemistry, 95, 41–61. doi:10.1007/698_2020_447

Ragusa, A., Svelato, A., Santacroce, C., Catalano, P., Notarstefano, V., Carnevali, O., Papa, F., Rongioletti, M. C. A., Baiocco, F., Draghi, S., D'Amore, E., Rinaldo, D., Matta, M., & Giorgini, E. (2021). Plasticenta: First evidence of microplastics in human placenta. *Environment International, 146*, 106274. doi:10.1016/j.envint.2020.106274 PMID:33395930

Rehm, R., Zeyer, T., Schmidt, A., & Fiener, P. (2021). Soil erosion as transport pathway of microplastic from agriculture soils to aquatic ecosystems. *The Science of the Total Environment, 795*, 148774. doi:10.1016/j.scitotenv.2021.148774 PMID:34328923

Rios Mendoza, L. M., Karapanagioti, H., & Álvarez, N. R. (2018). Micro(nanoplastics) in the marine environment: Current knowledge and gaps. *Current Opinion in Environmental Science & Health, 1*, 47–51. doi:10.1016/j.coesh.2017.11.004

Rist, S., Baun, A., Almeda, R., & Hartmann, N. B. (2019). Ingestion and effects of micro- and nanoplastics in blue mussel (Mytilus edulis) larvae. *Marine Pollution Bulletin, 140*, 423–430. Advance online publication. doi:10.1016/j.marpolbul.2019.01.069 PMID:30803663

Rist, S., Carney Almroth, B., Hartmann, N. B., & Karlsson, T. M. (2018). A critical perspective on early communications concerning human health aspects of microplastics. *The Science of the Total Environment, 626*, 720–726. doi:10.1016/j.scitotenv.2018.01.092 PMID:29396337

Roblin, B., & Aherne, J. (2020). Moss as a biomonitor for the atmospheric deposition of anthropogenic microfibres. *The Science of the Total Environment, 715*, 136973. doi:10.1016/j.scitotenv.2020.136973 PMID:32018105

Rodrigues, M. O., Abrantes, N., Gonçalves, F. J. M., Nogueira, H., Marques, J. C., & Gonçalves, A. M. M. (2018). Spatial and temporal distribution of microplastics in water and sediments of a freshwater system (Antuã River, Portugal). *The Science of the Total Environment, 633*, 1549–1559. doi:10.1016/j.scitotenv.2018.03.233 PMID:29758905

Sana, S. S., Dogiparthi, L. K., Gangadhar, L., Chakravorty, A., & Abhishek, N. (2020). Effects of microplastics and nanoplastics on marine environment and human health. *Environmental Science and Pollution Research International, 27*(36), 44743–44756. doi:10.100711356-020-10573-x PMID:32876819

Scheurer, M., & Bigalke, M. (2018). Microplastics in Swiss Floodplain Soils. *Environmental Science & Technology*, *52*(6), 3591–3598. doi:10.1021/acs.est.7b06003 PMID:29446629

Schwabl, Köppel, S., Königshofer, P., Bucsics, T., Trauner, M., Reiberger, T., & Liebmann, B. (2019). Detection of Various Microplastics in Human Stool: A Prospective Case Series. *Annals of Internal Medicine*, *171*(7), 453–457. doi:10.7326/M19-0618 PMID:31476765

Selvam, S., Jesuraja, K., Venkatramanan, S., Roy, P. D., & Jeyanthi Kumari, V. (2021). Hazardous microplastic characteristics and its role as a vector of heavy metal in groundwater and surface water of coastal south India. *Journal of Hazardous Materials*, *402*(August), 123786. doi:10.1016/j.jhazmat.2020.123786

Singh, B., & Sharma, N. (2008). Mechanistic implications of plastic degradation. In Polymer Degradation and Stability (Vol. 93, Issue 3, pp. 561–584). doi:10.1016/j.polymdegradstab.2007.11.008

Stanton, T., Johnson, M., Nathanail, P., MacNaughtan, W., & Gomes, R. L. (2019). Freshwater and airborne textile fibre populations are dominated by 'natural', not microplastic, fibres. *The Science of the Total Environment*, *666*, 377–389. doi:10.1016/j.scitotenv.2019.02.278 PMID:30798244

Su, L., Nan, B., Craig, N. J., & Pettigrove, V. (2020). Temporal and spatial variations of microplastics in roadside dust from rural and urban Victoria, Australia: Implications for diffuse pollution. *Chemosphere*, *252*, 126567. doi:10.1016/j.chemosphere.2020.126567 PMID:32443265

Sujathan, S., Kniggendorf, A. K., Kumar, A., Roth, B., Rosenwinkel, K. H., & Nogueira, R. (2017). Heat and Bleach: A Cost-Efficient Method for Extracting Microplastics from Return Activated Sludge. *Archives of Environmental Contamination and Toxicology*, *73*(4), 641–648. doi:10.100700244-017-0415-8 PMID:28550340

Talvitie, J., Mikola, A., Koistinen, A., & Setälä, O. (2017). Solutions to microplastic pollution – Removal of microplastics from wastewater effluent with advanced wastewater treatment technologies. *Water Research*, *123*, 401–407. doi:10.1016/j.watres.2017.07.005 PMID:28686942

Thiele, C. J., Hudson, M. D., Russell, A. E., Saluveer, M., & Sidaoui-Haddad, G. (2021). Microplastics in fish and fishmeal: An emerging environmental challenge? *Scientific Reports*, *11*(1), 1–12. doi:10.103841598-021-81499-8 PMID:33479308

Toussaint, B., Raffael, B., Angers-Loustau, A., Gilliland, D., Kestens, V., Petrillo, M., Rio-Echevarria, I. M., & Van den Eede, G. (2019). Review of micro- and nanoplastic contamination in the food chain. In Food Additives and Contaminants - Part A Chemistry, Analysis, Control, Exposure and Risk Assessment (Vol. 36, Issue 5, pp. 639–673). doi:10.1080/19440049.2019.1583381

Trainic, M., Flores, J. M., Pinkas, I., Pedrotti, M. L., Lombard, F., Bourdin, G., Gorsky, G., Boss, E., Rudich, Y., Vardi, A., & Koren, I. (2020). Airborne microplastic particles detected in the remote marine atmosphere. *Communications Earth & Environment*, *1*(1), 1–9. doi:10.103843247-020-00061-y

Van den Berg, P., Huerta-Lwanga, E., Corradini, F., & Geissen, V. (2020). Sewage sludge application as a vehicle for microplastics in eastern Spanish agricultural soils. *Environmental Pollution*, *261*, 114198. doi:10.1016/j.envpol.2020.114198 PMID:32097788

Veerasingam, S., Ranjani, M., Venkatachalapathy, R., Bagaev, A., Mukhanov, V., Litvinyuk, D., Verzhevskaia, L., Guganathan, L., & Vethamony, P. (2020). Microplastics in different environmental compartments in India: Analytical methods, distribution, associated contaminants and research needs. *Trends in Analytical Chemistry*, *133*, 116071. doi:10.1016/j.trac.2020.116071

Vianello, A., Jensen, R. L., Liu, L., & Vollertsen, J. (2019). Simulating human exposure to indoor airborne microplastics using a Breathing Thermal Manikin. *Scientific Reports*, *9*(1), 8670. Advance online publication. doi:10.103841598-019-45054-w PMID:31209244

Wang, C., Zhao, J., & Xing, B. (2021). Environmental source, fate, and toxicity of microplastics. *Journal of Hazardous Materials*, *407*, 124357. doi:10.1016/j.jhazmat.2020.124357 PMID:33158648

Wang, J., Peng, J., Tan, Z., Gao, Y., Zhan, Z., Chen, Q., & Cai, L. (2017). Microplastics in the surface sediments from the Beijiang River littoral zone: Composition, abundance, surface textures and interaction with heavy metals. *Chemosphere*, *171*, 248–258. Advance online publication. doi:10.1016/j.chemosphere.2016.12.074 PMID:28024210

WHO. (2019). *Microplastics in drinking-water: World Health Organization.* Geneva: World Health Organization.

Wright, S. L., & Kelly, F. J. (2017). Plastic and Human Health: A Micro Issue? *Environmental Science & Technology*, *51*(12), 6634–6647. doi:10.1021/acs.est.7b00423 PMID:28531345

Xu, Y., Chan, F. K. S., Stanton, T., Johnson, M. F., Kay, P., He, J., Wang, J., Kong, C., Wang, Z., Liu, D., & Xu, Y. (2021). Synthesis of dominant plastic microfibre prevalence and pollution control feasibility in Chinese freshwater environments. *The Science of the Total Environment*, *783*, 146863. doi:10.1016/j.scitotenv.2021.146863 PMID:33872912

Yang, L., Zhang, Y., Kang, S., Wang, Z., & Wu, C. (2021). Microplastics in soil: A review on methods, occurrence, sources, and potential risk. *The Science of the Total Environment*, *780*, 146546. doi:10.1016/j.scitotenv.2021.146546 PMID:33770602

Yaranal, N. A., Subbiah, S., & Mohanty, K. (2021a). Identification, extraction of microplastics from edible salts and its removal from contaminated seawater. *Environmental Technology and Innovation*, *21*, 101253. Advance online publication. doi:10.1016/j.eti.2020.101253

Yaranal, N. A., Subbiah, S., & Mohanty, K. (2021b). Distribution and characterization of microplastics in beach sediments from Karnataka (India) coastal environments. *Marine Pollution Bulletin*, *169*, 112550. doi:10.1016/j.marpolbul.2021.112550 PMID:34091249

Yukioka, S., Tanaka, S., Nabetani, Y., Suzuki, Y., Ushijima, T., Fujii, S., Takada, H., Van Tran, Q., & Singh, S. (2020). Occurrence and characteristics of microplastics in surface road dust in Kusatsu (Japan), Da Nang (Vietnam), and Kathmandu (Nepal). *Environmental Pollution*, *256*, 113447. doi:10.1016/j.envpol.2019.113447 PMID:31679875

Zbyszewski, M., Corcoran, P. L., & Hockin, A. (2014). Comparison of the distribution and degradation of plastic debris along shorelines of the Great Lakes, North America. *Journal of Great Lakes Research*, *40*(2), 288–299. Advance online publication. doi:10.1016/j.jglr.2014.02.012

Zhang, K., Xiong, X., Hu, H., Wu, C., Bi, Y., Wu, Y., Zhou, B., Lam, P. K. S., & Liu, J. (2017). Occurrence and Characteristics of Microplastic Pollution in Xiangxi Bay of Three Gorges Reservoir, China. *Environmental Science & Technology*, *51*(7), 3794–3801. doi:10.1021/acs.est.7b00369 PMID:28298079

Zhang, Y., Kang, S., Allen, S., Allen, D., Gao, T., & Sillanpää, M. (2020). Atmospheric microplastics: A review on current status and perspectives. Earth-Science Reviews. doi:10.1016/j.earscirev.2020.103118

Zhang, Z., & Chen, Y. (2020). Effects of microplastics on wastewater and sewage sludge treatment and their removal: A review. In Chemical Engineering Journal (Vol. 382). doi:10.1016/j.cej.2019.122955

Zhou, B., Wang, J., Zhang, H., Shi, H., Fei, Y., Huang, S., Tong, Y., Wen, D., Luo, Y., & Barceló, D. (2020). Microplastics in agricultural soils on the coastal plain of Hangzhou Bay, east China: Multiple sources other than plastic mulching film. *Journal of Hazardous Materials*, *388*, 121814. doi:10.1016/j.jhazmat.2019.121814 PMID:31843412

Zhou, Q., Zhang, H., Zhou, Y., Li, Y., Xue, Y., Fu, C., Tu, C., & Luo, Y. (2016). Separation of microplastics from a coastal soil and their surface microscopic features. *Kexue Tongbao. Chinese Science Bulletin*, *61*(14), 1604–1611. doi:10.1360/N972015-01098

Zhou, Y., Wang, J., Zou, M., Jia, Z., Zhou, S., & Li, Y. (2020). Microplastics in soils: A review of methods, occurrence, fate, transport, ecological and environmental risks. In *Science of the Total Environment* (Vol. 748, p. 141368). Elsevier. doi:10.1016/j.scitotenv.2020.141368

Zhu, J., Zhang, Q., Li, Y., Tan, S., Kang, Z., Yu, X., Lan, W., Cai, L., Wang, J., & Shi, H. (2019). Microplastic pollution in the Maowei Sea, a typical mariculture bay of China. *The Science of the Total Environment*, *658*, 62–68. doi:10.1016/j.scitotenv.2018.12.192 PMID:30577027

Chapter 4
Microplastics and Nanoplastics in Aquatic Environment:
Challenges and Threats to Aquatic Organisms

Aayushi Kundu
SCBC, Thapar Institute of Engineering and Technology, Patiala, India

Soumen Basu
SCBC, Thapar Institute of Engineering and Technology, Patiala, India

ABSTRACT

Marine trash can be found all around the oceans. Debris enters oceans through a variety of sources, including but not limited to sources onshore, vessels, and other marine infrastructure. Plastics are often the most significant component of marine debris, contributing up to 100% of floating trash. Microplastics (MPs) or nanoplastics (NPs), which are fragmented or otherwise minute plastic materials, have remained a source of environmental concern. This chapter traces the different avenues of NPs and MPs in an aquatic setting along with their origin. The toxic impacts of NPs and MPs on the marine ecosystem have been discussed in detail. This chapter also highlights the toxicity comparison of MPs/NPs and the brief analytical techniques for their mitigation. The available data suggests that the prolonged presence of NPs and MPs in the aquatic systems could have long-term repercussions. The more empirical and doctrinal study is pertinent for a better understanding of systemic toxicity caused by MPs/NPs, as well as the underlying mechanism.

INTRODUCTION

The world population is anticipated to expand from 7.7 billion in 2020 to 9.7 billion in 2050, and an increase of 11 billion by the end of the century (UNDESA, 2019). Transformation or the modification of natural conditions and processes leads to a succession of changes in the biotic and abiotic components of the environment (Surbhi Sharma, Kundu, et al., 2020). These factors have led to dangerous consequences

DOI: 10.4018/978-1-7998-9723-1.ch004

Figure 1. (a) Structures of non-degradable polymer, (b) major sources for MPs, (c) MPs from other substantial sources

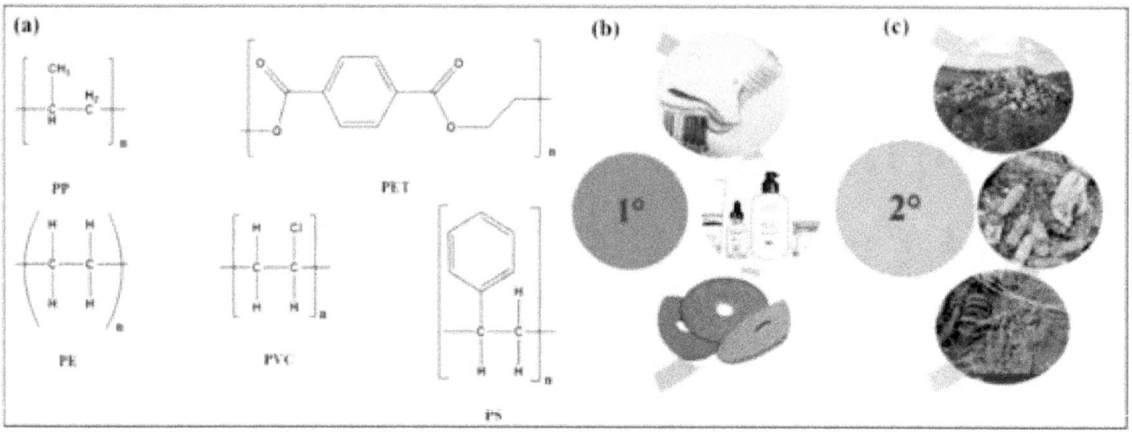

like environmental pollution (Garg et al., 2021; Kundu, Sharma, et al., 2021), increasing population as well as energy demands (Singla et al., 2022). Additionally, the reckless disposal of garbage's containing plastic items into natural bodies after domestic activities affect the quality of the water and also causes land pollution. The lives of aquatic organisms are affected, the alkalinity of the soil, the availability of magnesium is reduced, and the germination of the seeds is inhibited by the disposal of the garbage into the environment. Therefore, plastics have gained increased attention as a dominant large-scale pollutant.

Plastic debris pollution is a global environmental concern that has recently emerged as an emerging contaminant, with several research subjects focusing on its sources, origin, and ecological repercussions, as well as the prospective health implications. Plastic garbage output has risen at a yearly growth of 8.70% over the last five decades, with worldwide production standing at 9.1 billion tons (Rai et al., 2020). It has become a severe environmental issue as a result of the increased usage of plastic products, with an estimated 4.8-12.70 million tons of litter entering the marine ecosystem from land per year in 2010, and the number expected to rise to more than 100-250 million tons by 2025 (Peng et al., 2018). Merely a tiny chunk of 06-14% of plastics is refurbished and put to reuse, which indicates almost > 80% ultimately goes to landfills, in the natural environment, or water bodies through a variety of paths, posing a substantial threat to the atmosphere. Figure 1a depicts the chemical structure of the most common plastics. We have already (Kundu, Shetti, et al., 2021) reported that the breakdown of large-plastic waste produces macroplastics (>25 mm), mesoplastics (5-25 mm), microplastics (MPs) (5 mm), and nanoplastics (NPs) (100 nm).

NPs and MPs might have primary or secondary sources, dependent on their respective origins (Surbhi Sharma, Basu, et al., 2020). Primary MPs are made of plastics that are as small as pellets of any resinous material; hence virgin plastic production (usually ranging from 02-05 mm in diameter) can be called primary MPs (Mani et al., 2015). Primary MPs are mainly used as air blasting media or in facial cleansers and cosmetics. The best example of MPs are plastic beads utilized as an exfoliant in self-nourishment products, commercial, and factory used abrasives, and in involuntary and accidental spills (Kundu, Shetti, et al., 2021). Singh and Sharma stated that (Singh & Sharma, 2008) secondary MPs are small plastics fragments of bigger size, which result due to the disintegration of relatively larger plastic waste due to natural phenomena like sunshine, storm, rain, and other forms of geological wonder. Ropes, used plastic bottles, dysfunctional fishing nets, automobile tyres, plus agricultural mulches made up of plastic are some of the examples of secondary MPs (McDevitt et al., 2017). These two sources are primarily to blame for increased environmental pollution (Figure 1(b-c)). The absolute amount of secondary MPs emitted into the aquatic ecosystem is estimated to be between 68,500 to 275,000 tonnes per year (Alprol et al., 2021).

MPs are primarily found in wastewater treatment effluents (WWTE) and self-nourishment products such as cleaning chemicals, textile fibers, and, latterly in masks during the ongoing pandemic of COVID-19. As a result, these plastic residues are transferred to drainage systems, which haven't been much successful in removing these unwanted particles and therefore, ultimately landing into the oceans (Shivika Sharma & Chatterjee, 2017).

MP fibers also reach the aquatic ecosystem through natural fabrics or artificially produced fibers (both inorganic and organic) (Da Costa et al., 2019). Furthermore, the most common source of oceanic waste is overseas shipping, farming, allied activities, and several other sorts of industrial productions that dump their trash directly or indirectly into the water, whether on purpose or by accident. Furthermore, when sewage sludge is utilized as fertilizer on agricultural land, it contains microfibers and MPs, which can discharge into the terrestrial environment. Also, fishing rigs that have been lost, as well as nylon netting and plastic monofilament lines are some of the most regularly observed plastic trash products which might end up on the ocean floor (Horton et al., 2017).

NPs can come from various sources, including industrial uses and products. Polymeric nanoparticles, nanocapsules, and nanospheres are among the various nanoparticle applications used in drug delivery (Guterres et al., 2007). Thermic fragmentation of polystyrene foam reproduced polymer particles almost equal to the size of a nanometre. Engineered plastics are electro-pinned to create mats with nano-scale fibers which can distort further to the nanoscale (H. Zhang et. al., 2012). MPs break down to the 100 nm scale is another source of NPs. Synthetic fibers made of different polymers are the most critical NPs. Washing of synthetic cloths can produce >1900 fibers per wash in the sewage system (Mark Anthony Browne et. al., 2011).

The emergence of NPs and MPs scrutinizes the physical and chemical processes that lead to the production of MPs and then NPs. These processes are linked to the tendency of MPs/NPs to form single particles or agglomerates in water. Large plastic objects are fragmented by various mechanisms, which can occur separately or in combination, such as photo-oxidation by chemical reaction, mechanical shock, and ultraviolet light, resulting in biological assimilation by microorganisms and mechanical turbulence in water (Gewert et al., 2015). When exposed to ultraviolet radiation in soil and water environments, plastics pellets such as poly (lactic acid) (PLA), poly(styrene) (PS), terephthalate (PET), poly(ethylene) (PE), and poly (propylene) (PP) oxidize (Cai et al., 2018). Hydrolysis is one of the initial steps in the breakdown of heteroatom polymers such as poly(urethane) (PU) and poly (ethylene terephthalate) (PET) (Lambert & Wagner, 2016). The minor result of the air decomposition of certain hydrofluorocarbons as well as the pyrolysis of fluoropolymers, trifluoroacetic acid, is spread equally in seawater above 4000 m depth (González-Fernández et al., 2018). When an organic compounds bond is broken, a chemical group is formed, resulting in autocatalysis, which increases the hydrolysis rate in acidic environments. Both degradations of response and photo-oxidation cause break to divide and trap on the surface of things, resulting in plastics induction embrittlement. The plastic fragments are weakened to the point that mechanical stress such as abrasion or friction causes them to break down into MPs particles (Cai et al., 2018).

Figure 2. Dangers of MPs ingestion by marine creatures

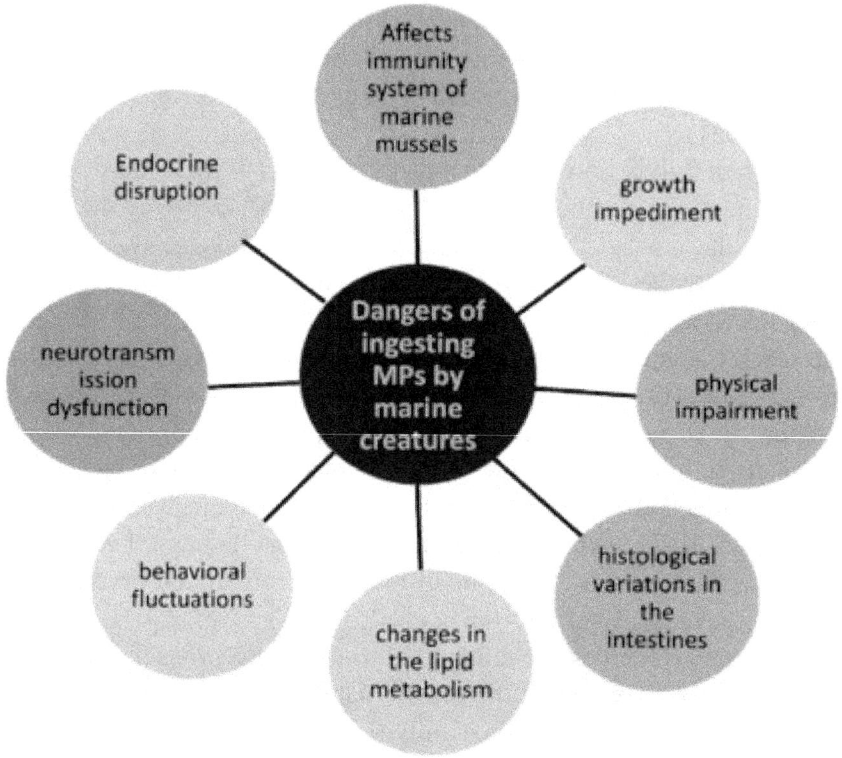

As shown in Figure 2, there are various threats of ingesting MPs by marine creatures. For instance, physical impairment, histological variations in the intestine, changes in the lipid metabolism, behavioral fluctuations, endocrine disruptions, dysfunctioning of neurotransmission, and growth impediment. MPs/NPs also affect the immunity systems of marine mussels.

Microplastics tend to agglomerate in aquatic media by a variety of species because of their minute-sized nature. Therefore, microplastics expand at various trophic levels through which they bioaccumulate in the human body as well. However, there are several analytical issues in identifying the microplastics, but the researchers have observed their enhanced false impacts (Q. Chen, Yin, et al., 2017). Owing to their small size, aquatic species are vulnerable to intake these MPs, sometimes for the sake of food resulting in the worst physical problems in this marine fauna. Persistent organic pollutants (POPs) can be absorbed by MPs which spreads the toxicity across the food chain. This, at the last stage, ends up bioaccumulating in humans. Desorption of POPs adds the concentration of the pollutant in water, enhancing the susceptibility of larger moieties to degradation. Several invertebrates and vertebrates such as zooplanktons, benthonic animals, fish, seabirds, amphibians, and others are prone to the adverse impacts of MPs. The primary impacts on zooplanktons occur via impediment of the digestive system, reduced appetite, eating impact, malnutrition, slow development, and also even death (Lee et al., 2013). Marine benthic organisms (oysters and mussels) are affected majorly because of their sedimental presence in the deep sea, which mussels move into the gastrointestinal system via endocytosis (Van Cauwenberghe et al., 2013). This further results in inflammation and reduction of lysosomal membrane stability. In the case of oysters, MPs increase mortality rate, poor growth, influence energy absorption, interfere with the progress of offspring, and reproductive issues. MPs also affect certain microorganisms harmfully, such as bacteria and fungus. For example, yeast cells are affected by polystyrene (PS) nanoparticles (Nomura et al., 2016).

Toxic Effects of NPs and MPs on Hydrosphere (Aquatic Species)

Aquatic species such as algae, ciliates, invertebrates, crabs, and fish have been used to test the toxicity of a variety of MPs of various sizes and features along with their lethal and sub-lethal impacts. Browne and co-workers (Mark A. Browne et al., 2008) analyzed the adverse effects of fluorescent polystyrene (PS) microspheres of different sizes upon cell viability, translocation, and uptake of *Mytilus edulis* (a model aquatic organism). The use of fluorescent particles enabled visual MPs examination. They inferred that small particle gets quickly accumulated in organisms and shorter interval of pulse exposure didn't generate substantial biological impacts. However, the authors recommended that more data and further analysis of the long-term effects were required. Graham and Thompson (Graham & Thompson, 2009) investigated the ingestion of different kinds of plastic waste [PVC fragments (polyvinyl chloride), pellets and fragments of nylon] which were gathered from sediments by sea cucumber (Echinodermata), particularly *Thyonella gemmata, Cucumaria frondose, Holothuria floridana, and Holothuria grisea*, during short term exposure (20-25 hours). The authors claimed that polychlorinated biphenyls (PCBs) adhered with the surface of plastics might have negative consequences and might pass across trophic chains from plastic consumers to predators and ultimately humans. In four-hour feeding trials, holothurians consumed between 2- and 20-fold more PVC pieces than expected and between 2- and 138-fold more nylon lines than expected. In addition, PVC pellets were ingested by two species with a diameter of 4 µm. Condition index, lysosomal membrane stability, uptake, lipofuscin, histological diagnosis, and neutral lipids were among the markers of exposure to high-density polyethylene (HDPE) particles in *Mytilus edulis* studied by Von Moos et al. (Von Moos et al., 2012) Despite the relatively short exposure time (96 hours), ingested microplastics (0-80 µm) had a considerable negative impact on M. edulis tissue and cells. Kaposi and co-workers (Kaposi et al., 2014) used luminous green polyethylene (PE) microspheres with a diameter measuring 10-45 µm to study the adverse effects of short-term PE exposure on the sea urchin, *Tripneustes gratilla*. The exposure periods varied between 15 minutes to 5 days. The microplastics were ejected from the stomach of T. gratilla larvae in some hours of intake. Ingested PE microplastics had some minor non-dose dependent influence over T. gratilla larvae development but did not affect their survival. The researchers found that microplastics concentration in the natural marine ecosystem poses harm to marine invertebrate larvae, including T. gratilla. Setälä et al., (Setälä et al., 2014) studied the ingestion of fluorescent polystyrene PS microspheres with a diameter of 10 µm by several zooplankton species. Prelabelled copepods and Marenzelleria sp. larvae were used to expose Mysis relicta and Mysis mixta to PS via food chain transmission. MPs could be transported from a lower trophic level to a higher level via the food chain. Hall et al. (Hall et al., 2015) tested the ingestion (over 48 h) and feeding rates (3 and 12 h) of the scleractinian coral *Dipsastrea pallida* using polypropylene microplastics (10-2 µm). Ingested MPs were discovered in mesenterial tissue within the coral gut cavity, showing that high levels of MPs can harm the corals' health. At concentrations 0 and 250 mL/L, Nobre et al., (Nobre et al., 2015) investigated the effects of virgin PE granules and beach-collected stranded pellets on the sea urchin *Lytechinus variegatus*. A pellet-water interface assay in interstitial water and an elutriate assay in the water column were used as test models. The embryonic development of L. variegatus was found to be more toxic to virgin PE pellets than beach-collected pellets in both models. The authors concluded that, plastics can act as a vector for pollutants and that leached chemicals from pellets can be toxic through various routes of exposure. Green and co-workers (Green et al., 2016) used polylactic acid (PLA) (235.7± 14.8 μm), PVC (130.6± 12.9 μm), and high-density polyethylene (HDPE) (102.6 ± 10.3 μm) microplastics in mesocosm investigation to examine the feeding activity, nitrogen cycling, bioturbation, and metabolic rate of *Arenicola marina* for 31 days. MPs were exposed at concentrations of 0.02%, 0.2%, and 2%, and A. marina generated fewer casts in MPs affected sediments. In the high-concentration exposure group, the metabolic rate was high and the microalgal biomass was low. According to the findings, various MPs compounds have varied effects on organisms. Toxicity investigation of MPs/NPs in marine habitats is summarised in Table 1.

Watts et al., (Watts et al., 2016) studied the effects of aminated, carboxylated, and neutral PS microplastics (8 μm) on the hemolymph function, absorption, and oxygen consumption of the marine crab C. maenas. After being swallowed into the gills and into the crab bodies, the MPS had a minor but substantial dose-response effect. The distribution of two distinct MPs with carboxyl (COOH) and amine (NH_2) functional groups in the gill surface was carried out, although neither had a significant influence. In more than 20 investigations, marine organisms were used in simulated marine habitats. Studies employing simulated freshwater habitats were not undertaken until recently because there is a larger interest in MPs pollution in the marine ecosystem. Only three studies on the effect of MPs on freshwater ecospecies have been reported, but active investigations on the effect of MPs on freshwater ecospecies are ongoing, and studies will be undertaken soon, owing to growing concerns about MPs utilized in personal care products.

Della Torre et al., (Della Torre et al., 2014) employed PS-NPs with carboxyl (40 nm) and amine (50 nm) functional group in the sea urchin *Paracentrotus lividus*. The organisms were toxic to embryos and had aberrant gene expression. Bergami and co-workers (Bergami et al., 2016) investigated sub-lethal effects and mortality on *Artemia franciscana* using amino-modified and carboxylated PS-NPs (40-50 nm). The motility, feeding, serial molting of A. franciscana were all adversely harmed by NPs. These findings suggest that NPs have an impact on the ecosystem as well as the organism and population. Besseling and co-workers (Ellen Besseling et al., 2014) studied the toxicity effects of PS-NPs functionalized with -COOH groups on S. obliquus and D. magna. The NPs had an impact on algae's photosynthetic capability and biomass, as well as the reproduction, body size, survival, and physical development of D. magna neonates. Cedervall and co-workers (Cedervall et al., 2012) and Mattsson and co-workers (Mattsson et al., 2015) conducted trophic transfer experiments on NPs. Cedervall and co-workers (Cedervall et al., 2012) investigated the trophic transmission of PS NPs (24 and 28 nm) in food chains that included Scenedesmus sp., *Carassius Carassius*, D. magna, as well as changes in cholesterol level in fish. More consumption of NPs causes disrupted lipid metabolism. Mattson et al. used the same food chain to study fish behavior and conduct NMR spectroscopy. They determined that PS-NPs influenced fish behavior and metabolism and that NPs were certainly transmitted up the food chain to higher trophic levels. NPs have a small volume and large surface area; they have tremendous potential for penetrating organisms' bodies and tissues. Ingestion of NPs by zebrafish (*Danio rerio*) larvae resulted in neurotoxicity in locomotor activity. MPs alone had no significant effects excluding upregulated zfrho visual gene expression, although NPs inhibited larval locomotion by 22% during the last darkness period and greatly reduced larvae body length by 6%. It also inhibits the acetylcholinesterase activity by 40%. Also, it significantly upregulated the zfblue, zfrho, and gfap gene expression (Q. Chen, Gundlach, et al., 2017).

Table 1. MPs/NPs have been used in ecotoxicity investigations in both freshwater and marine habitats

MPs/NPs	Size	Organisms studied	Conc.	Exposure time	Evaluation point	Ref.	Image of organisms studied
HDPE	0-80 μm	*Mytilus edulis*	For every 4-5ml, 1 drop	96 hours	Lysosomal Membrane, Lipofuscin, Lipids	(Von Moos et al., 2012)	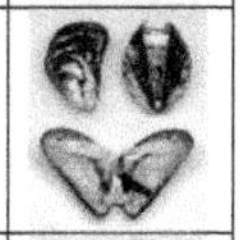
PS	7.3 μm 20.6 μm 30.6 μm	*Acartica clausi*	3000 beads/ml 2240 beads /ml 635 beads/ml	1/24 hours	Ingestion	(Cole et al., 2013)	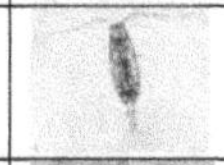
PVC	130 μm	*Arenicola marina*	0, 0.5% (w/w) 1, 5% (w/w) 0, 5% (w/w)	4 weeks 4 weeks 48 hours	Energy chronic reserves, Immunity Activity of feeding Egestion Gut residence	(Wright et al., 2013)	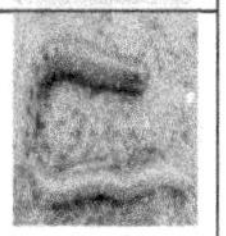
PE	10-45 μm	*Tripneustes gratilla*	0, 300 /mL 0, 1, 10, 100, 300 /mL 0, 500 /mL	1, 6 hours 5 days 1 hour-15 minutes	Ingestion	(Kaposi et al., 2014)	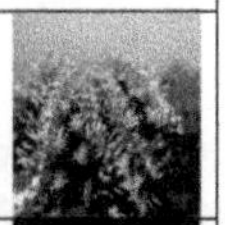
PS	8 μm	*Carcinus maenas*	10^7- 10^6 microspheres/mL	24 hours	Consumption of oxygen, analysis of hemolymph and uptake	(Watts et al., 2016)	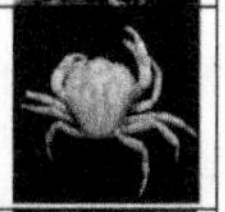
PP	20-75 mm in length	*Hyalella azteca*	0-90 MPs/mL	10 days	Ingestion of MPs, growth, and mortality	(Au et al., 2015)	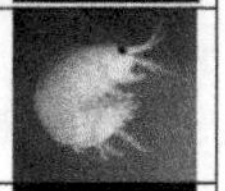
PS	10 μm	*Mysid Shrimps* *Monoporeia affins* *Gammarus sp* *Macoma balthica*	0, 5, 50, 250 Beads/mL	24 hours	Ingestion	Setälä *et al.*, 2016	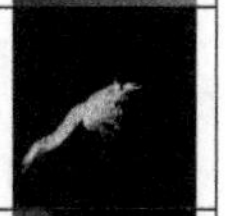
PS	90 μm	*Preca fluviatilis*	0, 10000, 80000 particles /m^3	3 weeks	Ingestion, Rate of hatching Rate of activity	(Lönnstedt & Eklöv, 2016)	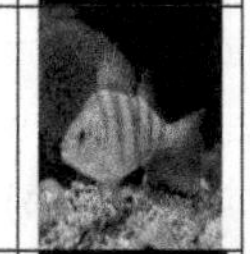
PLA	65.6 μm	*Ostrea edulis*	0.8, 80 μg/L	60 days	Rate of filtration, Respiration, Macro, and micro algal biomass	(Green, 2016)	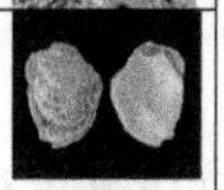
PP	500 μm	*Carcinus maenas*	0, 0.6, 1.2, 2.0 mg per 2 g of the month	1 month	Consumption of oxygen, Excretion rate of ammonia Food consumption	(Watts et al., 2015)	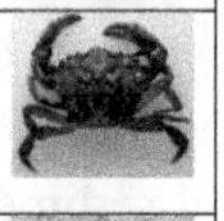
HDPE	102.6 μm	*Arenicola marina*	0.02, 0.2, 2 %	31 days	Nitrate and nitrite, metabolic rate, Bioturbation, the activity of feeding	(Green et al., 2016)	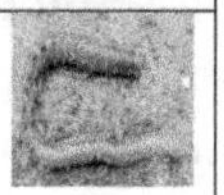

Due to the enormous surface area of MPs, they facilitate the transfer of hydrophobic substances HOCs by adsorbing a wide variety of organisms within the trophic level carrying those chemicals on the plastic's surface (Kowalski et al., 2016). These chemicals cause side effects for marine species like oil and alkanes, as well as bio-accumulative, persistent, and hazardous substances, including heavy metals and

Figure 3. MPs and NPs detritus in the seawater and their interactions with other contaminants and primary transport mechanism

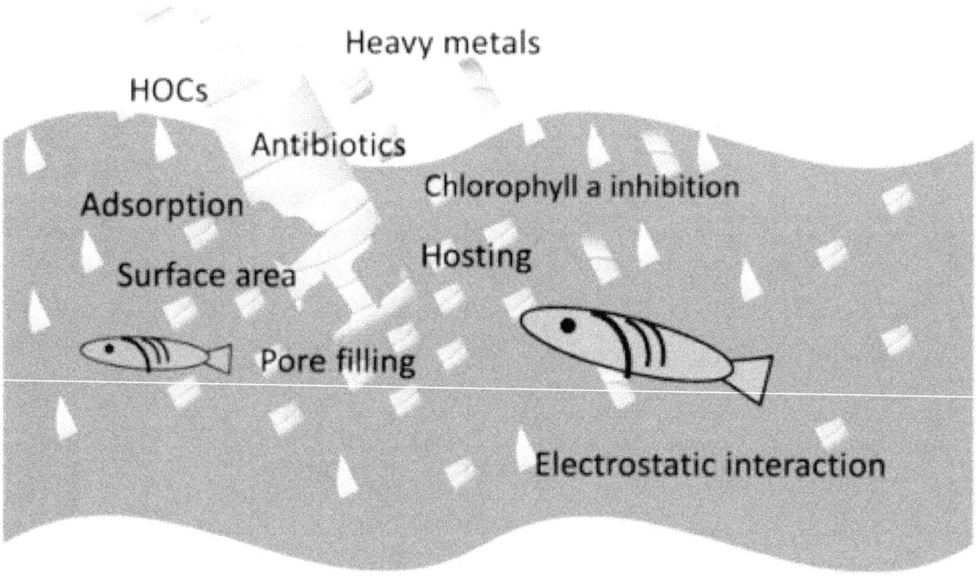

pesticides which are attached to the surface of plastic trash from the environment (J. Wang et al., 2016). According to Wang and co-workers (F. Wang et al., 2020), surface area (electrostatic interaction, van der wall force, and hydrogen bonding), pore filling, and partitioning are all important factors in the sorption behavior of various organic pollutants on MPs/NPs (Figure 3). Moreover, plastic additives and chemicals, such as bisphenol A (BPA), are mutagens and carcinogens, which leaked into the marine atmosphere or the digestive systems of marine animals, and proved to be a possible cause of mortality (Kowalski et al., 2016). This is because of their harmful effect on nutrition, reproduction, life span, growth, and development. Reactive oxygen species production and related inflammation, kidney and liver damage, secondary genotoxic effects, and immunological impacts are harmful consequences induced by NPs, according to a study by Bouwmeester and co-workers (Bouwmeester et al., 2009).

Plastic degradation into the atmosphere could spread toxic metals like (Pb, Cd, Zn, Cu, Cr) as discovered in MPs from the surface water in Thailand (Ta & Babel, 2020). MPs were found in surface water and sediments in a concentration of 48 ± 8 items/m^3 and 39 ± 14 items/kg, respectively. MPs having small sizes (0.05-0.3 mm) were dominant in all the samples. Polyethylene and polypropylene were present primarily in surface water and sediment, respectively (Ta & Babel, 2020).

Adu-Boahen and co-workers evaluated the environmental impacts of microplastics (< 5mm). The investigation discovered that MPs are prevalent in the river Akora and that some resident aquatic species uptake MPs, posing a threat to lives. The study also discovered favorable relationships between the number of fish present and MPs load in fish. They revealed that the primary sources are uncontrolled gutters that pour directly into the river. Running water and wind have been identified as potential sources of MPs entering the river (Adu-Boahen et al., 2020). In Code River, a particular region of Yogyakarta, Sulistyo et al. investigated the abundance of MPs in fishes. The collected samples were assessed utilizing

Wet Peroxide Oxidation (WPO) method. The results inferred that in comparison to the downstream area (3.25 particles/gram), fish samples collected from the upstream region had the highest abundance (4.33 particles/gram). Blue is the most common color, and fiber is the most common type of MPs (Sulistyo et al., 2020). Ding and co-workers (Ding et al., 2021) used zebrafish to evaluate the toxicity of MPs exposure. Here, PE-MPs in sphere shape having diameter 75-100 µm were exposed to zebrafish for 35 days showing that survival rate was not affected significantly but the growth rate. More investigation of oxidative stress-related enzyme activities revealed that exposure to MPs at lower concentrations (0.1 and 1 mg/L) stimulated the production of GSH, GSH-PX, and GST in the intestine, whereas exposure to those at 10 mg/L suppressed the production of SOD, CAT, GSH and GSH-PX. This investigation confirmed that the changes in intestinal enzyme activity of zebrafish, but found no evidence that persistent exposure to MPs cause higher mortality (Ding et al., 2021). Zhang and co-workers (C. Zhang et al., 2017) find a detrimental effect of micrometer-sized PVC MPs on microalgae *Skeletonema costatum* only at the highest and most ecologically unrealistic exposure concentration (50 mg/L). They inferred that aggregation and physical adsorption may have produced toxicity. After 96 h of exposure, it was shown that MPs (mPVC, average diameter 1 µm) had a significant inhibitory effect on microalgae development with a maximum growth inhibition ratio of 39.7%. The use of high concentrations of mPVC (50 mg/L) had a deleterious impact on algal photosynthesis, as both chlorophyll content and photosynthetic efficiency decreased (C. Zhang et al., 2017). Barboza and co-workers (Barboza et al., 2018) studied the single and combined effects of MPs and Hg on juveniles of the European seabass (*Dicentrarchus labrax*). They discovered the negative impacts on the swimming performance of seabass. MPs can cause some behavioral changes like reduction in swimming velocity and resistance time, erratic and lethargic swimming.

Plastic matters dominated in terms of several items (88% of 69 litter individual items) in the systematic survey of seafloor litter in the South African continental shelf. Of these plastic items, 38% were low-density polyethylene, 34% polypropylene, 12% polyamide, and 3% each of high-density polyethylene, and polyethylene terephthalate bottles. Floating and biofouling may cause these items to sink (Ryan et al., 2020). Marine filter feeders, i.e., baleen whale (Megaptera novaeangliae), are introduced to MPs because of their indiscriminate food source. The variety of plastic forms and shapes found in the intestine could be utilized to deduce the diversity of MPs and the non-selective way in which a baleen whale consumes them. Polymer kinds and shapes ranging from 1mm to 17 cm were discovered in this study (E Besseling et al., 2015).

Toxicity Comparison of MPs and NPs

Moving on to the toxicity comparison of MPs and NPs, Lee and co-workers (Lee et al., 2013) used fluorescent and plain MPs and NPs (50 nm, 500 nm, and 6 µm) in a toxicity test. The test species *Tigriopus japonicus* was studied for sex ratio, fecundity, ingestion, and mortality. T. japonicus fecundity was unaffected by the 50 nm polystyrene (PS) beads, however, all the PS beads physically hindered fertilization. There was no substantial difference in toxicity between NPs and MPs, on the other hand. Cole and Galloway (Cole & Galloway, 2015) employed fluorescently labeled PS MPs and NPs (70, 160, and 870 nm) (1.84, 4.1, 7.3, 10.2, and 20.3 µm), carboxylated and fluorescently labeled PS (940, 990 nm). The ingestion and growth of Crassostrea gigas larvae were studied using 1 and 10 µm MPs beads. The amount of plastic consumed during 24-hour exposure varied depending on the age of larvae, size of plastics. Aminated plastics were easier for larvae to absorb and keep in their bodies. Plastics had no discernible influence on the feeding or development of C. gigas. Utilizing fluorescently labeled

PS microbeads (50, 500 nm, and 6 µm), Jeong and co-workers (Jeong et al., 2016) studied the lifespan and fecundity of *Brachionus koreanus* in the presence of non-functionalized PS microbeads (50, 500 nm, and 6 µm) and analyzed ingestion, antioxidant enzymatic activity, ROS induction, and egestion. Plastic bead exposure was linked to an increase in oxidative stress and antioxidant enzymes, as well as a decrease in growth rate, body size, reproduction time, and lifespan. The study found that the toxicity of MPs and NPs is proportional to their size. Smaller plastics are more harmful than larger ones. *Danio reio* was used by Lu et al. (Lu et al., 2016), to test the toxicity of PS MPs and NPs. To study the uptake and accumulation, fluorescent PS particles (5, 20 µm) containing encapsulated fluorescent dyes were employed. Virgin PS particles (70 nm, 5 µm) were used to test catalase (CAT) activity and superoxide dismutase (SOD), metabolism, and histopathology of D. reio. Both larger and smaller MPs of size 20 µm and 5 µm, respectively were found in different parts of D. reio.

Brief of Analytical Methods for the Elimination of MPs and NPs

There have been different analytical techniques utilized to remove MPs and NPs (Figure 4), which will be discussed herein briefly. Biodegradation in which microorganisms have the potential for the breakdown of organic polymers into carbon dioxide, methane, water, and other inorganic products. This method is highly affected by environmental situations, such as temperature, humidity, and sunlight (Paço et al., 2017). Microorganisms are flexible to various environmental conditions and are also a factor for the revolution of soil-buried MPs. The microorganisms stick to the surface of the plastics to start the biodegradation by making biofilms. Since the MPs have hydrophobic nature but due to the interference with the groups of microbes as well as biofilm formation, microbial enzymes can enhance the incorporation of microorganisms on the surface of plastics by improving its hydrophilicity. Bacteria then act on plastics by excreting extracellular enzymes, further then accelerating the hydrolysis or oxidation processes (Helen Shnada Auta et al., 2018). The MPs biodegradation with the help of microorganisms is studied by various groups. Auta and co-workers (H S Auta et al., 2017) used *Bacillus cereus* to study polyethylene, polyethylene terephthalate, and polystyrene, and the polymer weight reduction observed was 1.6%, 6.6%, and 7.4%, respectively, in 40 days. This group also studied the biodegradation of polyethylene, polyethylene terephthalate, polystyrene, and polypropylene with the help of *Bacillus gottheilii* in 40 days. The weight reduction of respective polymers was observed to be 6.2%, 3.0%, 5.8%, and 3.6%. Paco et al., (Paço et al., 2017) used *Zalerionmaritimum* for the biodegradation of MP polyethylene in 14 days. The weight reduction of polyethylene was observed to be 56.7% ± 2.9%. Also, Chen et al., (Z. Chen et al., 2020) studied the degradation of polystyrene for 45 days using hyperthermophilic bacteria. The molecular weight reduction of polystyrene was found to be 43.7%. Park and Kim (Park & Kim, 2019) studied the biodegradation of polyethylene using *Bacillus sp.* and *Paenibacillus sp.* for 60 days. The molecular weight reduction of polyethylene was observed to be 14.7% and 22.8% for *Bacillus sp.* and *Paenibacillus sp,* respectively.

MPs adsorption by activated biochar and biochar was studied by Siipola et al. (Siipola et al., 2020). Kang and co-workers (Kang et al., 2019) developed magnetic N-doped carbon nano springs for accelerated sulphate oxidation of cosmetics MPs in hydrothermal conditions. After 8 hours of pyrolysis and hydrothermal temperatures of 800 and 160 °C, MPs lost ~54% of their weight. The hydrothermal conditions provided both high pressure and physical ripping of the polymer, causing it to degrade. Ye et al., (Ye et al., 2020) developed a method for eliminating adsorbed metals from MPs by using an advanced oxidation process triggered by $SO_4^{\cdot-}$ radicals to decompose an organic layer. This could help to reduce

Figure 4. Various techniques for the removal of MPs and NPs

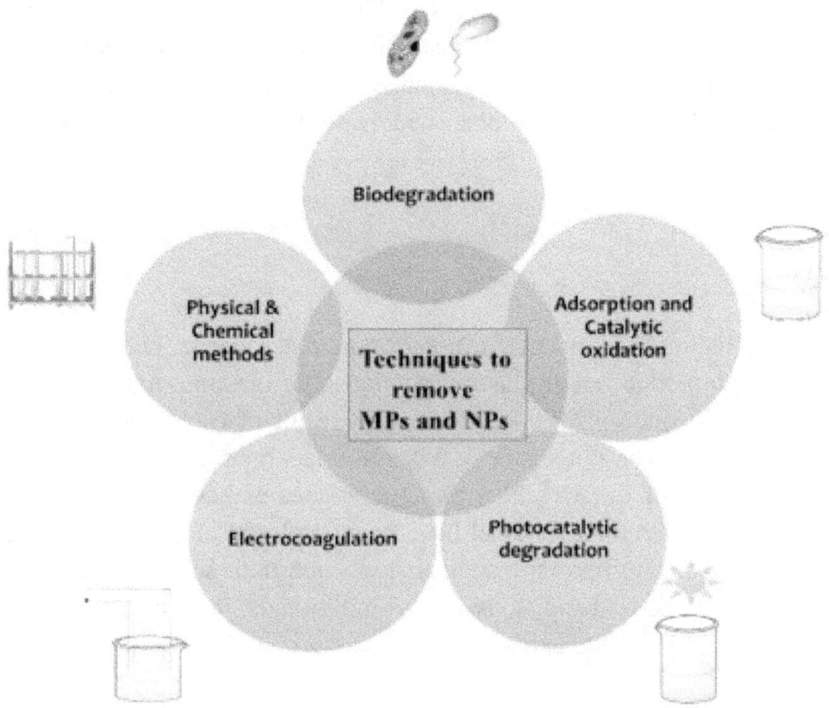

co-contamination by reducing the risk of MPs acting as vectors for harmful substances. The biochar-based catalyst with increased graphitization was capable of mineralizing organic contaminants into CO_2 and H_2O with the help of active sites of defects (P. Zhang et al., 2019). Thus, the adsorbent/catalysts' cost-effectiveness and reusability are the most important variables in assessing its practicality and utilization at large scale. To synthesize a versatile catalyst, more straight forward separation approaches and low-cost synthesis routes should be developed. To eliminate MPs and NPs, this methodology requires a thorough investigation.

Photocatalytic degradation is a reaction (redox) in which a semiconductor absorbs photons of a specific wavelength, and valence band (VB) electrons are driven to the conduction band (CB), leaving behind positive holes. Superoxide radicals and hydroxyl radicals are formed when electrons and holes react with adsorbed water and oxygen (Kundu, Sharma, et al., 2021; Rathi et al., 2019). TiO_2-embedment technique has been used to photocatalyzed the treatment of polyethylene, propylene, and polystyrene polymers under diverse light sources. The composite films were made by combining the polymers with TiO_2 in solvents like tetrahydrofuran or cyclohexane (Shang et al., 2003; Thomas et al., 2013; Verma et al., 2017). Sekino et al., (Sekino et al., 2012) used photocatalysis and TiO_2- based micro and nanodevices to explore the structure of MPs. Wang et al., (L. Wang et al., 2019) examined the use of Au@Ni@TiO_2 based micromotors to remove polystyrene MPs floating in freshwater using UV irradiation.

For the MPs and NPs removal, chemical procedures such as the sol-gel process, agglomeration, and ozonation, while physical techniques such as sedimentation and filtration are used. Chemical and physical methods are frequently utilized in conjugation with the wastewater treatment plant. Various researchers have used sol-gel to treat MPs from the aquatic environment (Herbort et al., 2018; Herbort & Schuhen, 2017; Ratola et al., 2016; Sturm et al., 2020). Coagulation allows for the creation of larger particles, making the separation process more accessible. Coagulants can bind minuscule particles using these strategies, which involve the ligand exchange mechanism (Ma et al., 2019). MPs coagulation by Al, Fe, and alum-based coagulants has been widely studied (Ma et al., 2019; Skaf et al., 2020; Y. Zhang et al., 2020).

CONCLUSIONS

The ubiquity of MPs/NPs poses a significant threat to the macrocosm. The primary MPs are purposefully produced for the preproduction of plastic granulates, air blasting, microbeads for cosmetics, and personal care products. Secondary MPs can form as a result of fragmentation in the terrestrial and aquatic environment. The micron range size of MPs/NPs lets them be swallowed by marine creatures and birds. The toxic effects of the MPs/NPs on aquatic species have been discussed in detail in the current chapter. Techniques for their removal have been explored in brief. Future research into MPs/NPs mitigation should focus on improving analysis tools and their source regulation. To eliminate the problems from their root, large-scale units, as well as individuals, must be aware of waste management and health dangers associated with plastics.

REFERENCES

Adu-Boahen, K., Dadson, I. Y., Mensah, D. K. D., & Kyeremeh, S. (2020). Mapping ecological impact of microplastics on freshwater habitat in the central region of Ghana: A case study of River Akora. *GeoJournal*, •••, 1–19. doi:10.100710708-020-10273-6

Alprol, A. E., Gaballah, M. S., & Hassaan, M. A. (2021). Micro and Nanoplastics analysis: Focus on their classification, sources, and impacts in marine environment. *Regional Studies in Marine Science*, *42*, 101625. doi:10.1016/j.rsma.2021.101625

Au, S. Y., Bruce, T. F., Bridges, W. C., & Klaine, S. J. (2015). Responses of Hyalella azteca to acute and chronic microplastic exposures. *Environmental Toxicology and Chemistry*, *34*(11), 2564–2572. doi:10.1002/etc.3093 PMID:26042578

Auta, H. S., Emenike, C. U., & Fauziah, S. H. (2017). Screening of Bacillus strains isolated from mangrove ecosystems in Peninsular Malaysia for microplastic degradation. *Environmental Pollution*, *231*, 1552–1559. doi:10.1016/j.envpol.2017.09.043 PMID:28964604

Auta, H. S., Emenike, C. U., Jayanthi, B., & Fauziah, S. H. (2018). Growth kinetics and biodeterioration of polypropylene microplastics by Bacillus sp. and Rhodococcus sp. isolated from mangrove sediment. *Marine Pollution Bulletin*, *127*, 15–21. doi:10.1016/j.marpolbul.2017.11.036 PMID:29475646

Barboza, L. G. A., Vieira, L. R., & Guilhermino, L. (2018). Single and combined effects of microplastics and mercury on juveniles of the European seabass (Dicentrarchus labrax): Changes in behavioural responses and reduction of swimming velocity and resistance time. *Environmental Pollution, 236*, 1014–1019. doi:10.1016/j.envpol.2017.12.082 PMID:29449115

Bergami, E., Bocci, E., Vannuccini, M. L., Monopoli, M., Salvati, A., Dawson, K. A., & Corsi, I. (2016). Nano-sized polystyrene affects feeding, behavior and physiology of brine shrimp Artemia franciscana larvae. *Ecotoxicology and Environmental Safety, 123*, 18–25. doi:10.1016/j.ecoenv.2015.09.021 PMID:26422775

Besseling, E., Foekema, E. M., Van Franeker, J. A., Leopold, M. F., Kühn, S., Rebolledo, E. L. B., Heße, E., Mielke, L., IJzer, J., & Kamminga, P. (2015). Microplastic in a macro filter feeder: Humpback whale Megaptera novaeangliae. *Marine Pollution Bulletin, 95*(1), 248–252. doi:10.1016/j.marpolbul.2015.04.007 PMID:25916197

Besseling, E., Wang, B., Lürling, M., & Koelmans, A. A. (2014). Nanoplastic affects growth of S. obliquus and reproduction of D. magna. *Environmental Science & Technology, 48*(20), 12336–12343. doi:10.1021/es503001d PMID:25268330

Bouwmeester, H., Dekkers, S., Noordam, M. Y., Hagens, W. I., Bulder, A. S., de Heer, C., ten Voorde, S. E. C. G., Wijnhoven, S. W. P., Marvin, H. J. P., & Sips, A. J. A. M. (2009). Review of health safety aspects of nanotechnologies in food production. *Regulatory Toxicology and Pharmacology, 53*(1), 52–62. doi:10.1016/j.yrtph.2008.10.008 PMID:19027049

Browne, M. A., Crump, P., Niven, S. J., Teuten, E., Tonkin, A., Galloway, T., & Thompson, R. (2011). Accumulation of microplastic on shorelines woldwide: Sources and sinks. *Environmental Science & Technology, 45*(21), 9175–9179. doi:10.1021/es201811s PMID:21894925

Browne, M. A., Dissanayake, A., Galloway, T. S., Lowe, D. M., & Thompson, R. C. (2008). Ingested microscopic plastic translocates to the circulatory system of the mussel, Mytilus edulis (L.). *Environmental Science & Technology, 42*(13), 5026–5031. doi:10.1021/es800249a PMID:18678044

Cai, L., Wang, J., Peng, J., Wu, Z., & Tan, X. (2018). Observation of the degradation of three types of plastic pellets exposed to UV irradiation in three different environments. *The Science of the Total Environment, 628–629*, 740–747. doi:10.1016/j.scitotenv.2018.02.079 PMID:29454214

Cedervall, T., Hansson, L.-A., Lard, M., Frohm, B., & Linse, S. (2012). Food chain transport of nanoparticles affects behaviour and fat metabolism in fish. *PLoS One, 7*(2), e32254. doi:10.1371/journal.pone.0032254 PMID:22384193

Chen, Q., Gundlach, M., Yang, S., Jiang, J., Velki, M., Yin, D., & Hollert, H. (2017). Quantitative investigation of the mechanisms of microplastics and nanoplastics toward zebrafish larvae locomotor activity. *The Science of the Total Environment, 584–585*, 1022–1031. doi:10.1016/j.scitotenv.2017.01.156 PMID:28185727

Chen, Q., Yin, D., Jia, Y., Schiwy, S., Legradi, J., Yang, S., & Hollert, H. (2017). Enhanced uptake of BPA in the presence of nanoplastics can lead to neurotoxic effects in adult zebrafish. *The Science of the Total Environment, 609*, 1312–1321. doi:10.1016/j.scitotenv.2017.07.144 PMID:28793400

Chen, Z., Zhao, W., Xing, R., Xie, S., Yang, X., Cui, P., Lü, J., Liao, H., Yu, Z., Wang, S., & Zhou, S. (2020). Enhanced in situ biodegradation of microplastics in sewage sludge using hyperthermophilic composting technology. *Journal of Hazardous Materials*, *384*, 121271. doi:10.1016/j.jhazmat.2019.121271 PMID:31611021

Cole, M., & Galloway, T. S. (2015). Ingestion of nanoplastics and microplastics by Pacific oyster larvae. *Environmental Science & Technology*, *49*(24), 14625–14632. doi:10.1021/acs.est.5b04099 PMID:26580574

Cole, M., Lindeque, P., Fileman, E., Halsband, C., Goodhead, R., Moger, J., & Galloway, T. S. (2013). Microplastic ingestion by zooplankton. *Environmental Science & Technology*, *47*(12), 6646–6655. doi:10.1021/es400663f PMID:23692270

Da Costa, J. P., Paço, A., Santos, P. S. M., Duarte, A. C., & Rocha-Santos, T. (2019). Microplastics in soils: Assessment, analytics and risks. *Environmental Chemistry*, *16*(1), 18–30. doi:10.1071/EN18150

Della Torre, C., Bergami, E., Salvati, A., Faleri, C., Cirino, P., Dawson, K. A., & Corsi, I. (2014). Accumulation and embryotoxicity of polystyrene nanoparticles at early stage of development of sea urchin embryos Paracentrotus lividus. *Environmental Science & Technology*, *48*(20), 12302–12311. doi:10.1021/es502569w PMID:25260196

Ding, N., Jiang, L., Wang, X., Wang, C., Geng, Y., Zhang, J., Sun, Y., Zhang, Y., Yuan, Q. & Liu, H. (2021). *The Toxicity of Polyethylene Microplastic Exposure and Its Concurrent Effect With Aeromonas Hydrophila Infection To Zebrafish*. Academic Press.

Garg, A., Basu, S., Shetti, N. P., & Reddy, K. R. (2021). 2D materials and its heterostructured photocatalysts: Synthesis, properties, functionalization and applications in environmental remediation. *Journal of Environmental Chemical Engineering*, *9*(6), 106408. doi:10.1016/j.jece.2021.106408

Gewert, B., Plassmann, M. M., & MacLeod, M. (2015). Pathways for degradation of plastic polymers floating in the marine environment. *Environmental Science. Processes & Impacts*, *17*(9), 1513–1521. doi:10.1039/C5EM00207A PMID:26216708

González-Fernández, C., Tallec, K., Le Goïc, N., Lambert, C., Soudant, P., Huvet, A., Suquet, M., Berchel, M., & Paul-Pont, I. (2018). Cellular responses of Pacific oyster (Crassostrea gigas) gametes exposed in vitro to polystyrene nanoparticles. *Chemosphere*, *208*, 764–772. doi:10.1016/j.chemosphere.2018.06.039 PMID:29902761

Graham, E. R., & Thompson, J. T. (2009). Deposit-and suspension-feeding sea cucumbers (Echinodermata) ingest plastic fragments. *Journal of Experimental Marine Biology and Ecology*, *368*(1), 22–29. doi:10.1016/j.jembe.2008.09.007

Green, D. S. (2016). Effects of microplastics on European flat oysters, Ostrea edulis and their associated benthic communities. *Environmental Pollution*, *216*, 95–103. doi:10.1016/j.envpol.2016.05.043 PMID:27239693

Green, D. S., Boots, B., Sigwart, J., Jiang, S., & Rocha, C. (2016). Effects of conventional and biodegradable microplastics on a marine ecosystem engineer (Arenicola marina) and sediment nutrient cycling. *Environmental Pollution*, *208*, 426–434. doi:10.1016/j.envpol.2015.10.010 PMID:26552519

Guterres, S. S., Alves, M. P., & Pohlmann, A. R. (2007). Polymeric Nanoparticles, Nanospheres and Nanocapsules, for Cutaneous Applications. *Drug Target Insights*, *2*. doi:10.1177/117739280700200002 PMID:21901071

Hall, N. M., Berry, K. L. E., Rintoul, L., & Hoogenboom, M. O. (2015). Microplastic ingestion by scleractinian corals. *Marine Biology*, *162*(3), 725–732. doi:10.100700227-015-2619-7

Herbort, A. F., & Schuhen, K. (2017). A concept for the removal of microplastics from the marine environment with innovative host-guest relationships. *Environmental Science and Pollution Research International*, *24*(12), 11061–11065. doi:10.100711356-016-7216-x PMID:27421855

Herbort, A. F., Sturm, M. T., Fiedler, S., Abkai, G., & Schuhen, K. (2018). Alkoxy-silyl induced agglomeration: A new approach for the sustainable removal of microplastic from aquatic systems. *Journal of Polymers and the Environment*, *26*(11), 4258–4270. doi:10.100710924-018-1287-3

Horton, A. A., Walton, A., Spurgeon, D. J., Lahive, E., & Svendsen, C. (2017). Microplastics in freshwater and terrestrial environments: Evaluating the current understanding to identify the knowledge gaps and future research priorities. *The Science of the Total Environment*, *586*, 127–141. doi:10.1016/j.scitotenv.2017.01.190 PMID:28169032

Jeong, C.-B., Won, E.-J., Kang, H.-M., Lee, M.-C., Hwang, D.-S., Hwang, U.-K., Zhou, B., Souissi, S., Lee, S.-J., & Lee, J.-S. (2016). Microplastic size-dependent toxicity, oxidative stress induction, and p-JNK and p-p38 activation in the monogonont rotifer (Brachionus koreanus). *Environmental Science & Technology*, *50*(16), 8849–8857. doi:10.1021/acs.est.6b01441 PMID:27438693

Kang, J., Zhou, L., Duan, X., Sun, H., Ao, Z., & Wang, S. (2019). Degradation of cosmetic microplastics via functionalized carbon nanosprings. *Matter*, *1*(3), 745–758. doi:10.1016/j.matt.2019.06.004

Kaposi, K. L., Mos, B., Kelaher, B. P., & Dworjanyn, S. A. (2014). Ingestion of microplastic has limited impact on a marine larva. *Environmental Science & Technology*, *48*(3), 1638–1645. doi:10.1021/es404295e PMID:24341789

Kowalski, N., Reichardt, A. M., & Waniek, J. J. (2016). Sinking rates of microplastics and potential implications of their alteration by physical, biological, and chemical factors. *Marine Pollution Bulletin*, *109*(1), 310–319. doi:10.1016/j.marpolbul.2016.05.064 PMID:27297594

Kundu, A., Sharma, S., & Basu, S. (2021). Modulated BiOCl Nanoplates with Porous g-C3N4 Nanosheets for photocatalytic degradation of Color/Colorless Pollutants in Natural Sunlight. *Journal of Physics and Chemistry of Solids*, *154*, 110064. doi:10.1016/j.jpcs.2021.110064

Kundu, A., Shetti, N. P., Basu, S., Reddy, K. R., Nadagouda, M. N., & Aminabhavi, T. M. (2021). Identification and removal of micro-and nano-plastics: Efficient and cost-effective methods. *Chemical Engineering Journal*, *421*, 129816. doi:10.1016/j.cej.2021.129816 PMID:34504393

Lambert, S., & Wagner, M. (2016). Formation of microscopic particles during the degradation of different polymers. *Chemosphere*, *161*, 510–517. doi:10.1016/j.chemosphere.2016.07.042 PMID:27470943

Lee, K. W., Shim, W. J., Kwon, O. Y., & Kang, J. H. (2013). Size-dependent effects of micro polystyrene particles in the marine copepod tigriopus japonicus. *Environmental Science & Technology*, *47*(19), 11278–11283. doi:10.1021/es401932b PMID:23988225

Lönnstedt, O. M., & Eklöv, P. (2016). Environmentally relevant concentrations of microplastic particles influence larval fish ecology. *Science*, *352*(6290), 1213–1216. doi:10.1126cience.aad8828 PMID:27257256

Lu, Y., Zhang, Y., Deng, Y., Jiang, W., Zhao, Y., Geng, J., Ding, L., & Ren, H. (2016). Uptake and accumulation of polystyrene microplastics in zebrafish (Danio rerio) and toxic effects in liver. *Environmental Science & Technology*, *50*(7), 4054–4060. doi:10.1021/acs.est.6b00183 PMID:26950772

Ma, B., Xue, W., Ding, Y., Hu, C., Liu, H., & Qu, J. (2019). Removal characteristics of microplastics by Fe-based coagulants during drinking water treatment. *Journal of Environmental Sciences (China)*, *78*, 267–275. doi:10.1016/j.jes.2018.10.006 PMID:30665645

Mani, T., Hauk, A., Walter, U., & Burkhardt-Holm, P. (2015). Microplastics profile along the Rhine River. *Scientific Reports*, *5*(1), 1–7. doi:10.1038rep17988 PMID:26644346

Mattsson, K., Ekvall, M. T., Hansson, L. A., Linse, S., Malmendal, A., & Cedervall, T. (2015). Altered behavior, physiology, and metabolism in fish exposed to polystyrene nanoparticles. *Environmental Science & Technology*, *49*(1), 553–561. doi:10.1021/es5053655 PMID:25380515

McDevitt, J. P., Criddle, C. S., Morse, M., Hale, R. C., Bott, C. B., & Rochman, C. M. (2017). Addressing the Issue of Microplastics in the Wake of the Microbead-Free Waters Act - A New Standard Can Facilitate Improved Policy. In Environmental Science and Technology (Vol. 51, Issue 12, pp. 6611–6617). ACS Publications. doi:10.1021/acs.est.6b05812

Nobre, C. R., Santana, M. F. M., Maluf, A., Cortez, F. S., Cesar, A., Pereira, C. D. S., & Turra, A. (2015). Assessment of microplastic toxicity to embryonic development of the sea urchin Lytechinus variegatus (Echinodermata: Echinoidea). *Marine Pollution Bulletin*, *92*(1–2), 99–104. doi:10.1016/j.marpolbul.2014.12.050 PMID:25662316

Nomura, T., Tani, S., Yamamoto, M., Nakagawa, T., Toyoda, S., Fujisawa, E., Yasui, A., & Konishi, Y. (2016). Cytotoxicity and colloidal behavior of polystyrene latex nanoparticles toward filamentous fungi in isotonic solutions. *Chemosphere*, *149*, 84–90. doi:10.1016/j.chemosphere.2016.01.091 PMID:26855210

Paço, A., Duarte, K., da Costa, J. P., Santos, P. S. M., Pereira, R., Pereira, M. E., Freitas, A. C., Duarte, A. C., & Rocha-Santos, T. A. P. (2017). Biodegradation of polyethylene microplastics by the marine fungus Zalerion maritimum. *The Science of the Total Environment*, *586*, 10–15. doi:10.1016/j.scitotenv.2017.02.017 PMID:28199874

Park, S. Y., & Kim, C. G. (2019). Biodegradation of micro-polyethylene particles by bacterial colonization of a mixed microbial consortium isolated from a landfill site. *Chemosphere*, *222*, 527–533. doi:10.1016/j.chemosphere.2019.01.159 PMID:30721811

Peng, G., Xu, P., Zhu, B., Bai, M., & Li, D. (2018). Microplastics in freshwater river sediments in Shanghai, China: A case study of risk assessment in mega-cities. *Environmental Pollution*, *234*, 448–456. doi:10.1016/j.envpol.2017.11.034 PMID:29207296

Rai, P. K., Lee, J., Brown, R. J. C., & Kim, K.-H. (2020). Micro-and nanoplastic pollution: Behavior, microbial ecology, and remediation technologies. *Journal of Cleaner Production*, •••, 125240.

Rathi, A., Basu, S., & Barman, S. (2019). Adsorptive removal of fipronil from its aqueous solution by modified zeolite HZSM-5: Equilibrium, kinetic and thermodynamic study. *Journal of Molecular Liquids*, *283*, 867–878. doi:10.1016/j.molliq.2019.02.140

Ratola, N., Ramos, S., Homem, V., Silva, J. A., Jiménez-Guerrero, P., Amigo, J. M., Santos, L., & Alves, A. (2016). Using air, soil and vegetation to assess the environmental behaviour of siloxanes. *Environmental Science and Pollution Research International*, *23*(4), 3273–3284. doi:10.100711356-015-5574-4 PMID:26490903

Ryan, P. G., Weideman, E. A., Perold, V., Durholtz, D., & Fairweather, T. P. (2020). A trawl survey of seafloor macrolitter on the South African continental shelf. *Marine Pollution Bulletin*, *150*, 110741. doi:10.1016/j.marpolbul.2019.110741 PMID:31785848

Sekino, T., Takahashi, S., & Takamasu, K. (2012). Fundamental study on nanoremoval processing method for microplastic structures using photocatalyzed oxidation. *Key Engineering Materials*, *523*, 610–614. doi:10.4028/www.scientific.net/KEM.523-524.610

Setälä, O., Fleming-Lehtinen, V., & Lehtiniemi, M. (2014). Ingestion and transfer of microplastics in the planktonic food web. *Environmental Pollution*, *185*, 77–83. doi:10.1016/j.envpol.2013.10.013 PMID:24220023

Shang, J., Chai, M., & Zhu, Y. (2003). Solid-phase photocatalytic degradation of polystyrene plastic with TiO2 as photocatalyst. *Journal of Solid State Chemistry*, *174*(1), 104–110. doi:10.1016/S0022-4596(03)00183-X

Sharma, S., Basu, S., Shetti, N. P., Nadagouda, M. N. & Aminabhavi, T. M. (2020). Microplastics in the environment: Occurrence, perils, and eradication. *Chemical Engineering Journal*, *127317*. Advance online publication. doi:10.1016/j.cej.2020.127317 PMID:34017217

Sharma, S., & Chatterjee, S. (2017). Microplastic pollution, a threat to marine ecosystem and human health: A short review. *Environmental Science and Pollution Research International*, *24*(27), 21530–21547. doi:10.100711356-017-9910-8 PMID:28815367

Sharma, S., Kundu, A., Basu, S., Shetti, N. P., & Aminabhavi, T. M. (2020). Sustainable environmental management and related biofuel technologies. *Journal of Environmental Management*, *273*, 111096. doi:10.1016/j.jenvman.2020.111096 PMID:32734892

Siipola, V., Pflugmacher, S., Romar, H., Wendling, L., & Koukkari, P. (2020). Low-cost biochar adsorbents for water purification including microplastics removal. *Applied Sciences (Basel, Switzerland)*, *10*(3), 788. doi:10.3390/app10030788

Singh, B., & Sharma, N. (2008). Mechanistic implications of plastic degradation. *Polymer Degradation & Stability*, *93*(3), 561–584. doi:10.1016/j.polymdegradstab.2007.11.008

Singla, S., Shetti, N. P., Basu, S., Mondal, K., & Aminabhavi, T. M. (2022). Hydrogen production technologies-Membrane based separation, storage and challenges. *Journal of Environmental Management, 302*, 113963. doi:10.1016/j.jenvman.2021.113963 PMID:34700079

Skaf, D. W., Punzi, V. L., Rolle, J. T., & Kleinberg, K. A. (2020). Removal of micron-sized microplastic particles from simulated drinking water via alum coagulation. *Chemical Engineering Journal, 386*, 123807. doi:10.1016/j.cej.2019.123807

Sturm, M. T., Herbort, A. F., Horn, H., & Schuhen, K. (2020). Comparative study of the influence of linear and branched alkyltrichlorosilanes on the removal efficiency of polyethylene and polypropylene-based microplastic particles from water. *Environmental Science and Pollution Research International, 27*(10), 10888–10898. doi:10.100711356-020-07712-9 PMID:31953766

Sulistyo, E. N., Rahmawati, S., Putri, R. A., Arya, N., & Eryan, Y. A. (2020). Identification of the Existence and Type of Microplastic in Code River Fish, Special Region of Yogyakarta. *EKSAKTA: Journal of Sciences and Data Analysis, 20*(1), 85–91.

Ta, A. T., & Babel, S. (2020). Microplastics pollution with heavy metals in the aquaculture zone of the Chao Phraya River Estuary, Thailand. *Marine Pollution Bulletin, 161*, 111747. doi:10.1016/j.marpolbul.2020.111747 PMID:33091841

Thomas, R. T., Nair, V., & Sandhyarani, N. (2013). TiO2 nanoparticle assisted solid phase photocatalytic degradation of polythene film: A mechanistic investigation. *Colloids and Surfaces. A, Physicochemical and Engineering Aspects, 422*, 1–9. doi:10.1016/j.colsurfa.2013.01.017

Van Cauwenberghe, L., Vanreusel, A., Mees, J., & Janssen, C. R. (2013). Microplastic pollution in deep-sea sediments. *Environmental Pollution, 182*, 495–499. doi:10.1016/j.envpol.2013.08.013 PMID:24035457

Verma, R., Singh, S., Dalai, M. K., Saravanan, M., Agrawal, V. V., & Srivastava, A. K. (2017). Photocatalytic degradation of polypropylene film using TiO2-based nanomaterials under solar irradiation. *Materials & Design, 133*, 10–18. doi:10.1016/j.matdes.2017.07.042

Von Moos, N., Burkhardt-Holm, P., & Köhler, A. (2012). Uptake and effects of microplastics on cells and tissue of the blue mussel Mytilus edulis L. after an experimental exposure. *Environmental Science & Technology, 46*(20), 11327–11335. doi:10.1021/es302332w PMID:22963286

Wang, F., Zhang, M., Sha, W., Wang, Y., Hao, H., Dou, Y., & Li, Y. (2020). Sorption behavior and mechanisms of organic contaminants to nano and microplastics. *Molecules (Basel, Switzerland), 25*(8), 1827. doi:10.3390/molecules25081827 PMID:32316227

Wang, J., Tan, Z., Peng, J., Qiu, Q., & Li, M. (2016). The behaviors of microplastics in the marine environment. *Marine Environmental Research, 113*, 7–17. doi:10.1016/j.marenvres.2015.10.014 PMID:26559150

Wang, L., Kaeppler, A., Fischer, D., & Simmchen, J. (2019). Photocatalytic TiO2 micromotors for removal of microplastics and suspended matter. *ACS Applied Materials & Interfaces, 11*(36), 32937–32944. doi:10.1021/acsami.9b06128 PMID:31429262

Watts, A. J. R., Urbina, M. A., Corr, S., Lewis, C., & Galloway, T. S. (2015). Ingestion of plastic microfibers by the crab Carcinus maenas and its effect on food consumption and energy balance. *Environmental Science & Technology*, *49*(24), 14597–14604. doi:10.1021/acs.est.5b04026 PMID:26529464

Watts, A. J. R., Urbina, M. A., Goodhead, R., Moger, J., Lewis, C., & Galloway, T. S. (2016). Effect of microplastic on the gills of the shore crab Carcinus maenas. *Environmental Science & Technology*, *50*(10), 5364–5369. doi:10.1021/acs.est.6b01187 PMID:27070459

Wright, S. L., Rowe, D., Thompson, R. C., & Galloway, T. S. (2013). Microplastic ingestion decreases energy reserves in marine worms. *Current Biology*, *23*(23), R1031–R1033. doi:10.1016/j.cub.2013.10.068 PMID:24309274

Ye, S., Cheng, M., Zeng, G., Tan, X., Wu, H., Liang, J., Shen, M., Song, B., Liu, J., Yang, H., & Zhang, Y. (2020). Insights into catalytic removal and separation of attached metals from natural-aged microplastics by magnetic biochar activating oxidation process. *Water Research*, *179*, 115876. doi:10.1016/j.watres.2020.115876 PMID:32387922

Zhang, C., Chen, X., Wang, J., & Tan, L. (2017). Toxic effects of microplastic on marine microalgae Skeletonema costatum: Interactions between microplastic and algae. *Environmental Pollution*, *220*, 1282–1288. doi:10.1016/j.envpol.2016.11.005 PMID:27876228

Zhang, H., Kuo, Y. Y., Gerecke, A. C., & Wang, J. (2012). Co-release of hexabromocyclododecane (HBCD) and nano- and microparticles from thermal cutting of polystyrene foams. *Environmental Science & Technology*, *46*(20), 10990–10996. doi:10.1021/es302559v PMID:23013539

Zhang, P., Tan, X., Liu, S., Liu, Y., Zeng, G., Ye, S., Yin, Z., Hu, X., & Liu, N. (2019). Catalytic degradation of estrogen by persulfate activated with iron-doped graphitic biochar: Process variables effects and matrix effects. *Chemical Engineering Journal*, *378*, 122141. doi:10.1016/j.cej.2019.122141

Zhang, Y., Diehl, A., Lewandowski, A., Gopalakrishnan, K., & Baker, T. (2020). Removal efficiency of micro-and nanoplastics (180 nm–125 μm) during drinking water treatment. *The Science of the Total Environment*, *720*, 137383. doi:10.1016/j.scitotenv.2020.137383 PMID:32325555

Chapter 5
Current Status and Future Challenges of Microplastics in the Agroecosystems

Huadong Zang
China Agricultural University, China

Jie Zhou
China Agricultural University, China

Yihan Lv
China Agricultural University, China

Yaddong Yang
China Agricultural University, China

Zhaohai Zeng
China Agricultural University, China

ABSTRACT

It is unavoidable that microplastics (MPs; <5 mm in diameter) are becoming widespread in agroecosystem. However, these changes act upon the agroecosystem with far-reaching but poorly understood consequences on ecosystem functions and subsequent plant-soil health. MPs could change a broad of essential soil biogeochemical processes by effecting soil properties, forming specific microbial hotspots, inducing diversed influences on microbial functions. The physical damage or chemical toxicity on soil organisms and plants caused by MPs may influence plant health. Due to the C contained in MPs, it contributes to the accumulation of soil organic matter as well dissolved organic matter. This further stimulates microbial activity and consequently CO2 and N2O emissions. Enhanced soluble C released from the decomposition of bioplastics increases microbial nutrient immobilizatization and thus causes competition between plants and microbes. Although MPs may confer some benefits in agroecosystems, it is thought that these will be far outweighed by the potential disbenefits.

DOI: 10.4018/978-1-7998-9723-1.ch005

INTRODUCTION

Nowadays, we live in a plastic world as various types, shapes, and sizes of plastics are everywhere (Jamieson et al., 2019). The high demand for plastics from the second industrial revolution has mainly been met by a high supply from the plastic industries, which reached up to 359 million tonnes in 2018 (PlasticsEurope, 2019). Since 79% would be landfilled or abandoned on Earth (de Lorenzo et al., 2018), these contaminants are thus considered as a global concern (Rillig et al., 2020). Due to the constant release but lower degradability of plastic debris in the environment, it causes a large accumulation of plastics in the environment (Geyer et al., 2017).

Plastics' final sinks are the ocean, therefore, scientists have been showing the environmental fates, potential ecological risks, and analytical methods for plastic determination in the past decades (Galloway et al., 2017; Sharma et al., 2022; Zhou et al., 2022). However, around 80% of plastic debris comes from the terrestrial ecosystem, which could be much more compared with the ocean (Nizzetto et al., 2016). When released into the soil, plastic wastes would be fragmented into particles with smaller sizes such as microplastics (MPs, <5 mm) or even nanoplastics (<100 nm) by mechanical abrasion, UV exposure, and biological weathering (He et al., 2018). Because of their inert polymer chains, MPs are ubiquitous in soils and eventually would drive alterations in soil quality, microbial community and structure, ecosystem function, and plant health (Rillig and Lehmann, 2020; Zhou et al., 2021b). Although recent studies have answered many questions, there are no consistent results on the effects of MPs on plant-microbe-soil interactions without systematic comparisons. It is also a big challenge to determine the ecological impacts of MPs in the agroecosystems where plants might uptake some of these tiny particles, inducing a potential risk in the food chain. Environmental risks with liberal petroleum-based plastic application have resulted in the requirement for biodegradable alternatives which are considered as eco-friendly plastics due to their easy degradability and lower ecotoxicity in ecosystems (Haider et al., 2019). The released monomers of this degradation can further be metabolized and incorporated into microbial biomass (Zumstein et al., 2018). However, such environmentally degradable plastics are not fully evaluated concerning their influences on plant-microbe-soil interactions and subsequent ecosystem functions in agroecosystems (Qi et al., 2020; Zhou et al., 2021a). As a consequence, it is crucial to assess the impacts of MPs on plant-microbe-soil interactions, soil biogeochemical cycles, and greenhouse gas emissions to gain a better understanding of this emerging contaminant in the agroecosystems.

Source and Mitigation

Agroecosystems have been determined as the most important source of MPs pollution. Based on literature reports, MPs can enter the soils either through primary or secondary pathways (Figure 1). The primary MPs mainly comes from the inputs of compost (Corradini et al., 2019), sludge (Crossman et al., 2020), irrigation (Sighicelli et al., 2018), while the secondary MPs mainly originate from plastic mulch films (Liu et al., 2014; Zhang and Liu, 2018). The fragmentation of secondary MPs can originate from agricultural practices, or environmental exposure to sunlight and temperatures (Horton et al., 2017). As a consequence, MPs in soils may appear in the form of particles, fibers, films, and beads, presenting a variety of shapes and compositions (Rillig et al., 2019b). Given that plastic mulching is intensively used to promote crop yields, agricultural lands would be highly influenced by microplastic films (Liu et al., 2014). It was reported that up to 550,800 tonnes of plastic film residues accumulated in agroecosystems from 1982 to 2011 based on a nationwide projection in China (Huang et al., 2020). The abundance of

MPs came up to 1.5×10^4 pieces kg^{-1} soil in the topsoil of a vegetable field from central China (Zhou et al., 2019). In Australia, the abundance of MPs reached 67.5 mg kg^{-1} in the topsoil (Fuller and Gautam, 2016). Likewise, the use of slow-release fertilizers is another source of MPs in soils (Stubenrauch and Ekardt, 2020). Previous studies also documented that the weight of plastic particles could be decreased by around 262,500 tonnes in the next 20 years in Europe without using plastics particles as fertilizer additives or coating (European Chemicals Agency, 2019). In addition, atmospheric deposition is another important source of MPs entering the agroecosystems (Liu et al., 2020). For example, around 29-280 particles m^{-2} per day of plastics were deposited in urban environment in 2014 in Paris (Dris et al., 2016).

After entering the soils, MPs can migrate to long distances from contaminated areas to remote places (Kundu et al., 2021; Sharma et al., 2021), and may leach into groundwater through biogenic activities and water infiltration (Figure 1) (Rillig et al., 2017; Chae and An, 2018). It has also been reported that MPs can accumulate in the food chain and become toxic to a wide array of organisms (de Souza Machado et al., 2019). The deposition and movement of MPs in soils are influenced by both biota activities and artificial disturbances (i.e. tillage). The main contribution to downward and horizontal transportation are biopores created by soil biota or soil cracking (Rillig et al., 2017) and farm management (e.g. harvesting and ploughing) (Paustian et al., 1997). Besides, this movement could also be influenced by the sizes and shapes of MPs (Rillig et al., 2017). Since nano-MPs have a larger ratio of surface area-to-volume and colloidal mobility compared to MPs, it would cause a stronger adsorption affinity to other pollutants and thus they serve as pollutant carriers to promote their transportation, consequently exhibiting a stronger toxic effect on soil organisms (Alimi et al., 2018). Therefore, MPs are ubiquitously present leaving almost no clean soil on Earth (Allen et al., 2019), which, in turn, raises concerns about the potential impacts of MPs on ecosystem functioning and plant-soil health (He et al., 2018).

Plant Health

The accumulated MPs in soils could migrate in plants, and then be transported into the food chain, ultimately posing risks to human health (Cole et al., 2016). So far, a diverse array of impacts has been documented within various plants species under MPs pollution, including stimulation or inhibition of plant growth and seed germination rate (Figure 2, 3; Table 1) (see review in Rillig et al., 2019b and Wang et al., 2022). This variation of individual plant responses could be explained by the direct physical and chemical effects, as well as the indirect alteration in soil physio-chemical properties and regulation of rhizosphere microorganisms (Rillig et al., 2019a; Zhou et al., 2021b).

The direct influences of MPs on plants are reported on two sides: physical damage and chemical toxicity (Rillig et al., 2019b; Lian et al., 2021). On the one hand, MPs can adhere to the root surface, establish obstruction in the space between root cells, and/or enter the plant tissues (Gao et al., 2019; Wang et al., 2020). In support of this, Bosker et al. (2019) found a 78% reduction in seed germination after 8 h exposure to MPs. On the other hand, various organic and inorganic additives are contained in the MPs, e.g., plasticizers, antioxidants, dyes, flame-retardants, and heavy metals (Cole et al., 2016; Hahladakis et al., 2018), which could be released into the soil. Additionally, MPs are considered as carriers or vectors of many chemical contaminants in soils (i.e. Cd^{2+}) (Bakir et al., 2016), which cause a chemical toxic to the plant and thus inhibit its' growth and performance. Specifically, nano-MPs are believed to not only obscure the connections between cells responsible for uptaking and transporting nutrients (Jiang et al., 2019), but also inhibit the disease resistance of crops (Lian et al., 2021).

The influence of MPs on plant is also attributed to the changes in soil properties, e.g., bulk density and soil moisture, due to the lower density (Lozano and Rillig, 2020). This, in turn, decreases the root penetration resistance and enhances aeration (de Souza Machado et al., 2019). Moreover, it facilitates resource (i.e. water and nutrient) supply to plants, thus increasing plant biomass (Rillig et al., 2019a), as proved by higher fine root length (Lehmann et al., 2021). On the contrary, MPs can affect the soil structure, reduce the soil O_2 diffusion and water evaporation, then inhibit crop growth (Zhang and Liu, 2018; Wan et al., 2019). Changes in soil porosity and water transport due to MPs could also inhibit aerobic microorganisms in the rhizosphere (Rubol et al., 2013), such as nitrogen (N) fixing bacteria, arbuscular mycorrhizal fungi (AMF) (Rillig et al., 2019a). The alteration in AMF colonization would then influence the interaction between carbon (C) allocation and nutrient uptake in the soil (Smith and Read, 2010; Zhou et al., 2020), consequently impacting crop growth. Moreover, the relatively high C content of biodegradable MPs would increase the soil C:N ratio, promote microbial N immobilization, and thereby inhibit the growth and nutrient uptake of other soil microorganisms and plants (Figure 3c). Therefore, these inconsistent results induced by MPs call for further studies to understand the intervention of MPs in the soil, and to clarify the underlying mechanism of MPs influence on plant growth and productivity.

Microbial Community and Functions

Soil microorganisms are indispensable players for food production and climate regulation. Previously, Zang et al. (2020a) showed that polyethylene (PE) and polyvinyl chloride (PVC) increased microbial biomass as indicated by the increased total amount of phospholipid fatty acids. However, Fei et al. (2020) showed that PE and PVC decreased the activity and diversity of soil bacterial community in the topsoil of farmland in China. This variation in the microbial activity and diversity induced by MPs could be explained in four main aspects (Table 2). One is by changing the soil physio-chemical properties during MPs degradation as mentioned above (Figure 1), thereby changing the microbial living environment, as a consequence driving alterations in microbial community structures and functions (Rillig et al., 2019b; Lozano et al., 2021). Secondly, MPs provide adsorption sites for microorganisms, allowing them to adsorb for a long time to form microbial hotspots (Zettler et al., 2013; Zhou et al., 2021a). Because of the large specific surface area of MPs, heavy metals, and organic pollutants as mentioned in section Plant Health will be adsorbed on the surface (Shen et al., 2019). These pollutants migrate with the MPs, thereby changing the soil microbial community and biodiversity (Wang et al., 2020). In addition, MPs may also become a transport carrier for pathogenic bacteria thus affecting soil quality (Huang et al., 2020). Thirdly, MPs are harmful to soil organisms directly due to toxic additives (Kim et al., 2021). Especially smaller or high concentrations of MPs can induce stress on plant growth and alter metabolic processes (Büks et al., 2020). MPs can further directly influence soil microbes via its' breakdown products. Since biodegradable MPs can be broken down into labile monomers, it serves as a C source and energy for microbes and thus stimulates microbial growth (Figure 3e). Finally, MPs could alter the root exudates and soil microbial metabolites to facilitate the new dominant microbial formation (Dong et al., 2021). Furthermore, the different characteristics of polymers used in different case studies could also alter the response of microbial activity to MPs. In line with this, beads and films caused stronger impacts on bacterial community compared to the naturally occurring shapes (i.e. fibers) (Sun et al., 2020). Because of the narrow studies, however, the magnitudes and directions of MPs with diverse types, sizes, concentrations, and shapes on soil microbial communities remain unclear.

The alterations in microbial communities may further influence the metabolic functional diversity (Feng et al., 2021). For instance, MPs-induced changes in metabolic functions may enhance the ability of bacteria to exploit polymers or additives as C sources (Kim et al., 2021), since the abundance of xenobiotics was affected by MPs (Feng et al., 2022). Also, soil C and N cycling were altered under MPs polluted soils, given that the lipid metabolism, amino acid metabolism, metabolism of terpenoids, and polyketides were increased (Neis et al., 2015). Although normally inert, MPs are mainly composed of C, which partly leaches as dissolved organic C (DOC) before being degraded by microorganisms (Romera-Castillo et al., 2018). This DOC could serve as an energy resource (Rillig, 2018), thus altering enzyme production as shown in Table 2. However, the impacts of MPs on soil enzyme activities show great differences. For example, while some studies showed that PVC and PE (1-20%, w/w) inhibit β-glucosidase and cellobiohydrolase (Zang et al., 2020a), others found that 28% of PP (polypropylene) stimulate the activities of phenol oxidase (Liu et al., 2017). Variations between studies can be explained by the different types, concentrations, sizes, and shapes of MPs used in the studies. Therefore, research about microbial metabolomics and functions are required to clarify the changes in soil ecosystem multifunctionality induced by MPs.

Soil Earthworm

Soil fauna, and in particular earthworm abundance, plays an important role in soil functions. Although lower concentrations of PE (less than 0.5%) did not affect the growth and survival of the earthworm *E. Foetida*, high levels of input (1-2%) resulted in a higher mortality rate and lower growth rate of earthworm (Cao et al., 2017). This was consistent with Huerta Lwanga et al. (2016) who found that a low amount of MPs had little influence on earthworms, but higher concentrations inhibited the growth of earthworms and increased their mortality. Taken together, the effects of MPs on earthworm was concentration-dependent. Given that earthworms can transport MPs in soil, incorporating MPs into soil via casts, burrows, and adherence to the earthworm's exterior thus leading to potential risks of exposure for other soil biotas (Huerta Lwanga et al., 2017; Rillig et al., 2017). Although bio-MPs are intrinsically less toxic than conventional plastics when applied at the same concentrations (1%, w/w), bio-MPs derived from starch-based films had more intensive effects on earthworm growth than conventional low-density polyethylene films (Qi et al., 2018). Although the exact damage to earthworms through ingestion of MPs is not yet clear, negative effects are inevitable.

Soil Biogeochemical Cycles

Soil Physical Properties

The existing evidence has revealed that the effect of MPs on soil properties depends on types, size, shape, and concentrations of MPs (Figure 3). For example, MPs with fibers significantly decreased soil bulk density and water-stable aggregates, as well as increased water-holding capacity and evapotranspiration, while other shapes of MPs, such as polyethylene fragments or polyamide beads had no effects on soil structures (de Souza Machadoet al., 2018, 2019). Similarly, Lozano et al. (2021) determined the impacts of MPs with different shapes on soil physical properties, and found that fibers increase water holding capacity, films decrease soil bulk density, while foams and fragments increase soil aeration and macroporosity. Not only shape-dependent, but the effect of MPs on soil properties is also size-dependent.

For example, Zhang et al. (2019) found that MPs (<5 μm) increased the volume of >30 μm pores and reduced the volume of <30 μm pores in clay soil. Also, water-stable aggregates significantly decreased with increasing polyester concentrations (de Souza Machado et al., 2018b). Likewise, higher concentrations of microfilms also reduced soil aggregation (de Souza Machado et al., 2019). In short, MPs with smaller sizes and higher concentrations pose stronger adverse effects on soil properties.

Soil Carbon Cycles

The MPs are high-C polymers with a C content of more than 90% (Rillig, 2018), which may induce a hidden contribution to soil organic matter (SOM) (Zhou et al., 2021b). Although SOM is closely associated with soil fertility and plant growth (Yan et al., 2021, 2022), the effects of MPs on SOM until now have only received limited attention (Zhang and Zhang, 2020). It has been reported that effects of MPs include SOM pool accumulation (Liu et al., 2017; Chen et al., 2020), inhibition (Dong et al., 2021), or no substantial changes (Zhou et al., 2021a). These inconsistent results indicated there are drivers regulating MPs effects on SOM. Firstly, MPs in soils vary soil physical properties, such as soil moisture, pH, and soil aggregation as discussed above. This, in turn, may facilitate the metabolism of specific microorganisms to accelerate the accumulation or inhibition of SOM (Wen et al., 2019; Figure 3). Although the majority of MPs-C is considered unavailable to microorganisms, previous studies have suggested that MPs present in soil might induce profound impacts on soil microorganisms due to the living plastic-degrading bacteria and pathogens in the MPs-polluted soils (Huang et al., 2020; Rillig, 2018). Besides SOM pools, soil dissolved organic matter (DOM), which is a sensitive indicator of soil quality changes, is more studied in the previous studies (Liu et al., 2017; Zhou et al., 2021a). In our literature review, we even found that the low amount of MPs increased the formation of DOC, while high-level of MPs had neutral impacts on DOC contents (Figure 3d, e). Moreover, rhizodeposition, as the main way for organic C to enter soils (Pausch and Kuzyakov, 2018; Zang et al., 2019), will be affected by the MPs in soils (Rillig et al., 2021b), either by the decreased plant growth and photosynthesis or the altered AMF colonization (Figure 2). In addition, MPs (especially bioplastics) can also be mineralized by some specific bacteria and then release soluble C into the soils. For instance, 10% (w/w) of PHBV enhanced the content of DOC (Zhou et al., 2021a). These findings suggest that MPs indeed affect the soil C pools, while the impact of MPs under environmental conditions is not well understood.

Soil Nutrient Cycles

The MPs also affected mineral nutrients (e.g., N and P), which are the foundation of plant growth and health (Achari and Kowshik, 2018; Wang et al., 2021). It has been shown that MPs increased, decreased, or did not affect soil nutrients (see Figure 3), which could be explained by two mechanisms. On the one hand, MPs occurring in the soil changed soil nutrient availability through absorption and accumulation due to the large specific surface area and strong hydrophobicity (Rillig et al., 2019b). For instance, PP fixed NH_4^+ through the carbonyl group (-C=O) and hydroxyl group (-OH) on the surface (Green et al., 2016). On the other hand, MPs also affected soil nutrient availability by mediating specific microbes (Rillig et al., 2019a). For example, AMF colonization was altered by MPs (Lehmann et al., 2020), thus indirectly influencing soil available P contents. However, these alterations in AMF colonization are dependent on the size, type, concentration, and shape of MPs. Specifically, the lower amount of MPs (<0-2%, w/w) stimulates the formation of AMF while higher amount of MPs (>2%, w/w) inhibited the

AMF colonization (Figure 3d, e). Lastly, the improved aggregation, changes in soil porosity, and aeration by MPs may accelerate O_2 diffusion in the soil, thus stimulating the nitrification of NH_4^+-N (Lozano et al., 2021). Different from the conventional polymers, the soluble C supply from biodegradable MPs to microorganisms stimulated the microbial N immobilization, as a consequence decreasing the nutrient availability in soils (Rillig et al., 2019a; Zhou et al., 2021a). In short, the effects of MPs on N and P cycles in agroecosystems vary greatly in different studies, and more studies are thus needed to clarify its regulatory mechanisms.

Greenhouse gases emissions

Soil respiration is a process that releases CO_2 from soil through microbial SOM decomposition and root respiration to a large extent (Pausch and Kuzyakov, 2018; Zhou et al., 2021c). That is, soil respiration mainly depends on soil microbial activity (Wen et al., 2020; Zang et al., 2020b), which is sensitive to soil environments, such as soil aggregation and water holding capacity, which can be affected by MPs as discussed above. Although MPs may inhibit the growth of microorganisms, it would increase DOC contents (Gao et al., 2021), which provides energy and resource for microbial SOM decomposition, and, as a consequence enhances the production of CO_2, regardless of low or high concentrations of MPs (Figure 3d, e). However, MPs can adsorb available C to their surfaces and then decrease the production of CO_2 (Rillig et al., 2021b). Furthermore, MPs may inhibit the activities of β-glucosidase and cellobiohydrolase, involved in C cycles (Zang et al., 2020a), and subsequently decrease soil microbial activity (de Souza Machado et al., 2018), as well as the emissions of CO_2. This could explain the neutral or negative response of CO_2 to MPs as shown in our meta-analysis (Figure 3).

Moreover, the presence of MPs herein induced alteration in the SOM, leading to changes in the N_2O emissions. For example, MPs increased soil DOC content, which also stimulated N_2O emissions (Figure 3a). Previous studies have documented that MPs can increase soil pH, which may favor nitrification (Qi et al., 2020; Lazano et al., 2021). MPs also decreased the utilization rate of O_2 due to the increased water content or reduced porosity (de Souza Machado et al., 2018; Boots et al., 2019), leading to incomplete denitrification process and inhibiting N_2O emissions (Jiang et al., 2016). When the O_2 diffusion in soils was enhanced by MPs, the soil oxidation ability would thus enhance (Seeley et al., 2020), which in turn increased oxidation-reduction potential and subsequently improve the oxidation of CH_4. Furthermore, studies have shown that PVC reduces CH_4 emissions by inhibiting hydrolysis, acidification, and methanation (Wei et al., 2019), and larger size of MPs may also reduce the cumulative absorption of CH_4 (Bettas et al., 2014). These deviations indicate that the presence of MPs could pose a potential threat to future climate change.

FUTURE RESEARCH DIRECTIONS

1. MPs are becoming universal in agroecosystems and their abundance is likely to increase in the next decades. Similar to climate warming, N deposition, MPs pollution thus has been a global change factor (Rillig, 2020). Given that global environmental change is a multifactorial phenomenon (Rillig et al., 2019c), there is further a fair chance of simultaneous interaction of MPs pollution and other global change factors, i.e. drought (Lozano et al., 2021). The co-occurrence of several global factors could intensify the impact of every single factor (Rillig et al., 2019c). Although soil microorganisms

are documented to contribute to resistance and resilience against drought and pathogens (Rillig et al., 2019a). This, however, can be challenged if soil microorganisms are influenced by MPs. This uncertainty about the potential for global change to modify the impact of MPs on plant-microbe-soil interactions requires urgent attention, if we would like to fully understand the current and future risks of MPs pollution on sustainable agroecosystems.

2. Although the physical properties of MPs (i.e. size, type, concentration, as well as shape) had variation in the impacts on terrestrial ecosystems (as reviewed by Zhou et al., 2021b), the research is still in the early stage. As shown from our literature review, most studies are focused on the MPs with the size of 1 μm to 5 mm, the effect of nanoplastics (<1 μm) on soil microorganisms, and soil quality and subsequent crop health are still unclear. Apart from that, due to the soluble C contained in the bioplastics, bioplastics may induce a stronger adverse effect on the plant-soil health because of the microbial nutrient immobilization. However, such environmentally degradable plastics are not fully evaluated concerning their effects on plant-microorganisms-soil interactions and subsequent ecosystem functions in agroecosystems. Therefore, further research about the effect of nanoplastics and bioplastics are required to perfect our knowledge gaps on the potential risks of MPs on agroecosystems.
3. Although previous studies documented that MPs may be a hidden contribution to SOM pools (Rillig, 2018), the analytical technology may limit our understanding of the impacts of MPs on SOM and DOM pools, since we could not discriminate the MPs-derived and soil-derived C (Rillig et al., 2021b). This further impedes our understanding and quantification of whether MPs could contribute to soil C pools. Therefore, more efforts are needed to develop analytical methods to trace and separate MPs-derived C from persistent soil-derived C.
4. Although it has been known that MPs can influence soil GHGs (Figure 3), this response depends on MPs' properties and soil conditions, with various magnitudes and directions. Therefore, more lab and field research is needed to focus on the underlying mechanisms for the major driving factors of GHG emissions under MPs.

CONCLUSIONS

Based on our current evidence, we found that MPs can impact plant growth and performance either by physical cell blocking or chemical toxic to soil organisms. The fact that MPs are particles that contain a lot of C, typically around 90%, makes them fairly unique to other pollutants, since they can drive diverse consequences for other element cycles (e.g., N and P). Alterations in structures and soil physical-chemical properties would be expected to change various microbial processes, including those related to N- and P-cycles. Also, the alterations in soil properties, such as controlling the availability of O_2 in the soil, may stimulate the processes of CO_2 and N_2O formations. The enhanced CO_2 and N_2O productions may also be induced by the increased microbial activity due to the increased dissolved organic C content by MPs. Specifically, the C atom contained in the bioplastics can provide soluble C to fuel microbial growth and enzyme activity, induce microbial nutrient immobilization, as a consequence aggravate the plant-microbe competition for essential nutrients (i.e. N and P), thereby inhibiting crop growth and performance. As MPs may transport into the soil with various types, sizes, shapes, and concentrations, a comprehensive understanding of their influences on plant-microbe-soil interactions is mandatory, especially considering the increasing use of plastic worldwide.

ACKNOWLEDGMENT

We are grateful for financial support from the Young Elite Scientists Sponsorship Program by CAST (2020QNRC001) and the earmarked fund for China Agriculture Research System (CARS07-B-5).

REFERENCES

Achari, G. A., & Kowshik, M. (2018). Recent developments on nanotechnology in agriculture: Plant mineral nutrition, health, and interactions with soil microflora. *Journal of Agricultural and Food Chemistry*, *66*(33), 8647–8661. doi:10.1021/acs.jafc.8b00691 PMID:30036480

Alimi, O. S., Farner Budarz, J., Hernandez, L. M., & Tufenkji, N. (2018). Microplastics and nanoplastics in aquatic environments: Aggregation, deposition, and enhanced contaminant transport. *Environmental Science & Technology*, *52*(4), 1704–1724. doi:10.1021/acs.est.7b05559 PMID:29265806

Allen, S., Allen, D., Phoenix, V. R., Le Roux, G., Duranteza, P., Simonneau, A., Stéphane, B., & Galop, D. (2019). Atmospheric transport and deposition of microplastics in a remote mountain catchment. *Nature Geoscience*, *12*(5), 339–344. doi:10.103841561-019-0335-5

Bakir, A., O'Connor, I. A., Rowland, S. J., Hendriks, A. J., & Thompson, R. C. (2016). Relative importance of microplastics as a pathway for the transfer of hydrophobic organic chemicals to marine life. *Environmental Pollution*, *219*, 56–65. doi:10.1016/j.envpol.2016.09.046 PMID:27661728

Bettas, A. G., Tosin, M., Barbale, M., & Degli-Innocenti, F. (2014). Biodegradation of plastics in soil and efects on nitrifcation activity. A laboratory approach. *Frontiers in Microbiology*, *5*, 710–723. PMID:25566223

Blöcker, L., Watson, C., & Wichern, F. (2020). Living in the plastic age - different short-term microbial response to microplastics addition to arable soils with contrasting soil organic matter content and farm management legacy. *Environmental Pollution*, *267*, 115468. doi:10.1016/j.envpol.2020.115468 PMID:32891047

Bolan, N. S., Hedley, M. J., & White, R. E. (1991). Processes of soil acidification during nitrogen cycling with emphasis on legume based pastures. *Plant and Soil*, *134*(1), 53–63. doi:10.1007/BF00010717

Bölscher, T., Paterson, E., Freitag, T., Thornton, B., & Herrmann, A. M. (2017). Temperature sensitivity of substrate-use efficiency can result from altered microbial physiology without change to community composition. *Soil Biology & Biochemistry*, *109*, 59–69. doi:10.1016/j.soilbio.2017.02.005

Boots, B., Russell, C. W., & Green, D. S. (2019). Effects of microplastics in soil ecosystems: Above and below ground. *Environmental Science & Technology*, *53*(19), 11496–11506. doi:10.1021/acs.est.9b03304 PMID:31509704

Bosker, T., Bouwman, L. J., Brun, N. R., Behrens, P., & Vijver, M. G. (2019). Microplastics accumulate on pores in seed capsule and delay germination and root growth of the terrestrial vascular plant Lepidium sativum. *Chemosphere*, *226*, 774–781. doi:10.1016/j.chemosphere.2019.03.163 PMID:30965248

Büks, F., Schaik, N. L. V., & Kaupenjohann, M. (2020). What do we know about how the terrestrial multicellular soil fauna reacts to microplastic? *Soil (Göttingen)*, *6*(2), 245–267. doi:10.5194oil-6-245-2020

Cao, D., Wang, X., Luo, X., Liu, G., & Zheng, H. (2017). Effects of polystyrene microplastics on the fitness of earthworms in an agricultural soil. *IOP C Ser. Earth Env.*, *61*, 012148.

Chae, Y., & An, Y. J. (2018). Current research trends on plastic pollution and ecological impacts on the soil ecosystem: A review. *Environmental Pollution*, *240*, 387–395. doi:10.1016/j.envpol.2018.05.008 PMID:29753246

Cole, M., Lindeque, P. K., Fileman, E., Clark, J., Lewis, C., Halsband, C., & Galloway, T. S. (2016). Microplastics alter the properties and sinking rates of zooplankton faecal pellets. *Environmental Science & Technology*, *50*(6), 3239–3246. doi:10.1021/acs.est.5b05905 PMID:26905979

Corradini, F., Meza, P., Eguiluz, R., Casado, F., Huerta-Lwanga, E., & Geissen, V. (2019). Evidence of microplastic accumulation in agricultural soils from sewage sludge disposal. *The Science of the Total Environment*, *671*, 411–420. doi:10.1016/j.scitotenv.2019.03.368 PMID:30933797

Crossman, J., Hurley, H. H., Futter, M., & Nizzetto, L. (2020). Transfer and transport of microplastics from biosolids to agricultural soils and the wider environment. *The Science of the Total Environment*, *724*, 138334. doi:10.1016/j.scitotenv.2020.138334 PMID:32408466

de Lorenzo, V. (2018). Environmental Microbiology to the Rescue of Planet Earth. *Environmental Microbiology*, *20*(6), 1910–1916. doi:10.1111/1462-2920.14105 PMID:29575463

de Souza Machado, A. A., Lau, C. W., Till, J., Kloas, W., Lehmann, A., Becker, R., & Rillig, M. C. (2018). Impacts of microplastics on the soil biophysical environment. *Environmental Science & Technology*, *52*(17), 9656–9665. doi:10.1021/acs.est.8b02212 PMID:30053368

de Souza Machado, A. A., Lau, C. W., Kloas, W., Bergmann, J., Bacheher, J. B., Faltin, E., Becker, R., Goerlich, A. S., & Rillig, M. C. (2019). Microplastics can change soil properties and affect plant performance. *Environmental Science & Technology*, *53*(10), 6044–6052. doi:10.1021/acs.est.9b01339 PMID:31021077

Dris, R., Gasperi, J., Saad, M., Mirande, C., & Tassin, B. (2016). Synthetic fibers in atmospheric fallout: A source of microplastics in the environment? *Marine Pollution Bulletin*, *104*(1-2), 290–293. doi:10.1016/j.marpolbul.2016.01.006 PMID:26787549

Dong, Y., Gao, M., Qiu, W., & Song, Z. (2021). Effect of microplastics and arsenic on nutrients and microorganisms in rice rhizosphere soil. *Ecotoxicology and Environmental Safety*, *211*, 111899. doi:10.1016/j.ecoenv.2021.111899 PMID:33453641

European Chemicals Agency (ECHA). (2019). *Annex XV Restriction Report. Proposal for a Restriction.* Intentionally Added Microplastics. ECHA.

Feng, X., Wang, Q., Sun, Y., Zhang, S., & Wang, F. (2022). Microplastics change soil properties, heavy metal availability and bacterial community in a Pb-Zn contaminated soil. *Journal of Hazardous Materials*, *424*, 127364. doi:10.1016/j.jhazmat.2021.127364 PMID:34879561

Fuller, S., & Gautam, A. (2016). A procedure for measuring microplastics using pressurized fluid extraction. *Environmental Science & Technology*, *50*(11), 5774–5780. doi:10.1021/acs.est.6b00816 PMID:27172172

Gao, M., Liu, Y., & Song, Z. (2019). Effects of polyethylene microplastic on the phytotoxicity of di-n-butyl phthalate in lettuce (*Lactuca sativa* L. *var. ramosa Hort*). *Chemosphere*, *237*, 124482. doi:10.1016/j.chemosphere.2019.124482 PMID:31398608

Gao, B., Yao, H., Li, Y., & Zhu, Y. (2021). Microplastic addition alters the microbial community structure and stimulates soil carbon dioxide emissions in vegetable-growing soil. *Environmental Toxicology and Chemistry*, *40*(2), 352–365. doi:10.1002/etc.4916 PMID:33105038

Galloway, T. S., Cole, M., & Lewis, C. (2017). Interactions of microplastic debris throughout the marine ecosystem. *Nature Ecology & Evolution*, *1*(5), 1–8. doi:10.103841559-017-0116 PMID:28812686

Geyer, R., Jambeck, J. R., & Law, K. L. (2017). Production, Use, and Fate of All Plastics Ever Made. *Science Advances*, *3*(7), e1700782. doi:10.1126ciadv.1700782 PMID:28776036

Green, D. S., Boots, B., Sigwart, J., Jiang, S., & Rocha, C. (2016). Effects of conventional and biodegradable microplastics on a marine ecosystem engineer (*Arenicola marina*) and sediment nutrient cycling. *Environmental Pollution*, *208*, 426–434. doi:10.1016/j.envpol.2015.10.010 PMID:26552519

Haider, T. P., Völker, C., Kramm, J., Landfester, K., & Wurm, F. R. (2019). Plastics of the future? The impact of biodegradable polymers on the environment and on society. *Angewandte Chemie International Edition*, *58*(1), 50–62. doi:10.1002/anie.201805766 PMID:29972726

Hahladakis, J. N., Velis, C. A., Weber, R., Iacovidou, E., & Purnell, P. (2018). An overview of chemical additives present in plastics: Migration, release, fate and environmental impact during their use, disposal and recycling. *Journal of Hazardous Materials*, *344*, 179–199. doi:10.1016/j.jhazmat.2017.10.014 PMID:29035713

He, L., Wu, D., Rong, H., Li, M., Tong, M., & Kim, H. (2018). Influence of nano- and microplastic particles on the transport and deposition behaviors of bacteria in quartz sand. *Environmental Science & Technology*, *52*, 11545–1155. doi:10.1021/acs.est.8b01673 PMID:30204419

Horton, A. A., Walton, A., Spurgeon, D. J., Lahive, E., & Svendsen, C. (2017). Microplastics in freshwater and terrestrial environments: Evaluating the current understanding to identify the knowledge gaps and future research priorities. *The Science of the Total Environment*, *586*, 127–141. doi:10.1016/j.scitotenv.2017.01.190 PMID:28169032

Hou, J., Xu, X., Yu, H., Xi, B., & Tan, W. (2021). Comparing the long-term responses of soil microbial structures and diversities to polyethylene microplastics in different aggregate fractions. *Environment International*, *149*, 106398. doi:10.1016/j.envint.2021.106398 PMID:33503554

Huang, Y., Zhao, Y., Wang, J., Zhang, M., Jia, W., & Qin, X. (2020). LDPE microplastic films alter microbial community composition and enzymatic activities in soil. *Environmental Pollution*, *254*, 112983. doi:10.1016/j.envpol.2019.112983 PMID:31394342

Huerta Lwanga, E., Gertsen, H., Gooren, H., Peters, P., Salanki, T., van der Ploeg, M., Besseling, E., Koelmans, A. A., & Geissen, V. (2017). Incorporation of microplastics from litter into burrows of Lumbricus terrestris. *Environmental Pollution*, *220*, 523–531. doi:10.1016/j.envpol.2016.09.096 PMID:27726978

Huerta Lwanga, E., Gertsen, H., Gooren, H., Peters, P., Salánki, T., Van, P. M., Besseling, E., Koelmans, A. A., & Geissen, V. (2016). Microplastics in the terrestrial ecosystem: Implications for Lumbricus terrestris (*Oligochaeta, Lumbricidae*). *Environmental Science & Technology*, *50*(5), 2685–2691. doi:10.1021/acs.est.5b05478 PMID:26852875

Jamieson, A. J., Brooks, L. S. R., Reid, W. D. K., Piertney, S. B., Narayanaswamy, B. E., & Linley, T. D. (2019). Microplastics and Synthetic Particles Ingested by Deep-Sea Amphipods in Six of the Deepest Marine Ecosystems on Earth. *Royal Society Open Science*, *6*(2), 180667. doi:10.1098/rsos.180667 PMID:30891254

Jiang, T., Ma, X., Tang, Q., Yang, J., Li, G., & Schuchardt, F. (2016). Combined use of nitrification inhibitor and struvite crystallization to reduce the NH_3 and N_2O emissions during composting. *Bioresource Technology*, *217*, 210–218. doi:10.1016/j.biortech.2016.01.089 PMID:26865057

Jiang, X., Chen, H., Liao, Y., Ye, Z., Li, M., & Klobučar, G. (2019). Ecotoxicity and genotoxicity of polystyrene microplastics on higher plant Vicia faba. *Environmental Pollution*, *250*, 831–838. doi:10.1016/j.envpol.2019.04.055 PMID:31051394

Judy, J. D., Williams, M., Gregg, A., Oliver, D., Kumar, A., Kookana, R., & Kirby, J. K. (2019). Microplastics in municipal mixed-waste organic outputs induce minimal short to long-term toxicity in key terrestrial biota. *Environmental Pollution*, *252*, 522–531. doi:10.1016/j.envpol.2019.05.027 PMID:31167160

Lehmann, A., Leifheit, E. F., Feng, L., Bergmann, J., Wulf, A., & Rillig, M. C. (2020). *Microplastic fiber and drought effects on plants and soil are only slightly modified by arbuscular mycorrhizal fungi*. Soil Ecology Letters., doi:10.100742832-020-0060-4

Lian, J., Liu, W., Meng, L., Wu, J., Zeb, A., Cheng, L., Lian, Y., & Sun, H. (2021). Effects of microplastics derived from polymer-coated fertilizer on maize growth, rhizosphere, and soil properties. *Journal of Cleaner Production*, *318*, 128571. doi:10.1016/j.jclepro.2021.128571

Lozano, Y. M., & Rillig, M. C. (2020). Effects of microplastic fibers and drought on plant communities. *Environmental Science & Technology*, *54*(10), 6166–6173. doi:10.1021/acs.est.0c01051 PMID:32289223

Lozano, Y. M., Aguilar-Trigueros, C. A., Onandia, G., Maaß, S., Zhao, T., & Rillig, M. C. (2021). Effects of microplastics and drought on soil ecosystem functions and multifunctionality. *Journal of Applied Ecology*, *00*(5), 1–9. doi:10.1111/1365-2664.13839

Liu, E., He, W. Q., & Yan, C. (2014). 'White revolution' to 'white pollution' - agricultural plastic film mulch in China. *Environmental Research Letters*, *9*(9), 091001. doi:10.1088/1748-9326/9/9/091001

Liu, H. F., Yang, X. M., Liu, G. B., Liang, C. T., Xue, S., Chen, H., Ritsema, C. J., & Geissen, V. (2017). Response of soil dissolved organic matter to microplastic addition in Chinese loess soil. *Chemosphere*, *185*, 907–917. doi:10.1016/j.chemosphere.2017.07.064 PMID:28747000

Liu, K., Wang, X., Song, Z., Wei, N., & Li, D. (2020). Terrestrial plants as a potential temporary sink of atmospheric microplastics during transport. *The Science of the Total Environment*, *742*, 140523.

Kim, S. K., Kim, J. S., Lee, H., & Lee, H. J. (2021). Abundance and characteristics of microplastics in soils with different agricultural practices: Importance of sources with internal origin and environmental fate. *Journal of Hazardous Materials*, *403*, 123997.

Kundu, A., Shetti, N. P., Basu, S., Reddy, K. R., Nadagouda, M. N., & Aminabhavi, T. M. (2021). Identification and removal of micro- and nano-plastics: Efficient and cost-effective methods. *Chemical Engineering Journal*, *421*, 129816.

Ng, E. L., Huerta Lwanga, E., Eldridge, S. M., Johnston, P., Hu, H. W., Geissen, V., & Chen, D. (2018). An overview of microplastic and nanoplastic pollution in agroecosystems. *The Science of the Total Environment*, *627*, 1377–1388.

Ng, E. L., Lin, S. Y., Dungan, A. M., Colwell, J. M., Ede, S., Lwanga, E. H., Meng, K., Geissen, V., Blackall, L. L., & Chen, D. (2021). Microplastic pollution alters forest soil microbiome. *Journal of Hazardous Materials*, *409*, 124606. doi:10.1016/j.jhazmat.2020.124606 PMID:33246819

Neis, E. P., Dejong, C. H., & Rensen, S. S. (2015). The role of microbial amino acid metabolism in host metabolism. *Nutrients*, *7*(4), 2930–2946. doi:10.3390/nu7042930 PMID:25894657

Nizzetto, L., Futter, M., & Langaas, S. (2016). Are agricultural soils dumps for microplastics of urban origin? *Environmental Science & Technology*, *50*(20), 10777–10779. doi:10.1021/acs.est.6b04140 PMID:27682621

Pausch, J., & Kuzyakov, Y. (2018). Carbon input by roots into the soil: Quantification of rhizodeposition from root to ecosystem scale. *Global Change Biology*, *24*(1), 1–12. doi:10.1111/gcb.13850 PMID:28752603

Paustian, K., Andrén, O., Janzen, H. H., Lal, R., Smith, P., Tian, G., Tiessen, H., Noordwijk, M. V., & Woomer, P. L. (1997). Agricultural soils as a sink to mitigate CO_2 emissions. *Soil Use and Management*, *13*(s4), 230–244. doi:10.1111/j.1475-2743.1997.tb00594.x

Plastics Europe. (2019). *Plastics-the facts*. https://www.plasticseurope.org/application/files/5515/1689/9220/2014plastics the_facts_PubFeb2015.pdf

Qi, Y., Ossowicki, A., Yang, X., Huerta Lwanga, E., Dini-Andreote, F., Geissen, V., & Garbeva, P. (2020). Effects of plastic mulch film residues on wheat rhizosphere and soil properties. *Journal of Hazardous Materials*, *387*, 121711. doi:10.1016/j.jhazmat.2019.121711 PMID:31806445

Qi, Y. L., Yang, X. M., Pelaez, A. M., Lwanga, E. H., Beriot, N., Gertsen, H., Garbeva, P., & Geissen, V. (2018). Macro- and micro- plastics in soil-plant system: Effects of plastic mulch film residues on wheat (*Triticum aestivum*) growth. *The Science of the Total Environment*, *645*, 1048–1056. doi:10.1016/j.scitotenv.2018.07.229 PMID:30248830

Rillig, M. C. (2020). Plastic and plants. *Nature Sustainability*, *3*(11), 1–2. doi:10.103841893-020-0583-9

Rillig, M. C. (2018). Microplastic disguising as soil carbon storage. *Environmental Science & Technology*, *52*(11), 6079–6080. doi:10.1021/acs.est.8b02338 PMID:29757627

Rillig, M. C., & Lehmann, A. (2020). Microplastic in terrestrial ecosystems. *Science*, *368*(6498), 1430–1431. doi:10.1126cience.abb5979 PMID:32587009

Rillig, M. C., Lehmann, A., Machado, A. A. D. S., & Yang, G. (2019a). Microplastic effects on plants. *The New Phytologist*, *223*(3), 1066–1070. doi:10.1111/nph.15794 PMID:30883812

Rillig, M. C., Lehmann, A., Ryo, M., & Bergmann, J. (2019b). Shaping up: Toward considering the shape and form of pollutants. *Environmental Science & Technology*, *53*(14), 7925–7926. doi:10.1021/acs.est.9b03520 PMID:31267727

Rillig, M. C., Ryo, M., Lehmann, A., Aguilar-Trigueros, C. A., Buchert, S., Wulf, A., Iwasaki, A., Roy, J., & Yang, G. (2019c). The role of multiple global change factors in driving soil functions and microbial biodiversity. *Science*, *366*(6467), 886–890. doi:10.1126cience.aay2832 PMID:31727838

Rillig, M. C., Ziersch, L., & Hempel, S. (2017). Microplastic transport in soil by earthworms. *Scientific Reports*, *7*(1), 1362. doi:10.103841598-017-01594-7 PMID:28465618

Rillig, M. C., Hoffmann, M., Lehmann, A., Liang, Y., Lück, M., & Augustin, J. (2021a). Microplastic fibers affect dynamics and intensity of CO_2 and N_2O fluxes from soil differently. *Microplastics and Nanoplastics*, *1*(1), 3. doi:10.118643591-021-00004-0

Rillig, M. C., Leifheit, E., & Lehmann, J. (2021b). Microplastic effects on carbon cycling processes in soils. *PLoS Biology*, *19*(3), e3001130. doi:10.1371/journal.pbio.3001130 PMID:33784293

Rochman, C. M. (2018). Microplastics research - from sink to source. *Science*, *360*(6384), 28–29. doi:10.1126cience.aar7734 PMID:29622640

Rubol, S., Manzoni, S., Bellin, A., & Porporato, A. (2013). Modeling soil moisture and oxygen effects on soil biogeochemical cycles including dissimilatory nitrate reduction to ammonium (DNRA). *Advances in Water Resources*, *62*, 106–124. doi:10.1016/j.advwatres.2013.09.016

Seeley, M. E., Song, B., Passie, R., & Hale, R. C. (2020). Microplastics affect sedimentary microbial communities and nitrogen cycling. *Nature Communications*, *11*(1), 2372. doi:10.103841467-020-16235-3 PMID:32398678

Sighicelli, M., Pietrelli, L., Lecce, F., Iannilli, V., Falconieri, M., Coscia, L., Vito, S. D., Nuglio, S., & Zampetti, G. (2018). Microplastic pollution in the surface waters of Italian Subalpine Lakes. *Environmental Pollution*, *236*, 645–651. doi:10.1016/j.envpol.2018.02.008 PMID:29433105

Sharma, S., Basu, S., Shetti, N. P., Nadagouda, M. N., & Aminabhavi, T. M. (2021). Microplastics in the environment: Occurrence, perils, and eradication. *Chemical Engineering Journal*, *408*, 127317.

Sharma, S., Shetti, N. P., Basu, S., Nadagouda, M. N., & Aminabhavi, T. M. (2022). Remediation of per- and polyfluoroalkyls (PFAS) via electrochemical methods. *Chemical Engineering Journal*, *430*, 132895.

Smith, S. E., & Read, D. J. (2010). *Mycorrhizal symbiosis*. Academic Press.

Stubenrauch, J., & Ekardt, F. (2020). Plastic pollution in soils: Governance approaches to foster soil health and closed nutrient cycles. *Environments*, *7*(5), 38. doi:10.3390/environments7050038

Sun, X. D., Yuan, X. Z., Jia, Y., Feng, L. J., Zhu, F. P., Dong, S. S., Liu, J., Kong, X., Tian, H., Duan, J. L., Ding, Z., Wang, S. G., & Xing, B. (2020). Differentially charged nanoplastics demonstrate distinct accumulation in Arabidopsis thaliana. *Nature Nanotechnology*, *15*(9), 755–760. doi:10.103841565-020-0707-4 PMID:32572228

Wan, Y., Wu, C., Xue, Q., & Hui, X. (2019). Effects of plastic contamination on water evaporation and desiccation cracking in soil. *The Science of the Total Environment*, *654*, 576–582. doi:10.1016/j.scitotenv.2018.11.123 PMID:30447596

Wang, X., Yang, Y. D., Pei, K., Zhou, J., Peixoto, L., Gunina, A., Zeng, Z., Zang, H., Rasmussen, J., & Kuzyakov, Y. (2020). Nitrogen rhizodeposition of legumes and its fate in agroecosystems: Field study and literature review. *Land Degradation & Development*, *32*(1), 410–419. doi:10.1002/ldr.3729

Wei, W., Huang, Q. S., Sun, J., Wang, J.-Y., Wu, S.-L., & Ni, B.-J. (2019). Polyvinyl chloride microplastics affect methane production from the anaerobic digestion of waste activated sludge through leaching toxic bisphenol-A. *Environmental Science & Technology*, *53*(5), 2509–2517. doi:10.1021/acs.est.8b07069 PMID:30758964

Wen, Y., Freeman, B., Ma, Q., Evans, C., Chadwick, D., Zang, H., & Jones, D. (2020). Raising the groundwater table in the non-growing season can reduce greenhouse gas emissions and maintain crop productivity in cultivated fen peats. *Journal of Cleaner Production*, *262*, 121179. doi:10.1016/j.jclepro.2020.121179

Wen, Y., Zang, H., Freeman, B., Musarika, S., Evans, C., Chadwick, D., & Jones, D. (2019). Microbial utilization of low molecular weight organic carbon substrates in cultivated peats in response to warming and soil degradation. *Soil Biology & Biochemistry*, *139*, 107629. doi:10.1016/j.soilbio.2019.107629

Yan, Z. J., Zhou, J., Nie, J. W., Yang, Y. D., Zhao, J., Zeng, Z. H., Marshall, M. R., Peixoto, L., & Zang, H. D. (2021). Do cropping system and fertilization rate change water-stable aggregates associated carbon and nitrogen storage? *Environmental Science and Pollution Research International*, *28*(46), 65862–65871. doi:10.100711356-021-15562-2 PMID:34322806

Yan, Z. J., Zhou, J., Yang, L., Gunina, A., Yang, Y. D., Peixoto, L., Zeng, Z. H., Zang, H. D., & Kuzyakov, Y. (2022). Diversified cropping systems benefit soil carbon and nitrogen stocks by increasing aggregate stability: Results of three fractionation methods. *The Science of the Total Environment*, *824*, 153878. doi:10.1016/j.scitotenv.2022.153878 PMID:35167890

Zang, H., Xiao, M., Wang, Y., Ling, N., Wu, J., Ge, T., & Kuzyakov, Y. (2019). Allocation of assimilated carbon in paddies depending on rice age, chase period and N fertilization: Experiment with $^{13}CO_2$ labelling and literature synthesis. *Plant and Soil*, *445*(1-2), 113–123. doi:10.100711104-019-03995-1

Zang, H., Zhou, J., Marshall, M. R., Chadwick, D. R., Wen, Y., & Jones, D. L. (2020a). Microplastics in the agroecosystem: Are they an emerging threat to the plant-soil system? *Soil Biology & Biochemistry*, *148*, 107926. doi:10.1016/j.soilbio.2020.107926

Zang, H., Blagodatskaya, E., Wen, Y., Shi, L., Cheng, F., Chen, H., Zhao, B., Zhang, F., Fan, M., & Kuzyakov, Y. (2020b). Temperature sensitivity of soil organic matter mineralization decreases with long-term N fertilization: Evidence from four Q_{10} estimation approaches. *Land Degradation & Development, 31*(6), 683–693. doi:10.1002/ldr.3496

Zettler, E. R., Mincer, T. J., & Amaral-Zettler, L. A. (2013). Life in the "plastisphere": Microbial communities on plastic marine debris. *Environmental Science & Technology, 47*(13), 7137–7146. doi:10.1021/es401288x PMID:23745679

Zhang, G. S., & Liu, Y. F. (2018). The distribution of microplastics in soil aggregate fractions in southwestern China. *The Science of the Total Environment, 642*, 12–20. doi:10.1016/j.scitotenv.2018.06.004 PMID:29894871

Zhang, G., & Zhang, F. (2020). Variations in aggregate-associated organic carbon and polyester microfibers resulting from polyester microfibers addition in a clayey soil. *Environmental Pollution, 258*, 113716. doi:10.1016/j.envpol.2019.113716 PMID:31831225

Zhou, B., Wang, J., Zhang, H., & Barceló, D. (2019) Microplastics in agricultural soils on the coastal plain of Hangzhou Bay, east China: multiple sources other than plastic mulching film. *Journal of Hazardous Materials, 388.*

Zhou, J., Zang, H., Loeppmann, S., Gube, M., Kuzyakov, Y., & Pausch, J. (2020). Arbuscular mycorrhiza enhances rhizodeposition and reduces the rhizosphere priming effect on the decomposition of soil organic matter. *Soil Biology & Biochemistry, 140*, 107641. doi:10.1016/j.soilbio.2019.107641

Zhou, J., Gui, H., Banfield, C. C., Wen, Y., Zang, H. D., Dippold, M. A., Charlton, A., & Jones, D. L. (2021a). The microplastisphere: Biodegradable microplastics addition alters soil microbial community structure and function. *Soil Biology & Biochemistry, 156*, 108211. doi:10.1016/j.soilbio.2021.108211

Zhou, J., Wen, Y., Marshall, M. R., Zhao, J., Gui, H., Zeng, Z. H., Jones, D. L., & Zang, H. D. (2021b). Microplastics as an emerging threat to plant and soil health in agroecosystems. *The Science of the Total Environment, 787*, 147444. doi:10.1016/j.scitotenv.2021.147444

Zhou, J., Wen, Y., Shi, L. L., Marshall, M. R., Kuzyakov, Y., Blagodatskaya, E., & Zang, H. D. (2021c). Strong priming of soil organic matter induced by frequent input of labile carbon. *Soil Biology & Biochemistry, 152*, 108069. doi:10.1016/j.soilbio.2020.108069

Zhou, J., Wen, Y., Cheng, H., Zang, H., & Jones, D. L. (2022). Simazine degradation in agroecosystems: Will it be affected by the type and amount of microplastic pollution? *Land Degradation & Development, 33*(7), 1128–1136. Advance online publication. doi:10.1002/ldr.4243

Zumstein, M. T., Schintlmeister, A., Nelson, T. F., Baumgartner, R., Woebken, D., Wagner, M., Kohler, H. P. E., McNeill, K., & Sander, M. (2018). Biodegradation of Synthetic Polymers in Soils: Tracking Carbon into CO_2 and Microbial Biomass. *Science Advances, 4*(7), eaas9024. doi:10.1126ciadv.aas9024 PMID:30050987

APPENDIX

Figures and Tables

Table 1. Effect of microplastics on plant growth and performance

Microplastics				Crop	Index	Effect	Location	Reference
Type	Shape	Size	Concentration					
PE	Beads	125 μm	1%, 5%, 10%, 20% (*w/w*)	Wheat	Shoot and root biomass	-	Gwynedd, Wales, England	Zang et al., 2020
	Beads	23μm	0.25, 0.5, 1 mg L^{-1}	Vegetable	Weight, height	-	/	Gao et al., 2019
	Beads	100-154 μm	0.1%, 1%, 1 0% (*w/w*)	Maize	Biomass	=	Qingdao, China	Wang et al., 2020
HDPE	Beads	<2 mm	0.1%, 0.25%, 0.5%, 1% (*w/w*)	Wheat	Seedling emergence, biomass	=	NSW, Australia	Judy et al., 2019
	Beads	102.6 μm	0.1% (*w/w*)	Perennial ryegrass	Shoot biomass, chlorophyll-a and chlorophyll-b content	=	Westland, Northern Ireland	Boots et al., 2019
					Root biomass, chlorophyll-a/ chlorophyll-b (chla-a/ chl-b) ratio	+		
PVC	Beads	125 μm	1%, 5%, 10%, 20% (*w/w*)	Wheat	Shoot and root biomass	-	Gwynedd, Wales, England	Zang et al., 2020
	Beads	<2 mm	0.01%, 0.1%, 0.25%, 0.5%, 1% (*w/w*)	Wheat	Seedling emergence, biomass	=	NSW, Australia	Judy et al., 2019
	Films	L: 0.5 mm W: 0.5 mm T: 0.008 mm	/	Rice	Biomass, tillers number	-	Haikou City, Hainan, China	Liu et al., 2021
PLA	Beads	65.6 μm	0.1% (*w/w*)	Perennial ryegrass	Germination percentage, plant height	-	Westland, Northern Ireland	Boots et al., 2019
					Shoot biomass (dry weight), chlorophyll-a and chlorophyll-b content	=		
					Chlorophyll-a/ chlorophyll-b (chla-a/ chl-b) ratio	+		
	Beads	100~154 μm	0, 0.1%, 1%, 10% (*w/w*)	Maize	Biomass, chlorophyll content of leaves	-	Qingdao, China	Wang et al., 2020
	Beads	53-1000μm	0.5-2.5% (*w/w*)	Vegetable	Biomass, leaf area	+	Netherlands	Meng et al., 2021
PS	Beads	87 nm	10 mg L^{-1}	Wheat	seedling emergence	+	/	Lian et al., 2020
PHBV	Beads	125μm	10% (*w/w*)	Wheat	Biomass	-	Gottingen, Germany	Zhou et al., 2021a
PET	Beads	<2 mm	0.1%, 0.25%, 0.5%, 1% (*w/w*)	Wheat	Seedling emergence, biomass	=	NSW, Australia	Judy et al., 2019

"+", "-", and "=" means microplastics addition has a positive, negative, and no effect, respectively. "/" means there is no information in the literature. "L" means length; "W" means width; "T" means thickness; unmarked letters mean particle size. PE: Polyethylene; HDPE: High-density polyethylene; LDPE: Low-density polyethylene; PP: Polypropylene; PS: Polystyrene; PVC: Polyvinyl chloride; PET: Polyethylene terephthalate; PLA: Polylactic acid; PHBV, 3-hydroxybutyrate-co-3-hydroxyvalerate.

Table 2. Effect of microplastics on microbial activity and community, as well as enzyme activity depending on the type, shape, size, and concentration of plastics

Microplastics				Microorganisms	Index	Effect	Location	Reference
Type	Shape	Size	Concentration					
PE	/	125 µm	1%, 5%, 10%, 20% (*w/w*)	Microbe	Biomass, carbon utilization efficiency	+	Gwynedd, Wales, England	Zang et al., 2020
	Beads	678 µm	1%, 5% (*w/w*)	Bacteria	Richness, diversity	-	Lin'an, Zhejiang, China	Fei et al., 2020
				BG, NAG, LAP	Activity	-		
				URE, ACP	Activity	+		
				FDAse	Activity	+		
	Beads	100-200 µm	1% (*w/w*)	Bacteria	Diversity and richness	-	/	Yu et al., 2021
LDPE	Films	0.01-2 mm	0.076 g kg^{-1}	Bacteria	Alpha diversities of the microbiota	=	Peking University, China	Huang et al., 2020
	Beads	200~630 µm	1% (*w/w*)	Microbe	Microbial biomass carbon	-	Kleve, Germany	Bl$_0$cker et al., 2020
	Films	0.01-2 mm	0.076 g kg^{-1}	Bacteria	Similarity	-	Peking University, China	Wang et al., 2020
	Beads	678 µm	1%, 5% (*w/w*)	Bacteria	*Nitrogen fixation*	+	Lin'an, Zhejiang, China	Fei et al., 2020
PVC	Beads	18 µm	5% (*w/w*)	Bacteria	Richness, diversity	-	China	Fei et al., 2020
			1% (*w/w*)		Richness, diversity	=		
			1%, 5% (*w/w*)		*Nitrogenfixation*	+		
	Beads	678 18 µm	1%, 5% (*w/w*)	URE, ACP	Activity	+		
				FDAse	Activity	-		
	Beads	<2 mm	0.01%, 0.1%, 0.25%, 0.5%, 1% (*w/w*)	Microbe	Community diversity	=	NSW, Australia	Judy et al., 2019
	Beads	125 µm	1%, 5%, 10%, 20% (*w/w*)	Microbe	Biomass, carbon utilization efficiency	+	Gwynedd, Wales, England	Zang et al., 2020
				BG, NAG, LAP	Activity	=		
PP	Beads	200~630 µm	1% (*w/w*)	Microbe	Activity, community composition	=	Kleve, Germany	Bl$_0$cker et al., 2020
	Beads	<250 µm	28% (*w/w*)	Microbe	Respiration	+	Ansai, Shaanxi, China	Yang et al., 2018
	Beads	100-200 µm	1% (*w/w*)	Bacteria	Diversity and richness	-	/	Yu et al., 2021
	Fibers	/	1%,0.1%,0.3%,1% (*w/w*)	BG	Activity	+	Kunming, China	Guo et al., 2021
				Bacteria	Richness	+		
PLA	Beads	20~50 µm	2% (*w/w*)	Bacteria	Diversity	=	Nanjing, Jiangsu, China	Chen et al., 2020
					Biomass	-		
PET	Beads	<2 mm	0.1%, 0.25%, 0.5%, 1% (*w/w*)	Microbe	Community diversity	=	NSW, Australia	Judy et al., 2019
	Beads	200 µm	0.1%,0.3%,1% (*w/w*)	Bacteria	Diversity	-	Jiangsu, China	Han et al., 2021
HDPE	Beads	<2 mm	0.1%, 0.25%, 0.5%, 1% (*w/w*)	Bacteria	Community diversity	=	NSW, Australia	Judy et al., 2019
PHBV	Beads	125µm	10% (w/w)	Microbe, BG, LAP, ACP	Activity	+	Goettingen, Germany	Zhou et al., 2021a
				Bacteria	*Acidbacteria, Bacteroidetes*	-		

"+", "-", and "=" means microplastics addition has a positive, negative, and no effect, respectively. "/" means there is no information in the literature. PE: Polyethylene; HDPE: High-density polyethylene; LDPE: Low-density polyethylene; PP: Polypropylene; PS: Polystyrene; PVC: Polyvinyl chloride; PET: Polyethylene terephthalate; PLA: Polylactic acid; PHBV, 3-hydroxybutyrate-co-3-hydroxyvalerate.
URE: Urease; ACP: Acid Phosphatase; FDAse: Fluorescein diacetate hydrolase; BG: β-glucosidase; NAG, chitinase; LAP, L-leucine aminopeptidase.

Figure 1. Conceptual figures about the source, mitigation, as well as the effects of microplastics on plant growth, microbes, soil organic matter decomposition, and greenhouse gases emissions

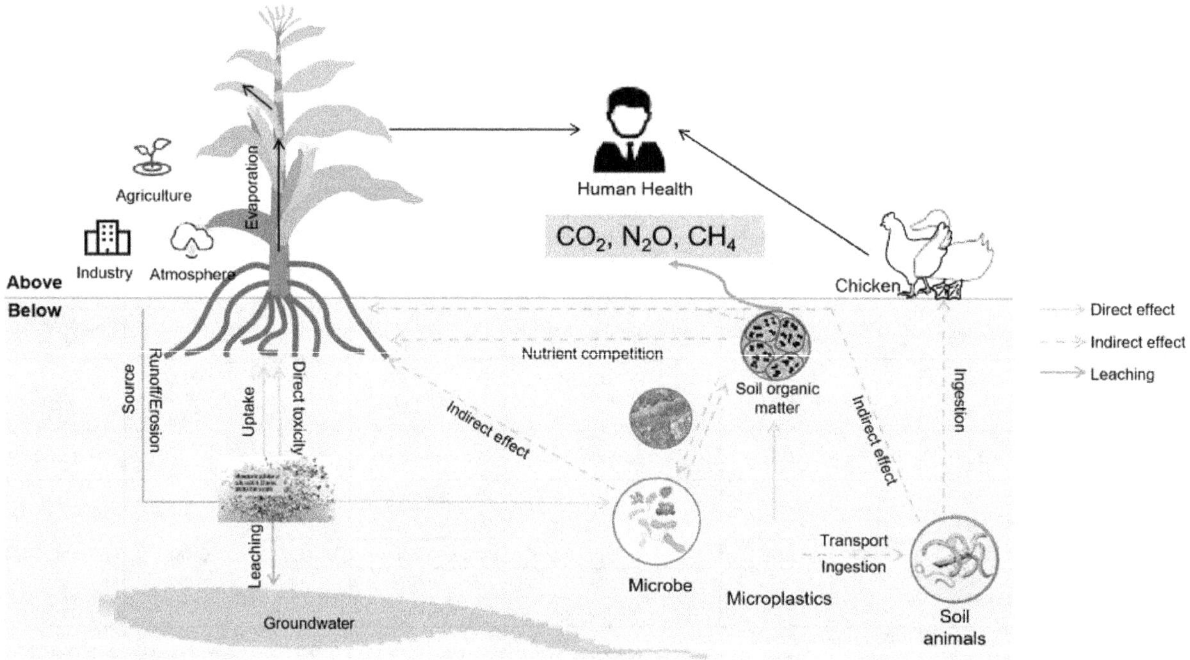

Figure 2. Observations from publications about the effects of microplastics types, shapes, sizes, and concentrations on plant biomass, soil nutrient, and greenhouse gases emissions. Publications we shown in this case were extracted before December 2021. PE: polyethene; PVC, polyvinyl chloride; PS, polystyrene; PET, polyethylene terephthalate; PP, polypropylene; PT, polytetrafluorethylene; PU, polyurethane; PC, polycarbonate; PA, polyamide; PES, poly(ether sulfones); Bioplastics includes polylactic acid (PLA), polylactic acid (PHA), and oly (butyleneadipate-co-terephthalate) (PBAT)

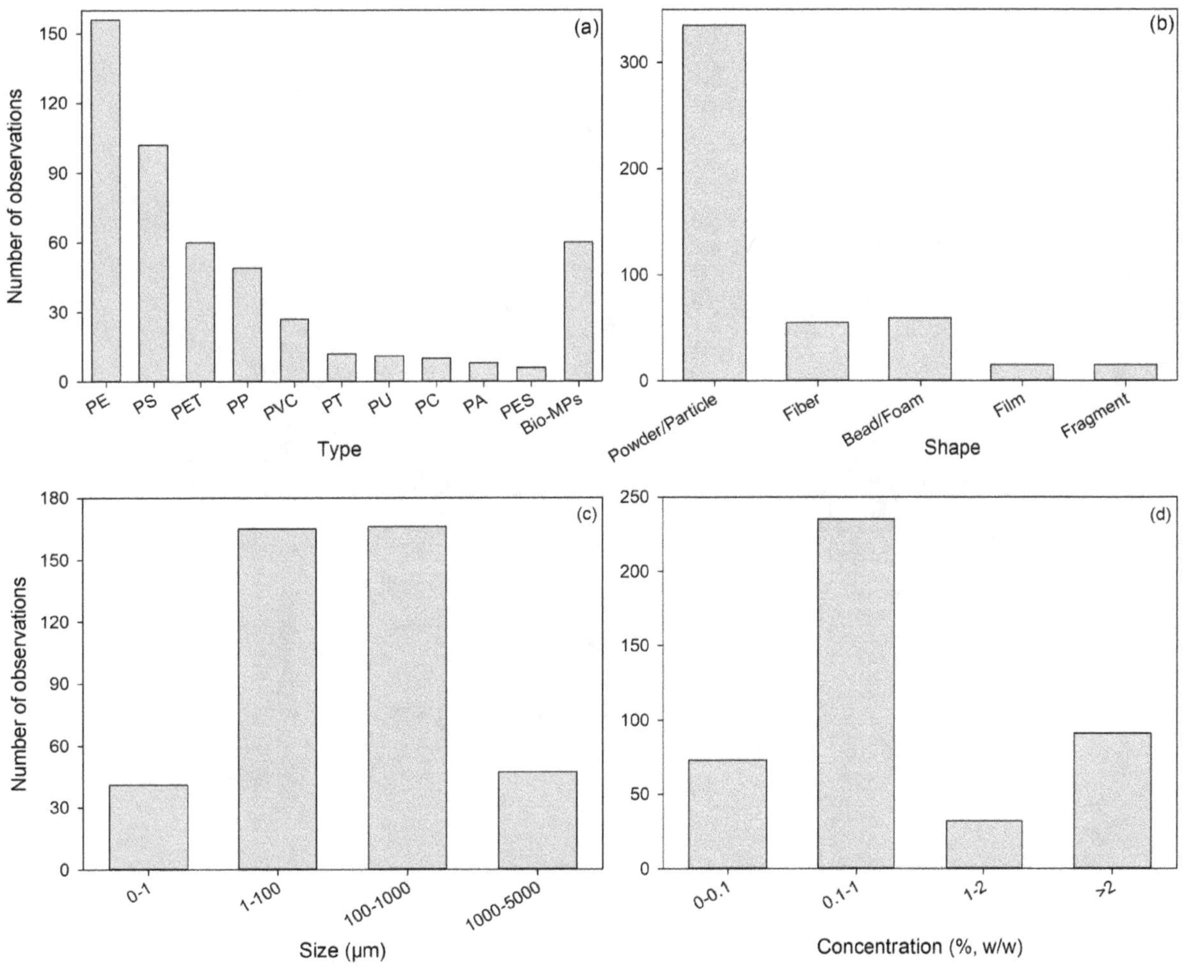

Figure 3. (a) Overall number of reported effects with a significant positive, negative, or neutral response to microplastics. Reported effects based on: microplastics types (conventional v. Biodegradable microplastics) (b, c); amount of microplastics (lower amount, 0-2%, w/w v. high amount, >2%, w/w) (d, e); as well as the microplastic shapes (powder v. fiber) (f, g). Here, the conventional microplastics were identified as polymer-based microplastics including PE, PVC, PS, PP, etc. And biodegradable microplastics identified as biodegradable bioplastics like PHA and PLA that can be broken down by a range of organisms and are not thought to produce any harmful by-products

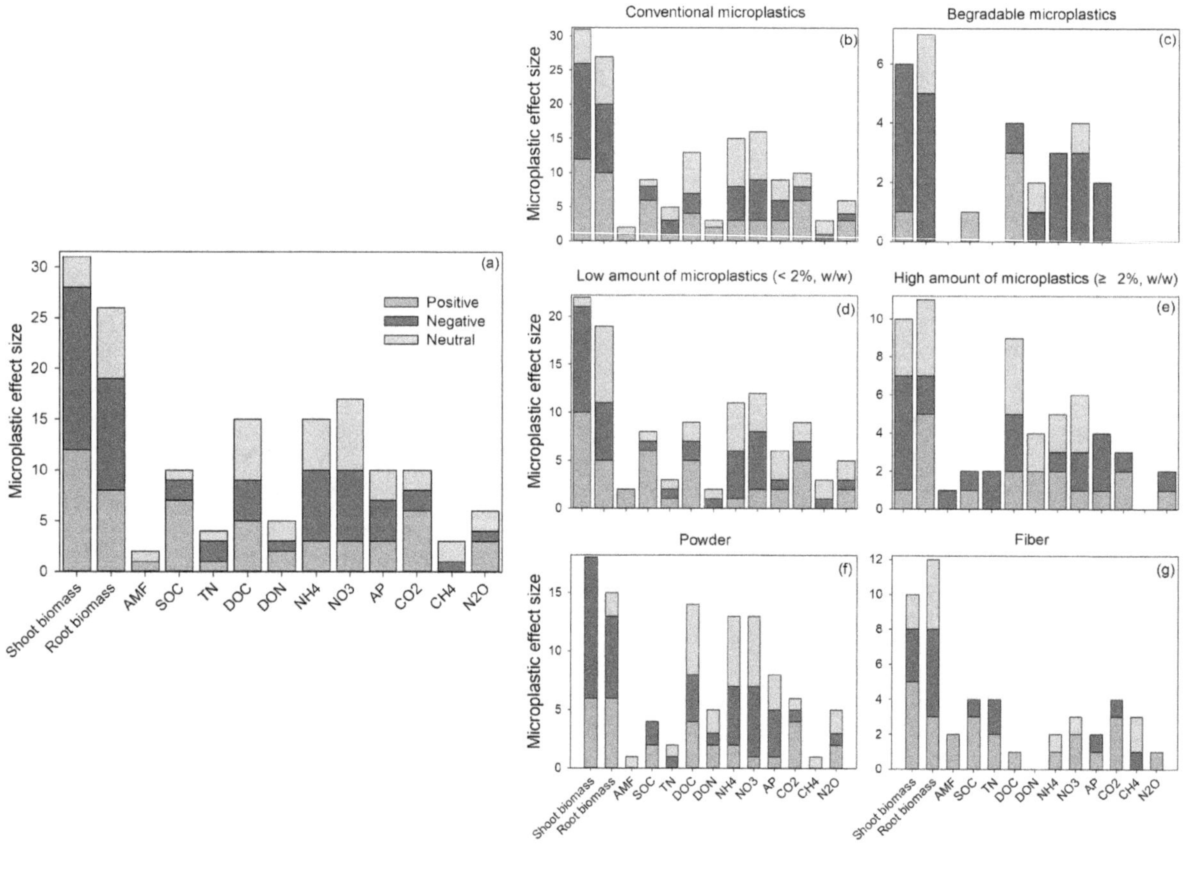

Chapter 6
Preventive Measures for Plastic Pollution

Bupe Getrude Mwanza
https://orcid.org/0000-0002-7456-5181
University of Zambia, Zambia

ABSTRACT

The production of plastics has rapidly overwhelmed the world's ability to manage it, hence the demanding environmental issues on plastics pollution. The negative effects of plastics have become omnipresent and prompted many studies to be conducted leading to a global treaty. This study focused on reviewing measures for preventing plastic pollution in the environment. Based on the literature review approach, seven key measures are identified: recycling prioritization, utilization of bio-based and biodegradable plastics, improvement of waste collection systems, awareness and education in communities, extended producer responsibility (EPR) enforcement, strengthen stakeholder engagement, and technology and innovations. The study concludes by providing practical recommendations that should be implemented contextually.

INTRODUCTION

Plastic pollution is the amassing of plastic particles and objects in the earth's environment thus affecting wildlife and human habitat. Plastic production continues to fuel the amassing of plastic wastes in the environment and this has continued to impact waste management practices globally. Changes in consumer preferences also continue to contribute to the design changes in the life-cycle of plastic products and thus contributing to plastic waste amassing. For example, the production of disposable plastic products is whelming the earth's ability to manage these wastes. Once a product such as 'mineral water' is bought and consumed, the plastic bottle reaches its end-of-life and it has to be disposed of sustainably or unsustainable. In most cases, the disposal is unsustainable and the plastic bottle ends up in the ocean or land. For example, 60 to 95% of marine litter account for plastic debris both in the deep-sea sediments and surface waters (Le Guern, 2018). Annually, between 4.8 and 12.7 million MT is approximated to

DOI: 10.4018/978-1-7998-9723-1.ch006

enter oceans (Jambeck, et al., 2015) while the rest is either landfilled, recycled, incinerated or ends up in other ecosystems (Geyer, 2017).

This study is significant because the production of plastics has continued to boom without a systematic management approach making it increasingly difficult to take away plastic from the environment. With the current challenges presented by plastic pollution, this research is relevant to all the stakeholders in the waste management arena such as the government, manufacturers, formal/informal waste management companies, households, etc. The research provides practical solutions for dealing with plastic wastes and at the same time, contributes theoretically to the body of knowledge. The research is also significant as it tries to use one of the waste management hierarchy aspects "prevention" but at the stage when waste has already been created. Research on preventive measures for plastic pollution is very important and comes at a time when the earth is trying to remedy all the processes and systems that are contributing to global warming. Therefore, there is an urgent need for studies that are focusing on the effects of emerging plastics on the environment and public health.

The objectives of this research are to review the current state of plastic pollution in the natural environment in developed and developing economies. With this general objective, the research establishes and discusses control measures for preventing plastic pollution. The development of bioplastics as a strategy for preventing plastic pollution is also discussed.

The rest of this chapter is organized as follows; the background of the study is discussed in section 2. The research methodology is discussed in section 3 while results and discussion is presented in section 4. Conclusion and recommendations are presented in the last section.

BACKGROUND OF THE STUDY

According to UN Environment Programme Report (2018), globally, every minute, 1.0 million plastic drinking bottles are sold while 5.0 trillion single-use plastic bags are utilized globally per annual. Research has estimated that, more than 8.3 million tons of plastics have been manufactured between 1950 and 2018 (Mortillaro, 2017) with 60% of these plastics having ended up in the natural environment or landfill (UN Environment Programme Report, 2018). Further, 79% of plastics ever produced has been disposed in the dumps, landfills or natural environment while only 9% has been recycled and 12% incinerated (Schmidt, Krauth, & Wagner, 2017; Geyer, 2017). According to Helinski, Poor & Wolfand (2021), plastic pollution prevention is heavily assigned on users through recycling but this is not working as only 9% of the plastics ever produced have been recycled. According to Surfers against sewage (2021) plastic pollution is having plastics where it should not be either in the ocean, bench or natural environment. With this definition and the statistics provided on the current state of plastics on the natural environment, there is an urgent need to prevent the current plastic pollution.

Plastic wastes present many problems once they enter the environment. They endanger and damage ships; cause animal death through ingestion and entanglement; structurally and visually damage freshwater, oceanic and coastal ecosystems; spread invasion diseases and species; and reduce economic gains (Krelling, Williams, & Turra, 2017). Plastics also impact human health in many ways such as, possible internal injury from ingestion of microplastics; accidents; water, air, and food contamination, and pathogen vectors from microplastics (Vethaak & Leslie, 2016; Thompson, Moore, vom Saal, & Swan, 2009).

To address plastic pollution from the environment, numerous strives have been made (¨ohr, et al., 2017) including research studies. Policy interventions and market-based strategies (i.e. levies, bans) have increased in the last 10 years (Schnurr, et al., 2018) and extended producer responsibility (EPR) is a prominent policy strategy that has been proposed for marine plastic pollution reduction (Tibbetts, 2015). Global ingenuities comprise Action Plans (APs) by the G20 and G7 countries (G7, Annex to the Leaders' Declaration, 2015.; G20, G20 Action Plan on Marine Litter, 2017); United Nations Law of the Sea Convention (Vince & Hardesty, 2018); the Honolulu Strategy (Shevealy, Courtney, & Parks, 2011); and the four Sustainable Development Goals important to marine wastes (Haward, 2018).

Despite the implementation of policies and strategic measures to combat the effect of plastic pollution on the environment, the challenges continue but the aspect of scientific research remains confident in pursuing more research for sustainable management of these plastic wastes. Helinski, Poor & Wolfand (2021) developed a framework to aid device capture selection for reducing plastic pollution in freshwater. The study concluded that, before device selection, community buy-in attainment and assessment of whether plastic pollution capture device is necessary should be considered first. Charitou, et al (2021) explored the attitudes and knowledge of the Greek public to marine plastic pollution and the EU Single-Use Plastics Directive. The study recommended the integration of topics on micro-plastics into formal education. Walther, Yen & Hu, (2021) reviewed the policies, strategies and actions for reducing plastic pollution and use as recommended by Taiwan's stakeholders. The study showed how Taiwan has become a comparatively successful example in terms of tackling plastic pollution related problems.

The reviewed studies above attempted to establish strategies or measures for managing plastic pollution. Helinski, Poor & Wolfand (2021) used a technological and innovative approach by indicating the relevance of engaging stakeholders. Charitou et al (2021) focused on the aspect of awareness and education as a measure for managing plastic wastes and Walther, Yen & Hu (2021) focused on policies as measures for reducing plastic pollution. These studies have shown that education and awareness, policy implementation, and technology and innovation are key measures for managing plastic pollution.

Harries, et al (2021) evaluated the influence of EPR packaging policy on shoreline pollution reduction and the study revealed no reduction in pollution from the introduction of EPR policy. To successfully evaluate plastic pollution prevention in the marine environment, it is proposed that, monitoring programs for plastic policy intervention should be tailored to their fixed requirements. Prata, et al (2019) reviewed and discussed strategies for improving waste management and the life-cycle of plastics for implementation to reduce environmental and health impacts caused by plastics as well as reduce plastic pollution. 10 recommendations to stakeholders were suggested for the reduction of plastic pollution. Flury & Narayan (2021) discussed the advantages of biodegradable plastics in integration with proper disposal systems. The study concluded that, while biodegradable plastics should be an essential part of strategies for minimizing environmental plastic pollution, their use and management should be specific to end-of-life scenarios, and disposal must never be an end-of-life option except for agricultural plastic mulches.

For the reviewed studies above, Harris, et al (2021), identified EPR as a key measure for controlling plastic pollution while Prata, et al (2019) recommends 10 strategies that embed the other strategies suggested by other authors such as Helinski, Poor & Wolfand (2021); Charitou et al (2021); Walther, Yen & Hu (2021), Harris, et al (2021) and Flury & Narayan (2021). Flury & Narayan (2021) showed that bio-based and biodegradable plastics should be considered as measures for managing plastic pollution.

Ponis, et al (2020) conducted a systematic meta-review analysis on papers that have used a review approach on the subject of marine plastic pollution (MMP). Based on the objectives that were set, the review identified the research gap that, land-based and water-based composition and sources including social and economic impacts of MMP are still under-reviewed areas despite the potential of the area. Ferraro & Failler (2020) dispenses the difficulties of marine plastic pollution by focusing on the policy feedback at the international level. The study presents many institutional problems in an effort to stop, manage and reduce marine plastic litter at universal level. Four aspects that are critical for an integrated, universal and holistic approach to the problem of plastic wastes management in the oceans are considered; science-policy interaction; harmonization of international laws; consistent across national policies; and coordination of international organizations.

Ponis, et al (2020) showed that there is a need for more research in the area of plastic pollution from a social and economic perspective. Ferraro & Failler (2020) showed that challenges are still existing in the area of managing plastic pollution and that universal and holistic approaches focus on science-policy interaction; harmonization of international laws; consistent across national policies; and coordination of international organizations should be considered.

The reviewed studies have shown that, there is a need for measures for managing plastic pollution to be considered at a universal level because the problem of plastic pollution is contributing to many difficulties that society is facing today. Difficulties of global warming, depletion of non-renewable resources and many others.

METHODOLOGY

In relation to, Mark (2018), review research types focus on synthesizing past work with the intend of assimilating recent knowledge and escalating its accumulation into the prevailing body of knowledge. Nevertheless, a broad range of review research types, conforming to disparate criteria are recognized in literature. To conduct this research, a literature review was conducted in order to answer the research questions. The questions that were answered focused attention on; (1) what are the measures that should be used for preventing plastic pollution? (2) has the development of bioplastics contributed to the prevention of plastic pollution?

To select the papers to use in the literature review, search engines such as Scopus and Science Direct were used. A query of keywords "plastic AND (pollution OR prevent measures) AND (bioplastics)" was entered in the search engine default tab (Document Search form). The inclusion and exclusion criteria for the consideration of articles for review demanded that, articles to be incorporated in the review process should be studies that should; (1) be affiliated to the "Environmental Science", "Social Sciences", "Engineering", and "Multidisciplinary"; (2) have been published in the English language, (3) incorporate the aforementioned keywords; and (4) be from published peer-reviewed journals. The articles that were found using the specified keywords from the specified database were précised and amount to 193. Further application of the inclusion and exclusion criteria resulted in a final review of 58 articles. After the review of the articles, themes emerging from the final reviewed articles were established. These themes formed the measures that were discussed in detail.

RESULTS AND DISCUSSION

This section discusses the measures that should be undertaken to prevent plastic pollution. Based on the studies that were reviewed, a number of preventative measures were identified. Seven major plastic pollution measures are discussed in detail by focusing on; what each prevention measure is; the applicability of each prevention measure and the benefits each pollution prevention measure offers. The following prevention measures are discussed; recycling prioritization; utilization of bio-based and biodegradable plastics; improvement of waste collections systems; awareness and education of communities; extended producer responsibility enforcement; strengthen stakeholder engagement and innovations and technologies. Further, a comparison between the amount of plastic waste littered from the land to the ocean in developed and developing countries is shown.

Recycling Prioritization

Recycling of plastic materials is complex and involves many processes such as sorting, collection, extrusion of polymers and selling of the recycled pellets to producers. According to Mwanza (2018) recycling involves processes in which unwanted waste materials are recovered for remanufacturing into new products. It is also classified into primary, secondary, tertiary and quaternary recycling depending on the nature of the recycling process. Primary recycling, also known as closed-loop recycling, produces high-grade plastics compared to secondary recycling. The products from primary recycling and secondary recycling are used in different applications and based on the grade of plastics, the majority of the products from secondary recycling are used in less demanding applications such as construction materials, concrete, composites and textiles etc. However, recycling should be applied in long term and durable applications (Walker & Xanthos, 2018).

Despite the several disadvantages of plastic recycling such as the low ability to substitute virgin plastics (Lazarevic, Aoustin, Buclet, & Brandt, 2010), there are several advantages. For instance, recycling is still preferred as a sustainable option for managing wastes. It decreases pollutant emissions, decreases the amount of wastes destined for the landfills, saves energy and resources, improves local economies and creates jobs, decreases the amount of imported resources and ultimately reduces plastic pollution. Despite recycling being expensive, the benefits it gives society outweigh the costs of other alternative waste management options. Therefore, countries need to prioritize recycling by improving recycling technologies, mandatory EPR policies, mandatory taxes and penalties associated with recycling. For the plastics that cannot be recycled because of contamination, other options such as tertiary or quaternary recycling should be encouraged.

Utilization of Bio-Based and Biodegradable Plastics

A clear definition of biodegradable plastics is necessary and according to Flury and Narayan (2021), they are plastics that are convertible to CO_2, CH_4 and microbial biomass through microbial action. They include additives that accelerate their decomposition rate in the presence of light and oxygen. The carbon substrate found in the plastic polymers is used by microorganisms for carbon assimilation and energy. It is a process that can occur under anaerobic and aerobic states, yet in terms of energy gain, aerobic is most efficient. Examples of biodegradable plastics include, polycaprolactone (PCL); polybutylene succinate (PBS); polybutyrate adipate terephthalate (PBAT) and polyvinyl alcohol (PVOH/PVA).

Bio-Based plastics are polymers extracted from renewable feedstocks (e.g. biomass) and are independent of biodegradability (i.e. bio-polyethylene) (Harding, Gounden, & Pretorius, 2017). These plastics are purely manufactured from natural substances such as corn starch and examples include; NatureWorks and EverCorns.

Despite the uncertainties found with the utilization of bio-based and biodegradable plastics, many benefits exist and include utilization in (i) single-use and packaging items and (ii) agricultural mulch films

(Flury and Narayan, 2021). Cellulose-based materials can replace conventional plastic packaging but in many situations plastic packaging is still in demand. For example, it is a challenge to replace plastics in food packaging because of standard stipulations for conserving food safety and quality. Nevertheless, research has affirmed that, biodegradable plastics functionality is equivalent to that of conventional plastics in terms of food packaging (Panseri, et al., 2018) and this presents a great opportunity for the usability of biodegradable plastics Guillard (2018).

From the circular economy model, utilization of biodegradable for non-packing single-use products is acceptable. For instance, many single-use products (i.e. straws, retail bags; toothpicks; cotton bud sticks) have been legally banned and are being replaced with non-plastic products. This has created an opportunity for the utilization of biodegradable plastics although not all single-use plastic products can be replaced.

Agricultural plastic films are manufactured from non-biodegradable plastics (polyethylene) and are critical parts of the agricultural production systems (i.e. fruits and vegetables). They control weeds, provide suitable microclimate and soil temperature, and preserve soil moisture. Despite their application and relevance in the agricultural production systems, they are non-biodegradable and become brittle because of weathering and fragments hence have to be removed. This is a tedious and expensive process and a majority of the time, it's not achievable. As a solution to the challenges presented by agricultural plastic films, biodegradable plastics are an alternative to polyethylene mulch films because of their ability to be tilled in the ground after use. This ability has resulted in no costly removal and equivalent agronomic performance between the two plastic mulch films (biodegradable and conventional) has been shown (Tofanelli & Wortman, 2020).

Bio-based and biodegradable plastics present many advantages that are comparable to conventional plastics. These advantages include; easy to recycle; consumption of less energy during manufacturing; reduction in the amount of waste produced; less petroleum consumption; compostability; carbon dioxide reduction; reduction of greenhouse gas emission levels; non-release of harmful products upon decomposition; ability to be broken by nature bacteria; ability to mix with other traditional products; and ability to compost under specific conditions.

Improvement of Waste Collection Systems

It is a fact that, human beings generate waste and will continue to generate it. This fact is evident from the amount of wastes that are generated and finally landfilled or illegally dumped. Wastes generated from plastic wastes continue to increase because of the many applications in which plastic products are used. As a result of this increase, it is necessary to discuss strategies for managing these plastic pollution problems. Based on the waste management hierarchy, final disposal of wastes to the landfills, should be the last option because wastes should be considered for reuse, recycling, and recovery.

Waste disposal is associated with collection, processing, recycling and deposition of generated waste materials. A number of methods exist for disposing of wastes. For example, plastic wastes can be recycled and this is one of the methods that is contributing to effective waste management of PSWs. Incineration and landfilling are but some of the methods that are currently used for disposing of PSWs. In as much as these methods exist, developed and developing economies, are still facing plastic pollution problems from plastic wastes. Globally, approximately 40% of waste is disposed of in the landfills (Chrisafis, 2016). These statistics indicate that, there need to improve waste disposal practices. According to Kaza, et al (2018) waste disposal actions alter remarkably by region and income level. For instance, in lower- income nations, open dumping is common since landfills are mostly unavailable. Almost 93% of the waste is dumped or burnt in roads, waterways or open land in lower-income nations, while in high-income nations, only 2% is dumped (Kaza, et al., 2018). These wastes are a composition of different waste types and plastic wastes account for 12% of the global waste composition. However, as the composition of waste alters greatly by income levels, organic waste which accounts for 44% of the global waste decreases as the income level rises. This means in higher-income nations, plastic wastes; paper and cardboard represent a high proportion compared to organic waste.

It is necessary for waste disposal practices such as waste collection to be improved both in developed and developing nations. The purpose of these improved collection systems is for improving waste disposal practices but it is suffice to mention, most developed nations have efficient waste collection systems but developing nations are still facing implementation challenges (Prata, et al., 2019). For example, in low-income nations, only 39% of generated waste is collected for disposal while in high-income nations, 96% is collected for disposal (Kaza, et al., 2018). To reduce the impact of plastic pollution in developing nations, it is necessary for suitable waste collection systems to be adopted.

The initial step in the implementation of effective waste disposal practices is the collection of waste by source or post-separation (Bing, Bloemhof-Ruwaard, & van der Vorst, 2014). It is a preferred practice because it is cheaper and decreases waste contamination. However, there are several waste collection systems that can be implemented as plastic pollution measures such as, door-to-door collection; curbside collection, buy-back-centers (purchasing litter); drop-off centers (not purchasing litter) (Liu, Adams, & Walker, 2018). These waste collection systems have a positive effect on reducing plastic pollution.

Awareness and Education in Communities

The majority of human activities result in waste generation and as such, everyone should have a structured and proper understanding of issues related to waste management. Otherwise, the absence of understanding waste management practices prevents the success of the best devised management plans. Hasan (2004) concluded that, the public should be made aware on the consequences of improper waste management and its effect on the well-being of living things. Mwanza and Mbohwa (2019) concluded that, there is an urgent call for society to be informed and educated on the importance of recycling/ waste management practices. Debrah, Vidal & Dinis (2021) affirmed that, to achieve environmental or waste sustainability in developing economies, environmental awareness, environmental knowledge and environmental attitude should be communicated to students from teachers using formal education. These studies show the relevance of awareness and education from different perspectives but all with the aim to achieve sustainable waste management that can result in less pollution.

Education has been recognized as a powerful tool for fighting plastic pollution (Potts, et al., 2011) and there are many strategies that can be used to provide awareness and education as a strategy for combating plastic pollution. The internet and social media platforms such as Facebook, Instagram, Twitter etc. can be exploited as tools for providing education and awareness on plastic pollution. Social media creates chances for engaging with information (Dabbagh & Kitsantas, 2012) and the majority of the population has access to these devices such as mobile phones to enable them to utilize the social media platforms. Awareness and education should focus on pragmatic actions such as boosting recycling rates; reducing harmful products consumption and reducing littering. In a study by Mwanza (2018), intensification of awareness on plastic recycling in households can be done through the provision of education on waste management in learning institutions particularly primary level institutions. Traditional methods of information dissemination such as radio, television, newspapers, billboards and magazines can be used to discuss prevention measures for plastic pollution. Promotion of public information campaigns for businesses and citizens on waste generation reduction, reuse, avoidance of littering and utilization of provided waste collection systems can be discussed in awareness campaigns.

There are many benefits to providing awareness and education as strategies for plastic pollution prevention. The benefits can include; creation of behavior change in the approach citizens have on garbage and this can result in instilling cultural responsibility on wastes (plastic) pollution. Other than focusing on the benefits, there are strategies that should be promoted to increase awareness on plastic pollution such as supporting local and international research collaborations, promotion of knowledge sharing through expert exchange and inclusion of technical and scientific aspects in measure related suggestions for plastic pollution prevention.

Extended Producer Responsibility Enforcement

Extended Producer Responsibility (EPR) is defined by the OECD as an environmental policy approach that extends the producer's responsibility for products manufactured to the post-consumer stage of that product's life cycle inclusive of final disposal (OECD, 2001; Widmer, Oswald-Krapf, Sinha-Khetriwal, & al., 2005). EPR has become an established environmental approach since the late 1980s and its mandate is to shift the environmental impacts of products on its producers throughout the product's life cycle inclusive of the post-consumer phase. The plan behind the establishment of EPR was to shift financial and/or physical responsibilities of managing waste to the upstream producers while calling for environmental deliberation during product designs. It was anticipated that, the approach can increase recycling rates and reduce amount of waste landfilled. EPR addresses authority for a cleaner and greener environment throughout the product's life cycle. Manufacturers of plastic packaging items and products are motivated to recycle end-of-life plastics using operational and funding activities towards EPR. It is among the best approaches for reducing plastic amassing rates (Thushari & Senevirathna, 2020).

As a policy approach, EPR can be implemented using policy and economic instruments. Walls (2011) discusses many policy tools that are used in OECD countries.

The policy instruments or tools center around; 'product take-back directive and recycling rate goals': this mandatory makes producers and/or retailers return EOL plastic products while setting recycling goals. It facilitates the formation of producer responsibility organization (PRO). 'Voluntary product take-back directive and recycling rate goals': this demands a completely voluntary take-back approach and penalties do not apply for unmet targets. 'Mandatory return and targets with tradable recycling plan': this tool enables producers to trade credits among themselves for target achievement even though it demands setting recycling goals and take-backs.

The economic instrument focuses on the following; 'advanced recycling fee': for the sale of the product, a tax is forced in order to cover the recycling cost of EOL products. Fees are charged during selling and are determined per unit of the product. Fees can also be assessed upstream on manufacturers and included in the retail price. 'Recycling fee merged with subsidy for recycling': it utilizes revenue made from advanced recycling fee or post-consumption recycling fee in order to subsidize recycling processes. Revenue created is used in many ways such as, subsidizing the upstream producer's enterprise of obtaining recycled waste or waste management cost inclusive of infrastructure cost. 'Deposit Refund System (DRS):' It merges the product's consumption tax with refund if the EOL product is returned for recycling. The deposit is the summation of the environmental cost related with recycling and the product's commercial cost.

There are several benefits associated with the implementation of EPR and these benefits apply to EOL plastic products. Surak (2018) mentions that, EPR benefits are environmental, social and economic. Environmental benefits include; increased product recyclability, decreased utilization of toxic components and reduced landfilling. Social benefits include increased demand by society for environmentally friendly products, increased product image and job creation. With the associated benefits of EPR, Lihndqvist (2000) has identified five responsibilities cardinal for EPR implementation and these are informative, liability, physical, economic and owner responsibility. These responsibilities are presented in a model and should be considered for successful implementation of EPR.

Strengthen Stakeholder Engagement

The waste management arena comprises of many stakeholders and these can be people and organizations that have a desire for proper management of wastes as well as to participate in possible activities. The stakeholders can consist of the public, city planners, NGOs/social workers, municipalities, academicians, vendors, households, hospitals, politicians and corporations (Vutivoradit & Jakkapattarawong, 2018). Structured approaches for the engagement of stakeholders is a cardinal measure for plastic pollution control because all stakeholders generate waste in one way or another. This entails they should be taking active steps to control the plastic pollution.

A number of strategies for encouraging stakeholder engagement and participation in waste management related activities should be developed. The G20 action plan on marine litter (G20 Germany, 2017) inspires a number of strategies for stakeholder engagement and these include; continue communicating among partners and third-parties; implementation and tracking of existing regional plans and development of new ones; acceptance of responsibilities among stakeholders for active and cooperative networks; continuous involvement of stakeholders; support a stimulation of Public Private Partnerships (PPP); development of integrated waste treatment and management solutions; and promotion of waste control subjects in high level focused economic forums. The implementation of these suggested strategies to the engagement of stakeholders can have a positive effect in terms of how plastic pollution is controlled.

Innovations and Technologies

Several technologies for managing plastic wastes exist. These technologies directly contribute to the reduction of plastic pollution. A study conducted in Zambia showed that, mechanical recycling is predominately used by a number of recycling companies (Mwanza, 2018) and this was the same outcome for a study conducted on low and medium-income countries on strategies for reducing marine plastic wastes (Gamaralalage & Onogawa, 2019). Despite the popular use of mechanical recycling, there are several technologies such as chemical recycling technologies (depolymerization) and energy recovery technologies (grate, Fluidized Bed and Two-Stage Incineration, Rotary and Cement Kiln Combustion). All these technologies directly contribute to the management of plastic wastes and should be promoted through the implementation of new ideas.

The implementation of new ideas for the purpose of introducing new products or services is innovation. This approach has contributed to the development of additional technologies. For example, the use of plastic wastes in road construction projects; the use of PSWs in co-processing (as an alternative raw

Table 1. Plastic pollution in developed and developing countries

Developed Country	HDI	Plastic Pollution	Developing Country	HDI	Plastic Pollution
Australia	0.944	13888.98	China	0.761	231157.42
Belgium	0.931	2742.975	Brazil	0.763	89582.315
Canada	0.929	7959.555	India	0.645	13728.015
France	0.901	24108.615	Indonesia	0.718	77821.65
Germany	0.947	31238.89	Mexico	0.779	14248.14
Italy	0.872	31238.89	Nigeria	0.539	20520.665
Japan	0.919	143120.88	Saudi Arabia	0.854	4075.225
Netherlands	0.944	27699.85	South Korea	0.919	33746.805
Poland	0.88	2302.42	Thailand	0.777	27262.945
Spain	0.904	45852.395	Turkey	0.82	52564.38

(Jambeck et al., 2015)

material) in industrial processes and the convention of PSWs to oil (Gamaralalage & Onogawa). All these innovations and technologies begin with the sorting and segregation of plastic wastes from other wastes, thus contributing to the reduction of plastic wastes that are disposed of. The benefits of advancing the technologies for managing PSWs is directly linked to the control of plastic pollution.

Comparative Analysis of Plastic Pollution in Developed and Developing Economies

Based on the study conducted by Jambeck et al (2015), the amount of plastic waste littered from the land into the oceans from developed and developing countries was determined (Table 1). The countries are categorized into developed and developing based on their Human Development Index of 2020 (The World Bank, 2021). Using this study, this chapter has compared the plastic waste littered from developed and developing economies. The results show that, developed countries litter less compared to developing countries. The difference in the amount littered can be attributed to the fact that, most developed countries have well-structured waste management systems compared to developing countries. Prata et al (2019) affirms that developing countries do not have efficient waste collection systems compared to developed countries. For example, 39% of generated waste is collected for disposal in developing countries compared to developed countries, 96% (Kaza, et al., 2018).

Figure 1 shows that, Japan is one of the developed countries with the highest plastic waste w littered from land into the oceans while Poland is the least. In Japan, 143120.88 MT of plastic waste was littered into the ocean compared to Poland which had 2,302.42 MT.

Figure 2 shows that, China is one of the developing countries with the highest plastic waste littered from land into the oceans while Saudi Arabia is the least. In China, 231157.42 MT of plastic waste was littered into the ocean compared to Saudi Arabia which had 4,075.225 MT.

Further analysis of the results shows that, China litters more compared to Japan. Similarly, Saudi Arabia also litters more compared to Poland.

Figure 1. Plastic pollution in developed countries

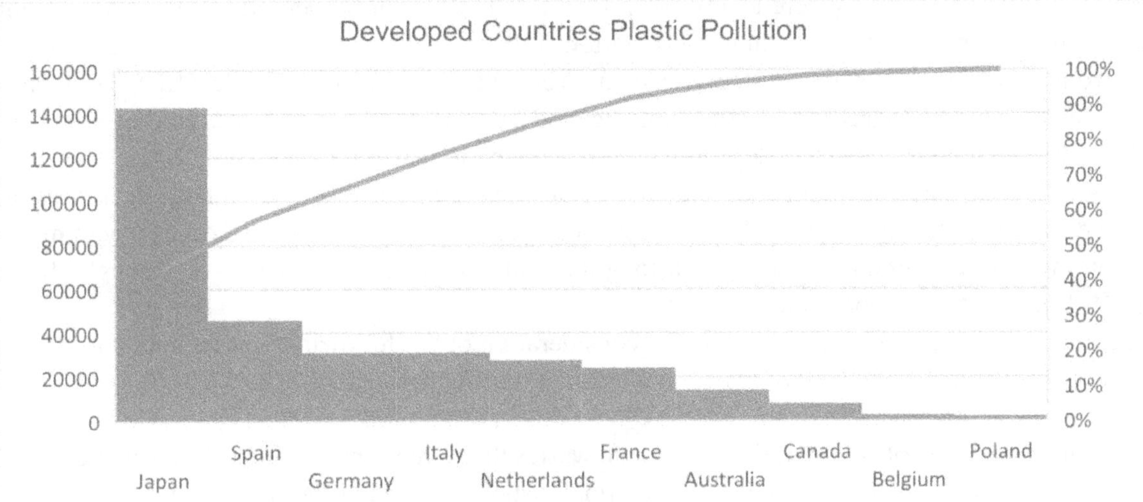

CONCLUSION AND RECOMMENDATIONS

Plastic is a widely used material because of the many applications in which it is utilized. Subsequently, the swift growth of the plastic manufacturing industry especially in the single-use plastics has contributed to plastic pollution related challenges in the environment. Thus, there are expanding international drives to resolve plastic pollution from the environment. The measures for controlling plastic pollution can be short and medium term but it depends on contextual implementation and acceptability.

Figure 2. Plastic pollution in developing countries

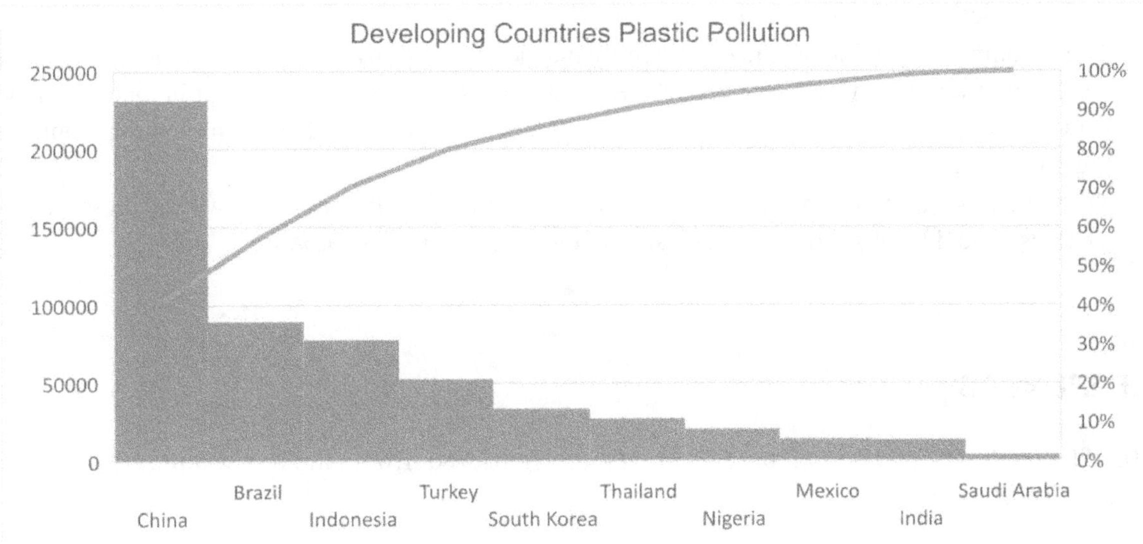

This study focused attention on reviewing measures for controlling plastic pollution from the environment. Several measures were identified in literature but the study focused attention on a detailed discussion of seven measures; recycling prioritization; utilization of bio-based and biodegradable plastics; improvement of waste collection systems; awareness and education in communities; ERP enforcement; strengthen stakeholder engagement and technologies and innovations. These measures can be implemented in the short, medium or long term depending on the context to which they are being implemented. The discussion around short, medium and long term implementation steps depend on how each measure is weighed by the implementing body. While these measures are proposed, it is also necessary to mention that, promotion of a circular economy is a long term strategy and can be achieved through effective implementation of the proposed measures.

In conclusion, this study recommends the consideration of the following crucial points for the successful control and management of plastic pollution in the environment.

- Comprehensive collection of data on plastic wastes throughout the product's lifecycle i.e. production, generation, collection, treatment and final disposal is needed for evidence-based monitoring performance, planning, coordination of waste management policies and systems. This information is cardinal for effective enforcement of EPR policies as well as prioritization of recycling. Therefore, the establishment of the necessary institutions at local, national and global levels to foresee the collection of data on plastic wastes should be a requirement.
- Despite the existence of several technologies and methods for managing plastic wastes, facilitation and identification of suitable technologies that are financially, technically and socially feasible to the local communities is important. Therefore, responsible stakeholders should be engaged in assessing key aspects such as characteristics and volume of plastic wastes, technology developments, commercial feasibility i.e. maintenance cost, operational costs, overall costs, social and environmental acceptability of the new technologies etc.
- Leadership from engaged stakeholders is required for the creation of integrated and holistic plastic wastes mitigation plans that focus on accelerating and addressing the plastic pollution challenges.
- To promote recycling and more innovations, suitable project-finance investments environment should be promoted for the private sectors. Nevertheless, risk management techniques should be set up to motivate investment from the private sector.
- Transitioning to sustainable and eco-friendly plastic manufacturing and consuming society is still challenging for most developing economies. However, strategies should be put in place on how to get there. In this case, the use of bio-based and biodegradable should be promoted in manufacturing companies.
- Waste disposal systems should be designed to fit the contextual needs. However, these disposal systems should be aligned to the drives for achieving the circular economy.

REFERENCES

G20. (2017). *G20 Action Plan on Marine Litter.* Retrieved from https://www.mofa.go.jp/mofaj/files/000272290.pdf

G20 Germany. (2017). *G20 Action Plan on Marine litter.* G20 Germany.

G7, Annex to the Leaders' Declaration. (2015.). *G7 Summit 7–8 June 2015. Think ahead Act together.* An morgen denken. Gemeinsam handeln.

Aretoulaki, E., Ponis, S., Plakas, G., & Agalianos, K. (2020). A systematic meta-review analysis of review papers in the marine plastic pollution literature. *Marine Pollution Bulletin, 161*, 111690. doi:10.1016/j.marpolbul.2020.111690 PMID:33039791

Aretoulaki, E., Ponis, S., Plakas, G., & Agalianos, K. (2021). A systematic meta-review analysis of review papers in the marine plastic pollution literature. *Marine Pollution Bulletin*, 111690. PMID:33039791

Bing, X., Bloemhof-Ruwaard, J., & van der Vorst, J. (2014). Sustainable reverse logistics network design for household plastic waste. *Flexible Services and Manufacturing Journal, 26*(1-2), 119–142. doi:10.100710696-012-9149-0

Boucher, J., & Friot, D. (2017). *Primary Microplastics in the Oceans: A Global Evaluation of Sources.* IUCN. doi:10.2305/IUCN.CH.2017.01.en

Charitou, A., Aga-Spyridopoulou, R., Mylona, Z., Beck, R., McLellan, F., & Addamo, A. (2021). Investigating the knowledge and attitude of the Greek public towards marine plastic pollution and the EU Single-Use Plastics Directive. *Marine Pollution Bulletin, 116*, 112182. doi:10.1016/j.marpolbul.2021.112182 PMID:33652246

Chrisafis, A. (2016). French Law Forbids Food Waste by Supermarkets. *The Guardian.* Retrieved from https://www.theguardian .com/world/2016/feb/04/french-law-forbids-food-waste-by-supermarkets

Dabbagh, N., & Kitsantas, A. (2012). Personal Learning Environments, social media, and self-regulated learning:A natural formula for connecting formal and informal learning. *Internet High Educ., 15*(1), 3–8. doi:10.1016/j.iheduc.2011.06.002

Debrah, J., Vidal, D., & Dinis, M. (2021). Raising Awareness on Solid Waste Management through Formal Education for Sustainability: Developing Countries Evidence Review. *Recycling, 6*(6).

Ferraro, G., & Failler, P. (2020). Governing plastic pollution in the oceans: Institutional challenges and areas. *Environmental Science & Policy, 112*, 453–460. doi:10.1016/j.envsci.2020.06.015

Flury, M., & Narayan, R. (2021). Biodegradable plastic as an integral part of the solution to plastic waste pollution of the environment. *Current Opinion in Green and Sustainable Chemistry, 30.*

Gamaralalage, P., & Onogawa, K. (2019). *Strategies to Reduce Marine Plastic Pollution from Land-based Sources in Low and Middle - Income Countries.* UNEP.

Geyer, R. J., Jambeck, J. R., & Law, K. L. (2017). Production, use, and fate of all plastics ever made. *Science Advances, 3*(7), 25–29. doi:10.1126ciadv.1700782 PMID:28776036

Guillard, V., Gaucel, S., Fornaciari, C., Angellier-Coussy, H., Buche, P., & Gontard, N. (2018). The next generation of sustainable food packaging to preserve our environment in a circular economy context. *Frontiers in Nutrition, 5*(121), 121. doi:10.3389/fnut.2018.00121 PMID:30564581

Harding, K., Gounden, T., & Pretorius, S. (2017). Biodegradable" plastics: A myth of marketing? *Procedia Manufacturing, 7*, 106–110. doi:10.1016/j.promfg.2016.12.027

Harris, L., Liboiron, M., Charron, L., & Mather, C. (2021). Using citizen science to evaluate extended producer responsibility policy to reduce marine plastic debris shows no reduction in pollution levels. *Marine Policy, 123*, 104319. doi:10.1016/j.marpol.2020.104319

Hasan, S. (2004). Public awareness is key to successful waste management. *Journal of Environmental Science and Health. Part A, Toxic/Hazardous Substances & Environmental Engineering, 39*(2), 483–492. doi:10.1081/ESE-120027539 PMID:15027831

Haward, M. (2018). Plastic pollution of the world's seas and oceans as a contemporary challenge in ocean governance. *National Commun.*, 667.

Helinski, K., Poor, J., & Wolfand, M. (2021). Ridding our rivers of plastic: A framework for plastic pollution capture device selection. *Marine Pollution Bulletin, 165*, 112095. doi:10.1016/j.marpolbul.2021.112095 PMID:33561713

Igarashi, M., de Boer, L., & Fet, A. (2013). What is required for greener supplier selection? A literature review and conceptual model development. *Journal of Purchasing and Supply Management, 19*(4), 247–263. doi:10.1016/j.pursup.2013.06.001

Jambeck, J., Geyer, R., Wilcox, C., Siegler, T., Perryman, M., Andrady, A., Narayan, R., & Law, R. (2015). Plastic waste inputs from land into the ocean. *Science, 347*(6223), 768–771. doi:10.1126cience.1260352 PMID:25678662

Kaza, S., Yao, L., Bhada-Tata, P., & Woerden, F. V. (2018). 2018. What a Waste 2.0: A Global Snapshot of Solid Waste Management to 2050. Urban Development Series. Washington, DC: World Bank. doi:10.1596/978-1-4648-1329-0

Krelling, A., Williams, A., & Turra, A. (2017). Differences in perception and reaction of tourist groups to beach marine debris that can influence a loss of tourism revenue in coastal areas. *Marine Policy, 85*, 87–99. doi:10.1016/j.marpol.2017.08.021

Lazarevic, D., Aoustin, E., Buclet, N., & Brandt, N. (2010). Plastic waste management in the context of a European recycling society: Comparing results and uncertainties in a life cycle perspective. *Resources, Conservation and Recycling, 55*(2), 246–259. doi:10.1016/j.resconrec.2010.09.014

Le Guern, C. (2018). *When the mermaids cry: The great plastic tide. Coastal Care.* Retrieved from https://coastalcare.org

Lindhqvist, T. (2000). *Extended Producer Responsibility in Cleaner Production' The International Institute for Industrial Environmental Economics.* Lund University.

Liu, Z., Adams, M., & Walker, T. (2018). Are exports of recyclables from developed to developing countries waste pollution transfer or part of the global circular economy? *Resources, Conservation and Recycling, 136*, 22–23. doi:10.1016/j.resconrec.2018.04.005

Mack, C. (2018). *How to Write a Good Scientific Paper.* SPIE. doi:10.1117/3.2317707

Mortillaro, N. (2017). *Humans have produced 8.3 billion tonnes of plastic, researchers say*. Retrieved from https://www.cbc.ca/amp/1.4210279

Mwanza, B. (2018). *An African Reverse Logistics Model for Plastic Solid Wastes* [PhD Thesis]. University of Johannesburg.

Mwanza, B. G. (2018). *An Afriacn Reverse Logistics Model for Plastic Solid Wastes*. University of Johannesburg.

Mwanza, B. G. (2020). Introduction to Recycling. In Recent Developments in Pastics Recycling (pp. 1-13). Springer.

Mwanza, B. G., & Mbohwa, C. (2019). Knowledge and awareness on Plastic Solid Waste (PSW) management in Zambia: where are we? Procs West Africa Built Environment Research (WABER) Conference, 749-756.

OECD. (2001). *Extended producer responsibility: A guidance manual for governments*. OECD.

¨ohr, A., Savelli, H., Beunen, R., Kalz, M., Ragas, A., & Van Belleghem, F. (2017). Solutions for global marine litter pollution. *Current Opinion in Environmental Sustainability*, *28*, 90–99. doi:10.1016/j.cosust.2017.08.009

Panseri, S., Martino, P., Cagnardi, P. C., & Tedesco, D. (2018). Feasibility of biodegradable based packaging used for red meat storage during shelflife:a pilot study. *Food Chemistry*, *249*, 22–29. doi:10.1016/j.foodchem.2017.12.067 PMID:29407927

Parker, L. (2019, June 7). *National Geographic*. Retrieved July 14, 2021, from https://www.nationalgeographic.com/environment/article/plastic-pollution

Ponis, S., Plakas, G., Agalianos, K., & Aretoulaki, E. (2020). A systematic meta-review analysis of review papers in the marine plastic pollution literature. *Marine Pollution Bulletin*, *161*, 111690. doi:10.1016/j.marpolbul.2020.111690 PMID:33039791

Potts, T., O'Higgins, T., Mee, L., & Pita, C. (2011). Public Perceptions of Europe's Seas: A Policy Brief. Brussels, Belgium: EU FP7 KNOWSEAS Project.

Prata, J., Silva, A., da Costa, J., Mouneyrac, C., Walker, T., Duarte, A., & Rocha-Santos, T. (2019). Solutions and Integrated Strategies for the Control and Mitigation of Plastic and Microplastic Pollution. *Int. J. Environ. Res. Public Health 2019, 2411*(16).

Schmidt, C., Krauth, T., & Wagner, S. (2017). Export of Plastic Debris by Rivers into the Sea. *Environmental Science & Technology*, *51*(21), 12246–12253. doi:10.1021/acs.est.7b02368 PMID:29019247

Schnurr, R., Alboiu, V., Chaudhary, M., Corbett, R., Quanz, M., Sankar, K., Srain, H. S., Thavarajah, V., Xanthos, D., & Walker, T. R. (2018). Reducing marine pollution from single-use plastics (SUPs): A review. *Marine Pollution Bulletin*, *137*, 157–171. doi:10.1016/j.marpolbul.2018.10.001 PMID:30503422

Sheveal, S., Courtney, K., & Parks, J. (2011). *The Honolulu Strategy: A global framework for prevention and management of marine debris*. United Nations Environment Programme. Retrieved December 13, 2021, from https://marinedebris.noaa.gov/sites/default/files/publications-files/Honolulu_Strategy.pdf

Surak, M. (2018). *Extended producer responsibility*. Encyclopedia Britannica. Retrieved November 17, 2021, from https://www.britannica.com/topic/extended-producer-responsibility

Surfers Against Sewage. (2021, July 16). Retrieved from www.sas.org.uk: https://www.sas.org.uk/our-work/plastic-pollution/plastic-pollution-facts-figures/

Thompson, R., Moore, C., vom Saal, F., & Swan, S. (2009). Plastics, the environment and human health: Current consensus and future trends. *Philosophical Transactions of the Royal Society of London. Series B, Biological Sciences*, *364*(1526), 2153–2166. doi:10.1098/rstb.2009.0053 PMID:19528062

Thushari, G., & Senevirathna, J. (2020). Plastic pollution in the marine environment. *Heliyon*, *6*(8), e04709. doi:10.1016/j.heliyon.2020.e04709 PMID:32923712

Tibbetts, J. (2015). Managing marine plastic pollution: Policy initiatives to address wayward waste. *Environmental Health Perspectives*, *123*(4), A90–A93. doi:10.1289/ehp.123-A90 PMID:25830293

Tofanelli, M., & Wortman, S. (2020). Benchmarking the agronomic performance of biodegradable mulches against polyethylene mulch film: A meta-analysis. *Agronomy (Basel)*, *2020*(10), 10. doi:10.3390/agronomy10101618

UN Environment Programme Report. (2018). *Banning single-use plastic: Lessons and experiences from countries.* UN Environment Programme.

UN Environment Programme Report. (2018). *Banning single-use plastic: Lessons and experiences from countries.* UN Environment Programme.

Vethaak, A., & Leslie, H. (2016). Plastic debris is a human health issue. *Environmental Science & Technology*, *50*(13), 6825–6826. doi:10.1021/acs.est.6b02569 PMID:27331860

Vince, J., & Hardesty, B. (2018). Governance solutions to the tragedy of the commons that marine plastics have become. *Frontiers in Marine Science*, *5*, 214. doi:10.3389/fmars.2018.00214

Vutivoradit, S., & Jakkapattarawong, S. (2018). Stakeholder Participation for sustainable waste management in Phranakorn District, Bangkok. *Proceedings of Academics World 92nd International Conference*, 103-107.

Walker, T., & Xanthos, D. (2018). A call for Canada to move toward zero plastic waste by reducing and recycling single-use plastics. *Resour. Conserv. Recycl.*, 99-100.

Walls, M. (2011). *Deposit–refund systems in practice and theory. Resources for the Future Discussion Paper No. 11–47.* Washington, DC: Resources for the Future.

Walther, A., Yen, N., & Hu, C.-S. (2021). Strategies, actions, and policies by Taiwan's ENGOs, media, and government to reduce plastic use and marine plastic pollution. *Marine Policy*, *126*, 104391. doi:10.1016/j.marpol.2021.104391

Widmer, R., Oswald-Krapf, H., Sinha-Khetriwal, A., Schnellmann, M., & Böni, H. (2005). Global perspectives on the e-waste. *Environmental Impact Assessment Review*, *25*(5), 436–458. doi:10.1016/j.eiar.2005.04.001

KEY TERMS AND DEFINITIONS

Awareness: Condition associated with being alert of something.

Education: The accession of personal development, values, knowledge, beliefs, skills, and habits.

Extended Producer Responsibility: A policy proposition in which producers are mandated to take responsibility (physical and financial) for the disposal of their end-of-life products.

Innovation: Is the pragmatic application of ideas that effect in the establishment of new services or goods or advancement in the offering of services or goods.

Plastic Wastes: Amassing of plastic objects in the Earth's environment with adverse effects on humans, wildlife, and wildlife habitat.

Prevention: The efforts of terminating something form arising or happening.

Measures: A scheme of action taken to attain a particular motive.

Strategies: A conventional plan to attain one or more long-term goals under uncertainty or certain circumstances.

Stakeholders: A person with a heed or care in something.

Technology: The summation of any processes, techniques, methods, and skills utilized in the manufacturing of goods and services.

Chapter 7
Study of the Potential Impact of Microplastics and Additives on Human Health

Ranjit Barua
https://orcid.org/0000-0003-2236-3876
Omdayal Group of Institutions, India

Debasish Banerjee
Omdayal Group of Institutions, India

Sumit Bhowmik
Omdayal Group of Institutions, India

ABSTRACT

The spreading and abundance of micro and nano plastics into the world are so wide that many researchers used them as main pointers of the modern and contemporary period defining a new historical era. However, the inferences of microplastics are not yet systematically understood. There is the significant difficulty involved to know their impact due to dissimilar physical-chemical characteristics that make micro-plastics complex stressors. Micro-plastics carry toxic chemicals in the ecosystems, therefore serving as vectors of transport, and, on the other hand, a combination of dangerous chemicals that are further voluntarily during their manufacture as additives to increase polymer properties and extend their life. In this chapter, the authors prominently discuss the different kinds of literature on micro and nano-plastic exposure pathways and their probable risk to human health to encapsulate present information with the target of enhanced attention, upcoming study in this area, and information gaps.

INTRODUCTION

Contagion by mass plastics and plastic waste is presently a severe environmental issue in the land, air, and marine ecosystems (Mato et al., 2001) (Gregory, 2009) (Dunlap et al., 1991) (Thompson et al., 2009)

DOI: 10.4018/978-1-7998-9723-1.ch007

(Rochman et al., 2013). Particularly, small-scale plastic waste for example micro and nano-plastics has become the most important supplier to the contamination of marine ecosystems. Researchers are investigating the effect of micro and nano-plastics on marine organisms and ecosystems globally. Plastics are widely used in our standard of living. Though, an important quantity of plastic waste is discharged into the environment openly or passing through inappropriate recycling or reusing. Degradation of plastic waste produces micro or nano-plastics which are named micro and nano-plastics or micro and nano-plastics (Lee et al., 2013) (Cole et al., 2015) (Kaposi et al., 2014) (Desforges et al., 2015). The range of Nanoplastics (NPS) diameter varies from 1 to 100 or 1000 nm (Koelmans et al., 2015) (Bergami et al., 2016), while the particles size of micro-plastics (MPs) diameter is less than 5 mm (Betts et al., 2008) (Barnes et al., 2009). In the present chapter, we initially summarize the environmental infectivity of micro and nano-plastics and then discuss their impacts on health derived from existing micro and nano-plastics studies. As plastics come in contact with marine water, the persistence and degradation rate of plastics differ by polymer, density, shape, and the purpose of it (Eriksen et al., 2014). These features also oversee wherein the water column plastics may be noticed. For instance, more floating plastics are expected to be passed by sea currents and wind across the marine environment (Eriksen et al., 2014). Moreover, while plastics are exposed to sunlight and wave action, they will degrade into MP (micro-plastics – the plastic particles <5 mm in size). The degree of plastic degradation relies on a few aspects including the type of polymer, environmental circumstances like pH, temperature, weathering, and irradiation (Akbay et al., 2016). Plastic particles pollute the aquatic environment and the food chain, as well as foods intended for human feeding (Smith et al., 2018). Our study signifies that micro and nano-plastics can be noticed in both land and marine ecosystems globally and be ingested and accrued by animals along the food chain. Data has suggested the injurious health impacts of micro and nano-plastics on marine animals. Latest studies found microplastics in human stool samples, suggesting that humans are exposed to microplastics throughout the food and drinking water chain (Rillig et al., 2012) (Cedervall et al., 2012) (Mattsson et al., 2014). Though, the impact of micro and nano-plastics on human health is barely investigated. Over and above the micro and nano-plastics themselves, these small plastic particles can discharge plastic additives or adsorb other environmental chemicals, a lot of which have been noticed to display endocrine disturbing and other toxic effects (Klein et al., 2015) (Cole et al., 2013). So far, there is a significant lack of knowledge on the main additives of concern applied in the plastic industry, their fate once micro-plastics dispose into the environment, and their resultant effects on human health when related to micro and nano-plastics. This chapter highlights the most dangerous and toxic chemical materials that are confined in all plastic goods to define the properties and effects of these harmful chemicals on human health, as long as a full summary of studies that have scrutinized their abundance in micro and nano-plastics.

TYPE AND USE OF PLASTICS

The most important categorization of plastics is based on the durability or non-durability of their natures, or whether they are thermoplastics or thermosets (Figure 1). Thermosets contain polyurethane, alkyd, and epoxy, and they are frequently applied as adhesives, insulators, and plywood. The thermosetting procedure is mainly based on heat-induced crosslinking to make new and irreparable covalent bonds, which makes the thermosets steady and not simple to decompose (Rudyak et al., 2018) (Jiang et al., 2020). In contrast, thermoplastics have no recently formed chemical bonds and can be recycled and remolded,

Figure 1. A schematic diagram of probable environmental degradation pathway of plastics

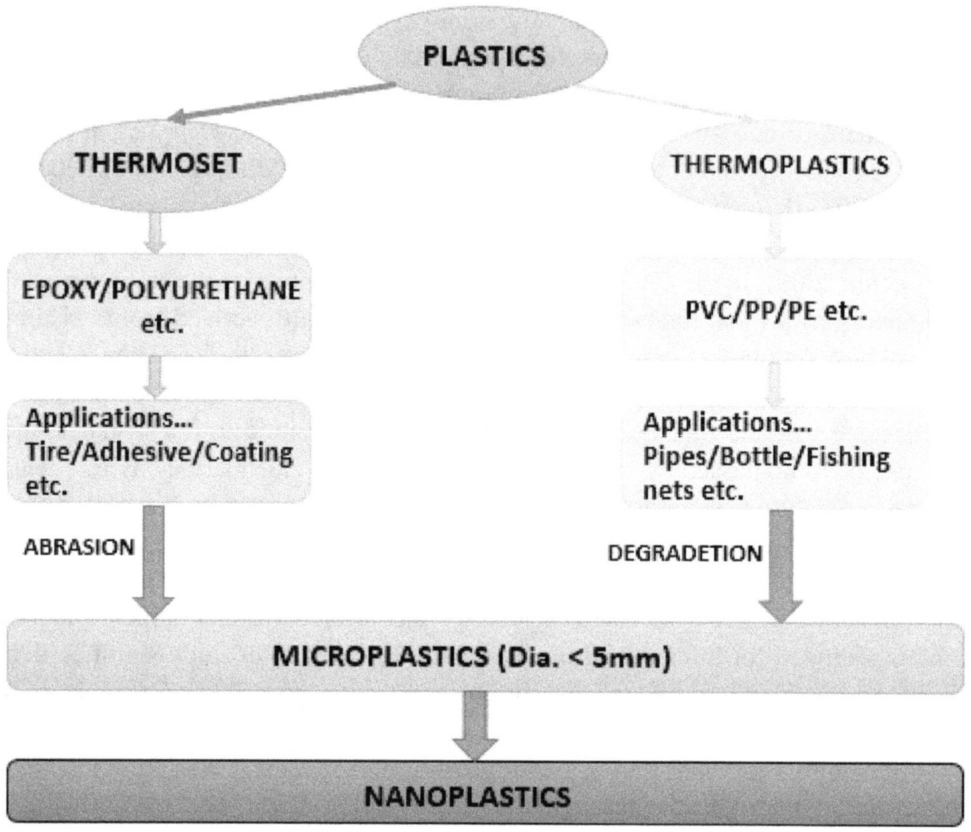

making them more extensively used than thermosets in customer goods (Mattsson et al., 2015) (Raddadi et al., 2019) (Xu et al., 2019) (Battulga et al., 2019). There are four special kinds of thermoplastics: polypropylene (PP), polyethylene (PE), polyvinyl chloride (PVC), and polystyrene (PS). Polyethylene (PE) is used in an extensive range of economical plastic products, as well as plastic bottles and bags. There are two regularly used subtypes of polyethylene (PE): (a) high-density polyethylene (HDPE), which is typically used in milk cans, and molded plastic cases; and (b) the low-density polyethylene (LDPE) used in siding, outdoor furniture, shower curtains, and floor tiles. Polypropylene (PP) is mainly used to create drinking straws, bottle caps, butter containers, fishing lines, car bumpers, appliances, and plastic pressure pipe systems. Polystyrene (PS) is the main chemical used to make CDs, food containers, cutlery, foam peanuts, disposable cups, plastic tableware, plates, and cassette boxes. Polyvinyl chloride (PVC) is the main element of shower curtains, plumbing pipes, window frames, and flooring. Over and above the usual plastic classifications listed above, microplastic fibers (MFs) are one of the most familiar types of microplastics found in the environment (Cole, 2016) (Hu et al., 2020). Micro-plastic fibers (MFs), are usually applied in a variety of fibrous materials, for example agricultural, clothing, industrial, as well as some textile products (Liu et al., 2019). Usually, polypropylene (PP), polyethylene (PE), and polyvinyl chloride (PVC) are the three main types of micro-plastics used in research. Polyethylene (PE) and polystyrene (PS) are the most accepted plastic materials applied in customer products. Moreover, polyvinyl

Figure 2. Human interaction and the pathway of micro and nano-plastic elements in the human body

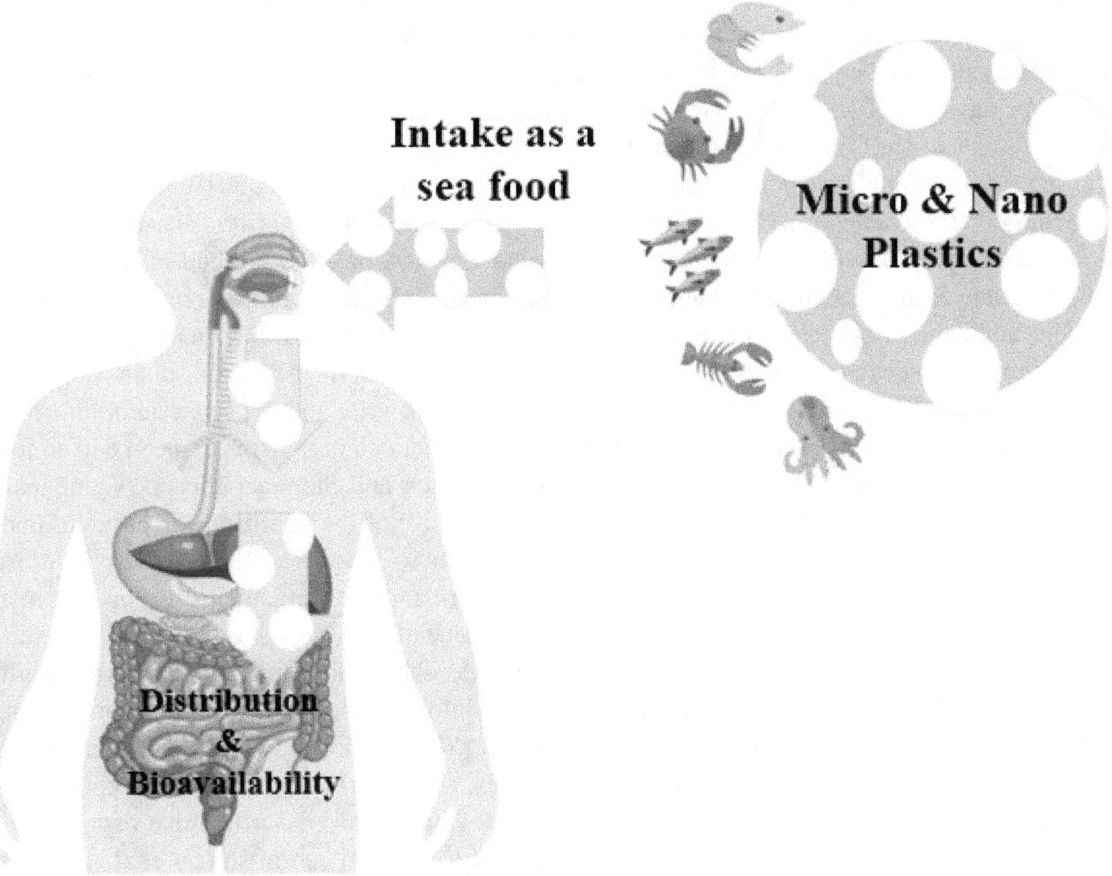

chloride (PVC) is mostly applied for plastic wire insulation or the cable jacket of data cables. When a cable's life span ends, only the inner metal wire is recycled but the outer PVC cover is usually thrown away into the environment as the separation cost is very high. It was informed that 15% is burned, only 3% is recycled, and 82% of PVC waste is thrown away in landfills (Suresh et al., 2017).

PLASTICS AND CO-CONTAMINANTS

Plastics are mainly synthetic components made of polymers and other chemical additives (like phthalates, bisphenols, and flame retardants) which add unique elements to plastic materials (Gigault et al., 2018). As plastics are cheaper, easier to manufacture, hydrophobic, and versatile, it is widely used in multiple profitable application. The production of plastics is rapidly growing each year, whereas, the policies of recycling, repurposing, and reusing are not effectively implemented in a few developing countries (Wang et al., 2019) (Avio et al., 2017). From the 1950s to 2015, almost 6.3 billion tons of plastic waste have been calculated to be generated globally (Geyer et al., 2017) (Kubowicz et al., 2017). This number might increase to 26 billion tons by 2050 if this continues (Guglielmi, 2017). Although only 21-26% of these wastes are prominently recycled and destroyed, the rest of the wastes are destroyed in open pits or dumped in an open environment, which leads to plastic pollution of the soil, water, air, etc. (Liu et al., 2016) (Rhodes et al., 2018). As the plastic comes in contact with nature, the communication between the natural elements and the plastic waste material can cut down the larger plastic pieces into smaller plastic trash (Waring et al., 2018). Additionally, smaller plastic elements are generally produced and added to customer kinds of stuff like personal care products which are thrown away after use, and this is another significant reason for plastic pollution in the environment (Hernandez et al., 2019) (Sharma et al., 2017). Depending on the diameter of the plastic particles, they can be classified into nano-plastics (NPS) and micro-plastics (MPs), with the diameter of NPs being 1 to 100 or 1000 nm and micro-plastics (MPs) being less than 5mm respectively (Jiang et al., 2020). Figure 2 shows the human contact and the pathway of micro and nano plastic elements in the human body. Presently, one of the major alarming factors is whether microplastics are a threat to human life and the ecosystem. Although, many improbabilities are related to this factor. To analyze the level of threat to human life and the ecosystem, information on disclosure and impact levels is required. The adversarial impact on organisms that came in contact with micro-plastics can be divided into two groups: physical impacts and chemical impacts (Campanale et al., 2020). It mainly depends on the shape, concentration, and size of the micro-plastic particles and lastly, it also depends on harmful chemicals which are related to micro-plastics. Although recently information on the disclosure level of micro-plastics in the atmosphere and with organisms has briskly increased, very restricted data is accessible about the chemicals related to micro-plastics (Zhang et al., 2018). Micro-plastic is comprised of two types of chemicals: (a) chemicals captivated from the neighboring atmosphere, and (b) additives and polymeric raw material (oligomers or monomers) originating from plastics (Figure 3). Therefore, micro and nano-plastics (MNPs) have been spotted worldwide in both oceanic and terrestrial environments including marines, rivers, drinking water, air, deposits, and diet (Bouwmeester et al., 2015) (Cózar et al., 2014). Earlier studies have described that exposure to micro and nano-plastics can cause propagative toxicity in liver toxicity in zebrafish (Lu et al., 2016), oysters (Sussarellu et al., 2016), and tissue bioaccumulation and possible organ harmfulness in mice (Yang et al., 2019) (Lu et al., 2018). These results designate that the affluence of micro and nano-plastics is extensive, and the biological harm of micro and nano plastics to both humans and other existing organisms cannot be overlooked. Though, the acquired experimental results are not convincing; the inferences given by dissimilar studies are rather contradictory, and the essential mechanisms of exposed toxicities are still unwell and unspoken. Furthermore, current studies have found microplastics in human feces, signifying that humans are uncovered to micro and nano-plastics over the food web or food chain (Huerta et al., 2017) (Prata et al., 2020). However, the influence of micro and nano-plastics on human health has been barely investigated. Moreover, in addition to the micro and nano-plastics themselves, these tiny plastic elements can release plastic additives and/or adsorb other eco-friendly chemicals, many of which have been exposed to display endocrine-disrupting and other toxic effects (Jin et al., 2019). Though, how micro and nano-plastics will influence the toxicities of these additives and adsorbents is still basically unidentified.

ADDITIVES OF CONCERN

Many elements that are categorized as harmful according to the European Union (EU) regulation on cataloging and classification (Regulation, E. C; 2008) are existing in everyday products as consistent

Figure 3. Micro and nano plastic

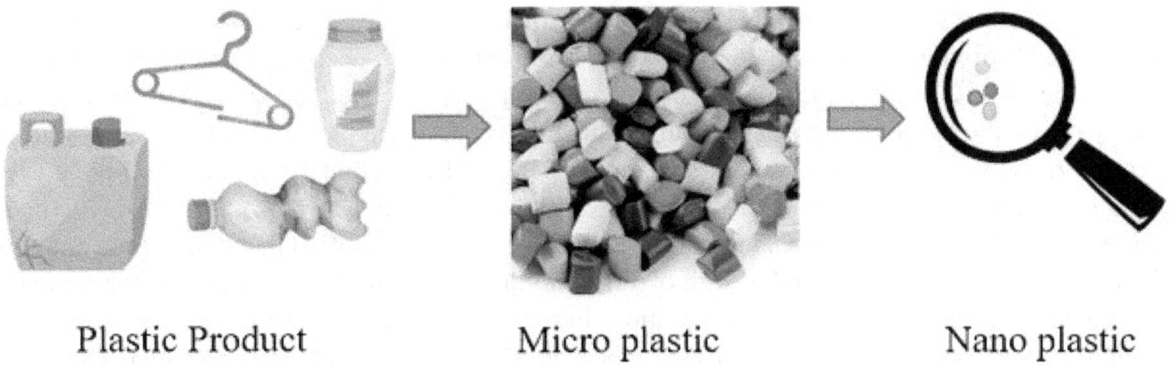

components. The toxicity of affluence is its capability to cause risky effects. These things can strike a particular cell or a total group of cells, an organ system, or the whole body. Elements that are measured as most injurious are those that cause mutations to DNA, cancer, have contaminated reproductive effects, are intractable into the environment, and other injurious properties, for example, disorderly hormones (Moyce et al., 2018). The vital organs that are most frequently affected are the kidneys, the liver, the nervous system (as well as the brain), the heart, and the reproductive system (Moyce et al., 2018) (Cingotti et al., 2019). Among these materials, numerous regularly used to create plastics are hazardous. Phthalates, BPA (Bisphenol-A), in addition to some of the brominated flame retardants, that are used to produce food packaging and household products, have been confirmed to be endocrine disruptors that can injure human health if inhaled or ingested (Cingotti et al., 2019).

EDC (Endocrine-disrupting chemicals), recognized as elements that are exogenous to the animal or human organism, have hormonal activity that modifies the homeostasis of the endocrine method, so they are of certain concern. These composites affect the growth of the endocrine system and affect the working of organs that reply to hormonal signals. The endocrinal and reproductive properties of endocrine disruptors may be a sign of their capability to (a) mimic normal hormones, (b) provoke their action, (c) modify their configuration of synthesis and metabolism, or (d) transform the expressions of exact receptors (Colborn et al., 1992) (Miyagawa et al., 2016) (Yu et al., 2008). Modern science has connected EDC (Endocrine-disrupting chemicals) with numerous infections and situations, for example, hormonal growths (prostate, breast, testes), reproductive complications (genital abnormalities, sterility), asthma, metabolic complaints (obesity, diabetes), and neurodevelopmental disorders (autism spectrum disorders, learning disorders). Together with the previously shown systematic proof, the concern occurs because of the increasing levels of many infections worldwide. Furthermore, people are extensively exposed to these chemicals from numerous sources (Cingotti et al., 2019).

IMPACTS ON FRESHWATER ORGANISMS

The micro and nano-plastics influence the organisms of freshwater habitat which leads to a major attraction. Research shows various concentrations of micro and nano-plastics in the terrestrial aquatic ecosystem, having numerous impacts on the growth, evolution, activities, reproduction, and fatality of aquatic animals (represented by Daphnia and zebrafish) (Chae et al., 2017). In toxicological research, an ornamental freshwater fish, mainly known as Zebrafish (Daniorerio) is generally used as a vertebrate model. The absorption and growth configurations of zebrafish have been observed using a seven-day acquaintance with 20 µm and 5 µm of polystyrene microplastics at concentrations of 20 mg/l, where, the toxicity of the liver was also examined using a three-day experience of 70-nm and 5-µm polystyrene microplastics at the concentrations of 20, 200, and 2000 mg/l. The outcomes indicated that 5-µm polystyrene microplastics can accrue in the liver, gills, and gut, but 20-µm polystyrene microplastics could not accrue in the gill tissue. The outcome of organ toxicity evaluation specified that both 70-nm and 5-µm PS MPs can persuade swelling and growth of fatty acid in the liver. In the meantime, by examining the rise and fall of certain enzyme actions, variations in oxidative anxiety and fat absorption were noticed (Lu et al., 2016). Another research states that microplastics do not impact or do not often cause death in zebrafish (Daniorerio) after a ten-day exposure to 0.001–10.0 mg/l microplastics. Nevertheless, after exposure to all four common MPs (polyamides (PA), PE, PP, and PVC), intestinal injuries, as well as cracking of villi and splitting of enterocytes were noticed (Lei et al., 2018). A small planktonic crustacean named Daphnia Magna (D. Magna) (adult length at 1.5–5.0 mm), is mostly used as fish food in aquaria and aquaculture and it is also analyzed as a biological research topic since the 18th century. Moreover, for examining chemicals in ecotoxicology, D. Magna is utilized as per OECD (Organization for Economic Co-operation and Development) guidelines. Recently, research on the impact of plastic wastes on marine organisms with the use of D. Magna has concentrated on the rate of survival after exposure, bioaccumulation of plastic elements in their intestinal tissues, and possible poisonous reproduction. One of research with exposure to four naturally applicable MPs at the concentration of 100 mg/l for 48 h was observed in the gut of D. Magna but no severe impacts were seen (Kokalj et al., 2018). Furthermore, after a short-term contact of 12.5–400 mg/l with diameters of 1 µm and 100 µm polyethylene microplastics for 96 h, Rehse et al., 2016 found that the effect of 1-µm plastic particles on D. Magna immobilization changed in a time- and dose-dependent manner. Although the 100-µm-sized plastic elements which could not be ingested or swallowed, have no major dangerous effect on the size of the plastic element. Another study used 100 nm and 2 µm fluorescent polystyrene microplastics to examine the consequence of microplastics on the feeding and reproduction rate of D. Magna.

IMPACTS ON MARINE ANIMALS

Nowadays, several studies are concentrating on the harmful effects of MNPs using non-mammalian marine animals for study material as the ocean act as the main storehouse for plastic waste (Guzzetti et al., 2018) (Franzellitti et al., 2019). Additionally, few organisms, like bivalves are used as it is a significant food source for humans, signifying one way which exposed humans directly to plastic elements. Bivalves are a group of animals that require some of the familiar molluscan organs, for example, the odontophore and radula, so they cannot chew up when they consume. All their ingested food goes openly into the digestive system and can be applied in micro and nano-plastic research (von Moos et al., 2012) (Magara et al., 2018) (Van Cauwenberghe et al., 2014). Mainly bivalves are filter feeders, as well as clams, oysters, mussels, shellfish, etc. Consequently, they consume an adequate amount of plastic particles to accrue in their bodies and cause dangerous impacts on health. Studies have shown that plastic particles lesser than 10 µm can gather in the gut and be engrossed into their circulatory system, and particles bigger than 4 μm can stay in the body of the blue mussel (Mytilusedulis) (Bouwmeester et al., 2015) (Riisgård et al., 1988). Moreover, another research found that when larvae of blue mussel (Mytilusedulis) were exposed with an equal mass of plastic particles, the consumption of 2 μm particles was more than the lesser particles with 100 nm diameter (Rist et al., 2019). Microplastics are consumed by marine creatures, which leads to their food chain. According to the International Atomic Energy Agency (IAEA), the volume of microplastics in the area, by 2030, it is predicted to rise to some 3.9 times as related to 2008 levels. This amount could almost double in 2050, and increase by 6.4 times related to 2008 levels, and again, the volume of plastics in the sea is predicted to be more than 10 times higher in 2100 compared to 2008 except act is taken to amend this trajectory (Figure 4). The discrepancy takes of dissimilar sized plastic particles may be because of the reality that the 2-μm particles were mistakenly consumed as food (1–9 μm), whereas the the100-nm particles float in the water and go through the gastrointestinal tract (GI) passively with the water. Consequences from the same study explained that while the blue mussel larvae growth was not exaggerated, irregular development increased, and irregularity showed in all treatment groups (0.42 g/L, 282 g/L, and 28.2 g/L) of both sizes of plastic particles (Rist et al., 2019). Another literature found that oyster larvae can usually consume plastic particles of 160–7.3 μm. Moreover, when oyster Crassostreagigas larvae (3–24 days post fertilization, d.p.f.) were uncovered to 1- and 10-μm Polystyrene (PS) particles for eight days at the concentrations of 0.11 × 10-3 μg/ml and 0.18 g/ml, correspondingly, there was no computable difficult effect on the development, growth, or feeding capacity (Cole et al., 2015). Another literature reported that mature oysters ate polystyrene (PS) microspheres and preferred 6 to 2–μm particles at the disclosure concentration of 0.023 mg/l (Sussarellu et al., 2016). It was assumed that the mature oysters preferred 6- to 2-μm plastic particles as 6-μm particles were more comparable in size and shape to their diet (Sussarellu et al., 2016). Microplastics were noticed to considerably decrease the number of sperm motility in oysters as well as the production and increase of offspring larvae after a 2-month maternal contact experiment (Sussarellu et al., 2016). Additionally, another study reported that exposure to 50 nm nano-plastics can cause an important reduction of overfertilization rates and embryo–larval growth, as well as many deformities, which consequences in the total stagnation of growth (Tallec et al., 2018).

CONSEQUENCES OF MICRO AND NANO-PLASTICS ON HUMAN HEALTH

In response to the studies signifying that micro-plastics are all over the place present in different environment mediums, their impacts on the health of both humans and other organisms have become one of the investigational focuses. Furthermore, the tropic move of plastic particles may be a general occurrence that arises at an equal time, creating the health impact of micro and nano-plastics extensive and multifarious (Au et al., 2017). A current study summarized the existence of micro and nano-plastics in animals and foods and explicated the extensive biological introduction of micro and nano-plastics (Toussaint et al., 2019), signifying that considering the health impacts of micro and nano-plastics is a critical and unmet requirement. A new piece of information from the WHO (World Health Organization) (Novotna et al., 2019) highlighted the everywhere micro-plastics existence in the surroundings and produced great alarm regarding the exhibition and belongings of micro and nano-plastics on human health (Revel et al., 2018) (Bradney et al., 2019) (Lehner et al., 2019). One of the most important micro and nano-plastic entrance positions into the human system is signified by the intake of unhygienic food (Silva-Cavalcanti et al., 2017). In a current study performed by (Cox et al., 2019), 0.44 MPs/g of micro and nano-plastics were

Figure 4. Microplastic abundance in Eastern Tropical Pacific
(Photo Curtsey to IAEA, 2020)

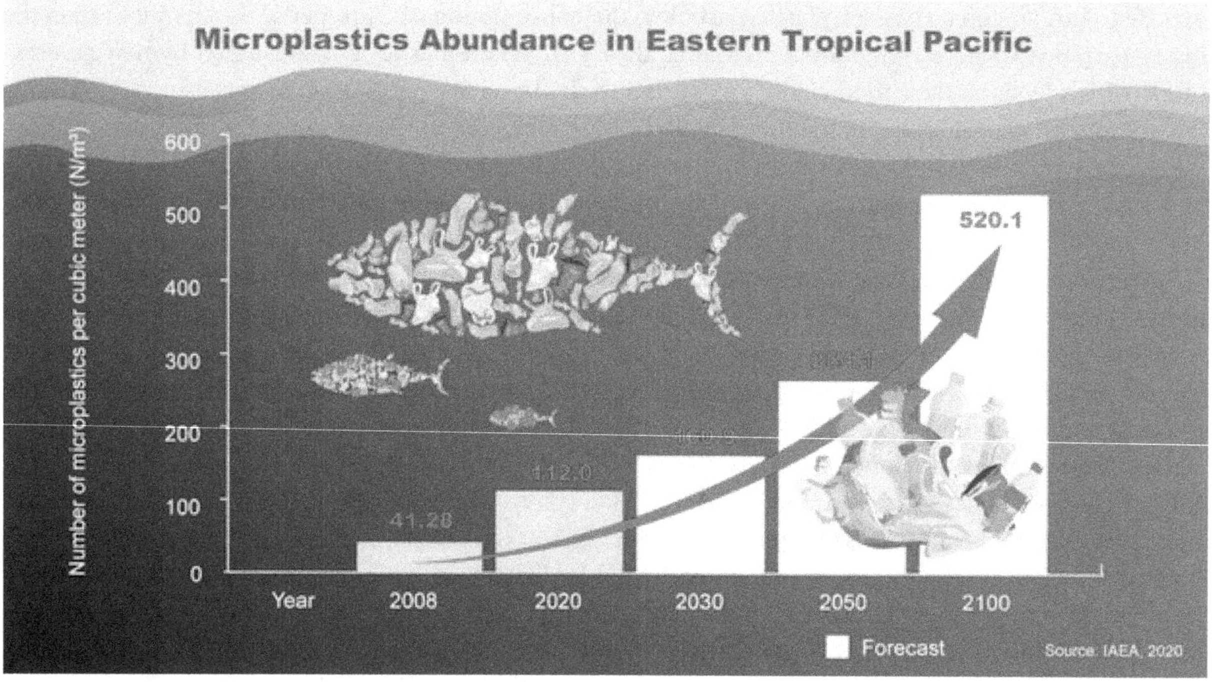

noticed in sugar, 0.11 MPs/g were noticed in salt, 0.03 MPs/g were noticed in alcohol, and 0.09 MPs/g were noticed in bottled water. Humans could also imagine the expected ingestion of 80 g per day of micro-plastics via vegetation and fruits which accrue micro-plastics during uptake from contaminated soil (Ebere et al., 2019). The existence of microplastics in the marine genus for human expenditure (bivalves, fish, and crustaceans) is now recognized (Smith et al., 2018). For example, in Mytilus gallo-provincialis and Mytilus edulis of five European countries, the micro-plastics number has been noticed to vary from 3 to 5 fibers per 10 g of mussels (Nelms et al., 2016). Consequently, subsequent experience through diet and uptake in humans is probable, as confirmed by the ability for synthetic particles lesser than 150 μm to pass the gastrointestinal (GI) epithelium in mammalian bodies that causes complete contact. Though, researchers consider that only 0.3% of these particles are estimated to be engrossed, at the same time a lower fraction (0.1%) which includes the particles that are larger than 10 μm should be able of getting both cellular and organs membranes and fleeting throughout the blood-brain barrier (BBB) and placenta (Barboza et al., 2018). Disclosure attentions are expected to be small, even though data about micro and nano-plastics in the atmosphere are still restricted because of the technical analytical difficulties to remove, differentiate, and measure them from ecological matrices (Stock et al., 2019). Another microplastic entrance point to the human body is the airborne one during inhalation (Gasperi et al., 2018). The authors of (Catarino et al., 2018) noticed how the intake of synthetic fibers from mussel consumption is fewer than that of the ones which are breathing in from domestic dust for the duration of the same food. The authors of (Wright et al., 2017) informed finding eighteen fibers and four fragments/L of rain throughout rainfall events. Microplastics are conceded by the wind or from atmospheric depositions and could also affect by the attrition of fertilized and agricultural lands, dried sludges, and crops from wastewater management, industrial emissions, synthetic clothes fabric, marine aerosol, and road dust. This increase could lead to respiratory suffering, inflammatory effects, cytotoxic, and autoimmune illness in humans (Rezaei et al., 2019) (Stock et al., 2019). Furthermore, the human lung has a reasonably spacious alveolation surface of ca. 150 m2, with a very lean tissue barrier that is smaller than 1 μm and which could permit nanoparticles to go through the bloodstream and all human body (Lehner et al., 2019). Figure 5 shows the effect of microplastic on human health. The 50 nm size of polystyrene particles has led to cytotoxic and genotoxic effects on cells and macrophages cells and pulmonary epithelial cells (Paget et al., 2015). More commonly, the reaction to breathing in particles, dependent on individual metabolism and vulnerability, maybe articulated as instantaneous bronchial effects (asthma-like), inflammatory and fibrotic changes in the bronchial and peribronchial tissue (chronic bronchitis), interalveolar septa lesions (pneumothorax), disseminate interstitial fibrosis and granulomas with fiber inclusions (extrinsic allergic alveolitis, chronic pneumonia) (Prata, 2018). For instance, comparable effects have been listed in workers in the textile industry in close contact with polyester, nylon, acrylic fibers, and polyolefin. The low deterioration of microfibers has been noticed in patients suffering from pulmonary cancer as a confirmation of the bio-persistence of these synthetic particles. As well as bio-persistence, fiber size has an impact on their toxicity (Wright et al., 2017); for instance, fibers of 15-20 μm cannot be effectively removed from macrophages to the lungs. Latest in-vitro studies about the properties of plastics on the human body have typically used engineered nano plastics which can manipulate their incorporation and also the translocation and manufacture of ROS due to their charge, dimension, and shape (Inkielewicz-Stepniak et al., 2018) (Forte et al., 2016). The application of metal nanoparticles (NPs) (ZrO2NPs, TiO2NPs, AuNP, CeO2NPs, AgNP, and Al2O3NPs), polyethylene (PE), carbon nanomaterials (C60 fullerene, graphene), and polystyrene (PS) micro-plastics has established that cytotoxic properties are stimulated on HeLa cell lines and T98G (human brain and epithelial cells) (Schirinzi et al., 2017). Furthermore, the employ of polypropylene (PP) particles has noticed dissimilar but dangerous impacts on different cell lines, based on the size (~20 μm and 25–200 μm) and the dissimilar applications used in the different tests. Consequently, the relations of micro-plastics with humans can create hypersensitivity, cytotoxicity, useless immune responses, and severe responses like hemolysis, therefore representing a possible threat to human health (Hwang et al., 2019).

CONCLUSION

Environmental pollution with plastics is a budding alarm, and due to the longevity of plastics, this trouble is estimated to continue for a long time. The production of plastic persists to produce noticeably, resulting in an increasingly raising amount of plastic waste. Therefore, microplastics will be all over the place nearby in the food chain for several years. One main distress is the impending destruction of microplastics into nanoparticles. Unlike nanoparticles, microplastics may attain and infiltrate all organs, as well as the brain and placenta. Though, it is possible that microplastics can be gradually eroded into the intestinal wall into the circulatory system and dispensed to different tissues and organs. If gathered ultimately, their toxic effects may create consequent injuries to the human body. These chapters focused on nanoparticles have just begun. Due to the inimitable size and shape-reliant characteristics of nanoparticles, they may display notably differential effects from microplastics. Upcoming studies on microplastics and nanoparticles should concentrate on the main critical topics, like a) the generational effects of microplastics and nanoplastics, and b) the connections between the surfaces of microplastics and nanoplastics and the atmosphere, aquatic organisms.

Figure 5. The impact of microplastic on human health

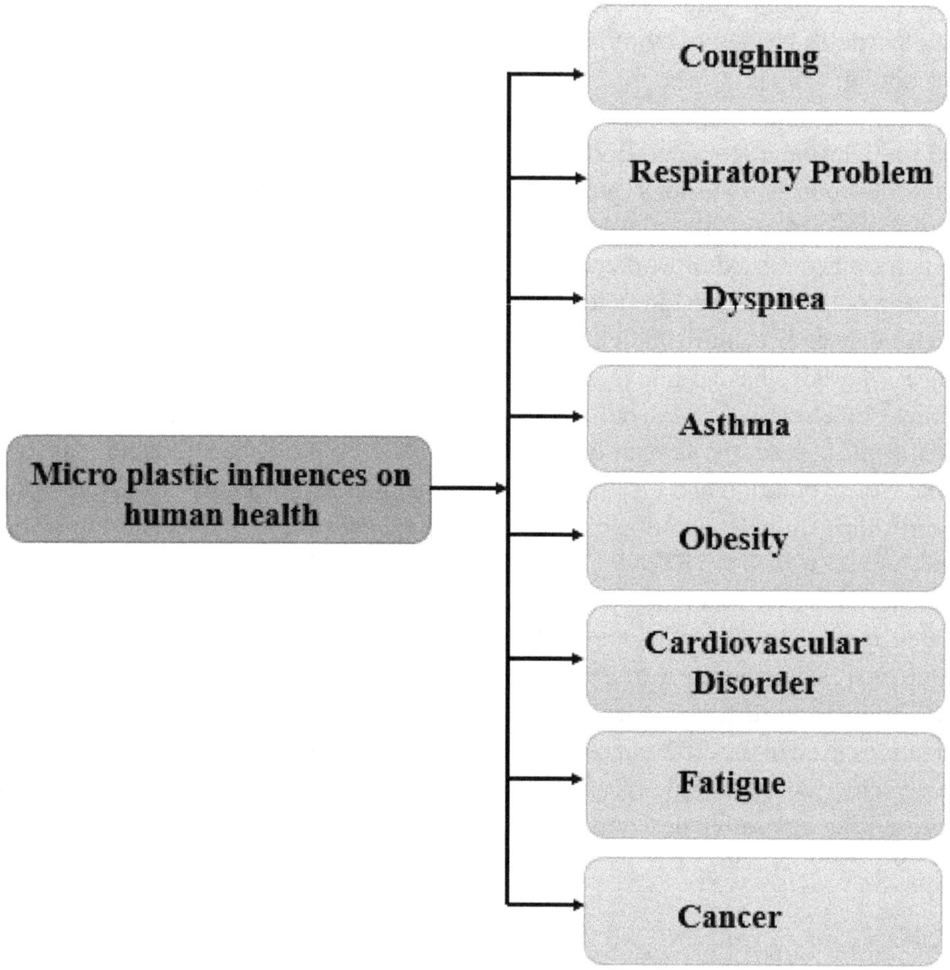

CONFLICTS OF INTEREST

The authors declare that there are no conflicts of interest regarding the publication of this chapter.

ADDITIONAL INFORMATION

Micro and nano-plastics are an evolving worldwide environmental pollutant that is distressing various domains. Despite their ubiquity in all provinces of life and ecosystem, little is identified about the health impacts of micro and nano-plastics contact with humans. This chapter searches the present substantiation on the possible human health effects of micro and nano-plastics and consequent information gaps. Human contact with micro and nano-plastics can happen through inhalation, drinking, eating, and dermal contact because of their existence in water, food, air, and different consumer products. Micro and nano-plastics exposure can cause harmfulness through inflammatory lesions, oxidative stress, increased uptake, etc. Numerous studies have confirmed the potentiality of neurotoxicity, metabolic disturbances, and cancer risk. Furthermore, micro and nano-plastics have been initiated to release their constituent compounds as well as those that are adsorbed onto their surface. Further research is needed to enumerate the properties of micro and nano plastics on human health.

ACKNOWLEDGMENT

The authors would like to thank Mechanical Engineering Department, Omdayal Group of Institutions, Uluberia, Howrah, and thanks to Mrs. Nibedita Bardhan for language proof reading.

REFERENCES

Akbay, İ. K., & Özdemir, T. (2016). Monomer migration and degradation of polycarbonate via UV-C irradiation within aquatic and atmospheric environments. Journal of Macromolecular Science. *Part A*, *53*(6), 340–345.

Au, S. Y., Lee, C. M., Weinstein, J. E., van den Hurk, P., & Klaine, S. J. (2017). Trophic transfer of microplastics in aquatic ecosystems: Identifying critical research needs. *Integrated Environmental Assessment and Management*, *13*(3), 505–509. doi:10.1002/ieam.1907 PMID:28440939

Avio, C. G., Gorbi, S., & Regoli, F. (2017). Plastics and microplastics in the oceans: From emerging pollutants to emerged threat. *Marine Environmental Research*, *128*, 2–11. doi:10.1016/j.marenvres.2016.05.012 PMID:27233985

Barboza, L., Dick Vethaak, A., Lavorante, B., Lundebye, A. K., & Guilhermino, L. (2018). Marine microplastic debris: An emerging issue for food security, food safety and human health. *Marine Pollution Bulletin*, *133*, 336–348. doi:10.1016/j.marpolbul.2018.05.047 PMID:30041323

Barnes, D. K., Galgani, F., Thompson, R. C., & Barlaz, M. (2009). Accumulation and fragmentation of plastic debris in global environments. *Philos. Trans. R. Soc. Lond. Ser. B Biol. Sci.*, *364*(1526), 1985–1998. PMID:19528051

Battulga, B., Kawahigashi, M., & Oyuntsetseg, B. (2019). Distribution and composition of plastic debris along the river shore in the Selenga River basin in Mongolia. *Environmental Science and Pollution Research International*, *26*(14), 14059–14072. doi:10.100711356-019-04632-1 PMID:30852749

Bergami, E., Bocci, E., Vannuccini, M. L., Monopoli, M., Salvati, A., Dawson, K. A., & Corsi, I. (2016). Nano-sized polystyrene affects feeding, behavior and physiology of brine shrimp Artemia franciscana larvae. *Ecotoxicology and Environmental Safety*, *123*, 18–25. doi:10.1016/j.ecoenv.2015.09.021 PMID:26422775

Betts, K. (2008). Why small plastic particles may pose a big problem in the oceans. *Environmental Science & Technology, 42*(24), 8995. doi:10.1021/es802970v PMID:19174862

Bouwmeester, H., Hollman, P. C., & Peters, R. J. (2015). Potential Health Impact of Environmentally Released Micro- and Nanoplastics in the Human Food Production Chain: Experiences from Nanotoxicology. *Environmental Science & Technology, 49*(15), 8932–8947. doi:10.1021/acs.est.5b01090 PMID:26130306

Bradney, L., Wijesekara, H., Palansooriya, K. N., Obadamudalige, N., Bolan, N. S., Ok, Y. S., Rinklebe, J., Kim, K. H., & Kirkham, M. B. (2019). Particulate plastics as a vector for toxic trace-element uptake by aquatic and terrestrial organisms and human health risk. *Environment International, 131*, 104937. doi:10.1016/j.envint.2019.104937 PMID:31284110

Campanale, C., Massarelli, C., Savino, I., Locaputo, V., & Uricchio, V. F. (2020). A Detailed Review Study on Potential Effects of Microplastics and Additives of Concern on Human Health. *International Journal of Environmental Research and Public Health, 17*(4), 1212. doi:10.3390/ijerph17041212 PMID:32069998

Catarino, A. I., Macchia, V., Sanderson, W. G., Thompson, R. C., & Henry, T. B. (2018). Low levels of microplastics (MP) in wild mussels indicate that MP ingestion by humans is minimal compared to exposure via household fibres fallout during a meal. *Environmental Pollution, 237*, 675–684.

Cedervall, T., Hansson, L. A., Lard, M., Frohm, B., & Linse, S. (2012). Food chain transport of nanoparticles affects behaviour and fat metabolism in fish. *PLoS One, 7*(2), e32254. doi:10.1371/journal.pone.0032254 PMID:22384193

Chae, Y., & An, Y. J. (2017). Effects of micro- and nanoplastics on aquatic ecosystems: Current research trends and perspectives. *Marine Pollution Bulletin, 124*(2), 624–632. doi:10.1016/j.marpolbul.2017.01.070 PMID:28222864

Cingotti, N., & Jensen, G. K. (2019). *Health and Environment Alliance (HEAL). Food contact materials and chemical contamination*. Health and Environment Alliance.

Colborn, T., & Clement, C. (1992). *Chemically-induced alterations in sexual and functional development: the wildlife/human connection*. Princeton Scientific Pub. Co.

Cole, M. (2016). A novel method for preparing microplastic fibers. *Scientific Reports, 6*(1), 34519. doi:10.1038rep34519 PMID:27694820

Cole, M., & Galloway, T. S. (2015). Ingestion of nanoplastics and microplastics by Pacific oyster larvae. *Environmental Science & Technology, 49*(24), 14625–14632. doi:10.1021/acs.est.5b04099 PMID:26580574

Cole, M., Lindeque, P., Fileman, E., Halsband, C., Goodhead, R., Moger, J., & Galloway, T. S. (2013). Microplastic ingestion by zooplankton. *Environmental Science & Technology, 47*(12), 6646–6655. doi:10.1021/es400663f PMID:23692270

Cox, K. D., Covernton, G. A., Davies, H. L., Dower, J. F., Juanes, F., & Dudas, S. E. (2019). Human Consumption of Microplastics. *Environmental Science & Technology, 53*(12), 7068–7074. doi:10.1021/acs.est.9b01517 PMID:31184127

Cózar, A., Echevarría, F., González-Gordillo, J. I., Irigoien, X., Ubeda, B., Hernández-León, S., Palma, A. T., Navarro, S., García-de-Lomas, J., Ruiz, A., Fernández-de-Puelles, M. L., & Duarte, C. M. (2014). Plastic debris in the open ocean. *Proceedings of the National Academy of Sciences of the United States of America, 111*(28), 10239–10244. doi:10.1073/pnas.1314705111 PMID:24982135

Desforges, J. P. W., Galbraith, M., & Ross, P. S. (2015). Ingestion of microplastics by zooplankton in the Northeast Pacific Ocean. *Archives of Environmental Contamination and Toxicology, 69*(3), 320–330. doi:10.100700244-015-0172-5 PMID:26066061

Dunlap, R. E., & Scarce, R. (1991). Poll trends: Environmental problems and protection. *Public Opinion Quarterly, 55*(4), 651–672. doi:10.1086/269288

Ebere, E. C., Wirnkor, V. A., & Ngozi, V. E. (2019). Uptake of microplastics by plant: A reason to worry or to be happy? *World Scientific News, 131*, 256–267.

Eriksen, M., Lebreton, L. C., Carson, H. S., Thiel, M., Moore, C. J., Borerro, J. C., Galgani, F., Ryan, P. G., & Reisser, J. (2014). Plastic Pollution in the World's Oceans: More than 5 Trillion Plastic Pieces Weighing over 250,000 Tons Afloat at Sea. *PLoS One, 9*(12), e111913. doi:10.1371/journal.pone.0111913 PMID:25494041

Forte, M., Iachetta, G., Tussellino, M., Carotenuto, R., Prisco, M., De Falco, M., Laforgia, V., & Valiante, S. (2016). Polystyrene nanoparticles internalization in human gastric adenocarcinoma cells. *Toxicology in Vitro: An International Journal, 31*, 126–136.

Franzellitti, S., Canesi, L., Auguste, M., Wathsala, R., & Fabbri, E. (2019). Microplastic exposure and effects in aquatic organisms: A physiological perspective. *Environmental Toxicology and Pharmacology, 68*, 37–51. doi:10.1016/j.etap.2019.03.009 PMID:30870694

Gasperi, J., Wright, S. L., Dris, R., Collard, F., Mandin, C., Guerrouache, M., Langlois, V., Kelly, F. J., & Tassin, B. (2018). Microplastics in air: Are we breathing it in? *Current Opinion in Environmental Science & Health, 1*, 1–5. doi:10.1016/j.coesh.2017.10.002

Geyer, R., Jambeck, J. R., & Law, K. L. (2017). Production, use, and fate of all plastics ever made. *Science Advances, 3*(7), e1700782. doi:10.1126ciadv.1700782 PMID:28776036

Gigault, J., Halle, A. T., Baudrimont, M., Pascal, P. Y., Gauffre, F., Phi, T. L., El Hadri, H., Grassl, B., & Reynaud, S. (2018). Current opinion: What is a nanoplastic? *Environmental Pollution, 235*, 1030–1034.

Gregory, M. R. (2009). Environmental implications of plastic debris in marine settings—Entanglement, ingestion, smothering, hangers-on, hitch-hiking and alien invasions. Philos. Trans. R. Soc. Lond. Ser. B Biol. *Sci., 364*(1526), 2013–2025. PMID:19528053

Guglielmi, G. (2017). *In the next 30 years, we'll make four times more plastic waste than we ever have*. https://www.sciencemag.org/news/2017/07/next-30-years-we-ll-make-four-times-more-plastic-waste-we-ever-have

Guzzetti, E., Sureda, A., Tejada, S., & Faggio, C. (2018). Microplastic in marine organism: Environmental and toxicological effects. *Environmental Toxicology and Pharmacology, 64*, 164–171. doi:10.1016/j.etap.2018.10.009 PMID:30412862

Hernandez, L. M., Xu, E. G., Larsson, H., Tahara, R., Maisuria, V. B., & Tufenkji, N. (2019). Plastic Teabags Release Billions of Microparticles and Nanoparticles into Tea. *Environmental Science & Technology*, *53*(21), 12300–12310. doi:10.1021/acs.est.9b02540 PMID:31552738

Hu, L., Chernick, M., Lewis, A. M., Ferguson, P. L., & Hinton, D. E. (2020). Chronic microfiber exposure in adult Japanese medaka (Oryzias latipes). *PLoS One*, *15*(3), e0229962. doi:10.1371/journal.pone.0229962 PMID:32150587

Huerta Lwanga, E., Mendoza Vega, J., Ku Quej, V., Chi, J., Sanchez Del Cid, L., Chi, C., Escalona Segura, G., Gertsen, H., Salánki, T., van der Ploeg, M., Koelmans, A. A., & Geissen, V. (2017). Field evidence for transfer of plastic debris along a terrestrial food chain. *Scientific Reports*, *7*(1), 14071. doi:10.103841598-017-14588-2 PMID:29074893

Hwang, J., Choi, D., Han, S., Choi, J., & Hong, J. (2019). An assessment of the toxicity of polypropylene microplastics in human derived cells. *The Science of the Total Environment*, *684*, 657–669. doi:10.1016/j.scitotenv.2019.05.071 PMID:31158627

Inkielewicz-Stepniak, I., Tajber, L., Behan, G., Zhang, H., Radomski, M. W., Medina, C., & Santos-Martinez, M. J. (2018). The Role of Mucin in the Toxicological Impact of Polystyrene Nanoparticles. *Materials (Basel, Switzerland)*, *11*(5), 724. doi:10.3390/ma11050724 PMID:29751544

Jiang, B., Kauffman, A. E., Li, L., McFee, W., Cai, B., Weinstein, J., Lead, J. R., Chatterjee, S., Scott, G. I., & Xiao, S. (2020). Health impacts of environmental contamination of micro- and nanoplastics: A review. *Environmental Health and Preventive Medicine*, *25*(1), 29. doi:10.118612199-020-00870-9 PMID:32664857

Jin, Y., Lu, L., Tu, W., Luo, T., & Fu, Z. (2019). Impacts of polystyrene microplastic on the gut barrier, microbiota and metabolism of mice. *The Science of the Total Environment*, *649*, 308–317. doi:10.1016/j.scitotenv.2018.08.353 PMID:30176444

Kaposi, K. L., Mos, B., Kelaher, B. P., & Dworjanyn, S. A. (2014). Ingestion of microplastic has limited impact on a marine larva. *Environmental Science & Technology*, *48*(3), 1638–1645. doi:10.1021/es404295e PMID:24341789

Klein, S., Worch, E., & Knepper, T. P. (2015). Occurrence and spatial distribution of microplastics in river shore sediments of the Rhine-main area in Germany. *Environmental Science & Technology*, *49*(10), 6070–6076. doi:10.1021/acs.est.5b00492 PMID:25901760

Koelmans, A. A., Bakir, A., Burton, G. A., & Janssen, C. R. (2016). Microplastic as a vector for chemicals in the aquatic environment: Critical review and model-supported reinterpretation of empirical studies. *Environmental Science & Technology*, *50*(7), 3315–3326. doi:10.1021/acs.est.5b06069 PMID:26946978

Kokalj, A. J., Kunej, U., & Skalar, T. (2018). Screening study of four environmentally relevant microplastic pollutants: Uptake and effects on Daphnia magna and Artemia franciscana. *Chemosphere*, *208*, 522–529. doi:10.1016/j.chemosphere.2018.05.172 PMID:29890490

Kubowicz, S., & Booth, A. M. (2017). Biodegradability of Plastics: Challenges and Misconceptions. *Environmental Science & Technology*, *51*(21), 12058–12060. doi:10.1021/acs.est.7b04051 PMID:29022342

Lehner, R., Weder, C., Petri-Fink, A., & Rothen-Rutishauser, B. (2019). Emergence of Nanoplastic in the Environment and Possible Impact on Human Health. *Environmental Science & Technology*, *53*(4), 1748–1765. doi:10.1021/acs.est.8b05512 PMID:30629421

Lei, L., Wu, S., Lu, S., Liu, M., Song, Y., Fu, Z., Shi, H., Raley-Susman, K. M., & He, D. (2018). Microplastic particles cause intestinal damage and other adverse effects in zebrafish Danio rerio and nematode Caenorhabditis elegans. *The Science of the Total Environment*, *619-620*, 1–8. doi:10.1016/j.scitotenv.2017.11.103 PMID:29136530

Liu, J., Lezama, N., Gasper, J., Kawata, J., Morley, S., Helmer, D., & Ciminera, P. (2016). Burn Pit Emissions Exposure and Respiratory and Cardiovascular Conditions Among Airborne Hazards and Open Burn Pit Registry Participants. *Journal of Occupational and Environmental Medicine*, *58*(7), e249–e255. doi:10.1097/JOM.0000000000000776 PMID:27218278

Liu, J., Yang, Y., Ding, J., Zhu, B., & Gao, W. (2019). Microfibers: A preliminary discussion on their definition and sources. *Environmental Science and Pollution Research International*, *26*(28), 29497–29501. doi:10.100711356-019-06265-w PMID:31444725

Lu, L., Wan, Z., Luo, T., Fu, Z., & Jin, Y. (2018). Polystyrene microplastics induce gut microbiota dysbiosis and hepatic lipid metabolism disorder in mice. *The Science of the Total Environment*, *631-632*, 449–458. doi:10.1016/j.scitotenv.2018.03.051 PMID:29529433

Lu, Y., Zhang, Y., Deng, Y., Jiang, W., Zhao, Y., Geng, J., Ding, L., & Ren, H. (2016). Uptake and Accumulation of Polystyrene Microplastics in Zebrafish (Danio rerio) and Toxic Effects in Liver. *Environmental Science & Technology*, *50*(7), 4054–4060. doi:10.1021/acs.est.6b00183 PMID:26950772

Magara, G., Elia, A. C., Syberg, K., & Khan, F. R. (2018). Single contaminant and combined exposures of polyethylene microplastics and fluoranthene: Accumulation and oxidative stress response in the blue mussel, Mytilus edulis. *Journal of Toxicology and Environmental Health. Part A.*, *81*(16), 761–773. doi:10.1080/15287394.2018.1488639 PMID:29969377

Mato, Y., Isobe, T., Takada, H., Kanehiro, H., Ohtake, C., & Kaminuma, T. (2001). Plastic resin pellets as a transport medium for toxic chemicals in the marine environment. *Environmental Science & Technology*, *35*(2), 318–324. doi:10.1021/es0010498 PMID:11347604

Mattsson, K., Ekvall, M. T., Hansson, L. A., Linse, S., Malmendal, A., & Cedervall, T. (2014). Altered behavior, physiology, and metabolism in fish exposed to polystyrene nanoparticles. *Environmental Science & Technology*, *49*(1), 553–561. doi:10.1021/es5053655 PMID:25380515

Mattsson, K., Hansson, L. A., & Cedervall, T. (2015). Nano-plastics in the aquatic environment. *Environmental Science. Processes & Impacts*, *17*(10), 1712–1721. doi:10.1039/C5EM00227C PMID:26337600

Miyagawa, S., Sato, T., & Iguchi, T. (2016). Handbook of Hormones. Academic Press.

Moyce, S. C., & Schenker, M. (2018). Migrant workers and their occupational health and safety. *Annual Review of Public Health*, *39*(1), 351–365. doi:10.1146/annurev-publhealth-040617-013714 PMID:29400993

Nelms, S. E., Duncan, E. M., Broderick, A. C., Galloway, T. S., Godfrey, M. H., Hamann, M., Lindeque, P. K., & Godley, B. J. (2016). Plastic and marine turtles: A review and call for research. *ICES Journal of Marine Science*, *73*(2), 165–181. doi:10.1093/icesjms/fsv165

Novotna, K., Cermakova, L., Pivokonska, L., Cajthaml, T., & Pivokonsky, M. (2019). Microplastics in drinking water treatment–Current knowledge and research needs. *The Science of the Total Environment*, *667*, 730–740. doi:10.1016/j.scitotenv.2019.02.431 PMID:30851606

Orayeva, J. (2020). *New Research on the Possible Effects of Micro-and Nano-plastics on Marine Animals.* IAEA. www.iaea.org/newscenter/news/new-research-on-the-possible-effects-of-micro-and-nano-plastics-on-marine-animals

Paget, V., Dekali, S., Kortulewski, T., Grall, R., Gamez, C., Blazy, K., Aguerre-Chariol, O., Chevillard, S., Braun, A., Rat, P., & Lacroix, G. (2015). Specific uptake and genotoxicity induced by polystyrene nanobeads with distinct surface chemistry on human lung epithelial cells and macrophages. *PLoS One*, *10*(4), e0123297. doi:10.1371/journal.pone.0123297 PMID:25875304

Prata J. C. (2018). Airborne microplastics: Consequences to human health? *Environmental Pollution, 234*, 115–126.

Prata, J. C., da Costa, J. P., Lopes, I., Duarte, A. C., & Rocha-Santos, T. (2020). Environmental exposure to microplastics: An overview on possible human health effects. *The Science of the Total Environment*, *702*, 134455. doi:10.1016/j.scitotenv.2019.134455 PMID:31733547

Raddadi, N., & Fava, F. (2019). Biodegradation of oil-based plastics in the environment: Existing knowledge and needs of research and innovation. *The Science of the Total Environment*, *679*, 148–158. doi:10.1016/j.scitotenv.2019.04.419 PMID:31082589

Regulation, E. C. (2008). No. 1272/2008 of the European Parliament and of the Council of 16 December 2008 on classification, labelling and packaging of substances and mixtures, amending and repealing Directives 67/548/EEC and 1999/45/EC, and amending Regulation (EC) No 1907/2006. *Official Journal of the European Union. 2008b L, 353.*

Rehse, S., Kloas, W., & Zarfl, C. (2016). Short-term exposure with high concentrations of pristine microplastic particles leads to immobilisation of Daphnia magna. *Chemosphere*, *153*, 91–99. doi:10.1016/j.chemosphere.2016.02.133 PMID:27010171

Revel, M., Châtel, A., & Mouneyrac, C. (2018). Micro (nano) plastics: A threat to human health? *Current Opinion in Environmental Science & Health*, *1*, 17–23. doi:10.1016/j.coesh.2017.10.003

Rezaei, M., Riksen, M., Sirjani, E., Sameni, A., & Geissen, V. (2019). Wind erosion as a driver for transport of light density microplastics. *The Science of the Total Environment*, *669*, 273–281. doi:10.1016/j.scitotenv.2019.02.382 PMID:30878934

Rhodes, C. J. (2018). Plastic pollution and potential solutions. *Science Progress*, *101*(3), 207–260. doi:10.3184/003685018X15294876706211 PMID:30025551

Riisgård, H. U. (1988). Efficiency of particle retention and filtration rate in 6 species of Northeast American bivalves. Marine ecology progress series. *Oldendorf*, *45*(3), 217–223. doi:10.3354/meps045217

Rillig, M. C. (2012). Microplastic in terrestrial ecosystems and the soil? *Environmental Science & Technology, 46*(12), 6453–6454. doi:10.1021/es302011r PMID:22676039

Rist, S., Baun, A., Almeda, R., & Hartmann, N. B. (2019). Ingestion and effects of micro- and nanoplastics in blue mussel (Mytilus edulis) larvae. *Marine Pollution Bulletin, 140*, 423–430. doi:10.1016/j.marpolbul.2019.01.069 PMID:30803663

Rochman, C. M., Hoh, E., Hentschel, B. T., & Kaye, S. (2013). Long-term field measurement of sorption of organic contaminants to five types of plastic pellets: Implications for plastic marine debris. *Environmental Science & Technology, 47*(3), 1646–1654. doi:10.1021/es303700s PMID:23270427

Rudyak, V. Y., Efimova, E. A., Guseva, D. V., & Chertovich, A. V. (2018). Thermoset Polymer Matrix Structure and Properties: Coarse-Grained Simulations. *Polymers, 11*(1), 36. doi:10.3390/polym11010036 PMID:30960020

Schirinzi, G. F., Pérez-Pomeda, I., Sanchís, J., Rossini, C., Farré, M., & Barceló, D. (2017). Cytotoxic effects of commonly used nanomaterials and microplastics on cerebral and epithelial human cells. *Environmental Research, 159*, 579–587. doi:10.1016/j.envres.2017.08.043 PMID:28898803

Sharma, S., & Chatterjee, S. (2017). Microplastic pollution, a threat to marine ecosystem and human health: A short review. *Environmental Science and Pollution Research International, 24*(27), 21530–21547. doi:10.100711356-017-9910-8 PMID:28815367

Silva-Cavalcanti, J. S., Silva, J., França, E. J., Araújo, M., & Gusmão, F. (2017). Microplastics ingestion by a common tropical freshwater fishing resource. *Environmental Pollution, 221*, 218–226.

Smith, M., Love, D. C., Rochman, C. M., & Neff, R. A. (2018). Microplastics in Seafood and the Implications for Human Health. *Current Environmental Health Reports, 5*(3), 375–386. doi:10.100740572-018-0206-z PMID:30116998

Stock, F., Reifferscheid, G., Brennholt, N., & Kostianaia, E. (2019). *Plastics in the Aquatic Environment-Part II: Stakeholders' Role Against Pollution*. Academic Press.

Suresh, S. S., Mohanty, S., & Nayak, S. K. (2017). Composition analysis and characterization of waste polyvinyl chloride (PVC) recovered from data cables. *Waste Management (New York, N.Y.), 60*, 100–111. doi:10.1016/j.wasman.2016.08.033 PMID:27594574

Sussarellu, R., Suquet, M., Thomas, Y., Lambert, C., Fabioux, C., Pernet, M. E., Le Goïc, N., Quillien, V., Mingant, C., Epelboin, Y., Corporeau, C., Guyomarch, J., Robbens, J., Paul-Pont, I., Soudant, P., & Huvet, A. (2016). Oyster reproduction is affected by exposure to polystyrene microplastics. *Proceedings of the National Academy of Sciences of the United States of America, 113*(9), 2430–2435. doi:10.1073/pnas.1519019113 PMID:26831072

Tallec, K., Huvet, A., Di Poi, C., González-Fernández, C., Lambert, C., Petton, B., Le Goïc, N., Berchel, M., Soudant, P., & Paul-Pont, I. (2018). Nanoplastics impaired oyster free living stages, gametes and embryos. *Environmental Pollution, 242*(Pt B), 1226–1235.

Thompson, R. C., Swan, S. H., Moore, C. J., & Vom Saal, F. S. (2009). Our plastic age. Philos. Trans. R. Soc. Lond. Ser. B Biol. *Sci., 364*(1526), 1973–1976.

Toussaint, B., Raffael, B., Angers-Loustau, A., Gilliland, D., Kestens, V., Petrillo, M., Rio-Echevarria, I. M., & Van den Eede, G. (2019). Review of micro- and nanoplastic contamination in the food chain. *Food Additives & Contaminants. Part A, Chemistry, Analysis, Control, Exposure & Risk Assessment, 36*(5), 639–673. doi:10.1080/19440049.2019.1583381 PMID:30985273

Van Cauwenberghe, L., & Janssen, C. R. (2014). Microplastics in bivalves cultured for human consumption. *Environmental Pollution, 193*, 65–70.

von Moos, N., Burkhardt-Holm, P., & Köhler, A. (2012). Uptake and effects of microplastics on cells and tissue of the blue mussel Mytilus edulis L. after an experimental exposure. *Environmental Science & Technology, 46*(20), 11327–11335. doi:10.1021/es302332w PMID:22963286

Wang, T., Li, B., Zou, X., Wang, Y., Li, Y., Xu, Y., Mao, L., Zhang, C., & Yu, W. (2019). Emission of primary microplastics in mainland China: Invisible but not negligible. *Water Research, 162*, 214–224. doi:10.1016/j.watres.2019.06.042 PMID:31276985

Waring, R. H., Harris, R. M., & Mitchell, S. C. (2018). Plastic contamination of the food chain: A threat to human health? *Maturitas, 115*, 64–68. doi:10.1016/j.maturitas.2018.06.010 PMID:30049349

Wright, S. L., & Kelly, F. J. (2017). Plastic and Human Health: A Micro Issue? *Environmental Science & Technology, 51*(12), 6634–6647. doi:10.1021/acs.est.7b00423 PMID:28531345

Xu, Y., He, Q., Liu, C., & Huangfu, X. (2019). Are Micro- or Nanoplastics Leached from Drinking Water Distribution Systems? *Environmental Science & Technology, 53*(16), 9339–9340. doi:10.1021/acs.est.9b03673 PMID:31393716

Yang, Y. F., Chen, C. Y., Lu, T. H., & Liao, C. M. (2019). Toxicity-based toxicokinetic/toxicodynamic assessment for bioaccumulation of polystyrene microplastics in mice. *Journal of Hazardous Materials, 366*, 703–713. doi:10.1016/j.jhazmat.2018.12.048 PMID:30583240

Yu, Z., Peldszus, S., & Huck, P. M. (2008). Adsorption characteristics of selected pharmaceuticals and an endocrine disrupting compound-Naproxen, carbamazepine and nonylphenol-on activated carbon. *Water Research, 42*(12), 2873–2882. doi:10.1016/j.watres.2008.02.020 PMID:18377945

Zhang, H., Zhou, Q., Xie, Z., Zhou, Y., Tu, C., Fu, C., Mi, W., Ebinghaus, R., Christie, P., & Luo, Y. (2018). Occurrences of organophosphorus esters and phthalates in the microplastics from the coastal beaches in north China. *The Science of the Total Environment, 616-617*, 1505–1512. doi:10.1016/j.scitotenv.2017.10.163 PMID:29089130

KEY TERMS AND DEFINITIONS

Additives: To inhibit plastic ingredients from becoming soft and sticky at high temperatures, or inflexible and brittle at low temperatures.

Atmospheric Pollutant: Atmospheric pollutants are elements that accrue in the air which is injurious to living organisms. Common air pollutants contain smog, smoke, and gases for example CO_2, CO, N_2, SO_2, and hydrocarbon fumes.

Micro Plastics: Microplastics are basically small plastic particles less than 5 mm long which can be injurious to our land and marine life. Microplastics originate from a multiplicity of sources, containing from higher plastic wreckage which degrades into smaller and smaller pieces. Additionally, micro beads, a type of micro plastic, are very small parts of manufactured polyethylene plastic which are supplementary as exfoliates to health and consumer products, for example some detergents and toothpaste.

Nano-Plastics: Nano plastics are elements caused by the degradation of plastic substances. It exhibits colloidal actions within size extending from 1 to 1μm.

Toxicity: Toxicity can denote the consequence on an entire organism, for example, bacterium, animal, or plant, other than the consequence on an arrangement of the organism, for example, a cell or an organ such as the heart, liver, etc.

Chapter 8
The Effects of (Micro and Nano) Plastics on the Human Body:
Nervous System, Respiratory System, Digestive System, Placental Barrier, Skin, and Excretory System

Sanchari Biswas
https://orcid.org/0000-0002-1159-5826
Salim Ali Centre for Ornithology and Natural History, India

Devarati Bagchi
GITAM Dental College and Hospital, India

Debjit Ghosh
GITAM Institute of Science, India

ABSTRACT

In the contemporary world, the menace of plastic pollution dovetailed with the current pandemic scenario is a globally rising concern which is affecting every life form on Earth. Plastics hold several properties like ductility that permit the material to be casted and given numerous shapes and forms for various commercial uses. When summed up, it has benefited mankind by becoming an indispensable part of our lives. But the negative impacts associated with it lurks behind silently. Most of the plastic polymers manufactured today are highly resistant to degradation, and the accumulation of these complex and persistent materials are not only causing serious damage to the environment, but also to human health. Additives are added during the manufacturing process to improve the life of these synthetic polymers. The excessive usage of plastic products has resulted in accumulation of the hazardous chemicals, associated with plastic polymers in human body about which this chapter discusses further.

DOI: 10.4018/978-1-7998-9723-1.ch008

INTRODUCTION

It was during the 1800s, when the term 'Plastic' was derived from a Greek Word. Owing to its cost benefit advantage, the terrestrial and aquatic ecosystem in the current times stand as the greatest witness and victim of emerging disposal of these synthetic and non-recyclable compounds. The particles or fragments of plastic which has dimension of £ 5 mm are termed as micro plastics (MPs). Often, these MPs end up being ingested by different phytoplankton, zooplanktons, corals, invertebrates and vertebrates, large sea mammals and ultimately find their fate through the food chain. Posing a direct threat not only to the marine biota but also to the ecosystems they propagate from, these plastic compounds have a property to adsorb other pollutants of marine origin. It can directly absorb hydrophobic pollutants, given its huge surface area to volume ratio.

The 20th century has been a revolutionary era with first advent of technology wherein plastic manufacturing industry had a major breakthrough, but it's after effects can only be observed in the 21st century. Inaccurate management, negligence of over exploitative usage, lack of scientific research and unconditioned discarding of the same into the ecosystem are few of the factors responsible for their increasing presence. One of the major reasons contributing to this factor is human conscience that is programmed into the concept of "out of sight out of mind". Continuous and uncontrolled disposal of plastics have led to its humongous accumulation into the environment. Given their size which is invisible to the naked eye, fragments of MPs easily enhance their bioavailability and the ability of being ingested by a vast batch of marine life forms which in turn impacts their survival, pacing its way up through the food chain, affecting the top predators in the food chain, nonetheless other than humans.

Thus, in this Chapter, we discuss the various facets of research that has been carried out regarding the effects of Micro and Nano-plastic concerning human health, their impacts on bodily systems with respect of nervous system, respiratory system, placental barrier, digestive system, excretory system and skin and the various research gaps that exists and hasn't been addressed yet.

BACKGROUND

It is just occasionally, that researchers have carried out studies on impacts of MPs on environment and human health. Initial studies in the past two decades dealt with consequences of MP's on circulatory system of bivalve (Mussels) which concluded effects on their immune responses. Various studies suggest that the bottom feeders, filter feeders, primary producers are primarily affected due to the size of MPs. Future research on this prospect is a strong need of the hour to understand such interactions. Investigations on the effects of MPs on marine mammals occurring as a result of contaminated food source (through small fishes) have also been documented frequently. Thus, necessity to elucidate the background structure for probing the occurrence of MPs which affect apex predators (or top consumers in the food chain) is acutely important. Although, detailed research studies are required regarding the extent to which MPs are involved in changing species assemblages and how they influence survival of certain endemic species, but still MPs serve the purpose as modes of transport for invasive microbes to inaccessible regions.

MAIN FOCUS OF THE CHAPTER

The current day synthetic compounds are a result of the primitive evolution of plastic from various natural compounds. One of the most remarkable characteristics of plastic is its ductility which allows it to be moulded into a handful of shapes and forms, which are later utilised in the commercial sector for packaging materials, constructing buildings, sports equipment, art and craft, pharma and medical industry, etc. Apart from its anti-corrosive nature and durability, other properties of plastics include its social aspect of possessing less face value which makes it easily accessible in the production market.

As lack of research persists on the present day, it is very important to understand how plastics (MPs & NPs) impact life forms on a regular basis. Mankind has depended upon oceans since ages. And since the biofouling of plastics is all over the oceans, there is rich growth of fauna everywhere which prevents plastic degradation by UV rays or slows down the process. There is no proven result of plastic degradation in the darker zones. In the areas where surface fauna is removed, the plastic may re-float on the water surface which may further aid its pathway for food chain entry. As human lives are dependent on Oceans, hence, a major threat lurks in the background which are either consciously or unconsciously created through humans actions.

Issues, Controversies, Problems

During the initial investigations by various researchers in the 2000's, it was understood that the level of organic contaminant is about twice as higher than that of natural sediments, although circumstantial studies are required in this context. Research gaps of pollutants adhering to micro-plastics remains higher when compared to studies done on suspended matter adhesion to micro-plastics, or adhesion of micro-plastics to detritivores or phytoplankton. Adding up, research gaps prevail even in existence of research data concerning human beings, as secondary data have always aided in the amount of literature available on human study subjects. Effect of MPs on humans through examining stools, nails, hair, bodily fluids are available but so far, no direct study has been carried out on humans as a test subject itself. Rarely, cadavers have been used as a tool to study the effects of micro and nano-plastics on human health.

Although there are a handful of research articles available that include measuring sub-micrometre plastic particles and analytical methods associated with it, studying and investigating micro-plastics in soil, review articles on soil micro-plastic analysis, analysis and separation of MPs and NPs in complex samples from environment (Paul MB et al., 2020), yet there are various critical parameters that need to be taken under consideration for detecting plastic particles analytically and for obtaining information with regards to both chemical and morphological composition of the particles which stands alone vastly as a data deficient area.

Types of Micro-Plastics and their Classification

Different characteristics of plastic like durability, strength, light weight and anti-resistance and anti-corrosiveness makes it useful and most widely accepted polymer. Withstanding high electrical discharge and thermal compression and insulation, plastics hold high potential in industrial as well as commercial applications. Plastic production has drastically increased from 1950 (One point five million tonnes) to three hundred twenty-two tonnes in 2015. Often it is observed that small fragments of plastics are generated from larger debris of plastic upon degradation. And these fragments can range from meter to

Figure 1. Schematic diagram representing the six majorly used micro plastics that govern the commercial industry and markets

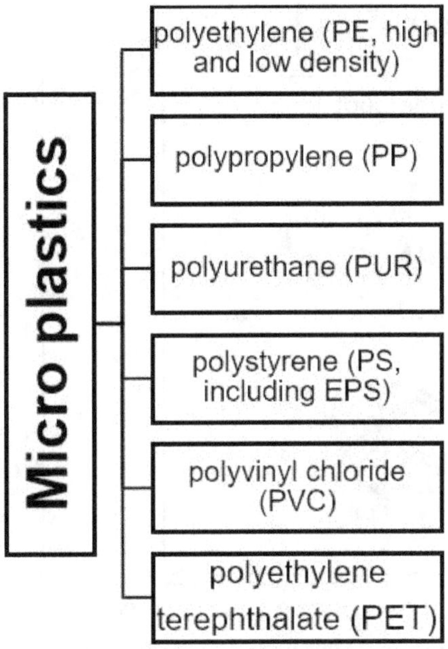

micro meter because of external conditions arising from the environment. Particles which are <5mm have been termed as micro plastics and they have the property to retain themselves in ecosystem and turn persistent with time. Certain criteria like shape, size, physical processes and chemical structures are considered while differentiating micro-plastics which are represented as follows:

Primary Micro Plastics

Primary micro plastics are generally composed of polypropylene (PP), polystyrene (PS) and polyethylene (PE) and are <2 mm in their size. They are composed of micro-sized synthetic polymers which are a result of various processes arising from chemical formations (or exfoliates), leachates (or by-products) of production processes, sand blasting and synthetic garment industries. Cosmetic products like Sunscreen, exfoliating scrubs are other contributors of micro plastics (<2mm) apart from health care related products. Industrial primary MPs are of different kinds, for example- 'industrial scrubbers' which are utilized for blast cleaning surfaces, plastics required in moulding related to industrial procedures. Additionally, virgin resin pellets (<5mm) which are either cylindrical or spherical have often found their usage in plastic manufacturing processes or during production of "feedstock" processes.

Secondary Micro-Plastics

When fragmentation occurs in primary micro-plastics because of weathering processes, it gives rise to what is called as secondary micro-plastics. Secondary micro-plastics are nothing but fragmented particles of macro/meso plastics arising under certain processes such as photo-degradation, thermal

Figure 2. Origin, source and various effects of micro and nano-plastic on human health

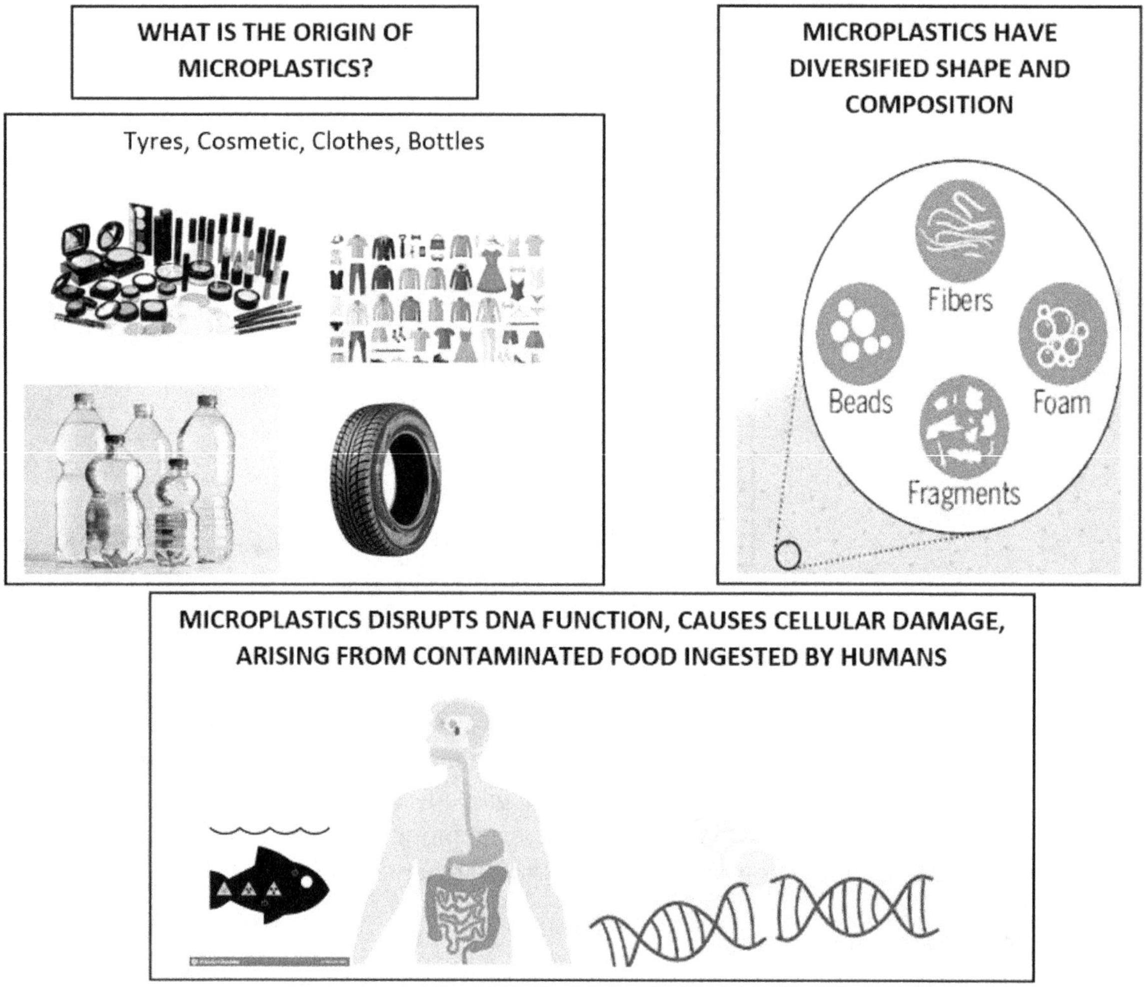

degradation, biodegradation, hydrolysis, emerging from different environmental processes. Secondary micro-plastics can further be divided again into Nano-plastics, (NPs). These are fragments of plastic < 1 µm size. Together MPs and NPs because of their particle size, have potential for inducing long term effects in the environment by bio-amplification/bio-magnification and bioaccumulation through the food chain. Examples which serve as secondary plastics arising from weather degradation processes include paints, tyres, rubber, textiles etc.

IMPACTS OF MICRO-PLASTICS AND NANO-PLASTICS ON DIGESTIVE SYSTEM

Marine organisms like Shellfish and those which are consumed whole, possesses major potential threat to human life. Toxicity, if imparted, are generally dose-dependent and lies on several factors like type of

Figure 3. Routes of entry of micro-plastics into human body through different pathways
Source: Joon, M. (2019). Trophic transfer of microplastics in zooplanktons towards its speculations on human health: A review. Journal of biomedical and therapeutic sciences, 6(1), 8-14.

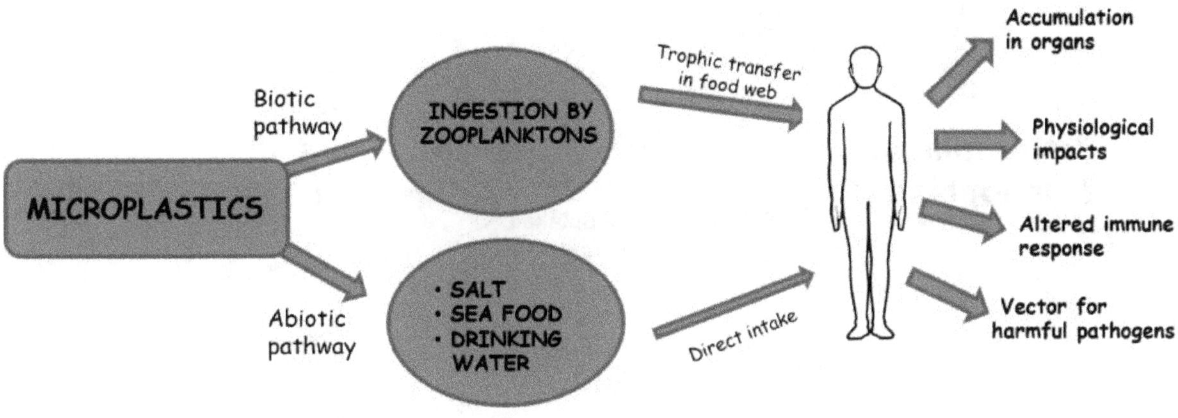

polymer, surface chemistry and its size, its property of hydrophobicity etc. Because of human-induced micro-plastic contamination, micro-plastics and nano-plastics are often ingested by shellfish.

Being a matter of global, governmental and public concern, MPs have less benefits when compared to the consequence it brings with its usage. According to Seltenrich, 2015, the main concerns about MPs include (1) non-conventional resource (2) its POP (Persistent Organic Pollutant) characteristic (3) It is degradation-resistant due to its property of durability (4) fragmenting vulnerability (5) Ingestion by living organisms leading to mortality (Wright et al. 2017).

Because of their size and structure, MPs are easily ingested by all organisms. Generally, it is because of trophic transfer by which direct or indirect intake of food takes place by micro-organisms. Documentation of MPs has been carried out in planktonic life or producers in food chain (Steer et al., 2017; Smith et al., 2018) in secondary consumers and invertebrates (Murray and Cowie 2011; Smith et al., 2018) as well as in fish (Lusher et al., 2017). Many studies have documented the presence of micro-plastic occurring in predatory Crucian carps (Smith et al., 2018). The presence of these MPs in every type of organisms makes contamination easily available, occurring via the food chain, thus affecting the top most consumers in the food chain. Because of whole consumption of small fishes and bivalves (which otherwise accumulate MPs and NPs), humans are easily susceptible to contamination occurring because of their diet (GESAMP 2016).

In studies carried out by Cauwenberghe and Janssen 2014, it was observed that mussels which were farmed, showed comparatively higher MP levels when compared to mussels that were caught in the wild. Apart from this, a study done by Rochman et al. 2015, concluded commercially sold fishes (> 500 µm) from Makassar, Indonesia contained MPs in tissues of dried fish and organs, gills, etc. Karami et al 2017 confirmed foreign particles of MPs in dried fishes which were later found to be polymers of plastics. Y Lu et al. 2016 investigated presence of MPs being translocated to gills from GI tract of many adult and juvenile fishes including that of Zebra fish (*Danio rerio)*. Few other fishes where MP translocation has been observed include Common Goby and European seabass (de Sá LC et al., 2015). Hence, summing up these studies together, it is evident that ingestion of sea food has a major role in contributing towards the continuous contamination and the ability to mitigate it remains the biggest challenge, given its ubiquitous nature in the environment. And hence, this makes humans more susceptible to its harmful effects.

Figure 4. Origin, uptake and pathway of micro and nano-plastic into digestive system
Source: Paul, M. B., Stock, V., Cara-Carmona, J., Lisicki, E., Shopova, S., Fessard, V., ... & Böhmert, L. (2020). Micro-and nanoplastics–current state of knowledge with the focus on oral uptake and toxicity. Nanoscale Advances, 2(10), 4350-4367.

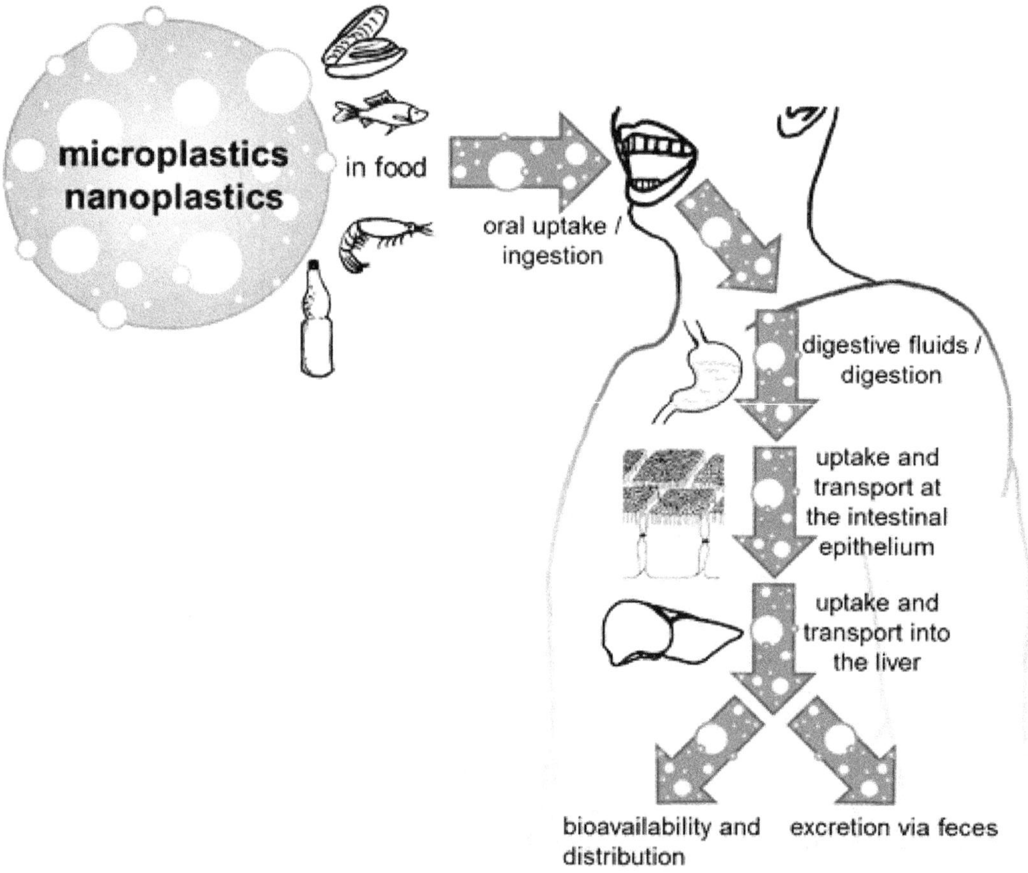

Researchers, worldwide has also investigated the chances of cross-contamination in products those are obtained from these substances. Few products which holds a record of being investigated with micro-plastic signatures include honey, beer, and ocean salt. (Smith et al., 2018). Potential sources which could be responsible for the former cause can be due to uptake of MP's by food products, or because of their presence in atmosphere, by-products arising from processing materials and packaging material contaminants, although other causes for their origin remains uncertain and cannot be ruled out (Liebezeit et al., 2014). On a different note, scientific evidence has demonstrated the increasingly growing history of MP exposure pathway which is arising via the food chain, thus contributing to increasing concern with regards to food safety and contamination of marine fisheries, globally (Lusher et al., 2017).

It was observed by researchers that annually, the intake of MPs on a total note, is thirty-seven particles per individual (Yang et al., 2015). It has been concluded by various studies that a consumer intakes approximately 11,000 particles of plastic, annually (Smith et al., 2018) of whose conclusion are still unknown. Further research is required for assessment, analysis and monitoring of MPs and its chemical association in sea food industry, especially in Shellfish industry. Apart from monitoring of rates of consumer consumption of sea food (for example: bivalves, shellfish), it is important to implement risk evaluation and management of the same and to elucidate the sources of MP contamination occurring in the background.

A common association that goes between biota and MPs involve "ingestion". Varying among the species and environment, micro-plastics have different kind of fate and effects on the environment (Lusher et al., 2017). Research across the world is still searching answers for the possible toxicological effects of MPs on humans and to what extent it can affect humans (Talsness et al., 2009), although in animals, there are significant differences. Often, localised toxicity to particle is exerted by MPs on their constituents, although when long term exposures are produced, can certainly lead to a matter of higher concern.

Research has shown that the reported values of MPs in packaged water and tap water generally varies between zero and hundred and four particles per litre thereby small-sized MPs constituting most of its component (Koelmans et al.,2019).. Some of the special concerns related to contamination occurring through MPs include direct intake of house-hold dust or particles settling on food, and also other sources like higher amount of indoor air exposure. (Vethaak et al., 2005). Other sources include direct exposures occurring through plastic containers and plastic bottles, food containers which also includes infant feeding containers containing polypropylene, etc. It is through faeces from where large particles of MPs are excreted apart from being disposed through respiratory tract/lungs or through clearance form muco-ciliary mechanism into the GI tract (gut) (Wright et al., 2017; Vethaak et al., 2005). Given, the limitations imposed by methodologies, and higher chances of passage of larger particles, existing research under determines the possibility of external human exposure to small size particles (which are <10mm) and are likely to pose greater danger in terms of toxicity (Yong. et al., 2020; Vethaak et al., 2005).

Notably, research is still being carried out in preliminary developmental stages regarding the effect of plastic particles inside human body. A superior idea and understanding are required to access the need to study the ability of MPs to cross GI tract and epithelial airway barriers which can aid in risk assessment studies of MPs on human health. It has been observed that only little portions of MPs which are administered (*in vitro* and *in vivo*) are able to cross epithelial lung and intestinal barriers with particular profiles of uptake and generally has shown greater uptake efficiency when particle size decreased. When considering long-term exposures which might affect organs and tissues, this particular point is important (Yong. et al., 2020; Vethaak et al., 2005). Sometimes, MPs act as vectors and are responsible for transferring of exogenous chemicals which are of hazardous nature to external or internal particles present in the body (Ribeiro et al., 2019; Vethaak et al., 2005). Various research studies suggest that MPs in the aquatic environment can also act as vectors of microbial toxicity which in turn carry associative opportunistic bio-film bacterial pathogens which in turn interferes with gut microbial fauna (Lu et al., 2019). A broader perspective of research is required to understand the potential toxicity effects, (short- and long-term effects) and underlying methods on life conditions.

Potentially toxic and hazardous as well as less explored and under-studied characteristic of MP is its presence of bio-corona (particles which are present on surface of MPs). This, directly or indirectly has an effect on the fate, impact and uptake of MPs (Vethaak et al., 2005). The determining factor of these bio-corona is based on its heterogeneous nature and the physicochemical properties it exerts with the human body and the nature of the environment (biomolecules, microbial fauna and chemical contaminants) (Ribeiro et al., 2019; Shi et al., 2021; Vethaak et al., 2005). Initially MPs get trapped in the lining of the mucus layer of the epithelial cells, before invading the intestine and lungs. Contrastingly, particles which are ingested have to pass under acidic conditions through the gut lining and stomach. The part of bio-corona composition, which MPs acquire externally to internally, arising across tissue barriers and their underlying toxicity mechanisms are very poorly recognised, hence, this requires further study.

POTENTIAL IMPACTS OF MICRO-PLASTICS AND NANO-PLASTICS ON EXCRETORY SYSTEM HEALTH

As liver and kidneys are the main excretory systems of our body and are responsible for filtering out most of the unwanted materials from our blood and other body fluids, hence, owing to their size, and easy transportability, the presence of NPs and MPs can have an adverse impact on the nephrotic tissue and overall excretory health. Long term exposure to MPs and polystyrene exposures possess a threat to kidney health. Studies done on vertebrates like mice have shown ER stress, internal inflammation, mitochondrial dysfunction, and autophagy in kidney tissues on being exposed to MPs. Not only kidneys but also organs and tissues such as the liver, intestine, and kidneys negatively respond to the presence of NPs and MPs. Adverse effects include alteration of the gut microbiota and induced inflammatory response of the small intestine. The impacts of liver include lipid accumulation, alterations in hepatic lipid expression, histopathological changes and changes in hepatic and serum markers. Certain signalling pathways like MAPK signalling pathways and AKT/mTOR signalling pathways are also altered at molecular level due to the presence of MPs and NPs. Further, kidney injury and alteration of creatinine levels due to presence of polystyrenes and NPs have also been observed in *in vitro* studies. Moreover, evidence gathered on autopsy of donated human cadavers strongly supports the presence of micro-plastics in spleen, kidneys and other organs.

Given the scenario of Sea food consumption globally, humans are the most susceptible to the effects of micro-plastics. It is known through literature that human being's excretory system removes MPs greater than 90% from the ingested Micro and Nano-Plastic through the waste they produce. The factors that affect retention and rate of clearance by human beings depend upon the shape, type of polymer, the additional chemicals of MPs which are used etc. (Lusher et al., 2017; Smith et al., 2018).

Preliminary research has led to the discovery of several potential harmful effects which include elevated inflammatory response, size-dependant toxicity of MPs, adsorbing tendency of plastic particle, thus causing disturbances and disruption of enzymes and microbiota of gut. Although, apart from this, there are several other physical effects of accumulated MPs which are less recognized. (Wright et al., 2017; Smith et al., 2018). Micro-plastic uptake is also dependant on size, surface charge, shape, functional groups on the surface and the charge it carries, buoyancy, and hydrophobicity (Anderson et al., 2016). It is because of mammalian systems modelling that has revealed that MPs with particular properties have the tendency to translocate across living cells of that which includes dendritic cells that have the capacity to translocate across lymphatic/circulatory system and get accumulated in secondary organs, which in turn can affect the internal organs and cell health (Brown et al., 2001; Smith et al., 2018). Pathways such as endocytic pathways and per-sorption through GI epithelium, has also been frequently reported to be disrupted functionally due to effects of Micro plastics (Smith et al., 2018). The dynamic movement of MPs in human beings which originates from various medical and surgical procedures, as medical literature suggests, provides information about their movement through human body (Lusher et al., 2017). For instance, MPs released from surgical substances and materials are only left to get absorbed in the tissue and bloodstream that gradually mimic the effects of enzymes/particles already absorbed in the blood stream, whereas particles those are inhaled interfere with similar epithelial tissue which are used during ingestion. Literature also suggests that microbes present in the surface of the ingested MP, can also serve as an active medium for harmful bacteria, especially when they are ingested, thus resulting in direct physiological effects that impacts developmental, nutritional, immunological, toxicological features on marine animals. MPs when ingested cause inflammatory tissue, necrosis, cellular proliferation

(Wright and Kelly, 2017) Studies carried out on Blue Crabs (*Callinectes sapidus*) have demonstrated instances of microspheres of plastic being ingested that stimulate hemocyte aggregation which in turn, reduces respiratory function (Johnson et al., 2011). Moreover, formation of Granulomas due to the same cause has been observed in Blue Mussels (Köhler et al., 2010). Apart from this, hepatic stress has also been experienced in several other organism like the Japanese Medaka (*Oryzias latipes*) after ingestion of virgin polyethylene fragments (Rochman et al., 2015).

THE EFFECTS OF MICRO- AND NANO-PLASTICS ON HUMAN PLACENTAL BARRIER

Most of the plastic polymers manufactured today are highly resistant to degradation and the accumulation of these highly complex and persistent materials is causing serious damage to both environment and humans as a whole. Several toxic substances and chemicals are added during the process of manufacturing which acts as additives, to improve the life of these synthetic polymers. Thus, the excessive usage of plastic products has resulted in accumulation of the hazardous chemicals associated with plastic polymers in human body (Pietroiusti, 2012). Prolonged exposure to these MPs may cause adverse effects such as inflammation, cellular proliferation, cellular necrosis, disrupt immune function, oxidative stress etc. Long term exposure to MPs and NPs may result in significant change in morphology and function (Rasmussen et al. 2010).

Presently the application of nanoparticles (NPs) in the consumer and industrial products is increasing gradually day by day. *In vitro* as well as epidemiological studies involving the use of engineered, naturally occurring as well as combustion-derived NPs have shown to jeopardise human health (Bell et al. 2012). However, nano-plastics need to overcome intricate and dense biological protective barriers in order to disrupt *in vivo* systems. Currently, various medical products like metal oxide particles (Oncogenic therapy) and contrast agents for imaging are equipped with NPs (Gupta and Gupta 2005). By the application of these medical products on the human body, NPs get infused into the blood circulation which further causes several adverse effects by crossing the protective barriers.

The feto-maternal organ which is an interface operating between mother and foetus is known as 'human placenta'. This disc-shaped organ deals with the gaseous exchange and the transfer of nutrients and waste products between maternal and foetal plasma. It also assists in the transfer of immunoglobulins from the mother to the foetus, thus providing immunity to the foetus. This organ secretes hormones which helps in maintaining the growth and development of the foetus. The only physical link between the mother and foetus is provided by the placenta. The placental growth takes place during pregnancy which provides an increase surface area for maternofoetal exchange (Enders and Blankenship 1999). The vascular projections of foetal tissue which are surrounded by chorion are known as the Villi. The chorion comprises of two cellular layers *viz.*, the outer syncytiotrophoblast through which maternal blood flows through out the intervillous space, and the inner cytotrophoblast. As the villi develops, significant reduction in the cytotrophoblast takes place, thereby separating only a single layer of syncytiotrophoblast from maternal blood and foetal capillary endothelium. The maternal blood supply to the uterus takes place through the uterine and ovarian arteries which form the arcuate arteries, and from which radial arteries penetrate the myometrium. The plasma membrane of the syncytiotrophoblast is highly polarised and comprises of two membranes *viz.*, the basal membrane and the brush border membrane. Furthermore, there is a large

Figure 5. Mechanism of micro and nano-plastic entering human-placental barrier
Source: Gruber, M. M., Hirschmugl, B., Berger, N., Holter, M., Radulović, S., Leitinger, G., & Wadsack, C. (2020). Plasma proteins facilitates placental transfer of polystyrene particles. Journal of nanobiotechnology, 18(1), 1-14.

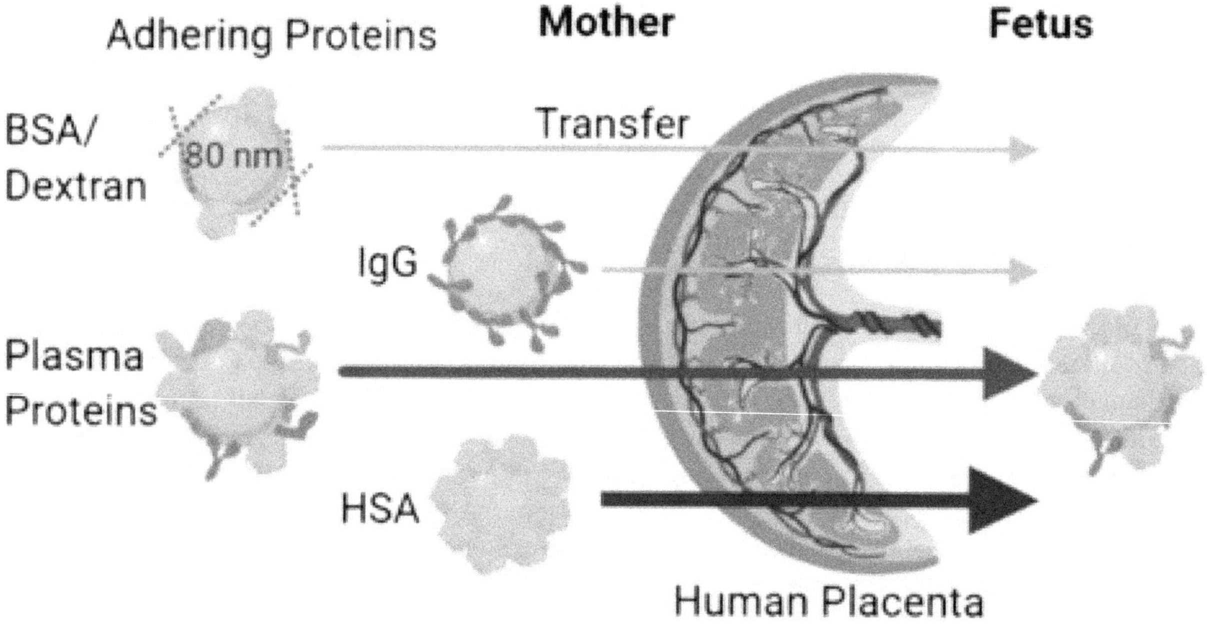

variety of transporters exporter and importer which ensure sufficient nutrient supply and proper efflux of waste products and harmful drugs at the right quantity (Ganapathy et al. 2000).

The placental transfer of these substances relies on four mechanisms, namely active transport, phagocytosis (or pinocytosis), passive diffusion & metabolic enzymes biotransformation (Syme et al. 2004). Various studies on animals, those were carried out *in vivo* revealed that several NPs like Si, Au or TiO_2 can bypass placental barrier and even damage foetal development (Semmler-Behnke et al. 2008; Yamashita et al. 2011). However, the placenta is also considered a species-specific organ and information that is obtained *in vivo* studies on experimental animals like rodents can never be extrapolated to the human placenta (Takata & Hirano 1997; Enders & Blankenship 1999). To investigate placental transport of the NPs as well as xenobiotics, an ethically validated model seems to be the *ex vivo* human placental perfusion (Grafmuller et al. 2013; Malek et al. 2009). Studies conducted in this model revealed that silica particles (25 - 50 nm) bypass human placental barrier while PEGylated gold particles (10 - 30 nm) remained intact in maternal circulation and placental tissue (Myllynen et al. 2008; Sonnegaard Poulsen et al. 2013). It has been observed that, the studies on *in vivo* and *in vitro* (about placental NP transport) has increased gradually, however, very less data is available on mechanism of transport across placental barrier (Buerki-Thurnherr et al. 2012). For understanding the mechanisms of transport of NPs, in the future, knowledge about their route/pathway bypassing placental barrier as well as physicochemical properties of the NPs, stands very important.

THE EFFECTS OF MICRO- AND NANO-PLASTICS ON RESPIRATORY SYSTEM

The process of respiration occurs through the exchange of gases between the cells and the blood. Respiratory system also known as pulmonary ventilation helps in delivering oxygen to the cells in the body. Nose, nasal cavity, larynx and pharynx constitute the upper respiratory tract system. Mucous membrane lining the tract trap foreign particles and prevent them from getting inhaled into the lungs. Situated in the thoracic cavity, the lungs look like two upside cones in the chest. The trachea (known as windpipe) connects larynx to bronchi of lungs and branch into primary bronchi and it is composed of 20 rings of cartilage. Although they are microscopic, alveoli are the workhorses of our respiratory system. They are made up of thin layer of epithelial cells and situated at the end of bronchioles where gaseous exchange takes place.

The pathway is through inhalation for the micro-plastics and nano-plastics that affect the respiratory system and cause adverse effect. Occupational exposure is when particles from synthetic textiles are inhaled unknowingly and unintentionally (Stapleton, 2019). Outdoor exposure occurs when fertilizer particles from wastewater treatments and contaminated aerosols pollute oceans. The barrier which is present (less than 1 μm) is sufficient enough for the penetration of nano particles into the respiratory system and blood stream circulation (Lehner et al., 2019). Absorption of various sized particles (MPs and NPs) leads to various harmful impacts on human health like chemical and particle toxicity thereby introducing vectors that of biological origin (pathogens/parasite) which often leads to mortality to humans (Vethaak and Leslie, 2016). Plastic particles which belong to this particular parameter embed themselves intricately inside lung and remain undisturbed on the alveolar surface or get transformed into various parts of the body (Stapleton, 2019; Porter et al., 2010). Apart from GI tract and skin, air-blood barrier happens to be a significant site for NP entry into the body. Both *in vitro* and *in vivo* invasion of NPs through this protective barrier has been observed in numerous research studies (Geiser et al. 2005; Kreyling et al. 2009). It is because of plastic particles, getting absorbed by lung tissues, which leads to serious damage caused to the lungs. The absorption of MP and NPs in lungs depends on several factors *viz.*, surface charge, hydrophobicity, protein surrounded coronas, surface functionalization, and the particle size. Additionally, literature (on rate of absorption by animals) suggests a positive correlation occurring among occupational exposures and increased inflammation and pulmonary cancer. (Prata, 2018).

Varela et al., 2012 observed that the size of the particle of plastic affected the absorption in alveolar epithelial cells. Recent studies on the inhalation of micro-plastics and nano-plastics particles showed that atmospheric fallout in the urban areas is a significant cause for the increase of these particulate pollutants which affects the air and thus enter the human body through inhalation. By considering the fibre dimensions, fibre densities average and the atmospheric flux of total fibres, an estimated 3–10 tons of MPs are deposited, in a year, because of atmospheric dust settling. The atmospheric flux recorded for the urban areas was double the average of the suburban areas. The observed depositions were also impacted with the amount of rainfall (Dris et al., 2016). A study conducted by Dris et al., 2017 to examine MP levels in outdoor & indoor setups of an office, in 2 private apartments revealed that concentration was between 1 and 60 fibres/m^3 in indoor samples whereas it was between 0.3 and 1.5 fibres/m^3 for outdoor samples indicating indoor samples had greater values when compared to outdoor samples.

Atmospheric dust and wind are the major carriers of micro-plastics. Others contributors of MPs are wastewater treatment plants, dried sludge, agricultural run offs containing fertilizer residues, industrial emissions, synthetic clothes fabric, marine aerosol, road-dusts etc. The accumulation of these MPs in the human body leads to major disruptive effects, thereby progressing into inflammation, cyto-toxicity,

Figure 6. Uptake and pathway of entry of micro and nano-plastic into respiratory system
Source: Facciolà, A., Visalli, G., Pruiti Ciarello, M., & Di Pietro, A. (2021). Newly Emerging Airborne Pollutants: Current Knowledge of Health Impact of Micro and Nanoplastics. International Journal of Environmental Research and Public Health, 18(6), 2997.

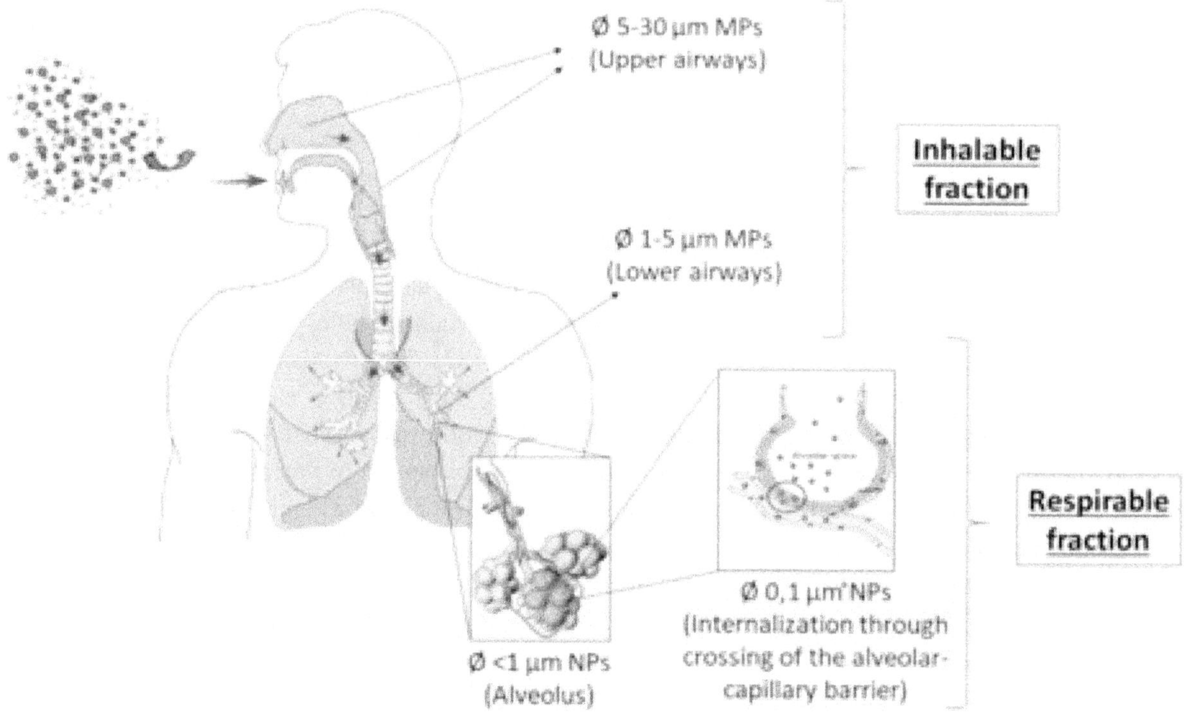

cell death, psycho-somatic ailments, including other respiratory diseases. Research has concluded that pulmonary epithelial cells (Calu-3 and THP-1) have faced cytotoxic and genotoxic effects and also, similar effects being caused to macrophages due to polystyrene particles (50 nm) (Paget et al., 2015). Responses to these particles those are inhaled, relies upon susceptibility of the particular individual and their metabolic rate, which, sometimes, may lead to asthma (or bronchial reactions), often progressing to chronic bronchitis (involving the peri-bronchial tissue), inflammatory responses, interstitial fibrosis. In various other cases, chronic pneumonia, pneumothorax (lesions in the interalveolar septa), and allergic alveolitis have also been observed (Da Costa, 2018). Very often, similar effects have been noticed in industrial workers (who were associated with working closely on polyolefin, polyester, nylon, acrylic fibres). Bio-persistence of synthetic particles has also been documented among patients with pulmonary cancer which in turn, depends upon the range of size of the fibres that can cause toxicity (Calafat et al., 2008). Also, a potential threat lingers in pathogen or microorganism transport suspended MPs in the air, where these pathogens get attached to the surface of MPs (usually for protecting themselves against UV radiation), which thereby could lead its way into lungs causing severe damaging effects (Da Costa, 2018).

THE EFFECTS OF MICRO- AND NANO-PLASTICS ON NERVOUS SYSTEM

The nervous system comprises of CNS (central nervous system) and PNS (peripheral nervous system). It helps in coordinating behaviour and transmission of signals between various parts of the body. The CNS contains brain and spinal cord. The PNS (peripheral nervous system) consists of nerves and enclosed in axons and connect the CNS to various body parts. Coordination of bodily movements and functions and transmission of sensory impulses are done by both the CNS and PNS. The brain and spinal cord act as the source of data centre as they receive information and impulses from various sensory organs and nerves and help in processing the information and transmitting the signals back to the source. The nerve endings carry the signals along the pathways. The spinal cord is a thin, long, tubular structure made of nervous tissue and extends from the medulla oblongata to the vertebral column. Primary function is to transmit nerve signals and coordinate and control reflexes.

The neurotoxic effects of MPs and Nano-plastics (NPs) on human brain is not familiar due to the lack of literature. But neurotoxicity in certain organisms have been documented where the immune system response of the brain was activated which caused oxidative stress. It could have been due to the direct contact with the transference plastic particles or else the pro-inflammatory cytokines which while circulating led to permanent neuron damage. (Waring et al., 2018). Due to lack of research data on human beings, different studies conducted on vertebrates like Zebra fish and European seabass (*Dicentrar chuslabrax*) have shown decrease in acetylcholinesterase (AChE) enzyme release, and increase in lipid peroxidation (LPO) levels which resulted in oxidative stress on being exposed to MPs like polystyrene and Bisphenol A (BPA) (Chen et al., 2017; Barboza et al., 2018). It was observed in the same species that the swimming ability had lowered due to affected neurotransmitter levels and disruption in locomotion. The findings were regarded as indication of neuronal behaviour. Damage of spatial recognition memory occurred due to oxidative damage cause of cell death which happened due to accumulation of MPs and NPs in the brain tissues of fishes. In vitro studies concluded that NPs and MPs can cross the blood brain barrier. Mammalian modelling studies put forward the ability of MNPs to transfer across dendritic cells and M cells accumulating internally, which compromised immunity and circulated in the lymphatic and circulatory system.

A study conducted by Shirinzi et al., 2017 on human brain & epithelial cells (T98G and HeLa cell lines) reported metal NPs, that of Ag, Au, CeO2, Al_2O_3, TiO_2, ZrO_2 and that of nanomaterials of Carbon (C60 fullerene, graphene) & polystyrene (PS) and polyethene (PE). The study concluded that MPs successfully induced effects (in cytotoxic origin) on T98G and HeLa cell lines. In addition, use of polypropylene (PP) particles indicated harmful effects on various cells according to the size (20 µm and 25–200 µm) together with the concentrations varying in each test. Hence as a result of human interaction with micro plastics were proven to cause hypersensitivity, haemolysis, cytotoxicity, standing as a potential risk to overall human health (Hwang et al., 2019).

Hence, monitoring of the exposure to MPs and NPs is indicative to neurotoxicity. In addition to exposure levels, route of exposure and nature of particles should also be determined. Various routes of exposure are through ingestion, inhalation, and retrograde transport. The weathering of the particles, size, shape and type should be determined along with the degree of inhalation through lungs or gills, nasal epithelium, gut, blood brain barrier crossing and translocating to various body parts. The above examinations will help in proving the mode of motion of MPs and NPs to the brain via taste nerve endings or olfactory nerve endings or via the blood stream. (Carbery et al., 2018).

POTENTIAL EFFECTS OF MICRO-PLASTICS AND NANO-PLASTICS ON THE SKIN

Being the largest part of the body and containing 15% of total adult body weight, the skin is one of the major components of human body. The skin helps against external biological assailants, thereby protecting us from various physical and chemical harm. Thermoregulation is also one of the major functions performed by the skin, thus, minimising excess loss of bodily water. Parallel with the mucous membranes underlining the body's surface, the skin can be divided into 3 layers *viz.,* the epidermis, the dermis, and subcutaneous tissue. Keratinocytes are the outermost layer (constellation of cells) that comprises of the epidermis, which are involved in synthesizing keratin, which is associated with a protective property. The middle layer constitutes dermis, and is mainly constituted of fibrillary structural protein which is called the 'collagen'. Lying on the subcutaneous tissue (panniculus), it consists of small lobes of fat cells known as lipocytes (James et al, 2006).

'Stratum corneum' is the outermost layer of the skin which fights against chemical, injuries and microbial agents that contains 'corneocytes' which are surrounded by lamellae of hydrophilic lipids. Some of these are Cholesterol, long-chain free fatty acids and ceramide (Bouwstra et al., 2001,). It is either through NP contaminated external sources like water or beauty & health products from where MPs and NPs are introduced. As MPs and NPs are of hydrophobic origin, hence, from contaminated sources like water, absorption through the stratum corneum is not possible, though sweat glands, skin wounds or hair follicles can give away a point of entry to plastic particles into human body (Facciolà et al., 2021). Washing scrubs are another major source of micro and nano-plastics entering human body. However, particles (MPs and NPs) those are lower than 100 nm are unable to penetrate into the corneous layer. Hence, it's not likely that micro-plastic absorption could take place through the skin, contradictorily, nano-plastic might hold a point of entry for the same cause (Revel et al., 2018).

Together, *in vivo* and *in vitro* studies have shown impacts of various beauty products being taken up by the human body via the skin barrier. Being hydrophobic in nature, when MPs and NPs transfer from contaminated water, they are unable to absorb via the stratum corneum (outermost layer of human skin), although high chances of MPs entering the body through sweat glands, hair follicles, open wounds can't be ruled out. Studies done on human skin have also concluded that polystyrene particles (20–200 nm) can penetrate only topical layer of the skin (2-3 μm). When certain products containing NPs are applied transcutaneously, they get absorbed by Langerhans cells. The mechanical processes involved in production of beauty products like facial scrub, containing microbeads also enhances the chances of fragmentation of these microbeads into more harmful NPs.

Key origin of NPs and MPs that affect human skin includes health and beauty products which are applied topically on skin and they are specifically found in body and facial scrubs. Another significant exposure route includes nano-carriers associated with drug delivery (through dermal applications). Incontrovertible data depicting the impacts on skin includes particle size(small) and skin in stress condition are critical parameters for skin penetration (Hernandez et al., 2017). Furthermore, no studies till date has been carried out which has intrinsically looked into the capability of NPs to invade skin topically. However, according to Som et al., 2011, it was proven likely that engineered nanoparticles arising from textiles were successful in penetrating the skin barrier, that too in very scarce quantity.

Alvarez-Roman et al. 2004 had made the use of fluorescent polystyrene particles (ranging from 20 - 200 nm diameter) and skin tissue from a pig to look into how plastic particles penetrate the body and get distributed thoroughly. The results concluded that more number of 20 nm polystyrene NPs were concentrated (compared to 200 nm Nano-plastics) in the hair follicles. However, it was observed that particles were unable to enter the stratum corneum and implant themselves in deeper skin tissue. Vogt et al. 2006 successfully differentiated 40 nm (diameter) fluorescent polystyrene NPs in the perifollicular tissue of skin explants which were treated with cyanoacrylate follicular stripping. Hence, this led to the conclusion that particles that were applied transcutaneously, got absorbed by Langerhans cells. Additionally, the mechanism involved in manufacturing the microbeads (used in facial and body scrubs) leads to chances of breaking NPs into even more harmful compounds that might continue to affect humans in the future.

FUTURE RESEARCH DIRECTIONS

Although several techniques are used scientifically for particle separation and size determination, procedures that remain available for material characterization are scanty and generally, it remains very challenging for extracting a suitable solution for the same. The two frequently available options available for identification of chemical structure and composition of plastic particles include micro-Raman spectroscopy and micro-FTIR spectroscopy. However, they are limited and bounded by the particle size in terms of applications. Given, their legal definitions, it gets obvious that the feasibility of these procedures does not include the size range of the NPs and MPs.

As currently, a lot of deficiency prevails in terms of nano-plastic quantification methods, hence detection of the same (micro and nano-plastics) through facades of analytical procedures gets difficult and remains very challenging in this field which is often overlooked. Often, localised particle toxicity is exerted by MPs on their constituents and is a matter of concern during long-term exposures. Summarizing this, future research techniques and technologies are the need of the hour, that are to be undertaken for estimating the exact dosage of toxicants (or chemicals) arising from contaminated biota irrespective of their particle size. Strong detection techniques are required in the future to address the ambiguity and research gaps in the present era of plastic particle research.

CONCLUSION

Summarizing it as a whole, as risk-assessment studies of MPs and NPs aren't possible practically because of data deficiency and research gaps, but nevertheless, various new outlooks have been opened up recently to question and target these gaps. As currently, there is lack of NP quantification methods, hence consumption of MPs and NPs through food remains a biggest inevitable challenge to mitigate. Other routes of exposures to MPs include bottled water as it contains leachates of PET (polyethylene terephthalate) or other materials. PET has also shown potential carcinogenic effects on humans. For accessing the exposure, the existing methods of analysis which are associated with nano-toxicological research, need to refined and adapted, specifically with respect to that of quantification of data from contaminated environments and particularly the food sector. Oral exposures of micro-plastic and transfer through food chain of the same also remain inevitable and challenging due to its particle size. Overall, numerous studies carried out still remain very less. *In vitro* studies have resulted in ambiguity of results and *in vivo* studies have often provided weak outputs which have frequently not allowed an evaluation and monitoring of standards, thereby over-looking several critical considerations.

Further, dose-dependent and dose-response relationship studies cannot be established, or neither can molecular tools and techniques be proclaimed that would otherwise permit generation of different pathways which would act as a tool to integrate data, mechanically into risk-assessment. As chronic and long-term studies have also been missing in terms of literature context, hence, continuous studies that bring about continuous evaluation, thereby obtaining relevant data and addressing the knowledge and research gaps that allow risk and hazard assessment of MPs and NPs on human health are the need of the hour today.

CONFLICTS OF INTEREST

The authors state that they do not have any conflict of interest.

REFERENCES

Anderson, J. C., Park, B. J., & Palace, V. P. (2016). Microplastics in aquatic environments: Implications for Canadian ecosystems. *Environmental Pollution*, *218*(Supplement C), 269–280. doi:10.1016/j.envpol.2016.06.074 PMID:27431693

Barboza, L. G. A., Vieira, L. R., Branco, V., Figueiredo, N., Carvalho, F., Carvalho, C., & Guilhermino, L. (2018). Microplastics cause neurotoxicity, oxidative damage and energy-related changes and interact with the bioaccumulation of mercury in the European seabass, *Dicentrarchus labrax* (Linnaeus, 1758). *Aquatic Toxicology (Amsterdam, Netherlands)*, *195*, 49–57. doi:10.1016/j.aquatox.2017.12.008 PMID:29287173

Bell, M. L., Belanger, K., Ebisu, K., Gent, J. F., & Leaderer, B. P. (2012). Relationship between birth weight and exposure to airborne fine particulate potassium and titanium during gestation. *Environmental Research*, *117*, 83–89. doi:10.1016/j.envres.2012.05.004 PMID:22705336

Bouwstra, J., Pilgram, G., Gooris, G., Koerten, H., & Ponec, M. (2001). New aspects of the skin barrier organization. *Skin Pharmacology and Physiology*, *14*(Suppl. 1), 52–62. doi:10.1159/000056391 PMID:11509908

Brown, D. M., Wilson, M. R., MacNee, W., Stone, V., & Donaldson, K. (2001). Size dependent proinflammatory effects of ultrafine polystyrene particles: A role for surface area and oxidative stress in the enhanced activity of ultrafines. *Toxicology and Applied Pharmacology*, *175*(3), 191–199. doi:10.1006/taap.2001.9240 PMID:11559017

Buerki-Thurnherr, T., von Mandach, U., & Wick, P. (2012). Knocking at the door of the unborn child: Engineered nanoparticles at the human placental barrier. *Swiss Medical Weekly*, *142*, w13559. doi:10.4414mw.2012.13559 PMID:22481566

Calafat, A. M., Ye, X., Wong, L.-Y., Reidy, J. A., & Needham, L. L. (2008). Exposure of the U.S. Population to Bisphenol A and 4- tertiary-Octylphenol: 2003–2004. *Environmental Health Perspectives*, *116*(1), 39–44. doi:10.1289/ehp.10753 PMID:18197297

Carbery, M., O'Connor, W., & Palanisami, T. (2018). Trophic transfer of microplastics and mixed contaminants in the marine food web and implications for human health. *Environment International*, *115*, 400–409. doi:10.1016/j.envint.2018.03.007 PMID:29653694

Chen, Q., Yin, D., Jia, Y., Schiwy, S., Legradi, J., Yang, S., & Hollert, H. (2017). Enhanced uptake of BPA in the presence of nanoplastics can lead to neurotoxic effects in adult zebrafish. *The Science of the Total Environment*, *609*, 1312–1321. doi:10.1016/j.scitotenv.2017.07.144 PMID:28793400

Da Costa, J. P. (2018). *Micro- and Nanoplastics in the Environment: Research and Policymaking* (Vol. 1). Elsevier.

de Sá, L. C., Luís, L. G., & Guilhermino, L. (2015). Effects of microplastics on juveniles of the common goby (Pomatoschistus microps): Confusion with prey, reduction of the predatory performance and efficiency, and possible influence of developmental conditions. *Environmental Pollution*, *196*, 359–362. doi:10.1016/j.envpol.2014.10.026 PMID:25463733

Dris, R., Gasperi, J., Mirande, C., Mandin, C., Guerrouache, M., Langlois, V., & Tassin, B. (2017). A first overview of textile fibers, including microplastics, in indoor and outdoor environments. *Environmental Pollution*, *221*, 453–458. doi:10.1016/j.envpol.2016.12.013 PMID:27989388

Dris, R., Gasperi, J., Saad, M., Mirande, C., & Tassin, B. (2016). Synthetic fibers in atmospheric fallout: A source of microplastics in the environment? *Marine Pollution Bulletin*, *104*(1-2), 290–293. doi:10.1016/j.marpolbul.2016.01.006 PMID:26787549

Enders, A. C., & Blankenship, T. N. (1999). Comparative placental structure. *Advanced Drug Delivery Reviews*, *38*(1), 3–15. doi:10.1016/S0169-409X(99)00003-4 PMID:10837743

Facciolà, A., Visalli, G., Pruiti Ciarello, M., & Di Pietro, A. (2021). Newly Emerging Airborne Pollutants: Current Knowledge of Health Impact of Micro and Nanoplastics. *International Journal of Environmental Research and Public Health*, *18*(6), 2997. doi:10.3390/ijerph18062997 PMID:33803962

Ganapathy, V., Prasad, P. D., Ganapathy, M. E., & Leibach, F. H. (2000). Placental transporters relevant to drug distribution across the maternal-fetal interface. *The Journal of Pharmacology and Experimental Therapeutics*, *294*, 413–420. PMID:10900213

Geiser, M., Rothen-Rutishauser, B., Kapp, N., Schurch, S., Kreyling, W., Schulz, H., Semmler, M., Im Hof, V., Heyder, J., & Gehr, P. (2005). Ultrafine particles cross cellular membranes by nonphagocytic mechanisms in lungs and in cultured cells. *Environmental Health Perspectives*, *113*(11), 1555–1560. doi:10.1289/ehp.8006 PMID:16263511

GESAMP. (2016). Sources, fate and effects of microplastics in the marine environment: part two of a global assessment. IMO/FAO/UNESCO-IOC/UNIDO/WMO/IAEA/UN/ UNEP/UNDP Joint Group of Experts on the Scientific Aspects of Marine Environmental Protection.

Grafmuller, S., Manser, P., Krug, H. F., Wick, P., & von Mandach, U. (2013). Determination of the transport rate of xenobiotics and nanomaterials across the placenta using the *ex vivo* human placental perfusion model. *Journal of Visualized Experiments*, *18*(76), 76. doi:10.3791/50401 PMID:23851364

Gruber, M. M., Hirschmugl, B., Berger, N., Holter, M., Radulović, S., Leitinger, G., & Wadsack, C. (2020). Plasma proteins facilitates placental transfer of polystyrene particles. *Journal of Nanobiotechnology*, *18*(1), 1–14. doi:10.118612951-020-00676-5 PMID:32907583

Gupta, A. K., & Gupta, M. (2005). Synthesis and surface engineering of iron oxide nanoparticles for biomedical applications. *Biomaterials*, *26*(18), 3995–4021. doi:10.1016/j.biomaterials.2004.10.012 PMID:15626447

Hernandez, L. M., Yousefi, N., & Tufenkji, N. (2017). Are There Nanoplastics in Your Personal Care Products? *Environmental Science & Technology Letters*, *4*(7), 280–285. doi:10.1021/acs.estlett.7b00187

Hwang, J., Choi, D., Han, S., Choi, J., & Honga, J. (2019). An assessment of the toxicity of polypropylene microplastics in human derived cells. *The Science of the Total Environment*, *684*, 657–669. doi:10.1016/j.scitotenv.2019.05.071 PMID:31158627

James, W. D., Berger, T. G., & Elston, D. M. (2006). *Andrews' diseases of the skin: Clinical dermatology* (10th ed.). Elsevier Saunders.

Johnson, N. G., Burnett, L. E., & Burnett, K. G. (2011). Properties of bacteria that trigger hemocytopenia in the Atlantic blue crab, Callinectes sapidus. *The Biological Bulletin*, *221*(2), 164–175. doi:10.1086/BBLv221n2p164 PMID:22042435

Joon, M. (2019). Trophic transfer of microplastics in zooplanktons towards its speculations on human health: A review. *Journal of Biomedical and Therapeutic Sciences*, *6*(1), 8-14.

Karami, A., Golieskardi, A., Ho, Y. B., Larat, V., & Salamatinia, B. (2017). Microplastics in eviscerated flesh and excised organs of dried fish. *Scientific Reports*, *7*(1), 5473. doi:10.103841598-017-05828-6 PMID:28710445

Koelmans, A. A., Nor, N. H. M., Hermsen, E., Kooi, M., Mintenig, S. M., & De France, J. (2019). Microplastics in freshwaters and drinking water: Critical review and assessment of data quality. *Water Research*, *155*, 410–422. doi:10.1016/j.watres.2019.02.054 PMID:30861380

Köhler, A. (2010). *Cellular fate of organic compounds in marine invertebrates.* Comparative Biochemistry and Physiology Part A: Molecular & Integrative Physiology; 27th Congress of the new European Society of Comparative Biochemistry and Physiology, Alessandria, Italy. 10.1016/j.cbpa.2010.06.020

Kreyling, W. G., Semmler-Behnke, M., Seitz, J., Scymczak, W., Wenk, A., Mayer, P., Takenaka, S., & Oberdörster, G. (2009). Size dependence of the translocation of inhaled iridium and carbon nanoparticle aggregates from the lung of rats to the blood and secondary target organs. *Inhalation Toxicology*, *21*(sup1, Suppl 1), 55–60. doi:10.1080/08958370902942517 PMID:19558234

Lehner, R., Weder, C., Petri-Fink, A., & Rothen-Rutishauser, B. (2019). Emergence of Nanoplastic in the Environment and Possible Impact on Human Health. *Environmental Science & Technology*, *53*(4), 1748–1765. doi:10.1021/acs.est.8b05512 PMID:30629421

Liebezeit, G., & Liebezeit, E. (2014). Synthetic particles as contaminants in German beers. *Food Additives & Contaminants. Part A, Chemistry, Analysis, Control, Exposure & Risk Assessment*, *31*(9), 1574–1578. doi:10.1080/19440049.2014.945099 PMID:25056358

Lu, L., Luo, T., Zhao, Y., Cai, C., Fu, Z., & Jin, Y. (2019). Interaction between microplastics and microorganism as well as gut microbiota: A consideration on environmental animal and human health. *The Science of the Total Environment*, *667*, 94–100. doi:10.1016/j.scitotenv.2019.02.380 PMID:30826685

Lu, Y., Zhang, Y., Deng, Y., Jiang, W., Zhao, Y., Geng, J., Ding, L., & Ren, H. (2016). Uptake and accumulation of polystyrene microplastics in zebrafish (*Danio rerio*) and toxic effects in liver. *Environmental Science & Technology*, *50*(7), 4054–4060. doi:10.1021/acs.est.6b00183 PMID:26950772

Lusher, A., Hollman, P., & Mendoza-Hill, J. (2017). Microplastics in fisheries and aquaculture: Status of knowledge on their occurrence and implications for aquatic organisms and food safety. *FAO Fisheries and Aquaculture Technical Paper*, 615.

lvarez-Román, R., Naik, A., Kalia, Y. N., Guy, R. H., & Fessi, H. (2004). Skin penetration and distribution of polymeric nanoparticles. *Journal of Controlled Release, 99*(1), 53-62.

Malek, A., Willi, A., Muller, J., Sager, R., Hanggi, W., & Bersinger, N. (2001). Capacity for hormone production of cultured trophoblast cells obtained from placentae at term and in early pregnancy. *Journal of Assisted Reproduction and Genetics*, *18*(5), 299–304. doi:10.1023/A:1016674503298 PMID:11464582

Mattsson, K., Hansson, L., & Cedervall, T. (2015). Nano-plastics in the aquatic environment. *Environmental Science. Processes & Impacts*, *17*(1), 1712–1721. doi:10.1039/C5EM00227C PMID:26337600

Murray, F., & Cowie, P. R. (2011). Plastic contamination in the decapod crustacean Nephrops norvegicus (Linnaeus, 1758). *Marine Pollution Bulletin*, *62*(6), 1207–1217. doi:10.1016/j.marpolbul.2011.03.032 PMID:21497854

Myllynen, P. K., Loughran, M. J., Howard, C. V., Sormunen, R., Walsh, A. A., & Vahakangas, K. H. (2008). Kinetics of gold nanoparticles in the human placenta. *Reproductive Toxicology (Elmsford, N.Y.)*, *26*(2), 130–137. doi:10.1016/j.reprotox.2008.06.008 PMID:18638543

Paget, V., Dekali, S., Kortulewski, T., Grall, R., Gamez, C., Blazy, K., Aguerre-Chariol, O., Chevillard, S., Braun, A., Rat, P., & Lacroix, G. (2015). Specific Uptake and Genotoxicity Induced by Polystyrene Nanobeads with Distinct Surface Chemistry on Human Lung Epithelial Cells and Macrophages. *PLoS One*, *10*(4), e0123297. doi:10.1371/journal.pone.0123297 PMID:25875304

Paul, M. B., Stock, V., Cara-Carmona, J., Lisicki, E., Shopova, S., Fessard, V., & Böhmert, L. (2020). Micro-and nanoplastics–current state of knowledge with the focus on oral uptake and toxicity. *Nanoscale Advances*, *2*(10), 4350–4367. doi:10.1039/D0NA00539H

Pietroiusti, A. (2012). Health implications of engineered nanomaterials. *Nanoscale*, *4*(4), 1231–1247. doi:10.1039/c2nr11688j PMID:22278373

Porter, D. W., Hubbs, A. F., Mercer, R. R., Wu, N., Wolfarth, M. G., Sriram, K., Leonard, S., Battelli, L., Schwegler-Berry, D., & Friend, S. (2010). Mouse pulmonary dose- and time course-responses induced by exposure to multi-walled carbon nanotubes. *Toxicology*, *269*(2-3), 136–147. doi:10.1016/j.tox.2009.10.017 PMID:19857541

Prata, J. C. (2018). Airborne microplastics: Consequences to human health? *Environmental Pollution*, *234*, 115–126. doi:10.1016/j.envpol.2017.11.043 PMID:29172041

Rasmussen, J. W., Martinez, E., Louka, P., & Wingett, D. G. (2010). Zinc oxide nanoparticles for selective destruction of tumor cells and potential for drug delivery applications. *Expert Opinion on Drug Delivery*, *7*(9), 1063–1077. doi:10.1517/17425247.2010.502560 PMID:20716019

Revel, M., Châtel, A., & Mouneyrac, C. (2018). Micro(nano)plastics: A threat to human health? *Current Opinion in Environmental Science & Health*, *1*, 17–23. doi:10.1016/j.coesh.2017.10.003

Ribeiro, F., O'Brien, J. W., Galloway, T., & Thomas, K. V. (2019). Accumulation and fate of nano-and micro-plastics and associated contaminants in organisms. *Trends in Analytical Chemistry*, *111*, 139–147. doi:10.1016/j.trac.2018.12.010

Rochman, C. M., Tahir, A., Williams, S. L., Baxa, D. V., Lam, R., Miller, J. T., Teh, F.-C., Werorilangi, S., & Teh, S. J. (2015). Anthropogenic debris in seafood: Plastic debris and fibers from textiles in fish and bivalves sold for human consumption. *Scientific Reports*, *5*(1), 14340. doi:10.1038rep14340 PMID:26399762

Schirinzi, G. F., Pérez-Pomeda, I., Sanchís, J., Rossini, C., Farré, M., & Barceló, D. (2017). Cytotoxic effects of commonly used nanomaterials and microplastics on cerebral and epithelial human cells. *Environmental Research*, *159*, 579–587. doi:10.1016/j.envres.2017.08.043 PMID:28898803

Seltenrich, N. (2015). New link in the food chain? Marine plastic pollution and seafood safety. *Environmental Health Perspectives*, *123*(2), A41. doi:10.1289/ehp.123-A34 PMID:25643424

Semmler-Behnke, M., Kreyling, W. G., Lipka, J., Fertsch, S., Wenk, A., Takenaka, S., Schmid, G., & Brandau, W. (2008). Biodistribution of 1.4- and 18-nm gold particles in rats. *Small*, *4*(12), 2108–2111. doi:10.1002mll.200800922 PMID:19031432

Shi, J., Wu, D., Su, Y., & Xie, B. (2021). Selective enrichment of antibiotic resistance genes and pathogens on polystyrene microplastics in landfill leachate. *The Science of the Total Environment*, *765*, 142775. doi:10.1016/j.scitotenv.2020.142775 PMID:33082042

Smith, M., Love, D. C., Rochman, C. M., & Neff, R. A. (2018). Microplastics in Seafood and the Implications for Human Health. *Current Environmental Health Reports*, *5*(3), 375–386. doi:10.100740572-018-0206-z PMID:30116998

Som, C., Wick, P., Krug, H., & Nowack, B. (2011). Environmental and health effects of nanomaterials in nanotextiles and facade coatings. *Environment International*, *37*(6), 1131–1142. doi:10.1016/j.envint.2011.02.013 PMID:21397331

Sonnegaard Poulsen, M., Mose, T., Leth Maroun, L., Mathiesen, L., Ehlert Knudsen, L., & Rytting, E. (2013). Kinetics of silica nanoparticles in the human placenta. *Nanotoxicology*. Advance online publication. doi:10.3109/17435390.2013.812259 PMID:23742169

Stapleton, P. (2019). Toxicological considerations of nano-sized plastics. *AIMS Environmental Science*, *6*(5), 367–378. doi:10.3934/environsci.2019.5.367 PMID:31745497

Steer, M., Cole, M., Thompson, R. C., & Lindeque, P. K. (2017). Microplastic ingestion in fish larvae in the western English Channel. *Environmental Pollution*, *226*, 250–259. doi:10.1016/j.envpol.2017.03.062 PMID:28408185

Takata, K., & Hirano, H. (1997). Mechanism of glucose transport across the human and rat placental barrier: A review. *Microscopy Research and Technique*, *38*(1-2), 145–152. doi:10.1002/(SICI)1097-0029(19970701/15)38:1/2<145::AID-JEMT15>3.0.CO;2-P PMID:9260845

Talsness, C. E., Andrade, A. J. M., Kuriyama, S. N., Taylor, J. A., & vom Saal, F. S. (2009). Components of plastic: Experimental studies in animals and relevance for human health. *Philosophical Transactions of the Royal Society of London. Series B, Biological Sciences*, *364*(1526), 2079–2096. doi:10.1098/rstb.2008.0281 PMID:19528057

Van Cauwenberghe, L., & Janssen, C. R. (2014). Microplastics in bivalves cultured for human consumption. *Environmental Pollution*, *193*, 65–70. doi:10.1016/j.envpol.2014.06.010 PMID:25005888

Varela, J. A., Bexiga, M. G., Åberg, C., Simpson, J. C., & Dawson, K. A. (2012). Quantifying size-dependent interactions between fluorescently labeled polystyrene nanoparticles and mammalian cells. *Journal of Nanobiotechnology*, *10*(1), 39. doi:10.1186/1477-3155-10-39 PMID:23006133

Vethaak, A. D., Lahr, J., Schrap, S. M., Belfroid, A. C., Rijs, G. B., Gerritsen, A., & de Voogt, P. (2005). An integrated assessment of estrogenic contamination and biological effects in the aquatic environment of The Netherlands. *Chemosphere*, *59*(4), 511–524. doi:10.1016/j.chemosphere.2004.12.053 PMID:15788174

Vethaak, A. D., & Leslie, H. A. (2016). Plastic Debris Is a Human Health Issue. *Environmental Science & Technology*, *50*(13), 6825–6826. doi:10.1021/acs.est.6b02569 PMID:27331860

Vogt, A., Combadiere, B., Hadam, S., Stieler, K. M., Lademann, J., Schaefer, H., Autran, B., Sterry, W., & Blume-Peytavi, U. (2006). 40 nm, but not 750 or 1,500 nm, nanoparticles enter epidermal CD1a+ cells after transcutaneous application on human skin. *The Journal of Investigative Dermatology*, *126*(6), 1316–1322. doi:10.1038j.jid.5700226 PMID:16614727

Waring, R. H., Harris, R. M., & Mitchell, S. C. (2018). Plastic contamination of the food chain: A threat to human health? *Maturitas*, *115*, 64–68. doi:10.1016/j.maturitas.2018.06.010 PMID:30049349

Wright, S. L., & Kelly, F. J. (2017). Plastic and human health: A micro issue? *Environmental Science & Technology*, *51*(12), 6634–6647. doi:10.1021/acs.est.7b00423 PMID:28531345

Yamashita, K., Yoshioka, Y., Higashisaka, K., Mimura, K., Morishita, Y., Nozaki, M., Yoshida, T., Ogura, T., Nabeshi, H., Nagano, K., Abe, Y., Kamada, H., Monobe, Y., Imazawa, T., Aoshima, H., Shishido, K., Kawai, Y., Mayumi, T., Tsunoda, S., ... Tsutsumi, Y. (2011). Silica and titanium dioxide nanoparticles cause pregnancy complications in mice. *Nature Nanotechnology*, *6*(5), 321–328. doi:10.1038/nnano.2011.41 PMID:21460826

Yang, D., Shi, H., Li, L., Li, J., Jabeen, K., & Kolandhasamy, P. (2015). Microplastic, pollution in table salts from China. *Environmental Science & Technology*, *49*(22), 13622–13627. doi:10.1021/acs.est.5b03163 PMID:26486565

Yong, C. Q. Y., Valiyaveetill, S., & Tang, B. L. (2020). Toxicity of microplastics and nanoplastics in mammalian systems. *International Journal of Environmental Research and Public Health*, *17*(5), 1509. doi:10.3390/ijerph17051509 PMID:32111046

ADDITIONAL READING

Facciolà, A., Visalli, G., Pruiti Ciarello, M., & Di Pietro, A. (2021). Newly Emerging Airborne Pollutants: Current Knowledge of Health Impact of Micro and Nanoplastics. *International Journal of Environmental Research and Public Health, 18*(6), 2997. doi:10.3390/ijerph18062997 PMID:33803962

Galloway, T. S. (2015). Micro-and nano-plastics and human health. In *Marine anthropogenic litter* (pp. 343–366). Springer. doi:10.1007/978-3-319-16510-3_13

Wang, Y. L., Lee, Y. H., Hsu, Y. H., Chiu, I. J., Huang, C. C. Y., Huang, C. C., Chia, Z.-C., Lee, C.-P., Lin, Y.-F., & Chiu, H. W. (2021). The Kidney-Related Effects of Polystyrene Microplastics on Human Kidney Proximal Tubular Epithelial Cells HK-2 and Male C57BL/6 Mice. *Environmental Health Perspectives, 129*(5), 057003. doi:10.1289/EHP7612 PMID:33956507

Yee, M. S. L., Hii, L. W., Looi, C. K., Lim, W. M., Wong, S. F., Kok, Y. Y., & Leong, C. O. (2021). Impact of microplastics and nanoplastics on human health. *Nanomaterials (Basel, Switzerland), 11*(2), 496. doi:10.3390/nano11020496 PMID:33669327

KEY TERM AND DEFINITIONS

Accumulation: The gradual gathering of mass/quantity of something.

Ambiguity: Anything possessing more than one interpretation.

Axons: The long threadlike portion of a nerve cell which conducts impulses from the cell body to other cells.

Bio-Persistent: Tending to stay inside any biological medium.

BioPET: Plastic based on 30% renewable raw material and 70% oil-based raw material.

Contamination: Turning impure by polluting or poisoning.

Degradation: The process of being degraded gradually.

Ecosystem: The sum total of the environment.

Exposure: The act of getting exposed or state of having protection from something harmful.

Histopathological: Examination of biological tissues in order to observe the appearance of diseased cells in microscopic detail.

Jeopardise: Put (someone or something) into a situation in which there is a danger of loss, harm, or failure.

Langerhans's Cell: Langerhans cells (LCs) reside in the epidermis as a dense network of immune system sentinels. These cells determine the appropriate adaptive immune response (inflammation or tolerance) by interpreting the micro-environmental context in which they encounter foreign substances.

Moulding: To give something a shape.

PEGylated: PEGylation (or pegylation) is the process of both covalent and non-covalent attachment or amalgamation of polyethylene glycol.

Persistent: Continuing firmly or obstinately in an opinion or course of action in spite of difficulty or opposition.

Phytoplankton: Phytoplankton, also known as microalgae, are similar to terrestrial plants in that they contain chlorophyll and require sunlight in order to live and grow.

Pollutant: A substance which is capable of polluting the environment physically, chemically or biologically.

Polymer: A substance which has a molecular structure built up chiefly or completely from a large number of similar units bonded together, e.g., many synthetic organic materials used as plastics and resins.

Spectroscopy: The branch of science concerned with the investigation and measurement of spectra produced when matter interacts with or emits electromagnetic radiation.

Toxic: Very harmful and unpleasant, capable of causing damage.

Transcutaneous: Existing, applied, or measured across the depth of the skin.

Translocate: Move from one place to another.

Uptake: The action of taking up or making use of something that is available.

Chapter 9
Impact of Micro and Nanoplastics in the Marine Environment

Gilberto Dias de Alkimin
Centre for Marine and Environmental Research, Portugal

Joanna M. Gonçalves
Centre for Marine and Environmental Research, Portugal

Justine Nathan
Centre for Marine and Environmental Research, Portugal

Maria João Bebianno
Centre for Marine and Environmental Research, Portugal

ABSTRACT

Plastic contamination in the ocean has recently received a lot of attention. Plastic production has been growing and its use spread to many sectors. More than 80% of plastic enters the ocean from land-based sources, with the remaining having ocean-based sources. Once in the ocean, plastic undergoes fragmentation and degradation that lead to the formation of microplastics (MPs) and nanoplastics (NPs), and their dimensions are becoming an environmental concern. Thus, this chapter provides an overview of the effects of MPs and NPs on marine organisms, from bacteria to fish. Plastic affects marine organisms from molecular to population levels but some knowledge gaps exist regarding the biogeochemical cycle of plastic, how it behaves and is distributed in the aquatic-sediment compartment and in deep-sea. Moreover, more attention is necessary concerning NPs ecotoxicological effects already detected and because not all polymer types and size effects have been investigated. In addition, risk assessment of plastic particles is needed to characterize their risks and for data to be comparable.

INTRODUCTION

DOI: 10.4018/978-1-7998-9723-1.ch009

Figure 1. Amount of global plastic production

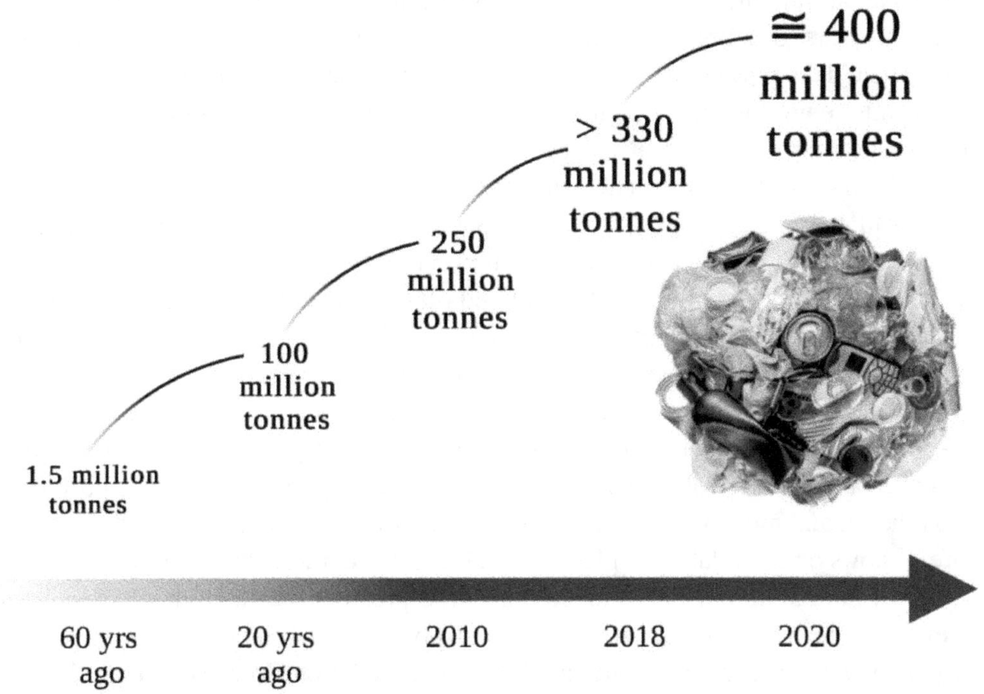

Plastic pollution in the ocean was first reported in the 1970s, yet in recent years, it has drawn tremendous attention from scientists and different parts of society (Law, 2017). In the middle of the 19th century, the first synthetic plastic, known as 'Bakelite', was invented and its countless properties have ever since led to different types of plastics shaping the world (PlasticsEurope, 2020). The increasing use of plastics in day-to-day life had world plastic production reaching 368 million tonnes in 2019 (Figure 1) (PlasticsEurope, 2020). In Europe, plastic production decreased between 2018 and 2019 by 3.9 million tonnes, representing 16% of the world's plastic production, whilst China alone is responsible for producing 31% of this amount (PlasticsEurope, 2020). Today, 60% of plastic products have a lifetime between 1 and 50 years, sometimes even more; however, a gap of information remains between the amount of plastic waste collected, and the quantity of plastic produced and/or consumed (PlasticsEurope, 2020).

The Plastics Europe Fact sheet (2020) states that the leading plastic polymers manufactured are polypropylene (PP; 19.4%), low-density polyethylene (LDPE; 17.4%), high-density polyethylene (HDPE; 12.4%), polyvinyl chloride (PVC; 10%), polyurethane (PUR; 7.9%), polyethylene terephthalate (PET; 7.9%), and polystyrene (PS; 6.2%). All these polymers have high demand in many industries, such as electronics, personal health care, food packaging, housing insulation, as well as in medical equipment and devices (PlasticsEurope, 2020).

The increasing use of plastics has incremented their release into the marine environment, where around 80% of plastic debris originates from land-based sources; illegal dumping and inadequate waste mismanagement, wastewater treatment plants inefficiency in filtering smaller particles, coastal littering, tourism, and industrial activity (Sebille et al., 2016). The remaining originates from ocean-based sources; fishing equipment, shipping, offshore oil and gas platforms, and undersea exploration (Sebille et al., 2016). Therefore, plastics are found in the atmosphere, ocean, lakes and rivers, soils, sediments, and animal biomass all around the world, being a ubiquitous problem (Lau et al., 2020). Despite expanded attempts in recent years to estimate the quantity of plastic pollution entering rivers and oceans (Tramoy et al. 2019), critical data gaps remain. Moreover, plastic particles can be detected in different compartments of freshwater environments, estuaries, and in the marine environment such as coastal beaches, water columns, and deep sediments (Ricciardi et al., 2021).

In the top 200 metres of the Atlantic Ocean, there is about 21.1 million metric tonnes of three main polymers (PE > PP > PS; 32-651 µm), which represents only 5.3% of the Atlantic Ocean volume, indicating that the problem is significantly worse than previously assumed (Pabortsava & Lampitt, 2020). Moreover, this does not include 44% of other littered plastic polymers or consider microplastics (MPs) below their detection limit and nanoplastics (NPs) are not included (Pabortsava & Lampitt, 2020).

In some areas, sediments are more contaminated by plastics than surface waters (Erni-Cassola et al., 2019). In intertidal sediments around $10^3 - 10^4$ plastic particles m^{-3} were detected, while in surface waters 0.1–1 particle m^{-3} were found with polyethylene (PE) being the most prevalent plastic polymer, accounting for 23% of relative abundance. The group PP&A (polyesters, PEST; polyamide, PA; and acrylics) was the second most prevalent polymers, accounting for 20%, followed by PP (13%), and PS (4%). Figure 2 shows data available on plastic detected in waters worldwide collected with a manta net (ranging from 0.15 to 3.0 mm in size) showing the widespread of plastic in the marine environment.

Once they reach the ocean, plastic particles are transported long distances by the currents and undergo two primary breakdown processes: fragmentation and degradation (Mattsson et al., 2018) (see Figure 3). The polymer itself is unaltered after fragmentation of larger plastic polymer chains into smaller pieces; nevertheless, during degradation processes, plastic polymers are vulnerable to bond-breaking mechanisms, altering the polymer characteristics. Five primary processes occur in the marine environment during the breakdown of plastics, namely, hydrolysis, mechanical/physical and thermal oxidative degradation, photo-degradation, and biodegradation (Andrady, 2011; Figure 3).

Plastics are quite resistant to decomposition and plastic debris is classified according to its size. Large plastic litter, known as mega (> 1m) macroplastics (25 mm – 1m) will breakdown to mesoplastics (5 – 25 mm), then to MPs (100 nm - 5 mm >) (GESAMP, 2016), and finally to NPs (1 – 100 nm) (Gigault et al., 2018) before full decomposition. MPs and NPs may enter the marine environment in two forms: as a primary micro/nanoplastics and as a secondary micro/nanoplastics. The difference between primary and secondary MPs/NPs is determined by whether the plastic particles were manufactured to that size from the start (primary), or if they were formed from the breakdown of bigger objects (secondary) (Kershaw, 2015). An example of primary MPs can be found in personal care items where they are added purposefully, such as glitter or microbeads found in scrubs, and account for less than 2% of total MPs discharged into the marine environment (Boucher & Friot, 2017). The bulk of MPs in the water come from inadvertently release of synthetic textile fibres (35%), tyre dust (28%), city dust (24%), road runoff (7%) and others (6%) (Boucher & Friot, 2017). Primary NPs, on the other hand, are found in specific applications and consumer products, such as cosmetics, clothing fibres, drug delivery and ink for 3D printers (Bergami et al., 2016; Canesi et al., 2015; Bessa et al., 2018; Tamminga et al., 2018; Wang et al., 2018), though it is assumed that most NPs in the marine environment are secondary. The existence of NPs in the ocean is known, and although quantification and several analytical methods remain challenging, Halle et al. (2017) managed to obtain a segment containing nano-scaled plastic polymers such as PVC, PET, PE, and PS in the North Atlantic Gyre.

Figure 2. (a) Particle count and (b) particle mass of plastic collected from 11,854 surface-towing plankton net trawls. The data were standardized using a generalized additive model to represent no-wind conditions. From Law (2017) and adapted from van Sebille et al. (2015)

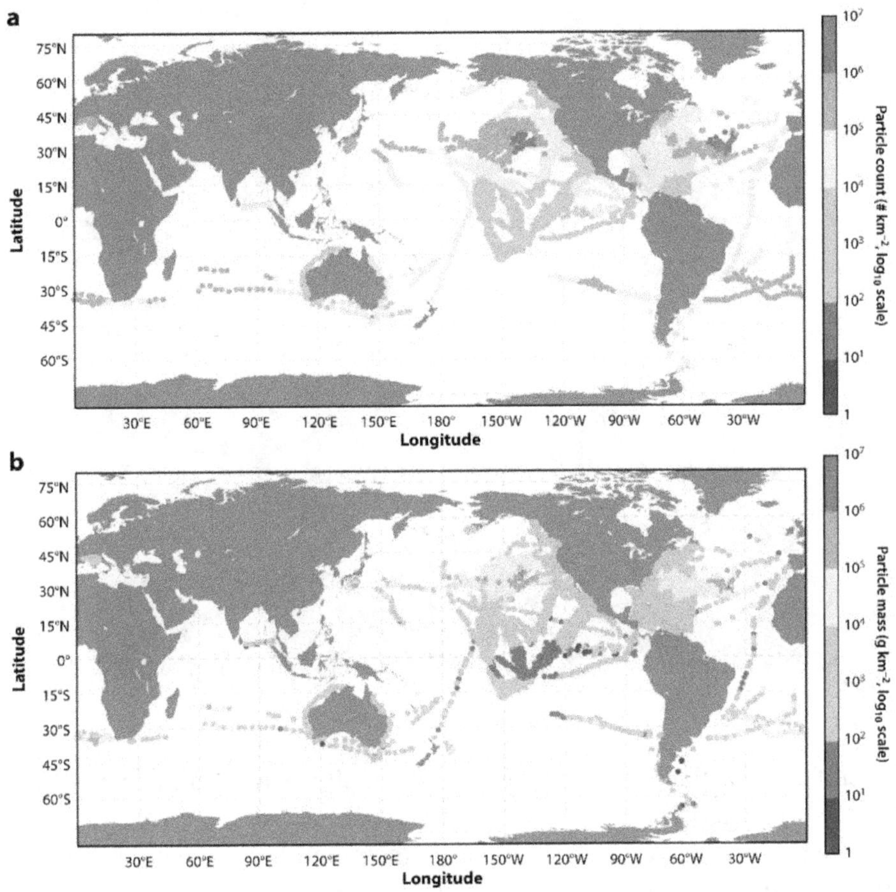

After entering the marine environment, plastic debris will migrate to other locations (Wang et al., 2016). Most synthetic polymers, such as PE and PP, float in seawater and can be carried for great distances due to ocean currents (Andrady et al., 2011). Even polymers that are denser than seawater (such as PVC) can be moved by underlying currents (Engler, 2012). During the permanence in the marine environment, the density of plastic can increase, which in turn increases plastic sedimentation (Morét-Ferguson et al., 2010). Moreover, marine plastic debris (MP/NPs) has also been shown to leach a "cocktail" of chemical compounds (Rochman, 2015) that also can cause additional effects on marine biota (Gunaalan et al., 2020; please see the specific section).

Moreover, the ability of plastics to adsorb other contaminants such as persistent organic compounds (POPs) and metals is a huge concern (O'Donovan et al., 2018, 2020; Islam et al., 2021). For POPs the adsorption is based on physical and chemical properties, the physical being mostly based on the large specific surface area and Van der Waals' force. Chemical adsorption is primarily based on organic contaminants' higher affinity for the hydrophobic surface of the plastic compared to saltwater (Wang et al., 2016). It is important to note that the surface area of plastic increases as the size decreases. Therefore,

Figure 3. Illustration of fragmentation/degradation of plastics in the marine environment

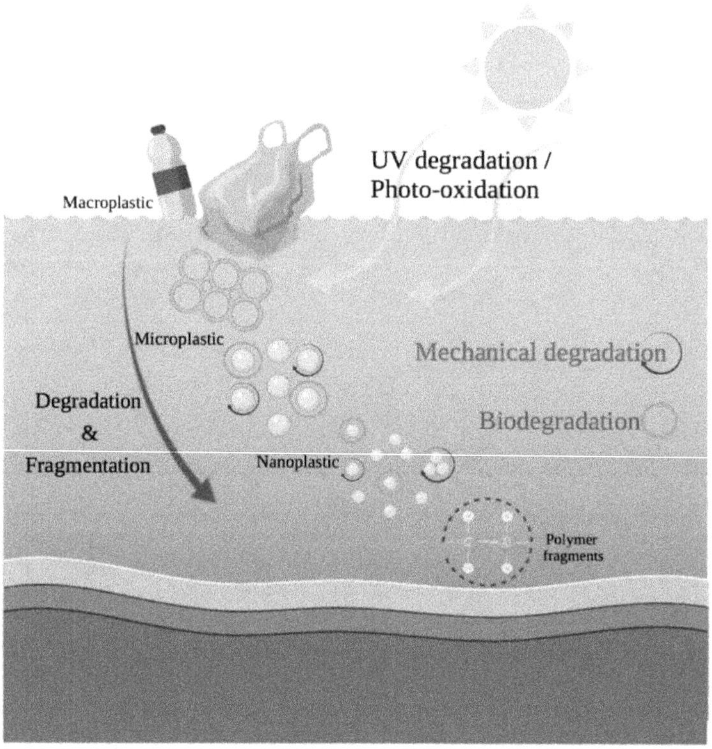

NPs have higher surface areas than MPs, making NPs potentially more harmful than MPs towards marine biota because of this characteristic.

Another factor that interferes in plastic behaviour is their ingestion by marine animals. Ingestion has been documented for a range of animals, from invertebrates, such as copepods, mussels, and jellyfish, to vertebrates such as fishes, turtles, and seabirds (Laist, 1997; Macali et al., 2018; Andrades et al., 2019; Sacova et al., 2021, Bai et al., 2021; Collard &Ask, 2021) (Tables 1-2). This ingestion by the animals is responsible for the spread of plastic particles to different locations from where it was ingested.

Overall, plastics in the marine environment can be a threat to living organisms. Thus, the aim of this chapter is to review the principal findings about MPs and NPs effects in marine organisms, from bacteria to fish.

IMPACT AND EFFECTS OF MICROPLASTICS ON MARINE ORGANISMS

In this section the impact and effects of MPs in different marine species will be described.

Bacteria

In marine ecosystems, bacteria and microbial communities play essential roles in critical ecosystem services such as biogeochemical cycling (Rotini et al., 2017). This group, however, can degrade pieces of (macro) plastic (Haritash & Kaushik, 2009), and this ability contributes to the MPs and NPs formation and dispersion in the environment (Rogers et al., 2020).

In bacterial communities, it has been noted that MPs toxicity leads to repercussions in growth and development, physiological and biochemical alterations, which ultimately can affect the whole ecosystem. For example, the toxicity of irregular shape and sized PE MPs (0 – 500 mg/L; 323.3 ± 51.8/656.8 ± 194.4 µm; 36 h) from commercially available toothpaste was tested in four different bacteria: two gram-positive (*Bacillus subtilis* and *Staphylococcus aureus*) and two gram-negative (*Pseudomonas aeruginosa* and *Escherichia coli*) (Ustabasi & Baysal, 2020). The PE-MPs caused significant growth inhibition of *B. subtilis* compared to the other three bacteria, presenting a species-specific effect. At a biochemical level, PE-MPs main toxicity pathway is related to oxidative damage and protein metabolism in *P. aeruginosa* and *B. subtilis,* whereas all species followed a similar increasing pattern in relation to extracellular carbohydrate levels (Ustabasi & Baysal, 2020). Physiological alterations and accumulation of MPs are also effects observed after exposure to MPs. For instance, the microbial composition in *Oryzias melastigma* internal organs, exposure to PE-MPs (100 µg/L; 2.5 µm; 30-d) reduced the diversity and abundance of the intestinal microbiota (Yan et al., 2020). This is highly concerning, as physiological alterations of an organism's organ can lead to unpredictable effects in species higher up in the trophic level.

There are several plastic polymers that end up as MPs in the ocean, however not all polymers' effects, and size, have been evaluated in some bacterial communities. Moreover, the effects they pursue are not comparable, as different polymers and/or sizes of MPs may act in a different way once in the ocean, thus incrementing the importance to assess differentiating MPs effects towards bacterial communities. Otherwise, it is impossible to get close to a conclusion about the real effects of MPs on these organisms.

Algae

A healthy aquatic environment starts at the beginning of the food chain with primary producers as key organisms. Algae are an important source of oxygen and many other nutrients (Mao et al., 2018), and their ecotoxicological importance is linked to their high-sensitivity response to toxic effects of low contaminant concentrations, which are unattainable by other marine organisms (Palumo & Mingazzini, 2011). Nonetheless, one of the main effects that is noticeable in algae is the presence of MPs accumulated in several species of macroalgae (Seng et al., 2020), microalgae, diatoms and cyanobacteria (Yokota et al., 2017) across freshwater, coastal, open ocean and even in sea ice (Hoffmann et al., 2020). Understanding the effects of MPs on algal species is still challenging, however negative impacts on growth (i.e., *Tetraselmis chuii*) (Davarpanah & Guilhermino, 2015), inhibition of photosynthesis and chlorophyll content (Besseling et al., 2014; Prata et al., 2018; Zhang et al., 2017) have been observed (Table 1). Additionally, in macroalgae populations, MPs have been shown to adhere to the surface of macroalgae and other macrophytes (i.e., seagrasses). MPs adhesion to algae can be explained by an electrostatic interation with cellulose, which is also seen later in this chapter in relation to NPs. Once MPs adhere to algae cell wall, these particles become more bioavailable to other organisms that feed on algae (Gutow et al., 2016; Seng et al., 2020). Thus, further ingestion and magnification of MPs may occur in higher trophic levels through direct or indirect consumption of macroalgae (Yang et al., 2021; see more about plastic magnification in the specific section). The effects that have been reported that MPs have on algae is alarming, as hindered photosynthesis, growth, and chlorophyll content rise severe implications for the whole ecosystem, and biomagnification of these particles through tropic transfer is even more apprehensive.

Rotifers

Rotifers, as zooplankton members, are relevantly important primary and secondary consumers that play a crucial role in the transference of energy from the bottom of the food chain to species higher up in the marine ecosystem (Wallace et al., 2006; Rico-Martínez et al., 2016). Additionally, rotifers are unable to digest MPs (Xue et al., 2020), therefore, rotifers are an important group of animals as they transport pollutants across the food web (Wallace et al., 2006). Different species of rotifers can ingest/uptake MPs from the water (Ronneberger, 1998), and through food (Setälä et al., 2014) (Table 1). Most rotifers are small (adults generally have a length of <200 µm; (Dahms et al., 2011)), the particle size ingestion and the palatability are limited, since they have preference for different particle sizes, according to the species, even when they have the same adult size, i.e., *Keratella cochlearis*, *Keratella quadrata*, and *Polyarthra dolichoptera* preferred 1– 2-µm diameter beads, whereas *Synchaeta pectinata* selected for 2–3-µm particles (Ronneberger, 1998). In addition, the ingestion of food-sized MPs by rotifers has not been completely explored (Lan et al., 2021).

The rotifer, *Brachionus plicatilis*, exposed to PS microbeads (6 µm; 1 and 2.5 µg/mL) had alterations in transcriptional expression levels of ATP-binding cassette genes related to multi-xenobiotic resistance function (Kang et al., 2021). MPs increase intracellular ROS levels of *B. plicatilis*, and, consequently, the activity of enzymes related to the antioxidant defence system (glutathione - GSH, superoxide dismutase - SOD and catalase - CAT activities), as well as the activity of biotransformation enzymes (glutathione-S-transferases - GSTs) this last one through the MP toxicity itself and/or the possible organic compounds released by the MPs. Similar results, at the biochemical level, were detected in *Brachionus koreanus,* exposed to PS microbeads (0.05 – 6 µm; 0.1 - 20 µg/mL), with ROS levels decreasing with the increase of microbeads size, indicating the size-dependent toxicity (Jeong et al., 2016). Also, this result suggests that the effects of the specific polymer (PS) can also be species-specific, as PS-MPs of similar size caused an increase in ROS production in *B. plicatilis* and a decrease in *B. koreanus*. Moreover, the status of phosphorylation of different mitogen-activated protein kinases (MAPK), a linking signal between extracellular signals to intracellular processes, associated with apoptosis and inflammation, increased, indicating the toxic effects of MP towards these species (Malik et al., 2015).

Additionally, MPs induce physiological alterations in rotifers, and can lead to significant repercussions on life cycle parameters. In reproduction terms, some MPs effects are associated with a delay in maturation time (appearance of the first batch of eggs in the brood pouch), thus producing offspring later but also decrease the total number of offspring per rotifer (Sun et al., 2018). In addition, growth is directly associated with rotifer maturation (Jeong et al., 2016), so, consequently, as population growth decreases, so does the reproduction rate, therefore, affecting animals' fecundity (Jeong et al., 2016; Sun et al., 2018; Xue et al., 2021).

Moreover, MPs cause swimming behaviour alterations (Kang et al., 2021: Xue et al., 2021), but these alterations can also be a hormetic response. *B. plicatilis* exposed to PS microbeads at low concentrations, resulted in a stimulatory effect, whilst an inhibitory one was noticeable at high concentrations (Gambardella et al., 2018). A decrease in swimming speed also decreases the ability of algae uptake and consequently affects survival, reproduction, and population growth negatively. MPs can also be lethal to rotifers by decreasing their lifespan (Jeong et al., 2016; Sun et al., 2018).

Indirectly, MPs can be lethal for this group of animals, as behaviour, physiology, molecular, a reproduction of rotifers is highly affected after exposure to MPs, and eventually jeopardizing the population. For rotifers, MPs toxicity is size-dependent and species-specific, though more information is necessary to confirm this. Moreover, the type, size and shape of the plastic polymer can have different effects, thus further studies need to be carried out to fully comprehend MPs toxicity towards different rotifers species.

Corals

Coral reef ecosystems are complex and diverse communities of animals that interact with one another and with their surroundings; coral, like hydroids, jellyfish, and sea anemones, is a type of colony (EPA, 2021). Corals live in shallow waters, produce reefs, and have a symbiotic interaction with photosynthetic algae known as zooxanthellae that dwell in their tissues. The coral provides a haven for zooxanthellae and the molecules they require for photosynthesis. In exchange, the algae provide the coral with carbohydrates as well as oxygen (NOAA, 2019).

In general, the first MP effect on marine animals is ingestion and this also occurs in corals (Table 1). In fact, corals can ingest different kinds (type, size, and shape) of MPs. High density PE (HDPE) microspheres, (≤1000 µm and >1.7 mm respectively) (Hankins et al., 2021), low density PE (LDPE) microspheres (90 µm–2.8 mm; <100 - 500 µm) (Syakti et al., 2019; Hall et al., 2015), shavings of blue PP (10 µm–2 mm) (Hall et al., 2015), PE microplastic beads (Hankins et al., 2018) and other polymers were detected in different tissues such as gastrovascular tissue and mesenterial filaments (Grillo et al., 2021). However, corals are also able to egest these particles (Axworthy et al., 2019; Hankins et al., 2018).

MPs in some coral species can be retained in the gut cavity (Hall et al., 2015) that induce the increase in mucus production, facilitating the adhesion of particles to the body surface (Martin et al., 2019). Furthermore, MP exposure can impair food intake (Chapron et al., 2018; Savinelli et al., 2020) and may be related to the decrease in polyps' activity (Chapron et al., 2018), consequently affecting the animal's fitness. For example, a forty-eight-hour exposure of fluorescent PE microbeads reduced the fitness of *Danafungia scruposa*, due to ingestion and tissue adhesion (Corona et al., 2020).

Growth parameters are another "group" of animals' responses that can be affected by MPs. Nine months of exposure to PE (175.5 ± 73.5 µm; 0.25 mg/L) decreased the surface area, volume, and calcification rate of *Acropora muricata* and *Heliopora coerulea* (Reichert et al., 2019). However, similar results were observed during a smaller exposure period. Hankins et al. (2021) exposed *Pseudodiploria clivosa* and *Acropora cervicornis* to HDPE microspheres and PE for 4 months and observed a decrease in tissue surface area and animal calcification.

At a biochemical level, changes can be seen at an earlier onset. A 6-hour exposure to 1 µm PS (50 mg/L) was enough to trigger the antioxidant system and increase SOD activity in *Pocillopora damicornis*, as well as a decrease of the immune system by decreasing alkaline phosphatase activity (AKP). After 12 hours, this exposure was also able to increase CAT activity and chlorophyll content and alter the detoxifying system by decreasing GSTs activity (Tang et al., 2019). On the other hand, when *Tubastrea aurea* was exposed to 300 mg/L of PVC, PE, PET, and PA-66, it decreased different enzymatic activity of the antioxidant and immune system, energy metabolism and calcification process (Liao et al., 2021) (*see* Table 1).

Another effect of MP exposure in coral species is bleaching, meaning that they expel the symbiotic algae living in their tissues, causing them to turn completely white (NOAA, 2021), decreasing, therefore, the access to carbohydrates and oxygen, which is seriously threatening for coral survival. This effect was observed in *Acropora formosa* after LDPE-14 days exposure (Syakti et al., 2019), in *Acropora humilis* and *Acropora millepora* after 4 weeks of pristine MPs (Reichert et al., 2018) and in *Pocillopora verrucose* after 6 months of exposure to PE (Reichert et al., 2019).

In reproduction terms, weathered PP MPs and spherical PE microbeads impair the success of gamete fertilization, embryo development and larval settlement in *Acropora tenuis* (Berry et al., 2019) and MP exposure can cause coral tissue necrosis (Reichert et al., 2018, 2019; Syakti et al., 2019) that can lead to problems at a populational level, as MPs can lead to a decreasing number of new coral generations.

Ultimately, coral communities are vital to many species as a source of food, shelter and/or nursery. The importance of these communities as part of the marine ecosystem is highly concerning when confronted with MPs effects. Coral bleaching has already significantly impacted the diversity of biota in coral regions, and inevitabley these effects are felt higher up the trophic levels. With the addition of the effects that MPs pursue on corals, MPs pollution may be devastating for the surrounding ecosystem. As priorly mentioned, there is still a vast array of unknown knowledge of MPs toxicity in corals, and different size and shape of MPs needs significant attention to fully understand MPs effects, not only towards corals, but how it impacts the surrounding environment. Moreover, as the detection of MPs has been reported in the deep sea (Peng et al., 2018), the coral communities at this depth and the impact of MPs still needs to be addressed.

Echinoderms

Echinodermata is the sole group of deuterostomes invertebrates in the animal kingdom, with roughly 6500 species, a unique phylogenetic position with a great diversity of forms and habitats (Ruppert et al., 2005). They are important key species since they help to reduce algae growth, feed other animals, and are an important food source in certain countries (Oney, 2015).

For more than a century, echinoderm embryos and larvae were employed as experimental model systems in a variety of fields (Micael et al., 2009), including MPs marine ecotoxicology. In general, different classes of echinoderm are capable of taking up MPs particles and this is the most studied "endpoint" in this animal group (Hart, 1991; Graham et al., 2009; Kaposi et al., 2014; Lizárraga et al., 2017) (*see* Table 1). MPs were detected in tissues, but also in the celomic fluid (Mohsen et al., 2019; 2021).

Holothuroid, asteroid, and echinoid larvae ingest PS divinylbenzene beads of different sizes that, within each species, the maximum size of edible beads increase with age and a variation according to species was detected, not exceeding >45 μm apart from *Astropecten armatus* (Lizárraga et al., 2017).

Morphological alterations in *Paracentrotus lividus*, exposed 48 h to PS (6 μm; 10^3, 10^4 and 10^5 microspheres PS/mL) microspheres and HPDE fluff (>0–80 μm; 0.005, 0.5 and 5 g HDPE fluff/L) reduced larval growth and increased larval abnormalities. These include undeveloped embryos, collapsed embryo development at early stages, thickening and abnormal proliferation of the ectodermal membrane and reduced arm length (Martínez-Gómez et al., 2017). After 72 h of exposure to spherical PS (10 μm), this species also presented alterations in body and arm length, and a decrease in body width (Messinetti et al., 2018). These alterations were related to the delay in their development (Richardson et al., 2021). For example, echinoderms, such as starfish, can regenerate and grow back arms. With the effects of MPs, this function is compromised, jeopardizing the animal's fitness, as the arms and rods of echinoderms are extremely important for locomotion, burrowing, and prey capture (Da, 2011). Moreover, MPs have also been found to increase swimming speed of echinoderms (Gambardella et al., 2018),

Additionally, biochemical parameters are also affected by MPs exposure. Spherical fluorescent green MPs (1–5 μm; 10 – 10000 MPs/mL) increase SOD, gluthatione peroxidase (GPx), CAT, protein carbonyl (PC) activities, and oxidative damage in *Pseudechinus huttoni* (Richardson et al., 2021). Moreover, *P. lividus*, exposed for 72 h to PS microbeads which caused an increase in intracellular ROS, reactive nitrogen species (RNS), and the total antioxidant capacity as well as immunological alterations (Murano et al., 2020).

Furthermore, molecular, and cytological alterations were also found in echinoderms after MPs exposure. PS and polymethyl methacrylate (PMMA) also cause an increase in cytogenetic aberrations and mitotic abnormalities in *Sphaerechinus granularis* (Trifuoggi et al., 2019). Alterations in a set of related metabolic and signal transduction pathways were also seen in *Apostichopus japonicus* after PE microsphere exposure (Mohsen et al., 2021). In a more concerning aspect, MPs can also cause a decrease in fertilization rates (Martínez-Gómez et al., 2017; Trifuoggi et al., 2019), and histological alterations revealed by injuries and loss of cell components in animal tissues (Mohsen et al., 2021), thus threatening the viability of future generations as well as populational dynamics.

Finally, exposure to MPs leads to impaired responses across a range of morphological, physiological, cytological, molecular, behavioural, growth and development, reproduction, and mortality endpoints for both larval and adult stages of echinoderms.

Crustaceans

Crustaceans contribute to a large proportion of commercial seafood; therefore, efforts have aimed to monitor the impacts of MPs on this group of organisms (Table 1). In the water column, copepods and amphipods ingest available plastic (Cole et al., 2013). Benthic crustaceans, including crabs, also show evidence of accumulating plastic in the gills, stomach, hepatopancreas and the brain from their environment (Brennecke et al., 2015; (Crooks et al., 2019). When crustaceans were exposed to MPs, they actively ingest particles causing behavioural changes in food consumption and swimming activity as well as physiological impacts on reproductive rates and enzyme activity (Cole et al., 2015; Gambardella et al., 2017). The behavioural changes of crustaceans can adversely impact their chance of survival by a reduction in feeding (Carrasco et al., 2019; Cole et al., 2015) and inhibited predator evasion responses as seen in European hermit crabs (*Pagurus bernhardus*) (Nanninga et al., 2020). Eventually, these impacts can cause a reduction in growth and higher mortality rates (Horn et al., 2020).

There is evidence of trophic transfer from prey items to crustaceans such as from mussels (*Mytilus edulis*) to crabs (*Carnicus maenas*) (Farrell & Nelson, 2013) and has been witnessed in other species (Crooks et al., 2019; Santana et al., 2017). In the Ria Formosa lagoon (Portugal) a green polypropylene MPs fragment (280 μm) was detected in the gills of the crab *C. maenas* (Vital et al., 2021). High levels (3 mg/g) of MPs accumulated in the hepatopancreas cause hepatic injury and reduce neural activity in the crab, *Charybdis japonica* (Wang et al., 2021). However, at lower concentrations (1-2 mg/g) crabs displayed a mitigated response to these foreign particles allowing physiological activity to remain normal (Wang et al., 2021).

Ingested particles are often expelled, and no obvious health impacts were observed as seen in the marine isopod, *Idotea emarginata* (Hämer et al., 2014). As MPs concentrations continue to increase in the ocean, the capacity of organisms to counteract MPs impact in their systems may collapse and cause increase damage to populations. This is especially relevant for intertidal and nearshore species living in the polluted coastal areas (Horn et al., 2020). Acute toxicity of MPs in crustaceans have been evaluated, however, there is a lack of information on the long-term effects of MPs exposure. Additionally, there is a need to evaluate more crustaceans species, as well as, other endpoints, such as histopathology, to increase the data spectrum of MPs effects for this group of organisms.

Molluscs

It is well known that bivalves are excellent sentinel species for ecotoxicological studies because of their wide geographical distribution and their natural filter-feeding habits, which allow these organisms to ingest MPs from the surrounding environment and therefore detect stressor levels in their tissues. Since they can ingest MPs particles (Xu et al., 2017; Guilhermino et al., 2018) these can, therefore, be detected in different organs, such as the haemolymph, gills and, especially, in digestive glands (Avio et al., 2015; Oliveira et al., 2018; Ribeiro et al., 2017; O'Donovan et al 2018, 2020; Islam et al. 2021) which, consequently, can jeopardize their biological functions (Table 1).

One of the first consequences of MPs in molluscs is related to feeding. MPs decrease the filtration rate of *Curbicula fluminea* after 8 and 14 days of exposure to 0.13 mg/L of a plastic of unknown composition (1-5 µm) (Oliveira et al., 2018). In addition, filtration by *M. edulis* was significantly decreased after 50 days of exposure to 25 µg/L of polylactic acid and HDPE (Green et al., 2017). Similarly, in *Scrobicularia plana,* after 14 d of exposure to LDPE (4-6 and 20-25 µm; 1 mg/L) the filtration rate also decreased (Islam et al., 2021). PS (between 63 µm and 250 µm) exposure for 10 d to 10 and 1000 particles/L decreased the clearance rate of *Atactodea striata* (Xu et al., 2017). Accordingly, even interspersed exposure periods (2-hour-time-periods per day for 3 months total), *Perna viridis* exposed to polyvinylchloride (PVC; 1 –50 µm) also caused a decrease in clearance rate (Rist et al., 2016). Overall, this effect can be allied with the decrease in valve opening duration after MPs exposure, in the bivalves' case (Bringer et al., 2021).

Morphological alterations were also observed in molluscs exposed to MPs. HDPE-MPs (20-25 µm) after 24-d exposure delayed shell growth in *Crassostrea gigas* (Bringer et al., 2021). However, the most analysed endpoints in molluscs are the biochemical ones, and the results are diverse according to the species, time of exposure and plastic type.

ROS are induced in MPs exposed mussels i.e., exposure of *Tegillarca granosa* to PS (30 and 500 µm; 0.26 and 0.29 mg/L) for 14 days (Shi et al., 2020; Sun et al., 2020; Zhou et al., 2021). The same material and time of exposure, though smaller in size (2 µm), caused an increase in ROS content in *Mytilus coruscus* (Huang et al., 2021). This, in most of the cases, triggered the antioxidant enzyme system, increasing the activity of enzymes such as CAT, SOD, GPx and others (Magara et al., 2018; O'Donovan et al., 2018; Cole et al., 2020; Wang et al., 2020; Teng et al., 2021). Ultimately, causing cellular damage, mostly through lipid peroxidation (Oliveira et al., 2018; Capolupo et al., 2021; Gu et al., 2021; Huang et al., 2021) in both the digestive gland and gills.

However, the effects can be more intense, and the antioxidant system is not capable of handling increasing ROS, which therefore decreases enzymatic activity (Paul-Pont et al., 2016; Teng et al., 2021). Besides the antioxidant enzyme system, GST is also affected by MPs, and its activity increases or decreases depending on tissue, time of exposure and material type (Ribeiro et al., 2017; Revel et al., 2019; Tlili et al., 2020).

Haematological effects can be related to a significant reduction in the total haemocyte count; decreased red granulocyte and hyalinocyte and increased basophil granulocyte; suppression of the phagocytic rate of haemocytes. This was observed after *T. granosa* was exposed to different concentrations of PS (Shi et al., 2020; Sun et al., 2020; Zhou et al., 2021).

In addition, even short exposure times (7 d) of PS and PE (20 µm and 75 µm) affect molluscs significantly, as shown in Trestrail et al. (2021), where MPs affect the activity of the digestive enzymes shown by the reduction in amylase, and xylanase activities, as well as increase cellulase and total protease activity.

Concerning reproduction, the total number of oocytes collected by stripping and oocyte diameter were significantly lower in *C. gigas* exposed to PS-MPs (Sussarellu et al., 2016) as well as increased larval mortality and delayed development time of the offspring in *Amphibalanus amphitrite* (Yu & Chan, 2020).

Genotoxic effects after PS-MP exposure (20 µm; 1 mg/L) for 14 d were observed in *S. plana* (Ribeiro et al., 2017). In addition, transcriptomic alterations in different genes of different systems, such as antioxidant, immune and energy balance (Gardon et al., 2020), immunotoxicity pathway (Sun et al., 2020) and carbon metabolism (Détrée and Gallardo-Escárate, 2017) were also affected by MPs in molluscs. Moreover, histopathological damage in gills and digestive glands can also be observed after MP exposure (Paul-Pont et al., 2016; Bråte et al., 2018; Alnajar et al., 2021; Teng et al., 2021). Overall, the toxicity of MPs towards molluscs is time, size, polymer type, shape, and concentration dependent. Thus, further studies should focus on the variety of plastic polymers type, shape, and size to gain a much deeper understanding of MPs impact and how it affects these filter-feeding organisms, as MPs can be biomagnified to higher trophic levels, including humans, due to the consumption of MP contaminated shellfish batches.

By far, molluscs is the group of marine organisms most evaluated in the marine environment concerning MPs toxicity. However, there is a lack of a standardized methodology, making the comparison between studies not always attainable. Thus, although there is extensive data on MPs effects in molluscs, the lack of a standardized method restricts decision-makers and authorities from developing risk-assessment and management policies for MPs pollution.

Fish

Many interactions between fish species and MPs in the ocean have been reported (Table 1). Due to the small nature of MPs, many species are exposed to them through ingestion (Boerger et al., 2010). The feeding behaviour of some fish species puts them directly at risk of ingesting MPs by mistake, and this has been documented extensively (Anastasopoulou et al., 2018; Boerger et al., 2010; Budimir et al., 2018; Chagnon et al., 2018; Collard et al., 2015; Davison & Asch, 2011; Foekema et al., 2013; Forrest & Hindell, 2018; Miranda & de Carvalho-Souza, 2016; Nelms et al., 2018). Surface feeders are likely to mistake floating microplastic for prey (Savoca et al., 2017) and benthic feeders will consume MPs that have sunk to the seafloor. The consequences of plastic ingestion include, but are not limited to, inflammation of the gut, starvation, and death (Rochman et al., 2016). Histopathological examinations of European seabass (*Dicentrarchus labrax*) fed with PVC have proven severe alterations to the structure and function after 90 days (Pedà et al., 2016). In more elevated cases of continued accumulation of plastic, stomachs can become full of plastic, and it is unable to be passed through the digestive system, causing gastric blockage, as seen in seabirds (Azzarello & Van Vleet, 1987). The plastic occupies important space in an animal's stomach, causing a feeling of false fullness and preventing them from absorbing enough nutrients to maintain growth. MPs were found in multiple wild fish organs including the digestive tract, gills and muscle (Barboza et al., 2020). Gills function is reduced as particles become stuck in gills, cause breakage, infection and oxidative stress (Barboza et al., 2018). Laboratory studies also show MPs to be easily eliminated from fish after ingestion (Mazurais et al., 2015).

MPs may cause long-term impacts on individuals and fish populations by reducing survival capabilities such as swimming speed, response time, predatory responses (Mattsson et al., 2015) and escape responses (Nanninga et al., 2021). This can cause knock-on effects by reducing growth (Critchell & Hoogenboom, 2018) and overall health of an animal. The cause of these behavioural changes can be seen in physiologi-

Table 1. Evidence of impact and effects of microplastics on marine organisms

Taxonomic group	Species	Particle type	Particle size	Concentration	Exposure time	Effects	Reference
Bacteria	*Bacillus subtilis*	PE	323.3 and 656.8 µm	10 - 500 mg/L	1-36 h	Growth inhibition; ↓ protein content and LPO; ↑ extracellular carbohydrate levels	Ustabasi et al., (2020)
	Escherichia coli					↑ extracellular carbohydrate levels	Ustabasi et al., (2020)
	Pseudomonas aeruginosa					↓ LPO; ↑ extracellular carbohydrate levels	Ustabasi et al., (2020)
	Staphylococcus aureus					↑ extracellular carbohydrate levels	Ustabasi et al., (2020)
Algae	*Chaetoceros gracilis*	PVC	1 µm	25, 50, 100, 200 mg/L	24, 48, 72, 96 h	↓ chlorophyll content, photochemical efficiency and photosynthesis	Wang et al., (2020)
	Chaetoceros neogracile	PS	2 µm	3.96 µg/L	30 d	Hetero-aggregation, little impact on algal physiology	Long et al., (2020)
	Dunaliella salina	PS (+ZnO)	-	1mg/L	72 h	MPs ↓harmful effects of ZnO	Gunasekazan et al., (2020)
	Dunaliella tertiolecta	PS	0.05, 0.5 and 6 µm	250 mg/L		Up to 45% ↓ of growth rate, smaller particles show higher ↓	Sjollema et al., (2016)
			0.04 µm	0.5 - 50 mg/L		Aggregation of MPs and inhibition of growth	Bergami et al., (2017)
	Heterocapsa triquetra		2 µm	3.96 µg/L	30 d	Little impact on algal physiology	Long et al., (2020)
	Karenia mikimotoi		65 nm, 100 nm, 1 µm	10 mg/L	72 h	Impaired cell viability, reduced cell membrane integrity and DNA concentration	Zhao et al., (2022)
	Platymonas helgolandica var. tsingtaoensis		1, 2, 3, 4, 5 µm	10mg/L		1 and 2 µm particles in algae, ↓ photosynthesis and density of algae	Chen et al., (2020)
	Phaeodactylum tricornutum	PS, PMMA	<100 µm	0.5, 50 mg/L	27 d	↓ in biomass and carbohydrate production	Cunha et al., (2020)
	Phaeodactylum tricornutum	PVC	1 µm	25, 50, 100, 200 mg/L	24, 48, 72, 96 h	↓ chlorophyll content, photochemical efficiency and photosynthesis	Wang et al., (2020)
	Pyropia yezoensis (Commercial Nori)	PET	100 - 2000 µm	0, 1000, 5000, 10,000 fibers/L	2 h	MP fibres adhere to surface of algae	Li et al., (2020)
	Rhodomonas baltica	PS	10 µm	75-7500 particles/L	264 h	Inhibition of cell count and ↓ chlorophyll content	Lyakurwa, (2017)
	Skeletonema costatum	PVC	1 µm	0-50 mg/L	96 h	40% ↓ in growth rate, up to 20% ↓ in chlorophyll content and photosynthetic rate	Zhang et al., (2017)
	Skeletonema costatum	mPVC (+Cu^{2+})		0, 3, 6, 10, 15, 20, 30 mg/L	24 h	Inhibited growth but ↓ toxicity of Cu particles	Zhu et al., (2020)
	Tetraselmis chuii	PE	1-5 µm	0.75 - 48 mg/L	96 h	↓ chlorophyll content at some concentrations	Prata et al., (2018)
				0.046 – 1.472 mg/L		No significant effects on population growth	Davarpanah & Guilhermino (2015)
	Thalassiosira sp.	PVC	1 µm	25, 50, 100, 200 mg/L	24, 48, 72, 96 h	↓ chlorophyll content, photochemical efficiency and photosynthesis	Wang et al., (2020)
	Tisochrysis lutea	PS	2 µm	3.96 µg/L	30 d	Little impact on algal physiology	Long et al., (2020)
Rotifers	*Brachionus calyciflorus*	PE-spherical	10–22 µm	0.5×10^3, 2.5×10^3, and 1.25×10^4 particles/mL	24 h-progenitors died	Ingestion; reproduction suppressed; ↓ swimming linear speed; ↓SOD and Na^+-K^+-ATPase activities, ↑ GPx activity	Xue et al., (2020)
	Brachionus koreanus	PS-beads	0.05 - 6 µm	1 - 20 g/L	24 h-12 d	↑ antioxidant enzymes activities; oxidative stress (ROS level) and phosphorylation status of MAPK); ↑ phosphorylation of c-Jun N-terminal kinase (p-JNK) and p38 (p-p38); ↓ growth rate, lifespan, fecundity, reproduction time and body size	Jeong et al., (2016)
	Brachionus plicatilis	PS-beads	6µm	1 and 2.5 g/L	24 h-6 d	↓ population growth rate and swimming behavior; ↑ ROS level, GSH, GSTs, SOD and CAT activities; ↓ calcein AM, Alterations in transcriptional expression levels of ATP-binding cassette genes related to multi xenobiotic resistance function.	Kang et al., (2021)
		PS	0.07 - 7 µm	1 - 20 g/L	initial maternal rotifers died or algae elimination	↓ rotifer survival and reproduction, prolonged the time to maturation, and reduced the body size at maturation; significantly delayed the elimination of phagocytosis by rotifers	Sun et al., (2019)
			10 µm	3 -5 mg/L	12, 24, 48 h	Ingestion	Laksono et al., (2021)
		PE	0.1 µm	0.001 -10 mg/L	48 h	Swimming speed stimulatory effect at low concentrations and an inhibitory at high concentrations; ingestion	Gambardella et al., (2018)
	Keratella cochlearis	latex beads	0.04 - 10 µm	-	5 min	Ingestion	Ronneberger (1998)
	Keratella quadrata						
	Polyarthra dolichoptera						
	Synchaeta pectinata						
	Synchaeta spp.	PS - spheres		1000 - 10 000 particles/mL	3 h	Ingestion from food web transfer	Setälä et al., (2014)
Corals	*Acropora cervicornis*	HDPE and PE	≤1000 µm and >1.7 mm	1560 mg/L	48 h and 12 w	ingestion and egestion until 1 mm; ↓ tissue surface area, calcification, and buoyant weight	Hankins et al., (2021)
	Acropora formosa	LDPE	<100 - 500 µm	0.05 - 0.15 g/L	0 - 14 d	Bleaching and necrosis; ingestion; ↓ Zooxanthellae abundance	Syakti et al., (2019)
	Acropora hemprichii	PE	53–63, 125–150, 215–250, 300–355 and 425–500 µm	0.2 g /L	28 h	ingestion; ↑ production of mucus	Lizárraga et al., (2017)
	Acropora humilis		37 - 163 µm	0.1 g/L	4 w	Bleaching; overgrowth of microplastic particle	Reichert et al., (2018)
	Acropora muricata		175.5 µm	0.25 mg/L	6 m	↓ growth parameters; ↑ photosynthesis	Reichert et al., (2019)
		weathered PP and PE beads	1 um - 2 mm²	5 - 200 pieces/L	2, 5 h and 24 h	↓ gamete fertilization, embryo development and larval settlement	Berry et al., (2019)
	Acropora sp.	PS spheres and microfibres	500–1000 µm,and 0.05–1 cm	0.1 mg/L	0-14 d	(Photo)physiology alterations according to temperature; ↓ gross photosynthesis (O_2 production) and ↑ net respiration (O_2 consumption)	Mendrik et al., (2021)
	Astroides calycularis	PE	2 and 3 mm	1.33 particles/L	30-90 min	Captures, ingests, and egests microplastics; ↓ food intake	Savinelli et al., (2021)
	Danafungia scruposa	fluorescent PE-beads	212–355, 600–710, and 850–1000 µm	0.38 g/L	48 h	↓ fitness	Corona et al., (2020)
	Dipsastrea pallida	shavings of blue PP	10 µm–2 mm	0.197 - 0.395 g/L	3 - 48 h	Ingestion, retainment within their gut cavity and egestion	Hall et al., (2015)
	Heliopora coerulea	PE	175.5 µm	0.25 mg/L	6 m	↓ growth parameters	Riechert et al., (2019)
	Lophelia pertusa	LDPE	500 µm	350 particles/L	2 m	↓ capture rates, percentage of active polyps and growth rates;	Chapron et al., (2018)
		LDPE	500 µm	350 particles/L	5 m	↓ growth rate and prey capture rates	Mouchi et al., (2019)
	Montastraea cavernosa	PE-beads and polyester microfibers	90 µm–2.8 mm	30 mg/L	48 h	Ingestion and egestion	Hankins et al., (2018)
	Montipora capitata	PE (green fluorescent)	150–180 µm	2000 particles/L	10 d	Ingestion and egestion	Axworthy et al., (2019)

continued on following page

Table 1. Continued

Taxonomic group	Species	Particle type	Particle size	Concentration	Exposure time	Effects	Reference
	Pocillopora damicornis	PS	1.0 µm	50 mg/L	6, 12, 24 h	↑ SOD and CAT activities and chlorophyll content; ↓ GSTs and AKP; 349 and 107 differentially expressed genes in the scleractinian coral and symbiotic zooxanthellae	Tang et al., (2018)
		PE	37 µm to 163 µm	0.1 g/L	4 w	Tissue necrosis	Reichert et al., (2018)
		PE (green fluorescent)	150–180 µm	2000 particles/L	10 d	Ingestion and egestion	Axworthy et al., (2019)
	Pocillopora verrucosa	PE	175.5 ± 73.5 µm	0.25 mg/L	6 m	↑ photosynthesis parameters; compromised coral health (i.e., bleaching, tissue necrosis, feeding scars from parasites)	Reichert et al., (2019)
			37 µm to 163 µm	0.1 g/L	4 w	Tissue necrosis	Reichert et al., (2018)
	Porites cylindrica		37 µm to 163 µm		4 w	Bleaching; overgrowth of microplastic particle	
	Porites lutea		37 µm to 163 µm		4 w	Mucus production; overgrowth of microplastic particle (energy coast)	
	Porites porites	PS	≤ 5µm	1 - 1000 mg/L	96 h	Ingestion	Grillo et al., (2021)
	Pseudodiploria clivosa	HDPE and PE	≤1000 µm and >1.7 mm respec	1560 mg/L	48 h and 12 w	Uptake and egestion until 2.8 mm; ↓ tissue surface area and calcification	Hankins et al., (2021)
	Seriatopora hystrix	PS spheres and microfibres	500–1000 µm and 0.05–1 cm	0.1 mg/L	0-14 d	(Photo)physiology alterations according to the temperature; ↑ gross photosynthesis (O_2 production) and ↓ net respiration (O_2 consumption)	Mendrik et al., (2021)
	Stylophora pistillata	PE	106–125 µm	5000 and 50,000 µg/L	28 d	↑ levels of phosphorylated sugars and pyrimidine nucleobases; ↑ photosynthetic efficiency	Lanctôt et al., (2020)
	Tubastrea aurea	PVC; PE; PET; PA66	1 to 20 µm	300 mg/L	24 h	Ingestion; ↓ GHS, CAT, SOD, TAC and Alkaline Phosphatase activities; ↓ Pyruvate Kinase and Na, K-ATP (energy metabolism) and Ca-ATP, Mg-ATP, and Ca, Mg-ATP activity (calcification process)	Liao et al., (2021)
	Zoanthus sociatus	LDPE and PVC	63–125 µm	1 and 10 mg/L (LDPE and PVC, respectively)	96 h	↑ adherence to coral epidermis, photosynthetic efficiency, LPO and CAT activity	Rocha et al., (2020)
Echinoderms	*Apostichopus japonicus*	PE-MFs	0.87 mm with a range of 0.13–2.54 mm	2 particles/mL	0.5 - 16 h		Mohsen et al., (2021)
			1–5 mm	3 - 6 mg/L (in water) 0.6 - 1.2 particles/g (in sediment)	72h/168h/60d	Ingestion and persistence in the coelomic fluid; ↑ lysozyme responses in the coelomic fluid;	Mohsen et al., (2019)
	Apostichopus parvimensis	PS-divinylbenzene beads	15–60 µm	25 - 100 beads/mL	5-16 d	Ingestion	Lizárraga et al., (2017)
	Astropecten armatus		45-120 µm	25 - 100 beads/mL	08-28 d	Ingestion	Lizárraga et al., (2017)
	Cucumaria frondosa	PVC fragments, nylon fragments, and PVC resin pellets	0.25 - 15 mm (PVC) and 0.25 - 1.5 mm nylon	10.0 g (wet) PVC shavings, 65.0 g (wet) PVC resin pellets, or 2.0 g (dry) nylon line	4 h	Ingestion	Graham and Thompson (2009)
	Dendraster excentricus	PS-divinylbenzene beads	15-60 µm	25 - 500 beads/mL	4-14 d	Ingestion	Lizárraga et al., (2017)
	Dermasterias imbricata	PS divinylbenzene microspheres	20 um	2.4 microplastics µL−1	-	Ingestion	Hart (1991)
	Holothuria cinerascens	PE	0.5–1 mm and 1–2 mm	50 - 150 particles/L	72 h	Ingestion	Iwalaye et al., (2021)
		PE fluorescent fragments	1–2 mm	1 mg/L		Microplastics in guts, coelomic fluid; digested respiratory trees and undigested respiratory trees	Iwalaye et al., (2020)
	Holothuria floridana	PVC fragments, nylon fragments, and PVC resin pellets	0.25 - 15 mm (PVC) and 0.25 - 1.5 mm nylon	10.0 g (wet) PVC shavings, 65.0 g (wet) PVC resin pellets, or 2.0 g (dry) nylon line	4 h	Ingestion	Graham and Thompson (2009)
	Holothuria grisea						
	Lytechinus pictus	PS - divinylbenzene beads	15-75 µm	25 - 500 beads/mL	5-21 d	Ingestion	Lizárraga et al., (2017)
	Paracentrotus lividus	PS and HPDE	6 µm (PS) and >0–80 µm (HPDE)	10^3, 10^4 and 10^5 particles/mL (PS) and 0.005 - 5 g/L (HDPE)	48 h	Reduce fertilization rate and larval growth; ↑ larvae abnormalities;	Martínez-Gómez et al., (2017)
		PS	10 µm and 45 µm	10 particles/mL	72 h	↑ total immune cells count, ratio between red (%) and white amoebocytes (%), intracellular ROS and RNS and total antioxidant capacity	Murano et al., (2020)
			10 µm	0.125 - 25 µg/ml microbeads	72 h	Ingestion; alterations ins body length and arm length; decrease body widths	Messinetti et al., (2018)
		PE	5.5 µm	1 mg/L	48 h	Ingestion; ↓ filtration rate	Beiras and Tato (2019)
			0.1 µm	0-0.001-0.01-0.1-1-10 mg L−1	24 h	↑ swimming speed	Gambardella et al., (2018)
	Patiria miniata	PS divinylbenzene beads	45-120 µm	25 - 100 beads mL−1	07-28 d	Ingestion	Lizárraga et al., (2017)
	Pseudechinus huttoni	spherical fluorescent green MPs	retention (1–5 µm), and short-term exposure effects (1–4 µm)	10 - 10,000 particles/mL	24 h/10 d	Ingestion ↑ SOD, GPx and CAT activities of protein carbonyl (PC) and lipid peroxides (LPx) concentrations, larval arm asymmetry	Richardson et al., (2021)
	Sphaerechinus granularis	PS and polymethyl methacrylate (PMMA)	10 - 230 µm (PS) and 10 - 50 µm (PMMA)	0.1 - 5 mg/L	72 h	Developmental morphological defects; ↑cytogenetic aberrations, mitotic abnormalities and developmental defects in offspring following sperm; ↓ fertilization rate;	Trifuoggi et al., (2019)
	Strongylocentrotus droebachiensis	PS - divinylbenzene microspheres	20 µm	2.4 particles/µL	-	Ingestion	Hart (1991)
					-		
	Strongylocentrotus purpuratus	PS divinylbenzene beads	15-100 µm	25 - 500 particles/mL	7-20 d		Lizárraga et al., (2017)
	Stylasterias forreri	PS divinylbenzene microspheres	20 µm	2.4 particles/µL	-		Hart (1991)

continued on following page

Table 1. Continued

Taxonomic group	Species	Particle type	Particle size	Concentration	Exposure time	Effects	Reference
	Thyonella gemmata	PVC fragments, nylon fragments, and PVC resin pellets	0.25 - 15 mm (PVC) and 0.25 - 1.5 mm nylon	10.0 g (wet) PVC shavings, 65.0 g (wet) PVC resin pellets, or 2.0 g (dry) nylon line	4 h	Ingestion	Graham and Thompson (2009)
	Tripneustes gratilla	PE microspheres	25–32 μm	1 - 300 particles/mL	27 h/5 d	Ingestion ↓ larvae body widths	Kaposi et al., (2014)
Crustaceans	*Acartia tonsa*	PE	10-90 μm	0-25000 MP/mL	48 h	ingestion, ↑ metabolic activity and mortality	Syberg et al., (2017)
	Amphibalanus amphitrite			0.001 - 10 mg/L	24 h and 48 h	Ingestion of MPs, alteration of swimming and enzyme activity indicating neurotoxic effects and oxidative stress	Gambardella et al., (2017)
	Artemia franciscana	PS beads	0.1 μm	0.001 – 10 mg/L	24 h and 48 h	Ingestion of MPs, alterations of swimming and enzyme activities indicating neurotoxic effects and oxidative stress	Gambardella et al., (2017)
	Calanus helgolandicus		20 μm	75 particles/L	24 h	↓ feeding and reproduction output	Cole et al., (2015)
	Callinectes ornatus	PVC	0.1-1 μm	0.5g/L from mussels as food	10 d	Trophic transfer but low particle resistance	Santana et al., (2017)
	Carcinus maenas	PP	1-5 mm	[0% (0 mg), 0.3% (0.6 mg), 0.6% (1.2 mg), 1% (2.0 mg	4 weeks	↓ food consumption, energy and growth	Watts et al., (2015)
	Charybdis japonica	PS	5μm	1 x 10^3 particles/mL	1 week	Capacity to counteract effects of low concentrations, hepatic injury, reduced neural activity	Wang et al., (2021)
	Emerita analoga	PP	1mm	3 pieces/L	71 d	↑ adult mortality, ↓ egg retention, variable embryonic development rates	Horn et al., (2020)
	Eriocheir sinensis		0.5μm	40000μg/L	7 d	↑ oxidative stress, negative effects on growth	Yu et al., (2018)
	Eriocheir sinensis		5μm	0, 0.04, 0.4, 4, 40 mg/L	7, 14, 21 days	↓ immune enzyme activity and immune gene expression.	Liu et al., (2019)
	Necora puber	PS	0.5μm	4.1 × 10^6 MPs/mussel as food	21 d	MPs in the brain, trophic transfer from mussels (Mytilus edulis)	Crooks et al., (2019)
	Orchestoidea tuberculata		8 μm	0%, 5% and 10% of artificial food source	24 h	↓consumption rate of algae	Carrasco et al., (2019)
	Pagurus bernhardus	PE	10-29 μm	0, 0.1, 1 mg/L	5 d	↓ startle response	Nanninga et al., (2020)
	Tigriopus japonicus		005, 0.5, 6μm	240 μm in 4mL	96 h	Acute toxicity, ↓ in fecundity and triggered mortality in next generation.	Lee et al., (2013)
	Uca rapax (Fidler crab)	PS	180 –250 μm	0.1-1% sediment volume	2 months	ingestion of fragments in gills, stomach and hepatopancreas	Brennecke et al., (2015)
Molluscs	*Amphibalanus amphitrite*		1.7 - 19 μm	1 - 1000 particles/mL	11 w	↑ larval mortality and delayed development time (offspring)	Yu and Chan (2020)
	Atactodea striata		63 - 250 μm	10 and 1000 particles/L	10 d	Ingestion and ↓ clearance rate	Xu et al., (2017)
	Corbicula fluminea	unknown composition	1 and 5 μm	0.13 mg/L	8 and 14 d	Ingestion; ↓ filtration rate and Che activity; ↑ LPO	Oliveira et al.; (2018)
			1–5 μm	0.2 and 0.7 mg/L	96 h	Ingestion; ↓ AChE activity	Guilhermino et al., (2018)
	Crassostrea gigas	PS	2 and 6 μm	2.06 and 118 particles/mL	2, 5, and 8 w	Ingestion; ↑ algal consumption; hyalinocytes and granulocytes size; ↓ total number and diameter of oocytes, D-larval yield, sperm velocity, larval growth; molecular alterations	Sussarellu, et al., (2016)
		HDPE	20-25 μm	10 and 30 μg/L	24 d	↑ valve micro-closures; ↓ valve opening duration and shell growth	Bringer et al., (2021)
		PS	6 μm	10^4, 10^5 and 10^6 particles/L	80 d	Ingestion; alterations in the condition index and shell length; ↑ weight; ↓ lysosomal membrane stability;	Thomas et al., (2020)
		PE and PET	irregularly shaped particles	10 and 1000 μg/L	21 d	Alterations in clearance, respiration rate, SOD and CAT activities, protein expression, expression levels of several genes from both intrinsic and extrinsic apoptosis pathways and aerobic and lipid metabolism	Teng et al., (2021)
			36.72 and 31.11 μm			Ingestion; ↓ hexokinase and glutamic pyruvic transaminase, total cholesterol, and triglyceride; histological damage; ↑ pyruvate kinase and glutamic pyruvic transaminase; metabolic alterations	
	Donax trunculus	PE and PP	100 - 400 μm	0.24 g of PP/PE mixture (0.06 g/Kg of sand)	3h, 1 -15 d	Ingestion; ↓ AChE activity; ↑ CAT and GSTs activities	Tlili et al., (2020)
	Mytilus coruscus	PS	2 μm	0, 10, 10^4, 10^6 particles/L	14 d	↑ ROS, LPO and MDA levels, acid phosphatase and alkaline phosphatase activity; metabolic alterations	Huang et al., (2021)
						↑ CAT, GSH and lysozyme activities; ↓ pepsin, trypsin, alpha-amylase, and lipase	Wang et al., (2019)
				2.5μg/L	21 d	↓ clearance rate; ↑ acid phosphatase, alkaline phosphatase activities and ROS content and MDA levels	Gu et al., (2020)
	Mytilus edulis	HDPE	0–80 μm	2.5 g/L	3 - 96 h	↑ granulocytoma formation;↓ LMS	Von Moos et al., (2012)
		Poly(l-lactide)	< 250 μm	10 and 100 μg/L	8 d	Metabolic alterations (Glycerophospholipids were down-regulated)	Khalid et al., (2021)
		PE	10 – 90 μm	100, and 1000 particles/mL	96 h	↑ CAT activity in gills and DG; ↑ SeGPx and GPx activities in gills; ↓ GPx activity in DG; alterations in total glutathione concentration	Magara et al., (2018)
	Mytilus edulis	Polylactic acid (PLA) and HDPE	65.6 μm - PLA and 102.6 μm - HDPE	2.5 and 25 μg/L	50 d	↓ filtration rate	Green et al., (2016)
	Mytilus galloprovincialis	PS and PE	20 μm and 75 μm	1 × 10^4 and 5 × 10^4 particles/L	7 d	↓ amylase and xylanase activities, ↑ cellulase activity and total protease activity	Trestail et al., (2021)
		PS	3 μm	1.5 - 150 ng/L	21 d	↓ LMS, lysozyme and hemocite phagocite activities; ↑ intra-lysosomal content of lipofuscin, LPO, CAT activity	Capolupo et al., (2021)
		PE	40–48 μm	1- 100 μg/L	14 d	↓ filtration rate, CAT and GST activities ;↑ LPO	Abidli et al., (2021)
		PE and PS	< 100 μm	1.5 g/L	7 d	Ingestion; ↑ DNA strand breaks in hemocytes; ↓ granulocytes versus hyalinocytes type cells, AChE, Se-GPX activities, LMS, lysosomal integrity and lipofucsin; molecular alterations	Avio et al., (2015)
	Mytilus galloprovincialis	PE	1–50 μm	1.5 x 10^7 particles/L	24 h	Up-regulation of genes relative to carbon metabolism, oxidative stress, immune response, and apoptosis; down-regulation of genes involve in carbon metabolism	Détrée and Gallardo-Escárate (2015)
		LDPE	20–25 μm	10 mg/L	28 d	Ingestion ↓ in phagocytosis activity and granulocytes/hyalinocytes ratio; ↑ micronuclei and heat shock protein 70(hps70) expression	Pittura et al., (2018)
		PS	3-μm	50–10,000 particles/mL	48 h	Ingestion: transcriptomic alterations in genes related with immune responses, alterations in lysosomal responses, neuroendocrine signaling, shell biogenesis, and antioxidant responses at the D-veliger stage	Capolupo et al., (2018)
		PE (virgin and weathered)	50-600 um	0.01 mg/mL	21 d	Ingestion; histopathological alterations in gills and digestive system;	Bråte et al., (2018)
		Lint microfibers	20 to 750 μm in length and were always <30 μm in thickness	56 - 180 mg/L	7 d	↑ DNA damage; histopathological alterations in gills and digestive gland	Alnajar et al., (2021)

continued on following page

Table 1. Continued

Taxonomic group	Species	Particle type	Particle size	Concentration	Exposure time	Effects	Reference
	Mytilus spp.	PS; Polyamide microfibres	20 µm; 10 ø × 30 µm	500 ng/mL	24 h or 7 d	↑ SOD activity	Cole et al., (2020)
		PS	2 and 6 µm	32 µg/L	7 d	Histopathological alterations; ↑ % of dead hemocytes and ROS production; ↓ CAT, GR activities and LPO; molecular alterations	Paul-Pont et al., (2016)
		mixture composed of PE and PP	0.4 and 720 µm - PE and 0.4 and 950 µm - PP	0.008 - 100 µg/L	10 d	Ingestion; alterations in enzymatic activity (CAT, SOD and GSTs); ↑ acid phosphatase activity, DNA damage	Revel et al., (2019)
	Ostrea edulis	PLA and HDPE	65.6 µm- PLA and 102.6 µm HDPE	2.5 and 25 µg/L	50 d	↑ filtration rate;	Green et al., (2016)
	Perna canaliculus	PE	38–45 µm	1 g/cc	48 h	↓ clearance rate, oxygen respiration and byssus production	Webb et al., (2020)
	Perna viridis	weathered-PE	<32 µm and 32 – 43 µm at the relative proportions of 15% and 85%,	1 - 3 µg/L	30 d	Ingestion; ↑ LPO and GSTs activity and decrease in CAT and GSH activities in intestine and gills; changes in the morphology of internal organs; ↓ locomotory behaviour and byssus production	Hariharan et al., (2021)
		PVC	1–50 µm	21.6 - 2160 mg/L	for two 2-hour-time-periods per day. 3 months total	↓ clearance and respiration rate; byssus production and survival	Rist et al., 2016)
	Pinctada margaritifera	PS	6 and 10 µm	0.25 - 25 µg/L	2 m	↓ assimilation efficiency, energy balance and gametogenesis alteration	Gardon et al., (2018)
		PS-beads	6 and 10 µm	0.25 - 25 µg/L	60 d	Alterations in gene expression of GCT 1, toll-like receptor 13, myeloid differentiation primary response 88, and HSP70. Transcriptomic alterations in different genes (antioxidant, immune and energy balance)	Gardon et al., (2020)
	Scrobicularia plana	LDPE	11–13 µm	1 mg/L	3 - 14 d	↑ CAT activity in gill and ↓ in digestive gland	O'Donovan et al., (2018)
			4-6 and 20-25 µm	1 mg/L	3 - 14 d	↓ filtration rate; ↑ SOD, GPx activities and MDA in the gills and SOD activity in digestive gland	Islam et al., 2021
		PS	20 µm	1 mg/L	14 d	PS microplastics in the hemolymph; alterarios in AChE, LPO, SOD, CAT, GPx and GSTs activities; genotoxic effects;	Ribeiro et al., (2017)
	Tegillarca granosa		30 µm and 500 nm	1 mg/L	4 d	↑ total hemocyte counts and ROS production; ↓ proportions of red granulocytes, phagocytic activity; intracellular concentrations of Ca^{2+} and LZM	Tang et al., (2019)
		PS	500 nm	0.26 mg/L	14 d	↓total hemocyte count, red granulocyte, hyalinocyte, lectin content in the serum of blood, phagocytic rate of hemocytes; cell viability, growth and gene expression (NFκB, IKKα, MAPK, GST and CYP1A2); ↑ basophil granulocyte, ROS content and DNA damage; molecular alterations	Zhou et al., (2021)
			30 µm			↓ total hemocyte count, red granulocyte, phagocytic activity and cell viability of hemocytes; ↑ basophil granulocyte, intracellular ROS content of hemocytes; alteration in genes from the immune-related NFκB signaling pathway; from the AHR-immunotoxicity pathway; from the apoptosis pathway	Sun et al., (2020)
			500 nm and 30 µm	0.29 mg/L		↑ caspase 3 activity, intracellular ROS, MDA and GABA content; ↓ total counts, phagocytosis of hemocytes, viability, ATP contents, pyruvate kinase activities, *in vivo* concentrations of CYP1A1; transcriptomic alterations	Shi et al., (2020)
Fish	*Acanthochromis polyacanthus* (Spiny chromis)	PET	1-2 mm	0, 0.025, 0.055, 0.083 and 0.1 mg/L	6 weeks	Negative effect on growth	Critchell & Hoogenboom, (2018)
	Dicentrarchus labrax (European seabass, juveniles)	Polymer (+Hg)	1-5µm	0.26 and 0.69 mg/L	96 h	↓ swimming velocity and resistance time, lethargic and erratic swimming behaviour	Barboza et al., (2018)
	Dicentrarchus labrax (European Seabass)	PE	10-45 µm	1, 10^4, 10^5 particles/g	43 d	Limited impact, slight ↑ in mortality	Mazurais et al., (2015)
		PVC, PE	40 – 150µm	0, 1, 10, 100 mg/mL	1, 24 h	Limited impact of MPs on immune system	Espinosa et al., (2018)
		PVC	-	1.4% body weight	90 d	Severe alterations to intestines and ↓ function	Pedà et al., (2016)
	Girella laevifrons	PS	8µm	0, 0.01, 0.1 g/feed	45 d	↑ crypt cell loss, leukocyte infiltration, hyperemia, lesions in intestine	Ahrendt et al., (2020)
	Oryzias latipes (Japanese medaka)	PE (+PCBs, PBDEs and PAHs)	<0.5 mm	0.3 mg/day	2 months	Glycogen ↓, fatty vacuolation, cellular necrosis, lesions in the gut and hepatic stress.	Rochman et al., (2013)
	Oryzias melastigma	PS	10µm	0, 2, 20, 200 µm/L	60 d	Oxidative stress, histological changes and adverse effects on reproduction	Wang et al., (2019)
	Pomatoschistus microps	PE	450-500 µm	100 items/L	96h	↓ of predatory performance and efficiency	de Sá et al., (2015)
		PE + pyrene	01-May	18.4-184 µm/L		Altered enzyme activity, ↓ energy production	Oliveira et al., (2013)
	Pomatoschistus microps	PE	1-5 µm	0.184mg/L		Mortality, ↓ predatory response	Fonte et al., (2016)
	Sebastes schlegelii	PS	15 µm	1 × 10^6 microspheres per L	14 d	↓ feeding activity, speed and movement, histopathological impact on gallbladder and liver, ↓ protein and lipid content	Yin et al., (2018)
	Sparus aurata (Gilt-head seabream)	PVC	40-150 µm	0, 100, 500 mg/kg feed	30 d	Altered gene expression, ↑ enzyme production	Espinosa et al., (2017)
		PVC, PE	40 – 150µm	0, 1, 10, 100 mg/mL	1, 24 h	Limited impact of MPs on immune system	Espinosa et al., (2018)
		PE	180–212 µm	4.1 mg/L	5 d	↓ escape response	Nanninga et al., (2021)

cal data on fish. The immune system can be significantly impacted by MP ingestion as they are foreign particles which initiate an immune response. The strain that MPs put on the immune system can alter the natural responses such as reducing phagocytic activity, increase lysosome activity and influence gene expression (Sharifinia et al., 2020). Populations may also be affected by the impacts on reproduction. Environmentally relevant levels of MPs are enough to cause reduced gonad development in female fish (*Oryzias melastigma*) and alter the production of hormones (Wang et al., 2019). The ingestion of MPs

Figure 4. (A) Microplastic effects in marine organisms; (B) Nanoplastic effects in marine organisms

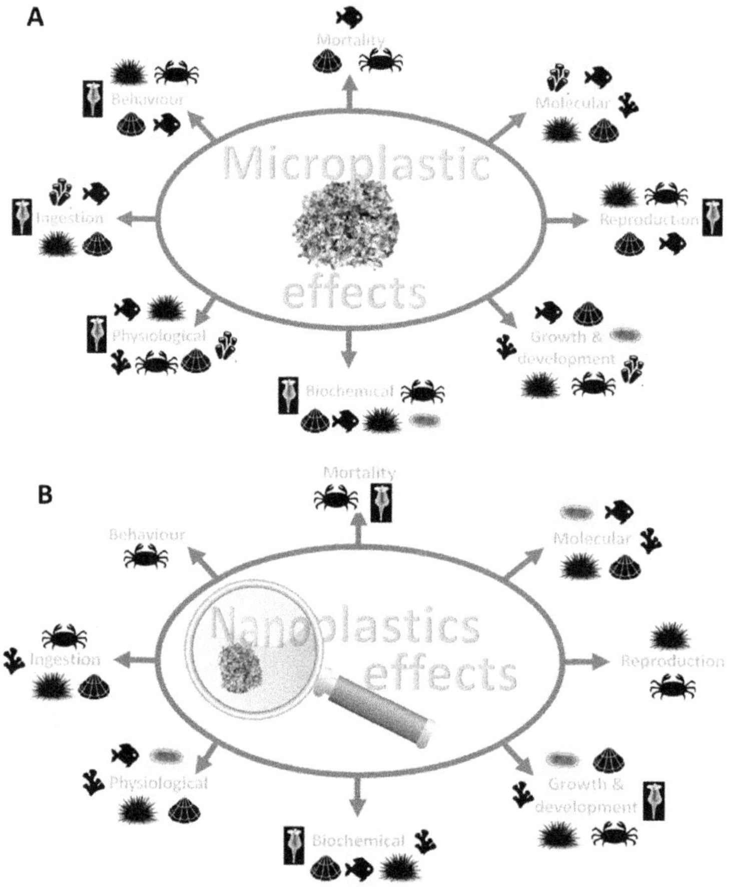

does not always cause obvious physiological or behavioural effects (Tosetto et al., 2017) but are very likely to contribute to long-term impacts. A summary of MPs effects can be found in Figure 4A.

IMPACT AND EFFECTS OF NANOPLASTICS ON MARINE ANIMALS

NPs possess properties facilitating their entry through biological barriers, accumulating in tissues, and consequently affecting the organism's metabolism and behaviour (Worm et al., 2017; Mattsson et al., 2018; Ramirez et al., 2019). These effects in different species will be described below.

Bacteria

In the presence of NPs, significant alterations in bacterial communities may occur (Table 2). NPs affect the biofilm formation of marine bacteria, being highly dependent on the polymer type, size, and concentration (Okshevsky et al., 2020). The surface charge of NPs, whether negative (-COOH) or positive (-NH2) have different properties and promotes differential effects in bacterial communities. PS-NPs with

Table 2. Evidence of impact and effects of nanoplastics on marine organisms

Taxonomic group	Species	Particle type	Particle size	Concentration (μg/mL)	Exposure time	Effects	Reference
Bacteria	*Marinobacter adhearens*	PS-NH2	20 nm	0 - 200	5 d	↑ aggregation; ↓ growth rate; ↓ OD600	Okshevsky et al., 2020
	Oceanobacter kriegii					↑ biofilm formation; ↑ aggregation; ↓ growth rate; ↓ OD600	
	Cobetia marina					↓ biofilm formation; ↑ aggregation; ↓ growth rate; ↓ OD600	
	Marinobacter algicola					↓ biofilm formation; ↑ aggregation; ↓ growth rate; ↓ OD600	
	Pseudoalteromonas carrageenovora					↓ biofilm formation; ↑ aggregation; ↓ growth rate; ↓ OD600	
	Phaeobacter inhibins					↓ biofilm formation; ↑ aggregation; ↓ growth rate; ↓ OD600	
	Marinobacter hydrocarbonoclasticus					↓ biofilm formation; ↑ aggregation; ↓ growth rate; ↓ OD600	
	Halomonas alkaliphilia		50 nm	20 - 320	2 h	⊥ growth rate; ↓ chlorophyll content; ↑ oxidative damage	Sun et al., 2018
	Marinobacter adhearens	PS-COOH	20 nm	0 - 200	5 d	↑ biofilm formation	Okshevsky et al., 2020
	Oceanobacter kriegii					↑ biofilm formation; ↓ growth rate; ↓ OD600	
	Cobetia marina					↑ biofilm formation; ↑ growth rate; ↑ OD600; ↑ aggregation	
	Marinobacter algicola					↑ biofilm formation	
	Pseudoalteromonas carrageenovora					↑ aggregation	
	Phaeobacter inhibins					↓ biofilm formation	
	Marinobacter hydrocarbonoclasticus					↑ biofilm formation	
	Halomonas alkaliphilia	PS (beads)	55 nm	20 - 320	2 h	↓ growth rate	Sun et al., 2018
	Escherichia coli	PS	30 nm	4, 8, 16 and 32	12 h	↑ ROS; ↑ Oxidative damage	Ning et al., 2022
Algae	*Tetraselmis chuii*	PMMA	40 nm	0 - 304.1	96 h	↓ growth rates; EC_{50} = 132.5 μg/mL; EC_{20} = 117.4 μg/mL	Venâncio et al., 2019
	Nannochloropsis gaditana					↓ growth rates	
	Isochrysis galbana					↓ growth rates	
	Thalassiosira weissflogii			0 - 293.0		⊥ growth rates; EC_{50}= 83.4 μg/mL; EC_{20} = 48.9 μg/mL	
	Rhodomonas baltica	PMMA	50 nm	0.5 - 100	72 h	↓ cell viability, ↑ cell size & complexity; ↑ ROS; ↑ LPO; ↓ DNA content; ↓ photosynthetic capacity; hyperpolarization of mitochondrial membrane; loss $_0$of membrane integrity; overproduction of pigments	Gomes et al., 2020
		PMMA-COOH				↓ growth; ⊥ cell cycle; ↓ cell viability; ↓ metabolic activity; ↓ photosynthetic capacity	
	Dunaliella tertiolecta	PS-COOH	50 nm	250		no effects	Bergami et al., 2017a
		PS-NH2	40 nm			⊥ growth rate (EC_{50} = 12.97 ± 0.57 μg/mL)	Bergami et al., 2017a
	Chaetoceros neogracile		50 nm	0.05 and 5	96 h	↓ cellular energy reserves; ↓ pigment composition; re-adjustment of galactolipids & triacylglycerol; re-adjustment of thylakoid membrane structures	González-Fernández et al., 2020

continued on following page

Table 2. Continued

Taxonomic group	Species	Particle type	Particle size	Concentration (µg/mL)	Exposure time	Effects	Reference
Rotifers	*Brachionus koreanus*	PS	50 nm	10	24 h	↑ mortality; NSW → EC_{50} = 6.62 ± 0.87 µg/mL; RSW → EC_{50} = 2.75 ± 0.67 µg/mL	Manfra et al., 2017
	Brachionus plicatilis	PS-COOH	40 nm	0.5 - 50	24 h & 48 h	↑ gut retention of PS-COOH	Manfra et al., 2017
		PS-NH2	50 nm	0.5 - 50	24 h &48 h	↑ mortality; NSW → EC_{250} = 6.62 ± 0.87 µg/mL; RSW → EC_{50} = 2.75 ± 0.67 µg/mL	Manfra et al., 2017
		PMMA	40 nm	4.7 - 75	96 h	⊥ survival (L-type > S-type); L-type → EC_{50} = 13.3 µg/mL; S-type → EC_{50} = 37.6 µg/mL	Venâncio et al., 2019
Crustaceans	*Amphibalanus amphitrite* (II stage of nauplius)	PS	100 nm	0.5 - 10	24 h & 48 h	↑ expression of *clap* and *cstb*; ↑ n° of molts	Bergami et al., 2017b
	Artemia franciscana (1st instar larvae)			0.001 - 10		⊥ swimming speed; Ingested and accumulated PS in gut	Gambardella et al., 2017
	Trigriopus japonicus		50 nm	0.125 - 25	96 h	↓ fecundity; ↑ embryo malformations; ↑ mortality larvae; mortality of parents at highest concentration	Lee et al., 2013
	Artemia franciscana	PS-COOH	40 nm	0.5 - 10	24 h & 48 h	no effects	Bergami et al., 2017b
	- upto instar III nauplius			5 - 100	72 h &14 d	Accumulated and retained in gut lumen	Bergami et al., 2016
	Euphausia superba		60 nm	2,5	48 h	No mortality; active swimming; waterborne ingestion and egestion	Bergami et al., 2020
	Artemia franciscana	PS-NH2	50 nm	0.5 - 10	24 h & 48 h	↑ expression of *clap* and *cstb*; ↑ n° of molts	Bergami et al., 2017b
	- upto instar III nauplius			5 - 100	72 and 14*	Ingested and retained in gut lumen; most toxic	Bergami et al., 2016
	Euphausia superba			2,5	48 h	no mortality; ↑ exuviae production; ↓ swimming activity	Bergami et al., 2020
	Amphibalanus amphitrite	PMMA	45 nm	25	24 h	↑ Ingestion	Bergami et al., 2017b
Echinoderms	*Paracentrotus lividus*	PS-NH2	50 nm	1 - 50	6, 24, 48 hpf	⊤ malformations in larvae; 24 hpf → EC_{50} = 3.82 µg/mL; 48 hpf → EC_{50} = 2.61 µg/mL	Della Torre et al., 2014
				3 and 4	24 h & 48 h	⊥ skeletal elongation; ⊤ malformations of skeletal rods and arms	Pinsino et al., 2017
	Sterechinus neumayeri			1 and 5	6 h & 24 h	*in vitro* assay; ↓ phagocytic capacity; ↓ gene modulation; ↑ cellular debris; ↑ inflammatory response; ↑ apoptosis	Bergami et al., 2019
	Paracentrotus lividus	PS-COOH	40 nm	2.5 - 50	6, 24, 48 hpf	Ingested in embryos; no malformations	Della Torre et al., 2014
	Sterechinus neumayeri			1 and 5	6 h & 24 h	*in vitro* assay; ↑ antioxidant response; ↑ apoptosis; ↑ phagocytic capacity; changes in modulation of genes related to external challenges; ↑ inflammatory response	Bergami et al., 2019
Molluscs	*Mytilus edulis*	PS	30 nm	100, 200 and 300	8 h	⊤ production of pseudofaeces → ↑ proportionally to concentration	Wegner et al., 2012
	Mytilus galloprovincialis		106 ± 10 nm	0.5 - 50	96 h	↓ enzymatic activity; ⊥ neurotransmission; ↑oxidative stress; ↑ LPO; ↑ genotoxicity; alterations in gene expression	Brandts et al., 2018b
		PS with carbamazepine (Cbz)		0.5 + 6.3 µg/L of Cbz		↑ genotoxicity; ↓gene expression	

continued on following page

Table 2. Continued

Taxonomic group	Species	Particle type	Particle size	Concentration (μg/mL)	Exposure time	Effects	Reference
	Crassostrea gigas (gametes)	PS-COOH	100 nm	0.1 - 100	1 h to 5 h	↑ cell size; ↑ spermatozoa complexity; ↓ nº spermatozoa; ↑ ROS (dose-response)	González-Fernández et al., 2018
		PS-NH2				↑ cell size; ↑ spermatozoa complexity; ↓ nº spermatozoa	González-Fernández et al., 2018
	Mytilus galloprovincialis		50 nm	0.0001 - 20	48 h	↑ malformations D-larvae; ↑ delay in development; ↓ shell length; EC_{50} = 0.142 μg/mL	Balbi et al., 2017
	Crassostrea gigas (gametes)	PS-COOH	100 nm	0.1 - 100	1 h to 5 h	↑ cell size; ↑ spermatozoa complexity; ↓ nº spermatozoa; ↑ ROS (dose-response)	González-Fernández et al., 2018
		PS-NH2				↑ cell size; ↑ spermatozoa complexity; ↓ nº spermatozoa	González-Fernández et al., 2018
	Mytilus galloprovincialis		50 nm	0.0001 - 20	48 h	↑ malformations D-larvae; ↑ delay in development; ↓ shell length; EC_{50} = 0.142 μg/mL	Balbi et al., 2017
	- haemocytes			1-50	30 m	↓ lysosomal membrane stability; ↑ ROS; ⊤ cellular damage	Canesi et al., 2016
	Mytilus galloprovincialis	PS		1.5, 15, and 150 ng/L	21 d	Gills: ↑ LPO; ↑ CAT; ↑ GST; ↓ Lysozyme activity; ↓ AChE Digestive gland: ↑ GST	Capolupo et al., 2021
				10 μg/L		Haemolymph: ↑ DNA damage Gills: ⊥ SOD; ⊥ CAT; ⊥ GPx; ⊥ GST; ↑ LPO Digestive gland: ↑ SOD; ⊥ CAT; ⊥ GPx; ↑ LPO	Gonçalves et al., 2022
Fish	*Dicentrarchus labrax*	PS	100 nm	0.001 - 10	24 h	↓ cell viability	Almeida et al., 2019
	Spaurus aurata			0.001 - 10	24 h	↓ cell viability; mild effects at higher concentrations	
		PMMA	45 nm	0 - 10	24 h & 96 h	↑ antioxidant defences; ⊤ alterations in lipid metabolism pathways; ↑ genotoxicity in blood cells; ↑ cholesterol and triglycerides in plasma; ↑ Erythrocytic nuclear abnormalities	Brandts et al., 2021
	Dicentrarchus labrax			0 - 20	96 h	↑ abundance of mRNA transcript; ⊥ fish immune system	Brandts et al., 2018
			100 nm	0.001 - 10	24 h	⊥ immune system; ↑ abundance of mRNA transcript; alterations in molecular signalling & pathways	Almeida et al., 2019

an attached amide group (PS-NH2; 20 nm; 200 ppm; 5 days) increase bacterial biofilm formation but generate a decrease in growth rate and optical density. On the other hand, NPs with an attached carboxyl group (PS-COOH; 20 nm; 200 ppm; 5 days) stimulate the aggregation of some bacterial species (e.g., *Marinobacter adherens, marinobacter algicola, cobetia marina, oceanobacter kriegii*) whilst decreasing the biofilm formation of others (e.g., *Phaeobacter inhibins*) (Okshevsky et al., 2020). Moreover, the size and functional modifications of NPs are crucial to comprehend NPs toxicity (Ning et al., 2022). In *Escherichia coli*, PS-NPs increase the generation of ROS and caused oxidative damage, and enhance antibiotic resistance mutations (Ning et al., 2022). Furthermore, NPs with a positive surface charge present synergistic effects when in contact with antibiotics (e.g., erythromycin) (Ning et al., 2022). NPs with a surface charge induce higher oxidative stress than NP beads, highlighting the importance of as-

Figure 5. Illustration of MPs biomagnification in the marine environment

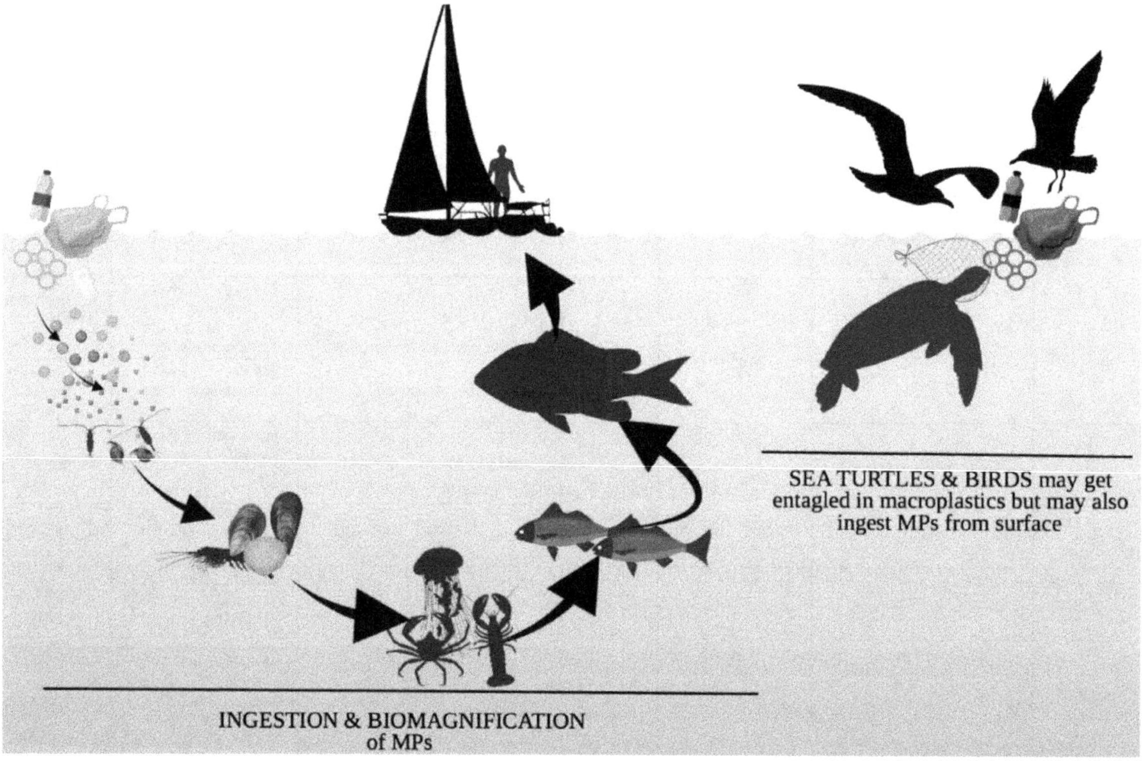

sessing polymer type, size, and shape. The main implications for bacteria are compromising cell growth, ammonia conversion efficiencies, and chemical composition, where the concentration of NPs is highly influential (Sun et al., 2018). The surface charge of NPs facilitates the adhesion to cells by electrostatic activity; however, overall toxicity of NPs is size, surface charge and concentration dependent.

Algae

The toxicity effects of NPs in algae (Table 2), with a focus on PS and PMMA with different surface charges and functional groups attached, include inhibition of cell growth, density, and development in microalgae (*Dunaliella tertiolecta, T. chuii, Nannochloropsis gaditana, Isochrysis galbana, Rhodomonas baltica*) (Sjollema et al., 2016; Bergami et al., 2017; Venâncio et al., 2019; González-Fernández et al., 2020; Gomes et al., 2020). The positively charged NPs can interact with cellulose by electrostatic interaction, explaining the high affinity of NPs to algae cell wall (Sjollema et al., 2016). This specific observation suggests that positively charged NPs are highly toxic when compared to negatively charged NPs. Thus, these interactions with microalgae are particle behaviour dependent, and the effects on cellular and physiological parameters of algae, consequently, can interrupt photosynthetic performance and hinder photosynthesis entirely, as NPs compromise algae cell wall and pigmentation (Gomes et al., 2020). As primary producers, the effects encountered in algae implement the importance of evaluating all polymer types, size and shape of NPs and raise concern about the repercussions that can affect the whole ecosystem. Comparing to MPs, the smaller size of NPs facilitates the entry through cellular barriers, however, the effects MPs and NPs pursue on algae are very similar. Future research is necessary to evaluate the accumulation of NPs in algae as seen for MPs, as well increase the number of analysed endpoints.

Rotifers

The effects of NPs in rotifers remains scarce (Table 2). Most evaluated polymer types of plastics are PS with amide group (-NH_2) or carboxyl group (-COOH) attached, and PMMA, being particles of a size range between 40 – 50 nm (Manfra et al., 2017; Jeong & Choi, 2019; Venâncio et al., 2019). NP mediated toxicity exerts difficulty for rotifers survival, and is highly dependent on polymer type and size, being that positively charged NPs are more toxic to rotifers than negatively charged, as seen for algae and bacteria. This is evidenced in Manfra et al. (2017), where PS-COOH (40 nm; 0.5 – 50 mg/L; 24 – 48 h) led to no acute toxicity, whereas PS-NH_2 (50 nm; 0.5 – 50 mg/L; 24 – 48 h) led to increase mortality of *B. plicatilis.* Also, after a 96 h exposure (PMMA; 40 nm; 4.7 – 75 mg/L), the survival of L and S type *B. plicatilis* was highly affected (LC_{50} = 13.3 mg/L and LC_{50} = 37.6 mg/L, respectively) (Venâncio et al., 2019), and comparing NPs with MPs, NPs present higher toxicity towards organisms as they accumulate a higher number of NPs. Their toxicity is associated with oxidative stress-induced damage to lipid membranes (Jeong & Choi, 2019). Not without mention, it is important to highlight that, as seen for MPs, more endpoints, such as at a molecular level and reproduction, needs to be evaluated, as well as the evaluation of the impacts of NPs in other rotifer species, in order to have a more deeper understanding on how plastic pollution affects this group of organisms.

Echinoderms

Not many data exist on NPs effects in echinoderms. Within this group, sea urchins are the most evaluated organism for the ecotoxicological evaluation of NPs effects, as they have high sensitivity to low concentrations of contaminants, especially during embryonic life stages (Sugni et al., 2007). PS-COOH and PS-NH_2 are the polymers of NPs that have been analysed (Table 2). Again, PS-NH_2 possess a more toxic threat to sea urchins than PS-COOH, suggesting a predominate association with the electrostatic cell membrane repulsion in relation to PS-COOH (Bhattacharya et al., 2010), though more evidence is necessary to confirm this. Malformations of skeletal rods and arms, and undeveloped embryos are the common effects observed by Della-Torre et al. (2014) and Pinsino et al. (2017). These were observed after exposure of NPs to *P. lividus* embryos and larvae for 6, 24 and 48 hours post fertilization (hpf) (PS-NH_2: 50 nm; 10 µg/mL) (PS-NH_2: 50 nm; 4 µg/mL), suggesting that this may be a specific effect of NPs exposure. Moreover, cellular phagocytosis, inflammatory response towards oxidative stress and apoptosis at a molecular level were incited in *Sterechinus neumayeri* after an *in vitro* exposure to PS-COOH and PS-NH_2 (40 and 50 nm, respectively; 6 and 24 h; 1 and 5 µg/mL) (Bergami et al., 2019). In summary, the toxicity of NPs are particle size and type dependent in echinoderms.

Crustaceans

PS, PS-COOH, PS-NH_2 and PMMA, ranging from 40 to 100 nm, are NPs polymers that have been studied in crustaceans (Bergami et al., 2017, 2020; Gambardella et al., 2017; Bhargava et al., 2018; Sendra et al., 2020; Table 2). As seen in other organisms, PS-COOH, although ingested, does not have adverse effects in crustaceans, whereas PS-NH_2 is highly toxic (Bergami et al., 2017). This suggests that NPs surface charge is an important factor determining the particles toxicity. On acute toxicity responses, (24, 48 and 72 h) NPs exposure led to an inhibitory effect on growth, development and mobility, and an increase accumulation of NPs as well as the mortality of larvae (Lee et al., 2013; Bergami et al., 2017, 2020; Gambardella et al., 2017; Bhargava et al., 2018; Sendra et al., 2020). The Antarctic krill, *Euphasia superba,* is a keystone species as they play an essential role in the Antarctic food chains and carbon cycling, and recently, after an exposure to PS-NH_2 (50 nm; 2.5 µg/L; 48 h), a reduction in swimming activity and increased moulting was observed (Bergami et al., 2020). In *Artemia franciscana* (PS-COOH and PS-NH_2; 40 and 50 nm, respectively; 0.5 – 10 µg/mL; 72 h and 14 d) (Bergami et al., 2017) and *A. nconsiste* (PS; 100 nm; 0.001 – 10 µg/mL; 24 and 48 h) (Gambardella et al., 2017) (PMMA; 45 nm; 5 – 25 ppm; 24h) NPs were ingested and retained in the gut. Therefore, NP ingestion is independent of polymer size, type, concentration, and exposure time. The evaluation of the ingestion of NPs in *A. franciscana* (PS; 100 nm; 0.006 and 0.6 mg/L; 24h) showed that more than 90% of NPs were ingested and accumulated in the mandible, stomach, gut, tail gut and appendages of the organism, and that the ingestion of microalgae in the presence of NPs was not affected (Sendra et al., 2020). There is an incrementing importance in understanding the toxicity of NPs towards crustaceans, especially in the Antarctic pelagic ecosystems, and how the biogeochemical cycle may be affected (Bergami et al., 2020), and what implications can surface at other trophic levels.

Molluscs

The effects of NPs in bivalves remain scarce, however the effects of both acute and chronic exposures have been evaluated. Wegner et al. (2012) suggests that mussels, *M. edulis*, recognize nPS (30 nm; 100 – 300 µg/mL) as non-or low-nutritional food and that the production of pseudofaeces was induced. The lysosomal membrane stability of haemocyte cells in *M. galloprovincialis* decreased after exposure to PS-NH_2 (50 nm; 1 – 50 mg/L; 30 mins) and increased the oxyradical generation (Canesi et al., 2015). In embryo-larval development, malformations of D-shaped veligers were observed in *M. galloprovincialis* (Balbi et al., 2017) and in *C. gigas* (Tallec et al., 2018) after exposure to PS-NH_2 (50 nm; 0.001 – 20 mg/L; 24 and 48 hpf) and PS-beads, PS-COOH and PS-NH_2 (50 nm; 0.1 – 25 µg/mL; 24 and 48 hpf), respectively. Moreover, in *M. galloprovincialis*, nPS-NH_2 (20 mg/L) led to complete inhibition of D-shaped veliger, being that 90% of larvae remained at the trocophore stage, with an EC_{50}= 0.142 mg/L (Balbi et al., 2017). In *C. gigas*, embryo-larval development success was completely inhibited (100% reduction) after exposure to nPS-NH_2 at an EC_{50} = 0.15 ± 0.4 µg/mL (Tallec et al., 2018). After a chronic exposure to nPS (50 nm; 1.5, 15 and 150 ng/L; 21 d) in comparison to PS-MPs (3 µm; 1.5, 15 and 150 ng/L; 21 d) in *M. galloprovincialis*, a change in overall greater health status of mussels was noticeable in nPS compared to nPS-MPs, being that PS elicited greater effects on lysosomal parameters and GST activity and impaired neurological functions of mussels (Capolupo et al., 2021). More recently, *M. galloprovincialis* exposed to nPS (50 nm; 10 µg/L; 21 d) led to genotoxicity after 3 days, overwhelmed antioxidant defences, and caused oxidative damage in gills and digestive gland, wherein the gills were the tissue most compromised (Gonçalves et al., 2022). However, after 21 days of exposure, an increase in enzymatic activity is observed in gills, and it was suggested that there is an activation repair mechanism such as autophagy (Gonçalves et al., 2022), though further investigation is necessary to confirm this. Additionally, Gonçalves et al. (2022) observed that NPs toxicity was tissue-specific and time-dependent, and that abiotic and biotic characteristics of seawater led to an increase in hydrodynamic diameter, and, consequently, the higher the concentration, the higher the probability that particle aggregates will fall within the µm spectrum rather than nm. However, this is true for the specific polymer characteristics evaluated in Gonçalves et al. (2022), thus for other nano-sized NPs, as well as other polymers, further attention is necessary in order to conclude that, in general, NPs aggregate/agglomerate in seawater conditions.

Fish

The metabolism of fish can also be affected by NPs as they move up trophic levels after being ingested by primary consumers (Mattsson et al., 2015) and/or by direct contact through water ingestion and filtration by fish gills. However, the knowledge of the effects of NPs in marine fish remain scarce (Table 2), and for ecotoxicological purposes, scientists are using marine continuous fish cell lines as a crucial tool to comprehend the molecular and physiological responses to stressors such as NPs (Langner et al., 2011; Villalba et al., 2017; Morcillo et al., 2017; Pannetier et al., 2018) as well as to avoid the use of animals in experiments as recommended by the European Union (Directive 2010/63 EU). An exposure of PS (100 nm; 0.001 – 10 mg/L; 24h) in two fish cell lines (*Sparus aurata*: SAF-1; *D. labrax*: DLB-1) led to a decrease in cell viability with oscillations observed at higher concentrations (Almeida et al., 2019). In *S. aurata* and *D. labrax* after exposure to PMMA (45 nm; 0 – 20 mg/L; 96 h), antioxidant defences were activated, lipid metabolism pathways suffered alterations, increased abundance of mRNA transcript, impaired fish's immune system and genotoxicity occurred in *S. aurata* blood cells (Brandts et al., 2018, 2021). With mRNA transcript being highly affected by the presence of NPs, the possibility for mutation increases, possibly leading to cellular malfunctions, henceforth its importance in understanding how different NPs polymers affect different species of fish, and what impact this may mean for the quality of aquaculture, effect on fisheries and, consequently, the effect on human beings. A summary of NPs effects can be found in Figure 4B.

Despite the emerging issue to reduce the use of large vertebrates in animal experimentation, for ethical reasons, a knowledge gap still remains in comprehending how NPs affect adult and juvenile fishes, and how NPs impact embryo-larval development. Additionally, more species need to be evaluated, as NPs toxicity may or may not differ from species to species. Moreover, additional endpoints, such as reproduction and histopathology, needs further attention, as this group of organisms is of high economic value and interest, due to human consumption.

MICRO- AND NANOPLASTICS IN THE FOOD WEB: IS THERE A BIOMAGNIFICATION PROBLEM?

Plastic debris has been found to impact more than 1400 marine species, through either ingestion or entanglement (Teuten et al., 2007, Galgani et al., 2021). MPs have the potential to enter the food chain; however, there is little evidence. Starting below and working our way up trophic levels, Setälä et al. (2014) shows for the first time the potential of MPs transfer via planktonic organisms from one trophic level (mesozooplankton) to a higher level (microzooplankton – mysid shrimp). Organisms were subjected to free-MPs and MPs coated with dichlorodiphenyltrichloroethane (DDT), where the authors highlight, in addition, the need to understand the transfer of MPs, and the ability to transfer compounds adsorbed to it or the release of compounds from the MPs themselves to other trophic levels. In a simplifying two-level trophic chain where copepod' nauplii (*T. fulvus*) was prey and the ephyrae stage of *Aurelia* sp.

A predator, feeding ephyrae with nauplii previously exposed to polyethylene MPs. MPs were detected clustered in the manubrium of the mouth and near gastric filaments of the jellyfish (Costa et al., 2020). Moreover, the common crab (*C. maenas*) was fed with blue mussel (*M. edulis*) previously exposed to PS-MPs. Although the number of MPs that transferred from one species to another was small, results demonstrate that trophic transfer occurs between mussels and crabs, and that MPs can translocate to the haemolymph and tissues (stomach, hepatopancreas, ovary and gills) of the crab (Farrel and Nelson, 2013). Complementary, the brown mussel (*P. perna*) was incubated with PVC microspheres and then supplied to two secondary consumers (fish – *Spheoeroides greeleyi* and crabs – *Callinectes ornatus*), in a first attempt to establish MP transmission through a multi-dimensional food web (Santana et al., 2017). Although MP translocation was demonstrated in both fish and crabs, it was suggested that the quick depuration of MPs posed no risk to higher trophic levels. In a laboratory perspective, Norway lobsters (*Nephrops norvegicus*) were fed with pieces of fish seeded with strands of PP, and after 24 hours, the plastic particles were detected in their stomachs (Murray & Cowie, 2011). Both examples show that MPs can be transferred from one trophic level to the next that could have negative consequences for accumulation and biomagnification.

Although, here, mammals were not the focus, in relation to biomagnification McMahon and colleagues (1999) made the first suggestion of this "event" when they discovered small plastic fragments in the scats of sea lions (*Phocartos hookeri*) together with otoliths of the *Electrona subaspera*, a Myctophid fish species. In addition, as previously shown, Myctophids constitute a large proportion of the diet of some fur seals cohabiting the same geographical location, being detected around 92% of all otoliths in the respective scats belonging to this fish species (Goldsworthy et al., 1997). Later, it was confirmed when Eriksson & Burton (2003) detected plastic particles in fur seals' (*Arctocephalus* spp) scat, were thus believed to have been ingested through the food web, that means, *E. subaspera* ingested the plastic particles, which were in turn eaten by the seals.

All factors that directly and/or indirectly can cause damage to the biota deserve greater attention, whether related to ingestion or biomagnification, where more research is crucial to comprehend these effects. Finally, the possible biomagnification of NPs up trophic levels is still unknown, and therefore future research should acknowledge this as an important matter due to their relatively small size and the facility in passing through cellular boundaries. An illustration of biomagnification of MPs can be found in figure 5.

IMPACT OF PLASTIC LEACHATE

As previously mentioned, the plastic classification follows their chemical structure, polarity, and application, thus, their fragmentation and degradation may accelerate the release of additive chemicals, the majority of which are not covalently bound to the polymers and so are prone to be released into the seawater (Teuten et al., 2009).

As a result of additives leaching from plastics discharged into seawater, wild animal species may be exposed to complex chemical mixtures including not just components controlled under existing environmental regulations, but also emerging contaminants of concern (Gunaalan et al., 2020). In general, the most common additives used in plastic production include metals, flame-retardants, polymerization solvents, dyes, UV stabilizers, antioxidants, and plasticizers (Hahladakis et al., 2018).

Two *Prochlorococcus* strains (the most abundant photosynthetic bacteria in the ocean) were subjected to leachate from common plastic products, including PVC matting and HDPE bags. Thus, the leachate exposure, *in vitro* of the two strains, reduces the growth and photosynthetic capacity, and causes genome-wide transcriptional alterations. Besides, the amount and timing of each strain's reaction to each leachate was significantly different, according to each observed effect with a leachate concentration range from 0.5 – 10% (PVC) and 6.25 – 50% (HDPE) produced from 5 min to 48 h (Tetu et al., 2019). On an environmental perspective, plastic leachates may have an impact on the composition of marine *Prochlorococcus* populations, as well as the overall composition and productivity of ocean phytoplankton communities.

Leachate effects on marine microalga *Skeletonema costatum* originated from car tire rubber PVC, PP and PS significantly inhibited the microalgae growth (EC_{50} in the range of 18–34% of leachate) (Capolupo et al., 2020). Chemical analysis of the leachate revealed a clear relationship between observed effects (growth) and relatively high concentrations (up to mg/L) of organic compounds (i.e plasticizers, antioxidants, antimicrobials, lubricants, and vulcanizers) and metals (notably Zn, Cu, Co, Sb and Pb), corroborating what was previously mentioned in relation to plastic components and additives.

Silva et al. (2016) observed that brown mussel embryo (*Perna perna*) development is sensitive to leachate from both virgin and beached pellets. However, the toxicity of leachate from beached pellets was higher than that of virgin pellets; suggesting that beached pellets' toxicity comes from the contaminants adsorbed onto the pellet surface, while the toxicity of leachate from virgin pellets was mainly due to plastic additives. However, there remains a lack of comparable information to reach a conclusion on the effects of plastic leachate. Thus, more evaluations of plastic debris from differentiating geographical locations are necessary to further understand the toxicity of plastic leachates.

The larval survival and settlement of barnacle *Amphibalanus (=Balanus) amphitrite* was affected by leachates of seven recyclable plastic categories (HDPE, LPDE, PP, PVC, polycarbonate-PC, PET, and PS) and the chemical analysis revealed a complex mixture of substances released in plastic leachates (Li et al., 2016).

Nitocra spinipes was also affected by plastic leachates. The species presented acute toxicity to different plastic products (i.e., DVD, garbage bags, gloves, phone covers and others) made of PE, PP, PVC, PS, PET, and polyurethane (PUR). The toxicity varies among the type of plastic (principal component), as well as the final product. Differences were also observed after plastic sunlight irradiation (attempt to simulate a natural process). However, no consistent trend in how toxicity of leachates from plastics changed as a function of irradiation time was observed (Bejgarn et al., 2015). Leachates from materials collected from a beach (natural weathering) was higher compared to matching new materials, which supports results obtained by Silva et al. (2016), as previously mentioned. Acute toxicity, i.e., PP, PS and PET pellets' leachates were higher when the leachate was obtained under sunlight irradiation compared with that obtained in the darkness. Meanwhile the raw leachate, obtained in the dark, caused no mortality in the organisms but increase to almost 100% after sunlight irradiation (Gewert et al., 2021).

Assessments of leachate toxicity on fish are much scarcer than on invertebrate species. In orchid dotty back (*Pseudochromis fridmani*) exposed to nonylphenol (surfactant) leached from Food Drug and Administration food-grade PE bags, nonylphenol leached up to about 160 µg/L after 48 h of plastic-water interaction and tended to accumulate in fish tissue at levels up to 369 µg/Kg. The leached concentration is very close to the fish lethal concentration ($LC_{50} = 175 \pm 14$ µg/L) (Hamlin et al., 2015).

Leachates from a new generation of compostable bags and conventional non-degradable bags (HDPE) was tested on the coastal dune plants *Thinopyrum junceum* and *Glaucium flavum*. Both plastic materials affected the timing of seed germination, led to alterations in seedling growth and seedling anomalies were observed in both species (Menicagli et al., 2019).

In addition, physiological impacts often result from compounds that have leached from ingested plastic such as plasticizers or colourants. Plasticizers such as dibutyl phthalate, diethylhexyl phthalate, dimethyl phthalate, butyl benzyl phthalate and bisphenol A (BPA) directly cause behavioural changes and can be toxic to crustaceans (Oehlmann et al., 2009).

In general, information about leachate toxicity is still scarce, and with many gaps, requiring more investigation. However, the available data suggests that MPs may be harmful even if ingestion is not the only pathway of interaction of marine organisms with contaminated plastic debris.

When considering leachates of plastic debris, there are some points that still need to be clarified. Leachates deriving from NPs needs significant attention, as to date, this class has not yet been evaluated. More importantly, it is crucial to understand the effects of leachates orginating from NPs as the smaller the particle size, the greater the surface area. Additonally, there is a lack in understanding the ability of NPs to release chemical compounds into the aquatic environment and produce toxic effects. On another note, the wide use of plastic materials in fishing gear should be a focus, as there is still scarcity on the effects of leachates orginating from fishing activities.

In this line of research, it is important to note that there is a lack in the diversity of species studied and in the standardization of methodology of how the leachate is obtained. Thus, the doubts within the scientific community in relation to plastic leachates leaves large knowledge gaps and reduces the possibility of comparisons to reach a conclusion. Finally, we recommend Gunaalan et al. (2020) review to attain a much deeper understanding of the matter.

CONCLUSIONS

The effects described throughout this chapter on different organism groups indicates that plastic particles, either MPs or NPs, are a threat to marine organisms. There is, by far, a vast amount of information on MPs in comparison to NPs. The complexity of analysed endpoints is also greater for MPs than NPs, wherein the effect at molecular and biochemical levels, growth and development, behaviour and reproduction raise a red signal on the topic and are classified as an emerging global environmental concern. NPs, on the other hand, a main focus has been growth, development and mortality, which nonetheless increments that NPs are also a threat, and may potentially be a bigger threat, however more attention is necessary concerning NPs ecotoxicology. On another note, the particle charge of NPs has been considered in comprehending the potential effects of NPs, though the same has not been evaluated for MPs, and may be an interesting approach to be explored. Although some data exist, not all polymer types and sizes have been investigated, remaining a huge knowledge gap in this research topic. Other gaps in the plastic research are related with the absence of a standard methodology for MP and NP detection and quantification in tissues, leading, sometimes to misinterpretation of the data, ensuring complexity in standardizing protocols for risk assessment of different particles (plastic size, polymers, type of exposure and the animals lifestage). A standard risk assessment should be proposed, as soon as possible, to facilitate data comparisons, so the scientific community can reach more effective and reliable conclusions. Additionally, this will aid politicians and decision makers with the legislation on this matter. Another crucial point is that most of the tested concentrations are quite high considering concentrations that have been detected in the marine environment, highlighting the necessity to use more realistic concentrations (environmentally relevant ones) to fully understand the biogeochemical cycle of plastic pollution as well the (possible) toxicity itself. Information relative to the biomagnification of plastic particles is almost inexistent, being most of the data on MPs, therefore biomagnification of NPs needs more attention. Concerning plastic leachates, there is still some inconsistency observed. The main breach in knowledge is due to the lack of a standardized methodology in the extraction of the leachates (i. e. light temperature, salinity, pH solar irradiation or note and etc). The use of micro and/or mesocosms approach, in a more integrative way, is suggested to interpret the possible effects of plastic particles in the marine environment. Finally, preventive, and legal measures should be considerable in terms of plastic use, disposal, ocean observation and care.

ACKNOWLEDGMENT

The authors would like to acknowledge the support of the RESPONSE project (FCT JPI OCEANS MICROPLAST/0005/2018) supported by national funding agencies in the framework of JPI Oceans and the projects (EMERGEMIX (02/SAICT/2017) funded by FCT and PlasticSea funded by Fundo Azul. J. M. Gonçalves would like to acknowledge the PhD grant (UI/BD/150758/2020) funded by FCT (Portugal). CIMA team further acknowledge the support from FCT through the grant UID/00350/2020 attributed to CIMA of the University of Algarve.

REFERENCES

Abidli, S., Pinheiro, M., Lahbib, Y., Neuparth, T., Santos, M. M., & Trigui El Menif, N. (2021). Effects of environmentally relevant levels of polyethylene microplastic on *Mytilus galloprovincialis* (Mollusca: Bivalvia): filtration rate and oxidative stress. *Environmental Science and Pollution Research International, 28*(21), 26643–26652. doi:10.100711356-021-12506-8 PMID:33495949

Abu-Hilal, A. H., & Al-Najjar, T. H. (2009). Plastic pellets on the beaches of the northern Gulf of Aqaba, Red Sea. *Aquatic Ecosystem Health & Management, 12*(4), 461–47. doi:10.1080/14634980903361200

Ahrendt, C., Perez-Venegas, D. J., Urbina, M., Gonzalez, C., Echeveste, P., Aldana, M., Pulgar, J., & Galbán-Malagón, C. (2020). Microplastic ingestion cause intestinal lesions in the intertidal fish *Girella laevifrons. Marine Pollution Bulletin, 151*(November), 110795. doi:10.1016/j.marpolbul.2019.110795

Alnajar, N., Jha, A. N., & Turner, A. (2020). Impacts of microplastic fibres on the marine mussel, *Mytilus galloprovinciallis. Chemosphere, 128290.* Advance online publication. doi:10.1016/j.chemosphere.2020.128290 PMID:33182139

Anastasopoulou, A., Kovač Viršek, M., Bojanić Varezić, D., Digka, N., Fortibuoni, T., Koren, Š., Mandić, M., Mytilineou, C., Pešić, A., Ronchi, F., Šiljić, J., Torre, M., Tsangaris, C., & Tutman, P. (2018). Assessment on marine litter ingested by fish in the Adriatic and NE Ionian Sea macro-region (Mediterranean). *Marine Pollution Bulletin, 133*(May), 841–851. doi:10.1016/j.marpolbul.2018.06.050 PMID:30041385

Andrades, R., dos Santos, R. A., Martins, A. S., Teles, D., & Santos, R. G. (2019). Scavenging as a pathway for plastic ingestion by marine animals. *Environmental Pollution, 248*, 159–165. Advance online publication. doi:10.1016/j.envpol.2019.02.010 PMID:30784834

Andrady, A. L. (2011). Microplastics in the marine environment. *Marine Pollution Bulletin, 62*(8), 1596–1605. doi:10.1016/j.marpolbul.2011.05.030 PMID:21742351

Avio, C. G., Gorbi, S., Milan, M., Benedetti, M., Fattorini, D., d'Errico, G., Pauletto, M., Bargelloni, L., & Regoli, F. (2015). Pollutants bioavailability and toxicological risk from microplastics to marine mussels. *Environmental Pollution, 198*, 211–222. doi:10.1016/j.envpol.2014.12.021 PMID:25637744

Axworthy, J. B., & Padilla-Gamiño, J. L. (2019). Microplastics ingestion and heterotrophy in thermally stressed corals. *Scientific Reports, 9*(1), 18193. Advance online publication. doi:10.103841598-019-54698-7 PMID:31796829

Azzarello, M., & Van Vleet, E. (1987). Marine birds and plastic pollution. *Marine Ecology Progress Series, 37*, 295–303. doi:10.3354/meps037295

Bai, Z., Wang, N., & Wang, M. (2021). Effects of microplastics on marine copepods. *Ecotoxicology and Environmental Safety, 217*, 112243. doi:10.1016/j.ecoenv.2021.112243 PMID:33915449

Balbi, T., Camisassi, G., Montagna, M., Fabbri, R., Franzellitti, S., Carbone, C., Dawson, K., & Canesi, L. (2017). Impact of cationic polystyrene nanoparticles (PS-NH2) on early embryo development of *Mytilus galloprovincialis*: Effects on shell formation. *Chemosphere, 186*, 1–9. doi:10.1016/j.chemosphere.2017.07.120 PMID:28759811

Barboza, L. G. A., Lopes, C., Oliveira, P., Bessa, F., Otero, V., Henriques, B., Raimundo, J., Caetano, M., Vale, C., & Guilhermino, L. (2020). Microplastics in wild fish from North East Atlantic Ocean and its potential for causing neurotoxic effects, lipid oxidative damage, and human health risks associated with ingestion exposure. *The Science of the Total Environment, 717*, 134625. doi:10.1016/j.scitotenv.2019.134625 PMID:31836230

Barboza, L. G. A., Lopes, C., Oliveira, P., Bessa, F., Otero, V., Henriques, B., Raimundo, J., Caetano, M., Vale, C., & Guilhermino, L. (2020). Microplastics in wild fish from North East Atlantic Ocean and its potential for causing neurotoxic effects, lipid oxidative damage, and human health risks associated with ingestion exposure. *Science of the Total Environment, 717*, 134625. doi:10.1016/j.scitotenv.2019.134625

Barboza, L. G. A., Vieira, L. R., & Guilhermino, L. (2018). Single and combined effects of microplastics and mercury on juveniles of the European seabass (*Dicentrarchus labrax*): Changes in behavioural responses and reduction of swimming velocity and resistance time. *Environmental Pollution, 236*, 1014–1019. doi:10.1016/j.envpol.2017.12.082

Barrett, J., Chase, Z., Zhang, J., Holl, M. M. B., Willis, K., Williams, A., Hardesty, B. D., & Wilcox, C. (2020). Microplastic Pollution in Deep-Sea Sediments From the Great Australian Bight. *Frontiers in Marine Science, 7*(October), 1–10. doi:10.3389/fmars.2020.576170

Beiras, R., & Tato, T. (2019). Microplastics do not increase toxicity of a hydrophobic organic chemical to marine plankton. *Marine Pollution Bulletin, 138*, 58–62. doi:10.1016/j.marpolbul.2018.11.029 PMID:30660309

Bejgarn, S., MacLeod, M., Bogdal, C., & Breitholtz, M. (2015). Toxicity of leachate from weathering plastics: An exploratory screening study with *Nitocra spinipes*. *Chemosphere, 132*, 114–119. doi:10.1016/j.chemosphere.2015.03.010 PMID:25828916

Benkendorff, K. (2010). Molluscan biological and chemical diversity: Secondary metabolites and medicinal resources produced by marine molluscs. *Biological Reviews of the Cambridge Philosophical Society, 85*(4), 757–775. doi:10.1111/j.1469-185X.2010.00124.x PMID:20105155

Bergami, E., Bocci, E., Vannuccini, M. L., Monopoli, M., Salvati, A., Dawson, K. A., & Corsi, I. (2016). Nano-sized polystyrene affects feeding, behaviour and physiology of brine shrimp *Artemia franciscana* larvae. *Ecotoxicology and Environmental Safety, 123*, 18–25. doi:10.1016/j.ecoenv.2015.09.021 PMID:26422775

Bergami, E., Krupinski Emerenciano, A., González-Aravena, M., Cárdenas, C. A., Hernández, P., Silva, J. R. M. C., & Corsi, I. (2019). Polystyrene nanoparticles affect the innate immune system of the Antarctic sea urchin *Sterechinus neumayeri*. *Polar Biology, 42*(4), 743–757. doi:10.100700300-019-02468-6

Bergami, E., Manno, C., Cappello, S., Vannuccini, M. L., & Corsi, I. (2020). Nanoplastics affect moulting and faecal pellet sinking in Antarctic krill (*Euphausia superba*) juveniles. *Environment International, 143*(July), 105999. doi:10.1016/j.envint.2020.105999 PMID:32763632

Bergami, E., Pugnalini, S., Vannuccini, M. L., Manfra, L., Faleri, C., Savorelli, F., Dawson, K. A., & Corsi, I. (2017). Long-term toxicity of surface-charged polystyrene nanoplastics to marine planktonic species *Dunaliella tertiolecta* and *Artemia franciscana*. *Aquatic Toxicology (Amsterdam, Netherlands), 189*, 159–169. doi:10.1016/j.aquatox.2017.06.008 PMID:28644993

Berry, K. L. E., Epstein, H. E., Lewis, P. J., Hall, N. M., & Negri, A. P. (2019). Microplastic Contamination Has Limited Effects on Coral Fertilisation and Larvae. *Diversity (Basel), 11*(12), 228. doi:10.3390/d11120228

Bessa, F., Barría, P., Neto, J. M., Frias, J. P. G. L., Otero, V., Sobral, P., & Marques, J. C. (2018). Occurrence of microplastics in commercial fish from a natural estuarine environment. *Marine Pollution Bulletin, 128*, 575–584. doi:10.1016/j.marpolbul.2018.01.044 PMID:29571409

Besseling, E., Wang, B., Lürling, M., & Koelmans, A. A. (2014). Nanoplastic affects growth of *S. obliquus* and reproduction of *D. magna*. *Environmental Science & Technology, 48*(20), 12336–12343. doi:10.1021/es503001d PMID:25268330

Bhargava, S., Chen Lee, S. S., Min Ying, L. S., Neo, M. L., Lay-Ming Teo, S., & Valiyaveettil, S. (2018). Fate of Nanoplastics in Marine Larvae: A Case Study Using Barnacles, *Amphibalanus amphitrite*. *ACS Sustainable Chemistry & Engineering, 6*(5), 6932–6940. doi:10.1021/acssuschemeng.8b00766

Bhattacharya, P., Lin, S., Turner, J. P., & Ke, P. C. (2010). Physical adsorption of charged plastic nanoparticles affects algal photosynthesis. *The Journal of Physical Chemistry C, 114*(39), 16556–16561. doi:10.1021/jp1054759

Boerger, C. M., Lattin, G. L., Moore, S. L., & Moore, C. J. (2010). Plastic ingestion by planktivorous fishes in the North Pacific Central Gyre. *Marine Pollution Bulletin, 60*(12), 2275–2278. doi:10.1016/j.marpolbul.2010.08.007 PMID:21067782

Boucher, J., & Friot, D. (2017). Primary microplastics in the oceans: A global evaluation of sources. In Primary microplastics in the oceans: A global evaluation of sources. doi:10.2305/IUCN.CH.2017.01.en

Brandts, I., Barría, C., Martins, M. A., Franco-Martínez, L., Barreto, A., Tvarijonaviciute, A., Tort, L., Oliveira, M., & Teles, M. (2021). Waterborne exposure of gilthead seabream (*Sparus aurata*) to polymethylmethacrylate nanoplastics causes effects at cellular and molecular levels. *Journal of Hazardous Materials, 403*(July), 123590. doi:10.1016/j.jhazmat.2020.123590

Brandts, I., Teles, M., Tvarijonaviciute, A., Pereira, M. L., Martins, M. A., Tort, L., & Oliveira, M. (2018). Effects of polymethylmethacrylate nanoplastics on *Dicentrarchus labrax. Genomics, 110*(6), 435–441. doi:10.1016/j.ygeno.2018.10.006 PMID:30316739

Bråte, I. L. N., Blázquez, M., Brooks, S. J., & Thomas, K. V. (2018). Weathering impacts the uptake of polyethylene microparticles from toothpaste in Mediterranean mussels (*M. galloprovincialis*). *The Science of the Total Environment, 626*, 1310–1318. doi:10.1016/j.scitotenv.2018.01.141 PMID:29898538

Brennecke, D., Ferreira, E. C., Costa, T. M. M., Appel, D., da Gama, B. A. P., & Lenz, M. (2015). Ingested microplastics (>100μm) are translocated to organs of the tropical fiddler crab *Uca rapax. Marine Pollution Bulletin, 96*(1–2), 491–495. doi:10.1016/j.marpolbul.2015.05.001 PMID:26013589

Bringer, A., Thomas, H., Dubillot, E., Le Floch, S., Receveur, J., Cachot, J., & Tran, D. (2021). Subchronic exposure to high-density polyethylene microplastics alone or in combination with chlortoluron significantly affected valve activity and daily growth of the Pacific oyster, *Crassostrea gigas. Aquatic Toxicology (Amsterdam, Netherlands), 237*, 105880. doi:10.1016/j.aquatox.2021.105880 PMID:34126365

Budimir, S., Setälä, O., & Lehtiniemi, M. (2018). Effective and easy to use extraction method shows low numbers of microplastics in offshore planktivorous fish from the northern Baltic Sea. *Marine Pollution Bulletin, 127*(December), 586–592. doi:10.1016/j.marpolbul.2017.12.054

Burke, L., Reytar, K., Spalding, M., & Perry, A. (2011). *Reefs at Risk: Revisted.* In World Resources Institute.

Canesi, L., Ciacci, C., Bergami, E., Monopoli, M. P., Dawson, K. A., Papa, S., Canonico, B., & Corsi, I. (2015). Evidence for immunomodulation and apoptotic processes induced by cationic polystyrene nanoparticles in the haemocytes of the marine bivalve *Mytilus. Marine Environmental Research, 111*, 34–40. doi:10.1016/j.marenvres.2015.06.008 PMID:26115607

Capolupo, M., Franzellitti, S., Valbonesi, P., Lanzas, C. S., & Fabbri, E. (2018). Uptake and transcriptional effects of polystyrene microplastics in larval stages of the Mediterranean mussel *Mytilus galloprovincialis. Environmental Pollution, 241*, 1038–1047. doi:10.1016/j.envpol.2018.06.035 PMID:30029311

Capolupo, M., Sørensen, L., Jayasena, K. D. R., Booth, A. M., & Fabbri, E. (2020). Chemical composition and ecotoxicity of plastic and car tire rubber leachates to aquatic organisms. *Water Research, 169*, 115270. doi:10.1016/j.watres.2019.115270 PMID:31731243

Capolupo, M., Valbonesi, P., & Fabbri, E. (2021). A Comparative Assessment of the Chronic Effects of Micro- and Nano-Plastics on the Physiology of the Mediterranean Mussel *Mytilus galloprovincialis. Nanomaterials (Basel, Switzerland), 11*(3), 649. doi:10.3390/nano11030649 PMID:33800064

Carrasco, A., Pulgar, J., Quintanilla-Ahumada, D., Perez-Venegas, D., Quijón, P. A., & Duarte, C. (2019). The influence of microplastics pollution on the feeding behavior of a prominent sandy beach amphipod, *Orchestoidea tuberculata* (Nicolet, 1849). *Marine Pollution Bulletin, 145*(December), 23–27. doi:10.1016/j.marpolbul.2019.05.018

Chae, Y., & An, Y. J. (2017). Effects of micro- and nanoplastics on aquatic ecosystems: Current research trends and perspectives. *Marine Pollution Bulletin, 124*(2), 624–632. doi:10.1016/j.marpolbul.2017.01.070 PMID:28222864

Chagnon, C., Thiel, M., Antunes, J., Ferreira, J. L., Sobral, P., & Ory, N. C. (2018). Plastic ingestion and trophic transfer between Easter Island flying fish (*Cheilopogon rapanouiensis*) and yellowfin tuna (*Thunnus albacares*) from Rapa Nui (Easter Island). *Environmental Pollution, 243*, 127–133. doi:10.1016/j.envpol.2018.08.042 PMID:30172118

Chapron, L., Peru, E., Engler, A., Ghiglione, J. F., Meistertzheim, A. L., Pruski, A. M., Purser, A., Vétion, G., Galand, P. E., & Lartaud, F. (2018). Macro- and microplastics affect cold-water corals growth, feeding and behaviour. *Scientific Reports, 8*(1), 15299. Advance online publication. doi:10.103841598-018-33683-6 PMID:30333567

Chen, Q., Yin, D., Jia, Y., Schiwy, S., Legradi, J., Yang, S., & Hollert, H. (2017). Enhanced uptake of BPA in the presence of nanoplastics can lead to neurotoxic effects in adult zebrafish. *The Science of the Total Environment, 609*, 1312–1321. doi:10.1016/j.scitotenv.2017.07.144 PMID:28793400

Chen, Y., Ling, Y., Li, X., Hu, J., Cao, C., & He, D. (2020). Size-dependent cellular internalization and effects of polystyrene microplastics in microalgae *P. helgolandica var. tsingtaoensis* and *S. quadricauda. Journal of Hazardous Materials, 399*(March), 123092. doi:10.1016/j.jhazmat.2020.123092 PMID:32531675

Chiba, S., Saito, H., Fletcher, R., Yogi, T., Kayo, M., Miyagi, S., Ogido, M., & Fujikura, K. (2018). Human footprint in the abyss: 30 year records of deep-sea plastic debris. *Marine Policy, 96*(March), 204–212. doi:10.1016/j.marpol.2018.03.022

Cole, M., Liddle, C., Consolandi, G., Drago, C., Hird, C., Lindeque, P. K., & Galloway, T. S. (2020). Microplastics, microfibres and nanoplastics cause variable sub-lethal responses in mussels (*Mytilus* spp.). *Marine Pollution Bulletin, 160*, 111552. doi:10.1016/j.marpolbul.2020.111552 PMID:32861936

Cole, M., Lindeque, P., Fileman, E., Halsband, C., & Galloway, T. S. (2015). The impact of polystyrene microplastics on feeding, function, and fecundity in the marine copepod *Calanus helgolandicus. Environmental Science & Technology, 49*(2), 1130–1137. doi:10.1021/es504525u PMID:25563688

Cole, M., Lindeque, P., Fileman, E., Halsband, C., Goodhead, R., Moger, J., & Galloway, T. S. (2013). Microplastic ingestion by zooplankton. *Environmental Science & Technology, 47*(12), 6646–6655. doi:10.1021/es400663f PMID:23692270

Cole, M., Lindeque, P., Halsband, C., & Galloway, T. S. (2011). Microplastics as contaminants in the marine environment: A review. *Marine Pollution Bulletin, 62*(12), 2588–2597. doi:10.1016/j.marpolbul.2011.09.025 PMID:22001295

Collard, F., Gilbert, B., Eppe, G., Parmentier, E., & Das, K. (2015). Detection of Anthropogenic Particles in Fish Stomachs: An Isolation Method Adapted to Identification by Raman Spectroscopy. *Archives of Environmental Contamination and Toxicology*, *69*(3), 331–339. doi:10.100700244-015-0221-0 PMID:26289815

Corona, E., Martin, C., Marasco, R., & Duarte, C. M. (2020). Passive and Active Removal of Marine Microplastics by a Mushroom Coral (*Danafungia scruposa*). *Frontiers in Marine Science*, *7*, 128. Advance online publication. doi:10.3389/fmars.2020.00128

Corsi, I., Bergami, E., & Caruso, G. (2021). Special issue plastics in polar regions. *Environment International*, *149*, 106203. doi:10.1016/j.envint.2020.106203 PMID:33121740

Costa, E., Piazza, V., Lavorano, S., Faimali, M., Garaventa, F., & Gambardella, C. (2020). Trophic Transfer of Microplastics From Copepods to Jellyfish in the Marine Environment. *Frontiers in Environmental Science*, *8*, 571732. Advance online publication. doi:10.3389/fenvs.2020.571732

Critchell, K., & Hoogenboom, M. O. (2018). Effects of microplastic exposure on the body condition and behaviour of planktivorous reef fish (*Acanthochromis polyacanthus*). *PLoS One*, *13*(3), 1–19. doi:10.1371/journal.pone.0193308 PMID:29494635

Crooks, N., Parker, H., & Pernetta, A. P. (2019). Brain food? Trophic transfer and tissue retention of microplastics by the velvet swimming crab (*Necora puber*). *Journal of Experimental Marine Biology and Ecology*, *519*(June), 151187. doi:10.1016/j.jembe.2019.151187

Cunha, C., Lopes, J., Paulo, J., Faria, M., Kaufmann, M., Nogueira, N., Ferreira, A., & Cordeiro, N. (2020). The effect of microplastics pollution in microalgal biomass production: A biochemical study. *Water Research*, *186*, 116370. Advance online publication. doi:10.1016/j.watres.2020.116370 PMID:32906034

Dahms, H. U., Hagiwara, A., & Lee, J. S. (2011). Ecotoxicology, ecophysiology, and mechanistic studies with rotifers. *Aquatic Toxicology (Amsterdam, Netherlands)*, *101*(1), 1–12. doi:10.1016/j.aquatox.2010.09.006 PMID:20961628

Das, D. (2011). *Echinoderm*. Available in: https://www.britannica.com/animal/echinoderm

Davarpanah, E., & Guilhermino, L. (2015). Single and combined effects of microplastics and copper on the population growth of the marine microalgae *Tetraselmis chuii*. *Estuarine, Coastal and Shelf Science*, *167*, 269–275. doi:10.1016/j.ecss.2015.07.023

Davison, P., & Asch, R. G. (2011). Plastic ingestion by mesopelagic fishes in the North Pacific Subtropical Gyre. *Marine Ecology Progress Series*, *432*, 173–180. doi:10.3354/meps09142

Davranche, M., Veclin, C., Pierson-Wickmann, A. C., El Hadri, H., Grassl, B., Rowenczyk, L., Dia, A., Ter Halle, A., Blancho, F., Reynaud, S., & Gigault, J. (2019). Are nanoplastics able to bind significant amount of metals? The lead example. *Environmental Pollution*, *249*, 940–948. doi:10.1016/j.envpol.2019.03.087 PMID:30965546 de Sá, L. C., Luís, L. G., & Guilhermino, L. (2015). Effects of microplastics on juveniles of the common goby (*Pomatoschistus microps*): Confusion with prey, reduction of the predatory performance and efficiency, and possible influence of developmental conditions. *Environmental Pollution, 196*, 359–362. doi:10.1016/j.envpol.2014.10.026 PMID:25463733

Della Torre, C., Bergami, E., Salvati, A., Faleri, C., Cirino, P., Dawson, K. A., & Corsi, I. (2014). Accumulation and embryotoxicity of polystyrene nanoparticles at early stage of development of sea urchin embryos *Paracentrotus lividus*. *Environmental Science & Technology, 48*(20), 12302–12311. doi:10.1021/es502569w PMID:25260196

Derraik, J. G. B. (2002). The pollution of the marine environment by plastic debris: A review. *Marine Pollution Bulletin, 44*(9), 842–852. doi:10.1016/S0025-326X(02)00220-5 PMID:12405208

Détrée, C., & Gallardo-Escárate, C. (2017). Polyethylene microbeads induce transcriptional responses with tissue-dependent patterns in the mussel *Mytilus galloprovincialis*. *The Journal of Molluscan Studies, 83*(2), 220–225. doi:10.1093/mollus/eyx005

Engler, R. E. (2012). Chemicals in the Ocean. *Environmental Science & Technology, 46*, 302–315. PMID:23088563

EPA. (2021). *EPA Research about Coral Reefs*. https://www.epa.gov/coral-reefs/epa-research-about-coral-reefs#Biological-Criteria

Eriksson, C., & Burton, H. (2003). Origins and biological accumulation of small plastic particles in fur seals from Macquarie Island. *Ambio, 32*(6), 380–384. doi:10.1579/0044-7447-32.6.380 PMID:14627365

Erni-Cassola, G., Zadjelovic, V., Gibson, M. I., & Christie-Oleza, J. A. (2019). Distribution of plastic polymer types in the marine environment; A meta-analysis. *Journal of Hazardous Materials, 369*, 691–698. Advance online publication. doi:10.1016/j.jhazmat.2019.02.067 PMID:30826562

Espinosa, C., Cuesta, A., & Esteban, M. Á. (2017). Effects of dietary polyvinylchloride microparticles on general health, immune status and expression of several genes related to stress in gilthead seabream (*Sparus aurata L.*). *Fish & Shellfish Immunology, 68*, 251–259. doi:10.1016/j.fsi.2017.07.006 PMID:28684324

Espinosa, C., García Beltrán, J. M., Esteban, M. A., & Cuesta, A. (2018). In vitro effects of virgin microplastics on fish head-kidney leucocyte activities. *Environmental Pollution, 235*, 30–38. doi:10.1016/j.envpol.2017.12.054 PMID:29274535

Europe, P. (2020). *Plastics – the Facts 2019, an Analysis of European Plastics Production, Demand and Waste Data.* https://www.plasticseurope.org/en/resources/market-data

Farrell, P., & Nelson, K. (2013). Trophic level transfer of microplastic: *Mytilus edulis* (L.) to *Carcinus maenas* (L.). *Environmental Pollution, 177*, 1–3. doi:10.1016/j.envpol.2013.01.046 PMID:23434827

Feng, Z., Zhang, T., Wang, J., Huang, W., Wang, R., Xu, J., Fu, G., & Gao, G. (2020). Spatio-temporal features of microplastics pollution in macroalgae growing in an important mariculture area, China. *The Science of the Total Environment, 719*, 137490. doi:10.1016/j.scitotenv.2020.137490 PMID:32143099

Ferreira, I., Venâncio, C., Lopes, I., & Oliveira, M. (2019). Nanoplastics and marine organisms: What has been studied? *Environmental Toxicology and Pharmacology*, *67*, 1–7. doi:10.1016/j.etap.2019.01.006 PMID:30685594

Foekema, E. M., De Gruijter, C., Mergia, M. T., Van Franeker, J. A., Murk, A. J., & Koelmans, A. A. (2013). Plastic in north sea fish. *Environmental Science & Technology*, *47*(15), 8818–8824. doi:10.1021/es400931b PMID:23777286

Fonte, E., Ferreira, P., & Guilhermino, L. (2016). Temperature rise and microplastics interact with the toxicity of the antibiotic cefalexin to juveniles of the common goby (*Pomatoschistus microps*): Post-exposure predatory behaviour, acetylcholinesterase activity and lipid peroxidation. *Aquatic Toxicology (Amsterdam, Netherlands)*, *180*, 173–185. doi:10.1016/j.aquatox.2016.09.015 PMID:27721112

Forrest, A. K., & Hindell, M. (2018). Ingestion of plastic by fish destined for human consumption in remote South Pacific Islands. *Australian Journal of Maritime and Ocean Affairs*, *10*(2), 81–97. doi:10.1080/18366503.2018.1460945

Fotopoulou, K. N., & Karapanagioti, H. K. (2012). Surface properties of beached plastic pellets. *Marine Environmental Research*, *81*, 70–77. doi:10.1016/j.marenvres.2012.08.010 PMID:23013745

Galgani, F., Brien, A. S., Weis, J., Ioakeimidis, C., Schuyler, Q., Makarenko, I., Griffiths, H., Bondareff, J., Vethaak, D., Deidun, A., Sobral, P., Topouzelis, K., Vlahos, P., Lana, F., Hassellov, M., Gerigny, O., Arsonina, B., Ambulkar, A., Azzaro, M., & Bebianno, M. J. (2021). Are litter, plastic and microplastic quantities increasing in the ocean? *Microplastics and Nanoplastics*, *1*(1), 8–11. doi:10.118643591-020-00002-8

Galgani, L., Engel, A., Rossi, C., Donati, A., & Loiselle, S. A. (2018). Polystyrene microplastics increase microbial release of marine Chromophoric Dissolved Organic Matter in microcosm experiments. *Scientific Reports*, *8*(1), 1–11. doi:10.103841598-018-32805-4 PMID:30279474

Gambardella, C., Morgana, S., Bramini, M., Rotini, A., Manfra, L., Migliore, L., Piazza, V., Garaventa, F., & Faimali, M. (2018). Ecotoxicological effects of polystyrene microbeads in a battery of marine organisms belonging to different trophic levels. *Marine Environmental Research*, *141*, 313–321. Advance online publication. doi:10.1016/j.marenvres.2018.09.023 PMID:30274720

Gambardella, C., Morgana, S., Ferrando, S., Bramini, M., Piazza, V., Costa, E., Garaventa, F., & Faimali, M. (2017). Effects of polystyrene microbeads in marine planktonic crustaceans. *Ecotoxicology and Environmental Safety*, *145*, 250–257. doi:10.1016/j.ecoenv.2017.07.036 PMID:28750293

Gardon, T., Morvan, L., Huvet, A., Quillien, V., Soyez, C., Le Moullac, G., & Le Luyer, J. (2020). Microplastics induce dose-specific transcriptomic disruptions in energy metabolism and immunity of the pearl oyster *Pinctada margaritifera. Environmental Pollution, 115180*. Advance online publication. doi:10.1016/j.envpol.2020.115180 PMID:32673975

Gardon, T., Reisser, C., Soyez, C., Quillien, V., & Le Moullac, G. (2018). Microplastics Affect Energy Balance and Gametogenesis in the Pearl Oyster *Pinctada margaritifera. Environmental Science & Technology*, *52*(9), 5277–5286. doi:10.1021/acs.est.8b00168 PMID:29620881

GESAMP Joint Group of Experts on the Scientific Aspects of Marine Environmental Protection. (2016). Sources, fate and effects of microplastics in the marine environment: part 2 of a global assessment. IMO, FAO/UNESCO-IOC/UNIDO/WMO/IAEA/UN/UNEP/UNDP.

Gewert, B., MacLeod, M., & Breitholtz, M. (2021). Variability in Toxicity of Plastic Leachates as a Function of Weathering and Polymer Type: A Screening Study with the Copepod *Nitocra spinipes. The Biological Bulletin*, *240*(3), 191–199. doi:10.1086/714506 PMID:34129442

Gigault, J., ter Halle, A., Baudrimont, M., Pascal, P. Y., Gauffre, F., Phi, T. L., El Hadri, H., Grassl, B., & Reynaud, S. (2018). Current opinion: What is a nanoplastic? *Environmental Pollution*, *235*, 1030–1034. doi:10.1016/j.envpol.2018.01.024 PMID:29370948

Goldsworthy, S. D., Hindell, M. A., & Crowley, H. M. (1997). *Diet and diving behaviour of sympatric fur seals Arctocephalus gazella and A. tropicalis at Macquarie Island, Marine Mammal Research in the Southern Hemisphere* (Vol. 1). Status, Ecology and Medicine.

Gomes, T., Almeida, A. C., & Georgantzopoulou, A. (2020). Characterization of cell responses in *Rhodomonas baltica* exposed to PMMA nanoplastics. *The Science of the Total Environment*, *726*, 138547. doi:10.1016/j.scitotenv.2020.138547 PMID:32320882

Gonçalves, J. M., Sousa, V. S., Teixeira, M. R., & Bebianno, M. J. (2022, January). Chronic toxicity of polystyrene nanoparticles in the marine mussel *Mytilus galloprovincialis. Chemosphere*, *287*, 132356. doi:10.1016/j.chemosphere.2021.132356 PMID:34600009

González-Fernández, C., Le Grand, F., Bideau, A., Huvet, A., Paul-Pont, I., & Soudant, P. (2020). Nanoplastics exposure modulate lipid and pigment compositions in diatoms. *Environmental Pollution*, *262*, 114274. Advance online publication. doi:10.1016/j.envpol.2020.114274 PMID:32135430

González-Fernández, C., Tallec, K., Le Goïc, N., Lambert, C., Soudant, P., Huvet, A., Suquet, M., Berchel, M., & Paul-Pont, I. (2018). Cellular responses of Pacific oyster (*Crassostrea gigas*) gametes exposed in vitro to polystyrene nanoparticles. *Chemosphere*, *208*, 764–772. doi:10.1016/j.chemosphere.2018.06.039 PMID:29902761

Graham, E. R., & Thompson, J. T. (2009). Deposit- and suspension-feeding sea cucumbers (Echinodermata) ingest plastic fragments. *Journal of Experimental Marine Biology and Ecology*, *368*(1), 22–29. doi:10.1016/j.jembe.2008.09.007

Green, D. S., Boots, B., O'Connor, N. E., & Thompson, R. (2016). Microplastics Affect the Ecological Functioning of an Important Biogenic Habitat. *Environmental Science & Technology*, *51*(1), 68–77. doi:10.1021/acs.est.6b04496 PMID:27936642

Greven, A. C., Merk, T., Karagöz, F., Mohr, K., Klapper, M., Jovanović, B., & Palić, D. (2016). Polycarbonate and polystyrene nanoplastic particles act as stressors to the innate immune system of fathead minnow (*Pimephales promelas*). *Environmental Toxicology and Chemistry*, *35*(12), 3093–3100. doi:10.1002/etc.3501 PMID:27207313

Grillo, J. F., Sabino, M. A., & Ramos, R. (2021). Short-term ingestion and tissue incorporation of Polystyrene microplastic in the scleractinian coral *Porites porites*. *Regional Studies in Marine Science*, *43*, 101697. doi:10.1016/j.rsma.2021.101697

Gu, H., Wei, S., Hu, M., Wei, H., Wang, X., Shang, Y., Li, L., Shi, H., & Wang, Y. (2020). Microplastics aggravate the adverse effects of BDE-47 on physiological and defence performance in mussels. *Journal of Hazardous Materials, 122909*, 122909. Advance online publication. doi:10.1016/j.jhazmat.2020.122909 PMID:32460126

Gu, Y. Y., Wei, Q., Wang, L. Y., Zhang, Z. M., Zhang, X. Q., Sun, A. L., Chen, J., & Shi, X. Z. (2021). A comprehensive study of the effects of phthalates on marine mussels: Bioconcentration, enzymatic activities and metabolomics. *Marine Pollution Bulletin, 168*(January), 112393. doi:10.1016/j.marpolbul.2021.112393 PMID:33932843

Guilhermino, L., Vieira, L. R., Ribeiro, D., Tavares, A. S., Cardoso, V., Alves, A., & Almeida, J. M. (2018). Uptake and effects of the antimicrobial florfenicol, microplastics and their mixtures on freshwater exotic invasive bivalve *Corbicula fluminea. The Science of the Total Environment, 622-623*, 1131–1142. doi:10.1016/j.scitotenv.2017.12.020 PMID:29890582

Gunaalan, K., Fabbri, E., & Capolupo, M. (2020). The hidden threat of plastic leachates: A critical review on their impacts on aquatic organisms. *Water Research, 116170*. Advance online publication. doi:10.1016/j.watres.2020.116170 PMID:32698093

Gunasekaran, D., Chandrasekaran, N., Jenkins, D., & Mukherjee, A. (2020). Plain polystyrene microplastics reduce the toxic effects of ZnO particles on marine microalgae *Dunaliella salina. Journal of Environmental Chemical Engineering*, *8*(5), 104250. doi:10.1016/j.jece.2020.104250

Gutow, L., Eckerlebe, A., Giménez, L., & Saborowski, R. (2016). Experimental Evaluation of Seaweeds as a Vector for Microplastics into Marine Food Webs. *Environmental Science & Technology*, *50*(2), 915–923. doi:10.1021/acs.est.5b02431 PMID:26654910

Hahladakis, J. N., Velis, C. A., Weber, R., Iacovidou, E., & Purnell, P. (2018). An overview of chemical additives present in plastics: Migration, release, fate and environmental impact during their use, disposal and recycling. *Journal of Hazardous Materials*, *344*, 179–199. doi:10.1016/j.jhazmat.2017.10.014 PMID:29035713

Hall, N. M., Berry, K. L. E., Rintoul, L., & Hoogenboom, M. O. (2015). Microplastic ingestion by scleractinian corals. *Marine Biology*, *162*(3), 725–732. doi:10.100700227-015-2619-7

Hämer, J., Gutow, L., Köhler, A., & Saborowski, R. (2014). Fate of microplastics in the marine isopod *idotea emarginata. Environmental Science & Technology*, *48*(22), 13451–13458. doi:10.1021/es501385y PMID:25289587

Hamlin, H. J., Marciano, K., & Downs, C. A. (2015). Migration of nonylphenol from food-grade plastic is toxic to the coral reef fish species *Pseudochromis fridmani. Chemosphere*, *139*, 223–228. doi:10.1016/j.chemosphere.2015.06.032 PMID:26134675

Hancock, L. (2019). *Our oceans are haunted by ghost nets: Why that's scary and what we can do.* WWF. https://www.worldwildlife.org/stories/our-oceans-are-haunted-by-ghost-nets-why-that-s-scary-and-what-we-can-do--23

Hankins, C., Duffy, A., & Drisco, K. (2018). Scleractinian coral microplastic ingestion: Potential calcification effects, size limits, and retention. *Marine Pollution Bulletin, 135*, 587–593. doi:10.1016/j.marpolbul.2018.07.067 PMID:30301077

Hankins, C., Moso, E., & Lasseigne, D. (2021). Microplastics impair growth in two atlantic scleractinian coral species, Pseudodiploria clivosa and Acropora cervicornis. *Environmental Pollution, 275*, 116649. doi:10.1016/j.envpol.2021.116649 PMID:33571858

Hariharan, G., Purvaja, R., Anandavelu, I., Robin, R. S., & Ramesh, R. (2021). Accumulation and ecotoxicological risk of weathered polyethylene (wPE) microplastics on green mussel (*Perna viridis*). *Ecotoxicology and Environmental Safety, 208*, 111765. doi:10.1016/j.ecoenv.2020.111765 PMID:33396084

Haritash, A. K., & Kaushik, C. P. (2009). Biodegradation aspects of Polycyclic Aromatic Hydrocarbons (PAHs): A review. *Journal of Hazardous Materials, 169*(1–3), 1–15. doi:10.1016/j.jhazmat.2009.03.137 PMID:19442441

Hart, M. W. (1991). Particle Captures and the Method of Suspension Feeding by Echinoderm Larvae. *The Biological Bulletin, 180*(1), 12–27. doi:10.2307/1542425 PMID:29303636

Hidalgo-Ruz, V., Gutow, L., Thompson, R. C., & Thiel, M. (2012). Thompson, R.C.; Thiel, M. Microplastics in the marine environment: A review of the methods used for identification and quantification. *Environmental Science & Technology, 2012*(46), 3060–3075. doi:10.1021/es2031505 PMID:22321064

Hoffmann, L., Eggers, S. L., Allhusen, E., Katlein, C., & Peeken, I. (2020). Interactions between the ice algae *Fragillariopsis cylindrus* and microplastics in sea ice. *Environment International, 139*(April), 105697. Advance online publication. doi:10.1016/j.envint.2020.105697 PMID:32334123

Hopewell, J., Dvorak, R., & Kosior, E. (2009). Plastics recycling: Challenges and opportunities. *Philosophical Transactions of the Royal Society of London. Series B, Biological Sciences, 364*(1526), 2115–2126. doi:10.1098/rstb.2008.0311 PMID:19528059

Horn, D. A., Granek, E. F., & Steele, C. L. (2020). Effects of environmentally relevant concentrations of microplastic fibers on Pacific mole crab (*Emerita analoga*) mortality and reproduction. *Limnology and Oceanography Letters, 5*(1), 74–83. doi:10.1002/lol2.10137

Hu, E., Shang, S., Fu, Z., Zhao, X., Nan, X., Du, Y., & Chen, X. (2020). Cotransport of naphthalene with polystyrene nanoplastics (PSNP) in saturated porous media: Effects of PSNP/naphthalene ratio and ionic strength. *Chemosphere, 245*, 125602. doi:10.1016/j.chemosphere.2019.125602 PMID:31864042

Huang, W., Wang, X., Chen, D., Xu, E. G., Luo, X., Zeng, J., Huan, T., Li, L., & Wang, Y. (2021). Toxicity mechanisms of polystyrene microplastics in marine mussels revealed by high-coverage quantitative metabolomics using chemical isotope labeling liquid chromatography mass spectrometry. *Journal of Hazardous Materials, 417*, 126003. doi:10.1016/j.jhazmat.2021.126003 PMID:33992921

Islam, N., Garcia da Fonseca, T., Vilke, J., Gonçalves, J. M., Pedro, P., Keiter, S., Cunha, S. C., Fernandes, J. O., & Bebianno, M. J. (2021). Perfluorooctane sulfonic acid (PFOS) adsorbed to polyethylene microplastics: Accumulation and ecotoxicological effects in the clam *Scrobicularia plana*. *Marine Environmental Research, 164*, 105249. doi:10.1016/j.marenvres.2020.105249 PMID:33477023

Iwalaye, O. A., Moodley, G. K., & Robertson-Andersson, D. V. (2020). The possible routes of microplastics uptake in sea cucumber *Holothuria cinerascens* (Brandt, 1835). *Environmental Pollution, 114644*. Advance online publication. doi:10.1016/j.envpol.2020.114644 PMID:32559857

Iwalaye, O. A., Moodley, G. K., & Robertson-Andersson, D. V. (2021). Water Temperature and Microplastic Concentration Influenced Microplastic Ingestion and Retention Rates in Sea Cucumber (*Holothuria cinerascens* Brandt, 1835). *Ocean Science Journal*, *56*(2), 141–155. doi:10.100712601-021-00013-3

Jambeck, J. R., Geyer, R., Wilcox, C., Siegler, T. R., Perryman, M., Andrady, A., Narayan, R., & Law, K. L. (2015). Plastic waste inputs from land into the ocean. *Science*, *347*(6223), 768–771. doi:10.1126cience.1260352 PMID:25678662

Jeong, C.-B., Won, E.-J., Kang, H.-M., Lee, M.-C., Hwang, D.-S., Hwang, U.-K., Zhou, B., Souissi, S., Lee, S.-J., & Lee, J.-S. (2016). Microplastic Size-Dependent Toxicity, Oxidative Stress Induction, and p-JNK and p-p38 Activation in the Monogonont Rotifer (*Brachionus koreanus*). *Environmental Science & Technology*, *50*(16), 8849–8857. doi:10.1021/acs.est.6b01441 PMID:27438693

Jeong, J., & Choi, J. (2019). Adverse outcome pathways potentially related to hazard identification of microplastics based on toxicity mechanisms. *Chemosphere*, *231*, 249–255. doi:10.1016/j.chemosphere.2019.05.003 PMID:31129406

Jovanović, B. (2017). Ingestion of microplastics by fish and its potential consequences from a physical perspective. *Integrated Environmental Assessment and Management*, *13*(3), 510–515. doi:10.1002/ieam.1913 PMID:28440941

Kang, H.-M., Byeon, E., Jeong, H., Lee, Y., Hwang, U.-K., Jeong, C.-B., Yoon, C., & Lee, J.-S. (2021). Arsenic exposure combined with nano- or microplastic induces different effects in the marine rotifer *Brachionus plicatilis*. *Aquatic Toxicology (Amsterdam, Netherlands)*, *233*, 105772. doi:10.1016/j.aquatox.2021.105772 PMID:33618324

Kaposi, K. L., Mos, B., Kelaher, B. P., & Dworjanyn, S. A. (2014). Ingestion of Microplastic Has Limited Impact on a Marine Larva. *Environmental Science & Technology*, *48*(3), 1638–1645. doi:10.1021/es404295e PMID:24341789

Kershaw, P. (2015). Sources, fate and effects of microplastics in the marine environment: A global assessment. *Reports and Studies GESAMP.*, *90*, 96.

Klaine, S. J., Koelmans, A. A., Horne, N., Carley, S., Handy, R. D., Kapustka, L., Nowack, B., & von der Kammer, F. (2012). Paradigms to assess the environmental impact of manufactured nanomaterials. *Environmental Toxicology and Chemistry*, *31*(1), 3–14. doi:10.1002/etc.733 PMID:22162122

Koelmans, A. A., Besseling, E., & Shim, W. J. (2015). *Marine anthropogenic litter* (M. A. Litter, Ed.). doi:10.1007/978-3-319-16510-3

Kögel, T., Bjorøy, Ø., Toto, B., Bienfait, A. M., & Sanden, M. (2020). Micro- and nanoplastic toxicity on aquatic life: Determining factors. *The Science of the Total Environment*, *709*(5817), 136050. doi:10.1016/j.scitotenv.2019.136050 PMID:31887526

Koller, M., & Braunegg, G. (2018). Advanced approaches to produce polyhydroxyalkanoate (PHA) biopolyesters in a sustainable and economic fashion. *The EuroBiotech Journal*, *2*(2), 89–103. doi:10.2478/ebtj-2018-0013

Laist, D. W. (1997). Impacts of marine debris: entanglement of marine life in marine debris including a comprehensive list of species with entanglement and ingestion records. In Marine Debris —Sources, Impacts and Solutions. SpringerVerlag. doi:10.1007/978-1-4613-8486-1_10

Lan, R., Wei, Y., & Xue, R. (2021). Uptake of polystyrene microplastics by marine rotifers under different experimental conditions. *IOP Conference Series. Earth and Environmental Science*, *687*(1), 012071. doi:10.1088/1755-1315/687/1/012071

Lanctôt, C. M., Bednarz, V. N., Melvin, S., Jacob, H., Oberhaensli, F., Swarzenski, P. W., Ferrier-Pagès, C., Carroll, A. R., & Metian, M. (2020). Physiological stress response of the scleractinian coral *Stylophora pistillata* exposed to polyethylene microplastics. *Environmental Pollution*, *114559*. Advance online publication. doi:10.1016/j.envpol.2020.114559 PMID:32325355

Langner, S., Rakers, S., Ciba, P., Petschnik, A. E., Rapoport, D. H., & Kruse, C. (2011). New cell line from adipopancreatic tissue of Atlantic herring *Clupea harengus*. *Aquatic Biology*, *11*(3), 271–278. doi:10.3354/ab00317

Lau, W. W. Y., Shiran, Y., Bailey, R. M., Cook, E., Stuchtey, M. R., Koskella, J., Velis, C. A., Godfrey, L., Boucher, J., Murphy, M. B., Thompson, R. C., Jankowska, E., Castillo Castillo, A., Pilditch, T. D., Dixon, B., Koerselman, L., Kosior, E., Favoino, E., Gutberlet, J., ... Palardy, J. E. (2020). Evaluating scenarios toward zero plastic pollution. *Science*, *369*(6510), 1455–1461. doi:10.1126cience.aba9475 PMID:32703909

Laville, S. (2019). Dumped fishing gear is biggest plastic polluter in ocean, finds report. *The Gardian*. https://www.theguardian.com/environment/2019/nov/06/dumped-fishing-gear-is-biggest-plastic-polluter-in-ocean-finds-report

Law, K. L. (2017). Plastics in the Marine Environment. *Annual Review of Marine Science*, *9*(1), 205–229. doi:10.1146/annurev-marine-010816-060409 PMID:27620829

Lee, H., Shim, W. J., & Kwon, J. H. (2014). Sorption capacity of plastic debris for hydrophobic organic chemicals. *The Science of the Total Environment*, *470–471*, 1545–1552. doi:10.1016/j.scitotenv.2013.08.023 PMID:24012321

Lee, K. W., Shim, W. J., Kwon, O. Y., & Kang, J. H. (2013). Size-dependent effects of micro polystyrene particles in the marine copepod *Tigriopus japonicus*. *Environmental Science & Technology*, *47*(19), 11278–11283. doi:10.1021/es401932b PMID:23988225

Lee, S., Gounley, J., Randles, A., & Vetter, J. S. (2019). Performance portability study for massively parallel computational fluid dynamics application on scalable heterogeneous architectures. *Journal of Parallel and Distributed Computing*, *129*, 1–13. doi:10.1016/j.jpdc.2019.02.005

Li, H.-X., Getzinger, G. J., Ferguson, P. L., Orihuela, B., Zhu, M., & Rittschof, D. (2015). Effects of Toxic Leachate from Commercial Plastics on Larval Survival and Settlement of the Barnacle *Amphibalanus amphitrite*. *Environmental Science & Technology*, *50*(2), 924–931. doi:10.1021/acs.est.5b02781 PMID:26667586

Li, Q., Feng, Z., Zhang, T., Ma, C., & Shi, H. (2020). Microplastics in the commercial seaweed nori. *Journal of Hazardous Materials*, *388*(December), 122060. doi:10.1016/j.jhazmat.2020.122060

Liao, B., Wang, J., Xiao, B., Yang, X., Xie, Z., Li, D., & Li, C. (2021). Effects of acute microplastic exposure on physiological parameters in *Tubastrea aurea* corals. *Marine Pollution Bulletin*, *165*, 112173. doi:10.1016/j.marpolbul.2021.112173 PMID:33621903

Lithner, D., Damberg, J., Dave, G., & Larsson, Å. (2009). Leachates from plastic consumer products - Screening for toxicity with *Daphnia magna*. *Chemosphere*, *74*(9), 1195–1200. doi:10.1016/j.chemosphere.2008.11.022 PMID:19108869

Liu, L., Fokkink, R., & Koelmans, A. A. (2016). Sorption of polycyclic aromatic hydrocarbons to polystyrene nanoplastic. *Environmental Toxicology and Chemistry*, *35*(7), 1650–1655. doi:10.1002/etc.3311 PMID:26588181

Liu, Z., Yu, P., Cai, M., Wu, D., Zhang, M., Chen, M., & Zhao, Y. (2019). Effects of microplastics on the innate immunity and intestinal microflora of juvenile *Eriocheir sinensis*. *The Science of the Total Environment*, *685*, 836–846. doi:10.1016/j.scitotenv.2019.06.265 PMID:31247433

Lizárraga, D., Danihel, A., & Pernet, B. (2017). Low concentrations of large inedible particles reduce feeding rates of echinoderm larvae. *Marine Biology*, *164*(5), 102. Advance online publication. doi:10.100700227-017-3134-9

Long, M., Paul-Pont, I., Hégaret, H., Moriceau, B., Lambert, C., Huvet, A., & Soudant, P. (2017). Interactions between polystyrene microplastics and marine phytoplankton lead to species-specific hetero-aggregation. *Environmental Pollution*, *228*, 454–463. doi:10.1016/j.envpol.2017.05.047 PMID:28558286

Lu, Y., Zhang, Y., Deng, Y., Jiang, W., Zhao, Y., Geng, J., Ding, L., & Ren, H. (2016). Uptake and Accumulation of Polystyrene Microplastics in Zebrafish (*Danio rerio*) and Toxic Effects in Liver. *Environmental Science & Technology*, *50*(7), 4054–4060. doi:10.1021/acs.est.6b00183 PMID:26950772

Luigi, P., Chiara, A., Elisabetta, G., Alessandra, S., & Luigi, M. G. (2012). Utilization of marine crustaceans as study models: A new approach in marine ecotoxicology for European (REACH) regulation. Academic Press.

Lyakurwa, D. J. (2017). *Uptake and effects of microplastic particles in selected marine microalgae species: Oxyrrhis marina* and *Rhodomonas baltica*. Academic Press.

Macali, A., Semenov, A., Venuti, V., Crupi, V., D'Amico, F., Rossi, B., Corsi, I., & Bergami, E. (2018). Episodic records of jellyfish ingestion of plastic items reveal a novel pathway for trophic transference of marine litter. *Scientific Reports*, *8*(1), 1–5. doi:10.103841598-018-24427-7 PMID:29666447

Magara, G., Elia, A. C., Syberg, K., & Khan, F. R. (2018). Single contaminant and combined exposures of polyethylene microplastics and fluoranthene: Accumulation and oxidative stress response in the blue mussel, *Mytilus edulis. Journal of Toxicology and Environmental Health. Part A., 81*(16), 761–773. do i:10.1080/15287394.2018.1488639 PMID:29969377

Malik, S., Suchal, K., Gamad, N., Dinda, A. K., Arya, D. S., & Bhatia, J. (2015). Telmisartan ameliorates cisplatin-induced nephrotoxicity by inhibiting MAPK mediated inflammation and apoptosis. *European Journal of Pharmacology, 748*, 54–60. doi:10.1016/j.ejphar.2014.12.008 PMID:25510231

Manfra, L., Rotini, A., Bergami, E., Grassi, G., Faleri, C., & Corsi, I. (2017). Comparative ecotoxicity of polystyrene nanoparticles in natural seawater and reconstituted seawater using the rotifer *Brachionus plicatilis. Ecotoxicology and Environmental Safety, 145*, 557–563. doi:10.1016/j.ecoenv.2017.07.068 PMID:28800530

Mao, Y., Ai, H., Chen, Y., Zhang, Z., Zeng, P., Kang, L., Li, W., Gu, W., He, Q., & Li, H. (2018). Phytoplankton response to polystyrene microplastics: Perspective from an entire growth period. *Chemosphere, 208*, 59–68. doi:10.1016/j.chemosphere.2018.05.170 PMID:29860145

Mao, Y., Li, H., Huangfu, X., Liu, Y., & He, Q. (2020). Nanoplastics display strong stability in aqueous environments: Insights from aggregation behaviour and theoretical calculations. *Environmental Pollution, 258*, 113760. doi:10.1016/j.envpol.2019.113760 PMID:31855670

Martin, C., Corona, E., Mahadik, G. A., & Duarte, C. M. (2019). Adhesion to coral surface as a potential sink for marine microplastics. *Environmental Pollution, 255*, 113281. doi:10.1016/j.envpol.2019.113281 PMID:31600700

Martínez-Gómez, C., León, V. M., Calles, S., Gomáriz-Olcina, M., & Vethaak, A. D. (2017). The adverse effects of virgin microplastics on the fertilization and larval development of sea urchins. *Marine Environmental Research, 130*, 69–76. doi:10.1016/j.marenvres.2017.06.016 PMID:28716299

Mattsson, K., Ekvall, M. T., Hansson, L. A., Linse, S., Malmendal, A., & Cedervall, T. (2015). Altered behaviour, physiology, and metabolism in fish exposed to polystyrene nanoparticles. *Environmental Science & Technology, 49*(1), 553–561. doi:10.1021/es5053655 PMID:25380515

Mattsson, K., Jocic, S., Doverbratt, I., & Hansson, L. A. (2018). Nanoplastics in the aquatic environment. In *Microplastic Contamination in Aquatic Environments: An Emerging Matter of Environmental Urgency*. Elsevier Inc. doi:10.1016/B978-0-12-813747-5.00013-8

Mazurais, D., Ernande, B., Quazuguel, P., Severe, A., Huelvan, C., Madec, L., Mouchel, O., Soudant, P., Robbens, J., Huvet, A., & Zambonino-Infante, J. (2015). Evaluation of the impact of polyethylene microbeads ingestion in European sea bass (*Dicentrarchus labrax*) larvae. *Marine Environmental Research, 112*, 78–85. doi:10.1016/j.marenvres.2015.09.009 PMID:26412109

McMahon, C. R., Holley, D., & Robinson, S. (1999). The diet of itinerant male Hooker's sea lions, *Phocarctos hookeri*, at sub-Antarctic Macquarie Island. *Wildlife Research, 26*(6), 839. doi:10.1071/WR98079

Mendrik, F. M., Henry, T. B., Burdett, H., Hackney, C. R., Waller, C., Parsons, D. R., & Hennige, S. J. (2021). Species-specific impact of microplastics on coral physiology. *Environmental Pollution, 269*, 116238. doi:10.1016/j.envpol.2020.116238 PMID:33321308

Menicagli, V., Balestri, E., & Lardicci, C. (2019). Exposure of coastal dune vegetation to plastic bag leachates: A neglected impact of plastic litter. *The Science of the Total Environment, 683*, 737–748. doi:10.1016/j.scitotenv.2019.05.245 PMID:31150894

Messinetti, S., Mercurio, S., Parolini, M., Sugni, M., & Pennati, R. (2018). Effects of polystyrene microplastics on early stages of two marine invertebrates with different feeding strategies. *Environmental Pollution, 237*, 1080–1087. doi:10.1016/j.envpol.2017.11.030 PMID:29146202

Miranda, D. de A., & de Carvalho-Souza, G. F. (2016). Are we eating plastic-ingesting fish? *Marine Pollution Bulletin, 103*(1–2), 109–114. doi:10.1016/j.marpolbul.2015.12.035 PMID:26763323

Mohsen, M., Sun, L., Lin, C., Huo, D., & Yang, H. (2021). Mechanism underlying the toxicity of the microplastic fibre transfer in the sea cucumber *Apostichopus japonicus. Journal of Hazardous Materials, 416*, 125858. doi:10.1016/j.jhazmat.2021.125858 PMID:34492807

Mohsen, M., Zhang, L., Sun, L., Lin, C., Wang, Q., & Yang, H. (2019). Microplastic fibers transfer from the water to the internal fluid of the sea cucumber *Apostichopus japonicus. Environmental Pollution, 113606*. Advance online publication. doi:10.1016/j.envpol.2019.113606 PMID:31761598

Moore, C. J. (2008). Synthetic polymers in the marine environment: A rapidly increasing, long-term threat. *Environmental Research, 108*(2), 131–139. doi:10.1016/j.envres.2008.07.025 PMID:18949831

Morcillo, P., Chaves-Pozo, E., Meseguer, J., Esteban, M. Á., & Cuesta, A. (2017). Establishment of a new teleost brain cell line (DLB-1) from the European sea bass and its use to study metal toxicology. *Toxicology In Vitro, 38*, 91–100. doi:10.1016/j.tiv.2016.10.005 PMID:27746373

Morét-Ferguson, S., Law, K. L., Proskurowski, G., Murphy, E. K., Peacock, E. E., & Reddy, C. M. (2010). The size, mass, and composition of plastic debris in the western North Atlantic Ocean. *Marine Pollution Bulletin, 60*(10), 1873–1878. doi:10.1016/j.marpolbul.2010.07.020 PMID:20709339

Mouchi, V., Chapron, L., Peru, E., Pruski, A. M., Meistertzheim, A.-L., Vétion, G., Galand, P. E., & Lartaud, F. (2019). Long-term aquaria study suggests species-specific responses of two cold-water corals to macro-and microplastics exposure. *Environmental Pollution, 253*, 322–329. Advance online publication. doi:10.1016/j.envpol.2019.07.024 PMID:31323615

Murano, C., Agnisola, C., Caramiello, D., Castellano, I., Casotti, R., Corsi, I., & Palumbo, A. (2020). How sea urchins face microplastics: Uptake, tissue distribution and immune system response. *Environmental Pollution, 114685*. Advance online publication. doi:10.1016/j.envpol.2020.114685 PMID:32402714

Murray, F., & Cowie, P. R. (2011). Plastic contamination in the decapod crustacean *Nephrops norvegicus* (Linnaeus, 1758). *Marine Pollution Bulletin, 62*(6), 1207–1217. doi:10.1016/j.marpolbul.2011.03.032 PMID:21497854

Nanninga, G. B., Horswill, C., Lane, S. M., Manica, A., & Briffa, M. (2020). Microplastic exposure increases predictability of predator avoidance strategies in hermit crabs. *Journal of Hazardous Materials Letters, 1*(October), 100005. doi:10.1016/j.hazl.2020.100005

Nanninga, G. B., Pertzelan, A., Kiflawi, M., Holzman, R., Plakolm, I., & Manica, A. (2021). Treatment-level impacts of microplastic exposure may be confounded by variation in individual-level responses in juvenile fish. *Journal of Hazardous Materials, 416*, 126059. doi:10.1016/j.jhazmat.2021.126059 PMID:34492894

Nelms, S. E., Galloway, T. S., Godley, B. J., Jarvis, D. S., & Lindeque, P. K. (2018). Investigating microplastic trophic transfer in marine top predators. *Environmental Pollution, 238*, 999–1007. doi:10.1016/j.envpol.2018.02.016 PMID:29477242

Ning, Q., Wang, D., An, J., Ding, Q., Huang, Z., Zou, Y., Wu, F., & You, J. (2022). Combined effects of nanosized polystyrene and erythromycin on bacterial growth and resistance mutations in Escherichia coli. *Journal of Hazardous Materials, 422*(August), 126858. doi:10.1016/j.jhazmat.2021.126858

NOAA. (2019). *Coral reef ecosystems*. NOAA.

O'Donovan, S., Mestre, N. C., Abel, S., Fonseca, T. G., Carteny, C. C., Cormier, B., Keiter, S. H., & Bebianno, M. J. (2018). Ecotoxicological Effects of Chemical Contaminants Adsorbed to Microplastics in the Clam *Scrobicularia plana. Frontiers in Marine Science, 5*, 143. Advance online publication. doi:10.3389/fmars.2018.00143

O'Donovan, S., Mestre, N. C., Abel, S., Fonseca, T. G., Carteny, C. C., Willems, T., Prinsen, E., Cormier, B., Keiter, S. S., & Bebianno, M. J. (2020). Effects of the UV filter, oxybenzone, adsorbed to microplastics in the clam *Scrobicularia plana. The Science of the Total Environment, 733*, 139102. doi:10.1016/j.scitotenv.2020.139102 PMID:32446057

Oehlmann, J., Schulte-Oehlmann, U., Kloas, W., Jagnytsch, O., Lutz, I., Kusk, K. O., Wollenberger, L., Santos, E. M., Paull, G. C., VanLook, K. J. W., & Tyler, C. R. (2009). A critical analysis of the biological impacts of plasticizers on wildlife. *Philosophical Transactions of the Royal Society of London. Series B, Biological Sciences, 364*(1526), 2047–2062. doi:10.1098/rstb.2008.0242 PMID:19528055

Okshevsky, M., Gautier, E., Farner, J. M., Schreiber, L., & Tufenkji, N. (2020). Biofilm formation by marine bacteria is impacted by concentration and surface functionalization of polystyrene nanoparticles in a species-specific manner. *Environmental Microbiology Reports, 12*(2), 203–213. doi:10.1111/1758-2229.12824 PMID:31997572

Oliveira, M., Ribeiro, A., Hylland, K., & Guilhermino, L. (2013). Single and combined effects of microplastics and pyrene on juveniles (0+ group) of the common goby *Pomatoschistus microps* (*Teleostei, Gobiidae*). *Ecological Indicators, 34*, 641–647. doi:10.1016/j.ecolind.2013.06.019

Oliveira, P., Barboza, L. G. A., Branco, V., Figueiredo, N., Carvalho, C., & Guilhermino, L. (2018). Effects of microplastics and mercury in the freshwater bivalve *Corbicula fluminea* (Müller, 1774): Filtration rate, biochemical biomarkers, and mercury bioconcentration. *Ecotoxicology and Environmental Safety, 164*, 155–163. doi:10.1016/j.ecoenv.2018.07.062 PMID:30107325

Oriekhova, O., & Stoll, S. (2018). Heteroaggregation of nanoplastic particles in the presence of inorganic colloids and natural organic matter. *Environmental Science. Nano, 5*(3), 792–799. doi:10.1039/C7EN01119A

Pabortsava, K., & Lampitt, R. S. (2020). High concentrations of plastic hidden beneath the surface of the Atlantic Ocean. *Nature Communications*, *11*(1), 4073. doi:10.103841467-020-17932-9 PMID:32811835

Palumbo, M. T., & Mingazzini, M. (2011). Toxicity Test With Algae: Evaluation of the Sensitivity Related To the Use of Biomass Versus Growth Rate Endpoint. *16th International MESAEP Symposium on Environmental Pollution*.

Pannetier, P., Fuster, L., Clérandeau, C., Lacroix, C., Gourves, P. Y., Cachot, J., & Morin, B. (2018). Usefulness of RTL-W1 and OLCAB-e3 fish cell lines and multiple endpoint measurements for toxicity evaluation of unknown or complex mixture of chemicals. *Ecotoxicology and Environmental Safety*, *150*, 40–48. doi:10.1016/j.ecoenv.2017.12.027 PMID:29268113

Paul-Pont, I., Lacroix, C., González Fernández, C., Hégaret, H., Lambert, C., Le Goïc, N., Frère, L., Cassone, A.-L., Sussarellu, R., Fabioux, C., Guyomarch, J., Albentosa, M., Huvet, A., & Soudant, P. (2016). Exposure of marine mussels *Mytilus* spp. to polystyrene microplastics: Toxicity and influence on fluoranthene bioaccumulation. *Environmental Pollution*, *216*, 724–737. doi:10.1016/j.envpol.2016.06.039 PMID:27372385

Pedà, C., Caccamo, L., Fossi, M. C., Gai, F., Andaloro, F., Genovese, L., Perdichizzi, A., Romeo, T., & Maricchiolo, G. (2016). Intestinal alterations in European sea bass *Dicentrarchus labrax* (Linnaeus, 1758) exposed to microplastics: Preliminary results. *Environmental Pollution*, *212*, 251–256. doi:10.1016/j.envpol.2016.01.083 PMID:26851981

Peng, L., Fu, D., Qi, H., Lan, C. Q., Yu, H., & Ge, C. (2020). Micro- and nano-plastics in marine environment: Source, distribution, and threats — A review. *The Science of the Total Environment*, *698*, 134254. doi:10.1016/j.scitotenv.2019.134254 PMID:31514025

Peng, X., Chen, M., Chen, S., Dasgupta, S., Xu, H. K., Ta, K., & Bai, S. (2018). Microplastics contaminate the deepest part of the world's ocean. *Geochemical Perspectives Letters*, *9*, 1–5. doi:10.7185/geochemlet.1829

Pinsino, A., Bergami, E., Della Torre, C., Vannuccini, M. L., Addis, P., Secci, M., Dawson, K. A., Matranga, V., & Corsi, I. (2017). Amino-modified polystyrene nanoparticles affect signalling pathways of the sea urchin (*Paracentrotus lividus*) embryos. *Nanotoxicology*, *11*(2), 201–209. doi:10.1080/17435390.2017.1279360 PMID:28091127

Pitt, J. A., Trevisan, R., Massarsky, A., Kozal, J. S., Levin, E. D., & Di Giulio, R. T. (2018). Maternal transfer of nanoplastics to offspring in zebrafish (*Danio rerio*): A case study with nanopolystyrene. *The Science of the Total Environment*, *643*, 324–334. doi:10.1016/j.scitotenv.2018.06.186 PMID:29940444

Pittura, L., Avio, C. G., Giuliani, M. E., d'Errico, G., Keiter, S. H., Cormier, B., Gorbi, S., & Regoli, F. (2018). Microplastics as Vehicles of Environmental PAHs to Marine Organisms: Combined Chemical and Physical Hazards to the Mediterranean Mussels, *Mytilus galloprovincialis*. *Frontiers in Marine Science*, *5*, 103. Advance online publication. doi:10.3389/fmars.2018.00103

Prata, J. C., & Lavorante, B. R. B. O. (2017, September). Maria da, M. da C., & Guilhermino, L. (2018). Influence of microplastics on the toxicity of the pharmaceuticals procainamide and doxycycline on the marine microalgae *Tetraselmis chuii. Aquatic Toxicology (Amsterdam, Netherlands), 197*, 143–152. doi:10.1016/j.aquatox.2018.02.015 PMID:29494946

Raisuddin, S., Kwok, K. W. H., Leung, K. M. Y., Schlenk, D., & Lee, J. S. (2007). The copepod *Tigriopus*: A promising marine model organism for ecotoxicology and environmental genomics. *Aquatic Toxicology (Amsterdam, Netherlands), 83*(3), 161–173. doi:10.1016/j.aquatox.2007.04.005 PMID:17560667

Ramirez, L., Gentile, R. S., Zimmerman, S., & Stoll, S. (2019). Drinking and Lake Geneva Waters. Impact of Water. *Water*.

Reichert, J., Arnold, A. L., Hoogenboom, M. O., Schubert, P., & Wilke, T. (2019). Impacts of microplastics on growth and health of hermatypic corals are species-specific. *Environmental Pollution, 254*, 113074. doi:10.1016/j.envpol.2019.113074 PMID:31473388

Reichert, J., Schellenberg, J., Schubert, P., & Wilke, T. (2018). Responses of reef building corals to microplastic exposure. *Environmental Pollution, 237*, 955–960. doi:10.1016/j.envpol.2017.11.006 PMID:29146203

Revel, M., Lagarde, F., Perrein-Ettajani, H., Bruneau, M., Akcha, F., Sussarellu, R., Rouxel, J., Costil, K., Decottignies, P., Cognie, B., Châtel, A., & Mouneyrac, C. (2019). Tissue-Specific Biomarker Responses in the Blue Mussel *Mytilus* spp. Exposed to a Mixture of Microplastics at Environmentally Relevant Concentrations. *Frontiers in Environmental Science, 7*, 33. Advance online publication. doi:10.3389/fenvs.2019.00033

Ribeiro, F., Garcia, A. R., Pereira, B. P., Fonseca, M., Mestre, N. C., Fonseca, T. G., Ilharco, L. M., & Bebianno, M. J. (2017). Microplastics effects in *Scrobicularia plana. Marine Pollution Bulletin, 122*(1-2), 379–391. doi:10.1016/j.marpolbul.2017.06.078 PMID:28684108

Ricciardi, M., Pironti, C., Motta, O., Miele, Y., Proto, A., & Montano, L. (2021). Microplastics in the Aquatic Environment: Occurrence, Persistence, Analysis, and Human Exposure. *Water (Basel), 13*(7), 973. doi:10.3390/w13070973

Richardson, C. R., Burritt, D. J., Allan, B. J. M., & Lamare, M. D. (2021). Microplastic ingestion induces asymmetry and oxidative stress in larvae of the sea urchin *Pseudechinus huttoni. Marine Pollution Bulletin, 168*, 112369. doi:10.1016/j.marpolbul.2021.112369 PMID:33932840

Rico-Martínez, R., Arzate-Cárdenas, M. A., Robles-Vargas, D., Pérez-Legaspi, I. A., Jesús, A.-F., & Santos-Medrano, G. E. (2016). Rotifers as Models in Toxicity Screening of Chemicals and Environmental Samples. In *Invertebrates - Experimental Models in Toxicity Screening* (pp. 57–99). Academic Press.

Rios, L. M., Moore, C., & Jones, P. R. (2007). Persistent organic pollutants carried by synthetic polymers in the ocean environment. *Marine Pollution Bulletin, 54*(8), 1230–1237. doi:10.1016/j.marpolbul.2007.03.022 PMID:17532349

Rist, S. E., Assidqi, K., Zamani, N. P., Appel, D., Perschke, M., Huhn, M., & Lenz, M. (2016). Suspended micro-sized PVC particles impair the performance and decrease survival in the Asian green mussel *Perna viridis. Marine Pollution Bulletin, 111*(1-2), 213–220. doi:10.1016/j.marpolbul.2016.07.006 PMID:27491368

Rocha, R. J. M., Rodrigues, A. C. M., Campos, D., Cícero, L. H., Costa, A. P. L., Silva, D. A. M., Oliveira, M., Soares, A. M. V. M., & Patrício Silva, A. L. (2020). Do microplastics affect the zoanthid *Zoanthus sociatus? The Science of the Total Environment, 713*, 136659. doi:10.1016/j.scitotenv.2020.136659 PMID:31955109

Rochman, C. M. (2015). *The complex mixture, fate and toxicity of chemicals associated with plastic debris in the marine environment.* In M. Bergmann, L. Gutow, & M. Klages (Eds.), *in Marine Anthropogenic Litter* (pp. 117–140). Springer. doi:10.1007/978-3-319-16510-3_5

Rochman, C. M., Hoh, E., Kurobe, T., & Teh, S. J. (2013). Ingested plastic transfers hazardous chemicals to fish and induces hepatic stress. *Scientific Reports, 3*(1), 1–7. doi:10.1038rep03263 PMID:24263561

Rogers, K. L., Carreres-Calabuig, J. A., Gorokhova, E., & Posth, N. R. (2020). Micro-by-micro interactions: How microorganisms influence the fate of marine microplastics. *Limnology and Oceanography Letters, 5*(1), 18–36. doi:10.1002/lol2.10136

Ronneberger, D. (1998). Uptake of latex beads as size-model for food of planktonic rotifers. *Hydrobiologia, 387*(387), 445–449. doi:10.1023/A:1017046711821

Rotini, A., Tornambè, A., Cossi, R., Iamunno, F., Benvenuto, G., Berducci, M. T., Maggi, C., Thaller, M. C., Cicero, A. M., Manfra, L., & Migliore, L. (2017). Salinity-based toxicity of CuO nanoparticles, CuO-bulk and Cu ion to *vibrio anguillarum. Frontiers in Microbiology, 8*, 2076. doi:10.3389/fmicb.2017.02076 PMID:29118743

Rouillon, C., Bussiere, P. O., Desnoux, E., Collin, S., Vial, C., Therias, S., & Gardette, J. L. (2016). Is carbonyl index a quantitative probe to monitor polypropylene photodegradation? *Polymer Degradation & Stability, 128*, 200–208. doi:10.1016/j.polymdegradstab.2015.12.011

Ryan, P. G. (1987). The effects of ingested plastic on seabirds: Correlations between plastic load and body condition. *Environmental Pollution, 46*(2), 119–125. doi:10.1016/0269-7491(87)90197-7 PMID:15092735

Sadri, S. S., & Thompson, R. C. (2014). On the quantity and composition of floating plastic debris entering and leaving the Tamar Estuary, Southwest England. *Marine Pollution Bulletin, 81*(1), 55–60. doi:10.1016/j.marpolbul.2014.02.020 PMID:24613232

Santana, M. F. M., Moreira, F. T., & Turra, A. (2017). Trophic transference of microplastics under a low exposure scenario: Insights on the likelihood of particle cascading along marine food-webs. *Marine Pollution Bulletin, 121*(1–2), 154–159. doi:10.1016/j.marpolbul.2017.05.061 PMID:28595982

Savinelli, B., Vega Fernández, T., Galasso, N. M., D'Anna, G., Pipitone, C., Prada, F., Zenone, A., Badalamenti, F., & Musco, L. (2020). Microplastics impair the feeding performance of a Mediterranean habitat-forming coral. *Marine Environmental Research, 155*, 104887. doi:10.1016/j.marenvres.2020.104887 PMID:32072989

Savoca, M. S., McInturf, A. G., & Hazen, E. L. (2021). Plastic ingestion by marine fish is widespread and increasing. *Global Change Biology*, *27*(10), 2188–2199. Advance online publication. doi:10.1111/gcb.15533 PMID:33561314

Savoca, M. S., Tyson, C. W., McGill, M., & Slager, C. J. (2017). Odours from marine plastic debris induce food search behaviours in a forage fish. *Proceedings of the Royal Society B: Biological Sciences, 284*(1860). 10.1098/rspb.2017.1000

Seng, N., Lai, S., Fong, J., Saleh, M. F., Cheng, C., Cheok, Z. Y., & Todd, P. A. (2020). Early evidence of microplastics on seagrass and macroalgae. *Marine and Freshwater Research*, *71*(8), 922–928. doi:10.1071/MF19177

Setälä, O., Fleming-Lehtinen, V., & Lehtiniemi, M. (2014). Ingestion and transfer of microplastics in the planktonic food web. *Environmental Pollution*, *185*, 77–83. doi:10.1016/j.envpol.2013.10.013 PMID:24220023

Setälä, O., Magnusson, K., Lehtiniemi, M., & Norén, F. (2016). Distribution and abundance of surface water microlitter in the Baltic Sea: A comparison of two sampling methods. *Marine Pollution Bulletin*, *110*(1), 177–183. doi:10.1016/j.marpolbul.2016.06.065 PMID:27339742

Sharifinia, M., Bahmanbeigloo, Z. A., Keshavarzifard, M., Khanjani, M. H., & Lyons, B. P. (2020). Microplastic pollution as a grand challenge in marine research: A closer look at their adverse impacts on the immune and reproductive systems. *Ecotoxicology and Environmental Safety*, *204*(July), 111109. doi:10.1016/j.ecoenv.2020.111109 PMID:32798751

Shen, M., Zhang, Y., Zhu, Y., Song, B., Zeng, G., Hu, D., Wen, X., & Ren, X. (2019). Recent advances in toxicological research of nanoplastics in the environment: A review. *Environmental Pollution*, *252*, 511–521. doi:10.1016/j.envpol.2019.05.102 PMID:31167159

Shi, W., Han, Y., Sun, S., Tang, Y., Zhou, W., Du, X., & Liu, G. (2020). Immunotoxicities of microplastics and sertraline, alone and in combination, to a bivalve species: Size-dependent interaction and potential toxication mechanism. *Journal of Hazardous Materials*, *122603*, 122603. Advance online publication. doi:10.1016/j.jhazmat.2020.122603 PMID:32289642

Silva, P. P. G. (2016). *Contaminação e toxicidade de microplásticos em uma área de proteção marinha costeira* [Master's Dissertation]. Escola de Engenharia de São Carlos, University of São Paulo, São Carlos. Retrieved 2021-11-12, from www.teses.usp.br doi:10.11606/D.18.2016.tde-27092016-084059

Sjollema, S. B., Redondo-Hasselerharm, P., Leslie, H. A., Kraak, M. H. S., & Vethaak, A. D. (2016). Do plastic particles affect microalgal photosynthesis and growth? *Aquatic Toxicology (Amsterdam, Netherlands)*, *170*, 259–261. doi:10.1016/j.aquatox.2015.12.002 PMID:26675372

Skjolding, L. M., Ašmonaitė, G., Jølck, R. I., Andresen, T. L., Selck, H., Baun, A., & Sturve, J. (2017). An assessment of the importance of exposure routes to the uptake and internal localisation of fluorescent nanoparticles in zebrafish (*Danio rerio*), using light sheet microscopy. *Nanotoxicology*, *11*(3), 351–359. doi:10.1080/17435390.2017.1306128 PMID:28286999

Sugni, M., Mozzi, D., Barbaglio, A., Bonasoro, F., & Candia Carnevali, M. D. (2007). Endocrine disrupting compounds and echinoderms: New ecotoxicological sentinels for the marine ecosystem. *Ecotoxicology (London, England), 16*(1), 95–108. doi:10.100710646-006-0119-8 PMID:17253161

Sun, S., Shi, W., Tang, Y., Han, Y., Du, X., Zhou, W., Hu, Y., Zhou, C., & Liu, G. (2020). Immunotoxicity of petroleum hydrocarbons and microplastics alone or in combination to a bivalve species: Synergic impacts and potential toxication mechanisms. *The Science of the Total Environment, 138852*. Advance online publication. doi:10.1016/j.scitotenv.2020.138852 PMID:32570313

Sun, X., Chen, B., Li, Q., Liu, N., Xia, B., Zhu, L., & Qu, K. (2018). Toxicities of polystyrene nano- and microplastics toward marine bacterium *Halomonas alkaliphila. The Science of the Total Environment, 642*, 1378–1385. doi:10.1016/j.scitotenv.2018.06.141 PMID:30045518

Sun, Y., Xu, W., Gu, Q., Chen, Y., Zhou, Q., Zhang, L., Gu, L., Huang, Y., Lyu, K., & Yang, Z. (2019). Small-sized microplastics negatively affect rotifers: Changes in the key life-history traits and rotifer-*Phaeocystis* population dynamics. *Environmental Science & Technology, 53*(15), 9241–9251. Advance online publication. doi:10.1021/acs.est.9b02893 PMID:31268695

Sussarellu, R., Suquet, M., Thomas, Y., Lambert, C., Fabioux, C., Pernet, M. E. J., Le Goïc, N., Quillien, V., Mingant, C., Epelboin, Y., Corporeau, C., Guyomarch, J., Robbens, J., Paul-Pont, I., Soudant, P., & Huvet, A. (2016). Oyster reproduction is affected by exposure to polystyrene microplastics. *Proceedings of the National Academy of Sciences of the United States of America, 113*(9), 2430–2435. doi:10.1073/pnas.1519019113 PMID:26831072

Syakti, A. D., Jaya, J. V., Rahman, A., Hidayati, N. V., Raza'i, T. S., Idris, F., Trenggono, M., Doumenq, P., & Chou, L. M. (2019). Bleaching and necrosis of staghorn coral (*Acropora formosa*) in laboratory assays: Immediate impact of LDPE microplastics. *Chemosphere, 228*, 528–535. Advance online publication. doi:10.1016/j.chemosphere.2019.04.156 PMID:31051356

Syberg, K., Nielsen, A., Khan, F. R., Banta, G. T., Palmqvist, A., & Jepsen, P. M. (2017). Microplastic potentiates triclosan toxicity to the marine copepod *Acartia tonsa* (Dana). *Journal of Toxicology and Environmental Health - Part A: Current Issues, 80*(23–24), 1369–1371. doi:10.1080/15287394.2017.1385046 PMID:29131715

Tallec, K., Huvet, A., Di Poi, C., González-Fernández, C., Lambert, C., Petton, B., Le Goïc, N., Berchel, M., Soudant, P., & Paul-Pont, I. (2018). Nanoplastics impaired oyster free living stages, gametes and embryos. *Environmental Pollution, 242*, 1226–1235. doi:10.1016/j.envpol.2018.08.020 PMID:30118910

Tamminga, M., Hengstmann, E., & Fischer, E. K. (2018). Microplastic analysis in the South Funen Archipelago, Baltic Sea, implementing manta trawling and bulk sampling. *Marine Pollution Bulletin, 128*, 601–608. doi:10.1016/j.marpolbul.2018.01.066 PMID:29571412

Tang, J., Ni, X., Zhou, Z., Wang, L., & Lin, S. (2018). Acute microplastic exposure raises stress response and suppresses detoxification and immune capacities in the scleractinian coral *Pocillopora damicornis. Environmental Pollution, 243*, 66–74. Advance online publication. doi:10.1016/j.envpol.2018.08.045 PMID:30172125

Tang, Y., Rong, J., Guan, X., Zha, S., Shi, W., Han, Y., ... Liu, G. (2019). Immunotoxicity of microplastics and two persistent organic pollutants alone or in combination to a bivalve species. *Environmental Pollution, 113845*. Advance online publication. doi:10.1016/j.envpol.2019.113845 PMID:31883493

Teng, J., Zhao, J., Zhu, X., Shan, E., & Wang, Q. (2021). Oxidative stress biomarkers, physiological responses, and proteomic profiling in oyster (*Crassostrea gigas)* exposed to microplastics with irregular-shaped PE and PET microplastic. *The Science of the Total Environment*, *786*, 147425. doi:10.1016/j.scitotenv.2021.147425

Teng, J., Zhao, J., Zhu, X., Shan, E., Zhang, C., Zhang, W., & Wang, Q. (2020). Toxic effects of exposure to microplastics with environmentally relevant shapes and concentrations: Accumulation, energy metabolism and tissue damage in oyster *Crassostrea gigas*. *Environmental Pollution*. Advance online publication. doi:10.1016/j.envpol.2020.116169 PMID:33302083

Ter Halle, A., Jeanneau, L., Martignac, M., Jardé, E., Pedrono, B., Brach, L., & Gigault, J. (2017). Nanoplastic in the North Atlantic Subtropical Gyre. *Environmental Science & Technology*, *51*(23), 13689–13697. doi:10.1021/acs.est.7b03667 PMID:29161030

Tetu, S. G., Sarker, I., Schrameyer, V., Pickford, R., Elbourne, L. D. H., Moore, L. R., & Paulsen, I. T. (2019). Plastic leachates impair growth and oxygen production in *Prochlorococcus*, the ocean's most abundant photosynthetic bacteria. *Communications Biology*, *2*(1), 184. doi:10.103842003-019-0410-x PMID:31098417

Teuten, E. L., Rowland, S. J., Galloway, T. S., & Thompson, R. C. (2007). Potential for Plastics to Transport Hydrophobic Contaminants. *Environmental Science & Technology*, *41*(22), 7759–7764. doi:10.1021/es071737s PMID:18075085

Teuten, E. L., Saquing, J. M., Knappe, D. R. U., Barlaz, M. A., Jonsson, S., Björn, A., Rowland, S. J., Thompson, R. C., Galloway, T. S., Yamashita, R., Ochi, D., Watanuki, Y., Moore, C., Viet, P. H., Tana, T. S., Prudente, M., Boonyatumanond, R., Zakaria, M. P., Akkhavong, K., ... Takada, H. (2009). Transport and release of chemicals from plastics to the environment and to wildlife. *Philosophical Transactions of the Royal Society of London. Series B, Biological Sciences*, *364*(1526), 2027–2045. doi:10.1098/rstb.2008.0284 PMID:19528054

Thiagarajan, V., Iswarya, V., P, A. J., Seenivasan, R., Chandrasekaran, N., & Mukherjee, A. (2018, October). Influence of differently functionalized polystyrene microplastics on the toxic effects of P25 TiO2 NPs towards marine algae *Chlorella* sp. *Aquatic Toxicology (Amsterdam, Netherlands)*, *207*, 208–216. doi:10.1016/j.aquatox.2018.12.014 PMID:30638491

Thomas, M., Jon, B., Craig, S., Edward, R., Ruth, H., John, B., Dick, V. A., Heather, L. A., & Matthew, S. (2020). The world is your oyster: Low-dose, long-term microplastic exposure of juvenile oysters. *Heliyon*, *6*(1), e03103. doi:10.1016/j.heliyon.2019.e03103 PMID:31909270

Thompson, R. C., Olson, Y., Mitchell, R. P., Davis, A., Rowland, S. J., John, A. W. G., McGonigle, D., & Russell, A. E. (2004). Lost at Sea: Where Is All the Plastic? *Science*, *304*(5672), 838. doi:10.1126cience.1094559 PMID:15131299

Thushari, G. G. N., & Senevirathna, J. D. M. (2020). Plastic pollution in the marine environment. *Heliyon*, *6*(8), e04709. doi:10.1016/j.heliyon.2020.e04709 PMID:32923712

Tlili, S., Jemai, D., Brinis, S., & Regaya, I. (2020). Microplastics mixture exposure at environmentally relevant conditions induce oxidative stress and neurotoxicity in the wedge clam *Donax trunculus*. *Chemosphere*, *127344*, 127344. Advance online publication. doi:10.1016/j.chemosphere.2020.127344 PMID:32554011

Tosetto, L., Williamson, J. E., & Brown, C. (2017). Trophic transfer of microplastics does not affect fish personality. *Animal Behaviour*, *123*, 159–167. doi:10.1016/j.anbehav.2016.10.035

Tramoy, R., Gasperi, J., Dris, R., Colasse, L., Fisson, C., Sananes, S., Rocher, V., & Tassin, B. (2019). Assessment of the Plastic Inputs From the Seine Basin to the Sea Using Statistical and Field Approaches. *Frontiers in Marine Science*, *6*, 151. Advance online publication. doi:10.3389/fmars.2019.00151

Trestrail, C., Walpitagama, M., Miranda, A., Nugegoda, D., & Shimeta, J. (2021). Microplastics alter digestive enzyme activities in the marine bivalve, *Mytilus galloprovincialis*. *The Science of the Total Environment*, *779*, 146418. doi:10.1016/j.scitotenv.2021.146418 PMID:33744572

Trifuoggi, M., Pagano, G., Oral, R., Pavičić-Hamer, D., Burić, P., Kovačić, I., Siciliano, A., Toscanesi, M., Thomas, P. J., Paduano, L., Guida, M., & Lyons, D. M. (2019). Microplastic-induced damage in early embryonal development of sea urchin *Sphaerechinus granularis*. *Environmental Research*, *108815*. Advance online publication. doi:10.1016/j.envres.2019.108815 PMID:31629182

Ustabasi, G. S., & Baysal, A. (2020). Bacterial interactions of microplastics extracted from toothpaste under controlled conditions and the influence of seawater. *The Science of the Total Environment*, *703*, 135024. doi:10.1016/j.scitotenv.2019.135024 PMID:31734496

Van Sebille, E., Gilbert, A., & Spathi, C. (2016). *The ocean plastic pollution challenge: towards solutions in the UK*. Grantham Institute Breifing Paper, 19(19), 3–4. www.imperial.ac.uk/grantham/publications

Venâncio, C., Ferreira, I., Martins, M. A., Soares, A. M. V. M., Lopes, I., & Oliveira, M. (2019). The effects of nanoplastics on marine plankton: A case study with polymethylmethacrylate. *Ecotoxicology and Environmental Safety*, *184*, 109632. doi:10.1016/j.ecoenv.2019.109632 PMID:31514077

Villalba, M., Pérez, V., Herrera, L., Stepke, C., Maldonado, N., Fredericksen, F., Yáñez, A., & Olavarría, V. H. (2017). Infectious pancreatic necrosis virus infection of fish cell lines: Preliminary analysis of gene expressions related to extracellular matrix remodeling and immunity. *Veterinary Immunology and Immunopathology*, *193–194*, 10–17. doi:10.1016/j.vetimm.2017.09.009 PMID:29129223

Vital, S. A., Cardoso, C., Avio, C., Pittura, L., Regoli, F., & Bebianno, M. J. (2021). Do microplastic contaminated seafood consumption pose a potential risk to human health? *Marine Pollution Bulletin*, *171*(April), 112769. doi:10.1016/j.marpolbul.2021.112769 PMID:34358788

Von Moos, N., Burkhardt-Holm, P., & Köhler, A. (2012). Uptake and Effects of Microplastics on Cells and Tissue of the Blue Mussel *Mytilus edulis* L. after an Experimental Exposure. *Environmental Science & Technology*, *46*(20), 11327–11335. doi:10.1021/es302332w PMID:22963286

Wallace, R. L., Snell, T. W., Ricci, C., & Nogrady, T. (2006). Rotifera. Biology, Ecology and Systematics. In Guides to the identification of the microinvertebrates of the continental waters of the world. Kenobi Productions and Backhuys Publishers.

Wang, J., Li, Y., Lu, L., Zheng, M., Zhang, X., Tian, H., Wang, W., & Ru, S. (2019). Polystyrene microplastics cause tissue damages, sex-specific reproductive disruption, and transgenerational effects in marine medaka (*Oryzias melastigma*). *Environmental Pollution*, *254*, 113024. doi:10.1016/j.envpol.2019.113024 PMID:31454586

Wang, J., Tan, Z., Peng, J., Qiu, Q., & Li, M. (2016). The behaviors of microplastics in the marine environment. *Marine Environmental Research*, *113*, 7–17. doi:10.1016/j.marenvres.2015.10.014 PMID:26559150

Wang, S., Wang, Y., Liang, Y., Cao, W., Sun, C., Ju, P., & Zheng, L. (2020). The interactions between microplastic polyvinyl chloride and marine diatoms: Physiological, morphological, and growth effects. *Ecotoxicology and Environmental Safety*, *203*(July), 111000. doi:10.1016/j.ecoenv.2020.111000 PMID:32736119

Wang, T., Hu, M., Xu, G., Shi, H., Leung, J. Y. S., & Wang, Y. (2021). Microplastic accumulation via trophic transfer: Can a predatory crab counter the adverse effects of microplastics by body defence? *The Science of the Total Environment*, *754*, 142099. doi:10.1016/j.scitotenv.2020.142099 PMID:32911152

Wang, W., Yuan, W., Chen, Y., & Wang, J. (2018). Microplastics in surface waters of Dongting Lake and Hong Lake, China. *The Science of the Total Environment*, *633*, 539–545. doi:10.1016/j.scitotenv.2018.03.211 PMID:29579665

Wardrop, P., Shimeta, J., Nugegoda, D., Morrison, P. D., Miranda, A., Tang, M., & Clarke, B. O. (2016). Chemical Pollutants Sorbed to Ingested Microbeads from Personal Care Products Accumulate in Fish. *Environmental Science & Technology*, *50*(7), 4037–4044. doi:10.1021/acs.est.5b06280 PMID:26963589

Watts, A. J. R., Urbina, M. A., Corr, S., Lewis, C., & Galloway, T. S. (2015). Ingestion of Plastic Microfibers by the Crab *Carcinus maenas* and Its Effect on Food Consumption and Energy Balance. *Environmental Science & Technology*, *49*(24), 14597–14604. doi:10.1021/acs.est.5b04026 PMID:26529464

Webb, S., Gaw, S., Marsden, I. D., & McRae, N. K. (2020). Biomarker responses in New Zealand green-lipped mussels *Perna canaliculus* exposed to microplastics and triclosan. *Ecotoxicology and Environmental Safety*, *201*, 110871. doi:10.1016/j.ecoenv.2020.110871 PMID:32559692

Wegner, A., Besseling, E., Foekema, E. M., Kamermans, P., & Koelmans, A. A. (2012). Effects of nanopolystyrene on the feeding behaviour of the blue mussel (*Mytilus edulis* L.). *Environmental Toxicology and Chemistry*, *31*(11), 2490–2497. doi:10.1002/etc.1984 PMID:22893562

Worm, B., Lotze, H. K., Jubinville, I., Wilcox, C., & Jambeck, J. (2017). Plastic as a Persistent Marine Pollutant. *Annual Review of Environment and Resources*, *42*(1), 1–26. doi:10.1146/annurev-environ-102016-060700

Xu, X.-Y., Lee, W. T., Chan, A. K. Y., Lo, H. S., Shin, P. K. S., & Cheung, S. G. (2017). Microplastic ingestion reduces energy intake in the clam *Atactodea striata*. *Marine Pollution Bulletin*, *124*(2), 798–802. doi:10.1016/j.marpolbul.2016.12.027 PMID:28038767

Xue, Y.-H., Sun, Z.-X., Feng, L.-S., Jin, T., Xing, J.-C., & Wen, X.-L. (2020). Algal density affects the influences of polyethylene microplastics on the freshwater rotifer *Brachionus calyciflorus*. *Chemosphere*, *128613*. Advance online publication. doi:10.1016/j.chemosphere.2020.128613 PMID:33131733

Yan, W., Hamid, N., Deng, S., Jia, P. P., & Pei, D. S. (2020). Individual and combined toxicogenetic effects of microplastics and heavy metals (Cd, Pb, and Zn) perturb gut microbiota homeostasis and gonadal development in marine medaka (*Oryzias melastigma*). *Journal of Hazardous Materials*, *397*(March), 122795. doi:10.1016/j.jhazmat.2020.122795 PMID:32388101

Yang, X., Wang, H., Zhang, L., Kong, L., Chen, Y., He, Q., Li, L., Grossart, H. P., & Ju, F. (2021). Marine algae facilitate transfer of microplastics and associated pollutants into food webs. *The Science of the Total Environment*, *787*, 147535. doi:10.1016/j.scitotenv.2021.147535 PMID:33991910

Yin, L., Chen, B., Xia, B., Shi, X., & Qu, K. (2018). Polystyrene microplastics alter the behaviour, energy reserve and nutritional composition of marine jacopever (*Sebastes schlegelii*). *Journal of Hazardous Materials*, *360*(August), 97–105. doi:10.1016/j.jhazmat.2018.07.110 PMID:30098534

Yokota, K., Waterfield, H., Hastings, C., Davidson, E., Kwietniewski, E., & Wells, B. (2017). Finding the missing piece of the aquatic plastic pollution puzzle: Interaction between primary producers and microplastics. *Limnology and Oceanography Letters*, *2*(4), 91–104. doi:10.1002/lol2.10040

Yu, P., Liu, Z., Wu, D., Chen, M., Lv, W., & Zhao, Y. (2018). Accumulation of polystyrene microplastics in juvenile *Eriocheir sinensis* and oxidative stress effects in the liver. *Aquatic Toxicology (Amsterdam, Netherlands)*, *200*(March), 28–36. doi:10.1016/j.aquatox.2018.04.015 PMID:29709883

Yu, S.-P., & Chan, B. K. K. (2020). Intergenerational microplastics impact the intertidal barnacle *Amphibalanus amphitrite* during the planktonic larval and benthic adult stages. *Environmental Pollution*, *115560*. Advance online publication. doi:10.1016/j.envpol.2020.115560 PMID:33254593

Zhang, C., Chen, X., Wang, J., & Tan, L. (2017). Toxic effects of microplastic on marine microalgae *Skeletonema costatum*: Interactions between microplastic and algae. *Environmental Pollution*, *220*, 1282–1288. doi:10.1016/j.envpol.2016.11.005 PMID:27876228

Zhang, Y., Chen, Y., Westerhoff, P., Hristovski, K., & Crittenden, J. C. (2008). Stability of commercial metal oxide nanoparticles in water. *Water Research*, *42*(8–9), 2204–2212. doi:10.1016/j.watres.2007.11.036 PMID:18164742

Zhao, T., Tan, L., Han, X., Wang, X., Zhang, Y., Ma, X., Lin, K., Wang, R., Ni, Z., Wang, J., & Wang, J. (2022). Microplastic-induced apoptosis and metabolism responses in marine Dinoflagellate, *Karenia mikimotoi*. *The Science of the Total Environment*, *804*(238), 150252. doi:10.1016/j.scitotenv.2021.150252 PMID:34798757

Zhou, W., Tang, Y., Du, X., Han, Y., Shi, W., Sun, S., Zhang, W., Zheng, H., & Liu, G. (2021). Fine polystyrene microplastics render immune responses more vulnerable to two veterinary antibiotics in a bivalve species. *Marine Pollution Bulletin*, *164*, 111995. doi:10.1016/j.marpolbul.2021.111995 PMID:33493858

Zhu, X., Zhao, W., Chen, X., Zhao, T., Tan, L., & Wang, J. (2020). Growth inhibition of the microalgae *Skeletonema costatum* under copper nanoparticles with microplastic exposure. *Marine Environmental Research*, *158*(April), 105005. doi:10.1016/j.marenvres.2020.105005 PMID:32501269

KEY TERMS AND DEFINITIONS

Biological Effects: Processes that occur in the body and cells of an organism.

Biomagnification: Or biological magnification is the process by which a a concentration of a pollutant (such as plastic particles) in organisms in a food chain increases towards the top of that chain.

Ecotoxicology: The branch of toxicology concerned with the effects of toxic chemicals on biological organisms, especially at the population, community, and ecosystem level.

Leachate: A solution resulting from leaching as a soluble constituent from a solid passing phase, or suspended solids, or any other component of the material.

Marine Pollution: Refers to diret or indirect introduction by humans of substances or energy into the marine environment (including estuaries) resulting in harm to living resources, hazards to human health, hundrances to marine actividies including fisheries, impairment of the quality of sea water and reduction of amenities.

Microplastics: Plastic particles, with size < 5 mm normally formed from the deterioration/degradation of plastic objects/products.

Nanoplastics: Particles with a colloidal characteristic, formed unintentionally (i.e. from the deterioration and production of plastic objects) and ranging in size from 1 to 100 nm.

Chapter 10
Impacts of Microplastics on the Hydrosphere (Aquatic Environment)

Alina Zehra
Ecotoxicology Laboratory, Regulatory Toxicology Group, Academy of Scientific and Innovative Research (AcSIR), Ghaziabad, India & CSIR-Indian Institute of Toxicology Research, Lucknow, India

Kavita Krishna
Ecotoxicology Laboratory, Regulatory Toxicology Group, Academy of Scientific and Innovative Research (AcSIR), Ghaziabad, India

Namrata Pandey
Ecotoxicology Laboratory, Regulatory Toxicology Group, Academy of Scientific and Innovative Research (AcSIR), Ghaziabad, India

S. Anbumani
Ecotoxicology Laboratory, Regulatory Toxicology Group, Academy of Scientific and Innovative Research (AcSIR), Ghaziabad, India & CSIR-Indian Institute of Toxicology Research, Lucknow, India

ABSTRACT

Pollution by microplastics is a recent global problem owing to their preponderance in various matrices like air, water, biota, sediment, or soil and has become a global concern for the future generation sustainability. The mushrooming concerns about the detrimental effects of microplastics (MPs) on biota in response to its crescive detection and quantification in the aqueous ecosystems is looming large since last few decades, and it's a need of the hour for a thorough ecological risk assessment. The chapter highlights the MP production, release, and transport pathways along with its detrimental impacts on the aquatic biota at different levels of biological organization with available degradation approaches.

DOI: 10.4018/978-1-7998-9723-1.ch010

INTRODUCTION

Plastic polymers have given a new definition to the comforts of human life from packaging, textiles, consumer & institutional products, electrical/electronics, constructions, industrial machinery, transportation, cosmetics to even the most important healthcare sector (Wang et al., 2021). These ironical necessities have instead demanded the health of the entire biosphere thereby coming back to the humankind in life threatening forms. With a whopping 368 million metric tons of plastics being produced by 2019 (PlasticsEurope -2019), even the quantity of plastic wastes (60 to 99 million metric tons by 2015) has been extrapolated to be reaching a figure of 155- 265 million metric tons/year by 2060 (Lebreton et al., 2019). These kind of macroplastics of sizes 1 cm or more (Hartmann et al., 2019) eventually results in the formation of micro- (<5 mm) and nano- (<100 nm) plastics respectively. The type of polymers includes Polypropylene (PP), Polystyrene (PS), Polyethylene (PE), Polyvinylchloride (PVC), Polymethyl methacrylate (PMMA), Polyethylene terephthalate (PET) etc. Their ubiquitousness, hydrophobicity and characteristic residence time in the various environmental matrices jeopardizes the biosphere to a greater extent (Chen et al., 2021). It has been largely reported that the number of plastics in certain stretches of the oceans have surpassed its planktonic abundances and is already on the way to transcend the fish populations in next thirty years (Jovanović et al., 2018). MPs as well as its nano-sized transformations have reached even the remote pristine areas of the world from the Challenger Deep, Mariana Trench (Peng et al., 2018), reaching heights of 8,848 m above the sea level to that of the Mount Everest (Napper et al., 2020). MPs internalization has been vastly reported from the microbial colonies and planktons to the aquatic mammals and is known to be exerting significant levels of adverse effects in near future. However, the environmental concentrations of MPs which elicit the adverse effects in the biota are largely unknown and highly debatable (Phuong et al., 2018).

The hydrological cycle governing the movement of water among the aqueous ecosystems such as oceans, lakes, rivers, ponds, snow, glaciers, ground water as well as soil moisture; plays an integral part in the climate change due to constant energy exchanges, depicting its pivotal role in the process of evolution (Gonçalves et al., 2011; Chahine, 1992). Any obstacles in the form of even a minute particle of plastic, provides functional friction in the entire mechanism that governs the ecological cycles over time. Water bodies act as the ultimate destination of plastic trash harbouring all shapes, sizes and types of the plastics constantly infiltrating into it with an anthropogenic lineage which themselves act as a sink to other contaminants (Amrutha et al., 2020; Liu et al., 2019). The movement of these plastic particles give rise to an imbalanced aquatic ecosystem that is unfit for the biota inhabitation. The physico-chemical factors such as water current, temperature, depth, biodiversity, density, and size of the MPs governs its transport across the water surface. Biofouling of the MPs and its ingestion by biota is also known to facilitate vertical displacement of plastics (Vecchi et al., 2021). The requisite to study, extrapolate, update as well as combat the hazardous effects of MPs in the aquatic environment is the need of the hour. The routes of MPs entry and transport in the hydrosphere and subsequent biota exposure is shown in figure1.

Over the last 4 decades, MPs in the form of fibres, pellets, fragments, beads, etc., have been filling in the environmental pockets taking away their natural essence and posing greater risks to the keystone species ranging from invertebrates to vertebrates. for instance, Everaert et al., 2018 highlights the surge of MPs from 2010 to 2100 by a 50-folds increase to 1.3E+08 MPs/m^3 in the worst-case scenario where the rate of production is greater than the rate of MPs removal or degradation. According to the UNEP, (2016) the global status of MPs from 2013 to 2016 across the continents was 41 million tonnes (Mt) in Asia (Excluding Japan and China), 11 Mt in Japan and 62 Mt in China alone, 18 Mt in Middle East

Africa, 12 Mt in South America, 60 Mt in Europe, 49 Mt in North America, and 7 Mt in Commonwealth states respectively. Since oceans are the ultimate sink for MPs, it is difficult to predict accurately the quantity owing to their continuous fragmentations, aggregation, transportations, etc., (Hale et al., 2020).

The present chapter deals with current trend of MPs pollution and its potential adverse impacts on the hydrosphere in terms of the ecophysiology of the biotic components as well as abiotic components. Specifically, the overall impact of MPs/NPs on the aquatic environment can be well assessed by studying the effects on:

1. Water quality and nutrient cycling of the biosphere
2. The entire biota inhabiting the aqueous ecosystems; and
3. Human beings

ROUTES OF INFILTRATIONS

Anthropogenic Sources (Production and Release Pathway)

In the forms of fibres from cloth to beaded or fragmentized particles from the most hygienic medical equipment and products, plastic has first largely infiltered human life than being evident in the environment. Occurrence of Primary MPs results from the use of ready-made products such as, pellets and beads used in common household items (toothpastes, personal care products, shaving creams (Leslie et al., 2014), makeups, and shower gels (Hintersteiner et al., 2015) etc. In a study by Lechner et al., (2015), MPs in the forms of pellets and flakes was found outnumber the larval fish in Austrian river Danube. Other primary sources include road markings, household dusts, decorative items such as glitters and beads (Yurtsever, 2019), architectural paint coatings, and marine coatings (Boucher & Friot, 2017). Textile effluents from the processing mills was found to be another source of MP fibres (MPFs) (Chan et al., 2020). Wang et al., (2019) have elaborated the sources of primary MPs into the water systems under four major categories such as from the 1) Domestic sewage pathway 2) Road wash-off pathway 3) Winds, and 4) Adjacent water pathway. Wastewater Treatment Plants (WWTPs) are a significant contributor of MPs releasing around 100 MPs/individual in a day (Murphy et al., 2016). The sampling of WWTPs by several authors have been reported between 0.0009 to 0.009 MPs/L in the secondary treatment wastewater and from 0.000002 to 1 MPs/L in the tertiary samples (Carr et al., 2016). Road markings and abrasions of the tyres were reported to be the largest source of MPs to the hydrosphere (42%) followed by textile polymers (29%), dusts (19%), and personal care products (10%) (Siegfried et al., 2017). Rillig et al., (2018) reported that approximately, 94500 microbeads are released into the environment leading to a nearby sewage by the cuticle removers in toothpastes (Tang et al., 2020; Praveena et al., 2018) and facial cleansers. Nonetheless, MPs from the aquaculture gears and activities are another potential secondary source of MPs (Tang et al., 2020; Krüger et al., 2020).

Natural Sources: (Transport Pathway)

MPs in the hydrosphere comprises of their presence and transport in the freshwater and marine ecosystems where the freshwater juggles between MPs riverine transport and deposition into the lakes and ponds whereas the marine ecosystem majorly acts as the sink (Petersen & Hubbart, 2020). The floating debris of the MPs on the surface water constitutes 1% of the total MP production (Sebille et al., 2015; Halle et al., (2017). The MP debris released into the hydrosphere undergoes natural processes of breakdown such as photo-oxidation, weathering, mechanical stress from the sediments, pebbles, waves, and water currents (Luo et al., 2022; Duan et al., 2021; Sun et al., 2020), heat irradiation, and biodegradation by ingestion and egestion phenomenon of the water inhabitants feeding unknowingly on the surrounding MPs thereby displacing them from one place to another.

Wind and Waves: Horizontal Transport

Allen et al., (2019) outlined MPs transport size ranging from 300 to 750 µm to about 100 kms through winds that are responsible for the contamination of pristine sites such as the Himalayas and the Mount Everest, the Italian Alps (Ambrosini et al., 2019) and Ross Sea. Bergmann et al., (2019), reported many MPs in the European snow where the explanation of transport was reported to be the global warming leading to melting of the glacial ice and subsequent transport of MPs to the nearby rivers and oceans. Storm water run-off was also regarded as a significant source of MPs to the aquifers (Horton et al., 2017). Siegfried et al., (2017), presented a model for the transport of MPs from land to sea for the European rivers. Total export of the MPs storm water ponds samples reported 3.44E+03 MPs from seven ponds as analysed by Liu et al., (2019). Water currents too rapidly transport MPs to significant distances from their source of origin and is the reason why MPs are discovered all over the surface of the earth. Nature, therefore, is found to redistribute the already existing load of MPs apart from the invasion of secondary MPs through various anthropogenic non-point sources.

Biofouling: Vertical Transport MPs

Biofilms are microorganisms' community surrounded by the extracellular macromolecules, increasing the sizes of MPs, and rendering some hydrophilic properties unlike its innate nature, also known as a Plastisphere. As MPs infiltrate the aquatic ecosystem and interact with the various abiotic factors such as water, pressure, salinity, pH, etc., it gets colonized by the diverse microbial lifeforms creating a biofilm corona (Rummel et al., 2017). The film covers the sharp and uneven edges of the MPs and changes the chemical as well as the physical properties such as crystallinity, molecular weight, hardness, and hydrophobicity and increases the density of the MPs (Luo et al., 2022). Aging of the MPs in water due to the physicochemical and biological processes, releases some additives and leachates which might act as a nutritional source to the microbial communities colonizing it enhancing their growth rate (Rummel et al., 2017). The phenomenon of formation of a biofilm is commonly referred to as biofouling (Ye et al., 1991) and it impacts the aquatic ecosystem by reducing the intensity of light, perturbed oxygen, and carbon production, and inhibits the exchange of gases etc. (Galgani et al., 2021). Kooi et al., (2017) has given an interesting size selective model of vertical transport of MPs showing particles either float, sink or reside in the water column over time depending on their size and density and hence their concentration at the surface water is highly variable. Sinking of MPs due to biofouling depends largely upon the aquatic ecosystem type as PE particles were found to sink within 6 weeks of incubation in coastal waters due macrofouling in the presence of blue mussels whereas no sinking was noted even after 14 weeks of incubation in an estuarine water of Germany (Kaiser et al., 2017), however their continuous dialogues with the inhabiting biota may superimpose their sinking patterns. The MPs transported to the seafloor becomes available for ingestion to the benthic communities (Vecchi et al., 2021).

MPs IN ABIOTIC COMPONENTS OF THE HYDROSPHERE

The Great Pacific Garbage Patch (Pacific Ocean between Hawaii and California) has accumulated 79 (45–129) thousand tonnes of ocean plastic inside an area of 1.6 million km^2 (Lebreton et al., 2018). Numerous reports are available on the occurrence of microplastics in the most deserted regions. For instance, microplastic concentration ranges from 1 to 3 items/m^3 were recorded in the sub-water off Northeast Greenland (Morgana et al., 2018). Nonetheless, samples of South Korean urban coastal seawater have the mean microplastic abundance as high as 1051 particles/m^3, compared to 560 particles/m^3 in rural coastal areas (Song et al., 2018). Microplastics evidence in freshwater ecosystems have been widely reported in variable concentration. Depending upon the location of sampling, the abundance of microplastics can vary from more than 1 million pieces /m^3 to less than 1 piece in 100 m^3. (Li et al., 2018). On the other hand, a noticeable high concentration of microplastic of around 172000 to 419000 particles/m^3 were detected in Saigon River, Vietnam (Lahens et al., 2018). This widely spaced range of microplastic in freshwater ecosystems is largely governed by factors like geographical locations, topography, seasons, hydrodynamic influences, and proximity to population rich areas (Vanapalli et al., 2020). Studies have reported positive correlation of microplastic abundance with population density and a negative corelation of MP abundance with velocity of water (Xiong et al., 2019). Microplastics in sediments were influenced by water flow rate, sediment depth, and distance from the shoreline. Compared to the inner depth, the abundance of microplastics near the shoreline is found to be in uptrend (Zhang et al., 2019). In a study of the sediments collected from the southeast coast of India, the high tide line was four times more polluted (MP abundance of 95 – 2551 mg/m^2) than low tide line (0 – 439 mg/m^2) (Vanapalli et al., 2021). Physiochemical characteristics of sediments in addition to spatial variation and flow rate of aquatic systems affects the abundance of microplastics in freshwater sediments. Elevated abundance of MPs was found to be in river Ganges at several locations, highest being at Frazergunj (500-600/Kg), 400-500 MP/Kg in Buxar, 300-400 MP/Kg at Godakhali and least in Patna, Bhagalpur, Nabadwip, and Barrackpore (100-200/Kg) respectively. The microplastic abundance was highly correlated with the phosphate content and electrical conductivity of the sediments (Sarkar et al., 2019).

EFFECTS AND OCCURRENCE OF MPs IN BIOTA

The occurrences of MPs cannot be listed on fingers and are rather increasing rapidly with every passing second of MPs disposal, their impacts on the biotic in terms of survivorship, fecundity, organ toxicity, cytotoxicity, have been reported at all the phylum level.

Aquatic Producers

Aquatic MPs affect the microalgae mostly in terms of growth dynamics however, the impact on physiological, biochemical responses, as well as gene expressions have been studied by (Mao et al., 2018; Lagarde et al., 2016). Zhang., (2017) exposed *Skeletonema costatum* to PVC-MPs (0.001 mm) and a 40% reduction in the growth rate was observed at 50 ppm due to blockage of the airways and surficial damage to the cells. A size dependent observation was noted where no effects were seen at larger MPs of size 1mm even up to 40 times higher concentration. Increased toxicity to decreasing size was also seen with *Chlorella vulgaris* and *Thalassiosira pseudonana* exposed to PS-MPs (Sjollema et al., 2015).

Chae et al., (2019) however demonstrated a positive impact of MPs where the growth rate of the algae was enhanced post exposure to PE MPs. Long et al., (2017) reported aggregation of MPs and algae cells. Another report of MP's minimal effects on aquatic vascular plants which were found to adsorb the particles on their surface due to electrostatic forces, and leaf structure. Reduced root-lengths, growth rate, photosynthesis of the freshwater plants is reported (Ge et al., 2021; Tang et al., 2021). Oxidative stress was reported in *Chlorella vulgaris* and Scenedesmus sp. (Prata et al., 2019).

Aquatic Invertebrates

MP uptake have been reported in Protozoans (Zhang et al., 2021; Geng et al., 2021-b) where the feeding experiments depicted a reduced biomass for the ciliates exposed to MPs. Ingestional experiments reported a significant MP induced toxicity in poriferans (Mendrik et al., 2021; Savinelli et al., 2020; Reichert et al., 2018; Martin et al., 2019). Apoptotic stress was reported in the corals after they were found to selectively enrich MPs where small-polyp corals *(Pocillopora damicornis)* were more affected by the MPs than their larger counterpart *Galaxea fascicularis*. The overall physiology, growth, and energy balance in the corals was found to be greatly affected by the presence of MPs (Huang et al., 2020). Coelenterate were affected by MPs majorly by the pathway of ingestion as depicted by Costa et al., (2019). Feeding behaviour in anthozoans is mediated significantly by the chemical cues which are in turn triggered by the release of the phagostimulants, present on the plastics as the core ingredients of the plastic production recipe or produced by the microorganisms during the biofouling of the MPs (Allen et al., 2017). Diana et al., (2020) observed that, sea anemones readily ingested pristine LDPE, HDPE II, and HDPE III plastic pellets without the presence of any supplementary food item, thereby undergoing physiological stress and sided with the hypotheses that the pristine plastics have 'flavour-molecules' which stimulate the chemoreceptor cells of the organism. Jeong et al., (2016) studies the effect of PS-MPs on monogonont rotifer, *Brachionus koreanus* depicting significant size dependent effects in terms of inhibited growth and reproduction, biomass, and elevated levels of antioxidant enzymes along with an activated MAPK signalling pathway up 20 mg/L. The bigger particles were found to be egested out faster than their smaller counterparts. Ingestion, accumulation, and translocation of MPs was studied in economically and ecologically significant Sydney rock oyster *Saccostrea glomerate* (Scanes et al., 2019). Translocation of MPs from the gut to the haemolymph and MP accumulations upon feeding exposures in the mussel *Mytilus edulis*, Pacific oyster *Magallana gigas,* freshwater pond snail *Lymnaea stagnalis*, Quagga Mussel *Dreissena bugensis* have been reported (Cauwenberghe et al., 2014; Weber et al., 2021; Pedersen et al., 2021). Inefficiency of the aquatic organisms to distinguish between the food and plastic particles leading to the unintentional or falsely selective consumption of the latter are reported, mostly in the case of filter feeders (Canniff et al., 2018; Hossain et al., 2019). *Paracentrotus lividus* was exposed to mechanically powdered MPs which exerted no adverse effects other than reducing the density of the faecal matters egested loaded with ingested MPs, affecting its ability to sink (Piarulli et al., 2020; Melkebeke et al., 2020). Reproductive toxicity leading adverse effects on the developing young one has been demonstrated to highlight the impact of MPs on an organism's fecundity. Life history stages of *Meretrix meretrix*, when exposed to PS-COOH and PS-NH_2 by Luan et al., (2019) exerted toxicity in the increasing order of the developmental stages where PS-NH_2 (164 nm) was found to be more toxic than PS-COOH (206 nm) in terms of its higher binding affinity towards negatively charged lipid bilayers of embryo. Similarly, PS-NH^2 caused inhibitory effects on the larvae movements in comparison to the PS-COOH at the end of 48 hours (Bergami et al., 2016). Hatching success of *Limecola balthica* varied between 68.5 and 86.2% when exposed to PS-MPs (Colen et al., 2020). Early life stages of *Sphaerechinus granularis* (sea urchins) when exposed to PS and PMMA from 10 min post-fertilisation to the pluteus larval stage resulted in a significant concentration dependent increase of developmental defects and MP uptake in the pluteus stage (Trifuoggi et al., 2019). Inhibition of brain neurotransmitters specifically AChE, and oxidative stress signifies MPs induced neurotoxicity in *Scrobicularia plana* and is known to be time dependent (Ribeiro et al., 2017). Other instances of neurotoxicity in invertebrates have been compiled by Deidda et al., 2021.

Aquatic Vertebrates

The first report of MP ingestion in fish was in 1972 (Carpenter et al., 1972). As false food particles MPs are ingested directly or indirectly by a range of fish thereby damaging and blocking their digestive tract (Setälä et al., 2014), besides acting as a pollution collector due to its high affinity towards a range of environmental organic contaminants. The dietary exposure of *Sparus aurata* resulted in altered growth rate, oxidative stress, and bioaccumulation. MPs were detected in the livers of some fish at an average rate of <1 particle per liver. Dantas et al. (2020), reported MPs in the stomach contents of the fish from an urban beach in Brazil. MPs have a species-specific distribution in terms its abundance, physical attributes, and polymeric units as reported by Zheng et al., (2019). The species-specific variation was significantly observed among the Redbelly Tilapia and the Common Carp where the former had the highest number of MPs retained in the GITs than the latter. Ingestion NPs/MPs in fish affects the metabolism of fish as well as their distribution in muscle and liver tissues (Cedervall et al., 2012). In a study on small spotted catshark (*Scyliorhinus canicular*) from the Mediterranean Sea, macroplastics (MaP) particles (> 1 cm in) composed of PP, PE, and PET, were found to be more toxic than the smaller MPs (1 μm to <1 mm) in terms of eliciting an immune response (Mancia et al., 2020). Incidental ingestion (Sun et al., 2019) is known to be a potential route of MPs in fishes of Yellow Sea, though the excretion happens over a short time (Mazurais et al., 2015), the vector properties of MPs cause harms. Ingestion NPs/MPs in fish affects the metabolism of fish through alteration of triglycerides and cholesterol in blood serum, as well as their distribution in muscle and liver tissues (Cedervall et al., 2012). Marine medaka (*Oryzias melastigma*) exposed to PS MPs for 60 days to elucidate the effects of MPs by Wang et al., (2019) corroborated not only into obvious oxidative stress and tissue damages after significant accumulations (5.8E+02 particles/L) in the liver gills and intestines, but also disrupted the reproductive endocrine system in a sex-dependent manner. Moreover, an exhibition of transgenerational effect was evident as the fertility (10%) and hatching rate (17.5%) decreased in the offspring derived from parents exposed to 20 mg/L MPs. Seizures are the abnormal involuntary movements of the body, elicited by the unprecedented firing of the neurons, often a precursor to the neurotoxicity. They are followed by the inflections of the neurotransmitters required for stimulation (Acetylcholine) and inhibition (GABA and glutamate). Neurotoxicity of 1–5 μm of red fluorescent MPs causing inhibition of brain acetylcholinesterase was reported at 0.69 ppm in European seabass (Barboza et al., 2019). Sarasamma et al., (2020) reported neurotoxicity in adult zebrafish when exposed to PS-NPs (70 nm) at 0.5, 1.5 and 5 ppm, to determine the neurobehavioral modifications, (where AChE, ACh, dopamine, GABA, Serotonin (5-HT), vasopressin, kisspeptin, prolactin, oxytocin and vasotocin were considered) accumulation, tissue NP retention. Genotoxic effects of PS (1 μm) on *Daphnia magna* and *Neocaridina davidi* were investigated by Berber, (2019), where the robust tail length and movement in the comet assay with increasing doses, signifying DNA damage in *N. Davidi*. Reactive Oxygen Species (ROS) is associated centrally to the toxic responses, and the imbalance between ROS production and antioxidant capacity results in oxidative stress leading to perturbed expressions of the stress related genes. DNA fragmentation, oxidative stress due to overproduction of ROS in the the early juvenile stage of Nile Tilapia (*Oreochromis niloticus*) exposed to 1-100 mg/L of MPs were studied by Hamed et al., (2020). Gilthead seabream (*S. aurata*) when exposed to PVC-MPs for a long-term observation, affected the expression of genes (*prdx5, ucp1, hsp90, coxIV*). The nuclear factor erythroid 2–related factor 2 (*nrf2*) gene, which is functional for the regulation of oxidative stress, was found to be up-regulated in exposed head-kidney leucocytes (Espinosa et al., 2018).

Trophic Transfer

MPs transitions from lower trophic levels towards the top, through freshwater ecosystem face a paucity of relevant and realistic data as compared to the marine food webs. Transfer of MPs from the contaminated brown seaweed to the periwinkle as they consume the former (Gutow et al., 2016), from artemia to zebrafish (Batel et al., 2016), mussels to crab (Farrell and Nelson 2013). Presence of MPs on the blades of the seagrass (*Thalassia testudinum*, a potential feed for the invertebrates) in natural environment has been shown by (Goss et al., 2018.) Santana et al., (2017) depicted a multilevel food web with brown mussel *(Perna perna*), fish (*Spheoeroides greeleyi*) and crabs (*Callinectes ornatus*) confirming Bio-transference. The unintentional ingestion of MPs transfers through the prey species of common minke (*Balaenoptera acutorostrata*) and sei whale (*B. borealis*) was explored by Burkhardt-Holm et al., (2019). Similarly, Nelms et al., (2018) suggested that the feeding pattern of the consumption of the whole prey represents an important route of MPs tropic transfer. Walkinshaw et al., (2019) suggested that the increase in the number of MPs is not directly dependent on the increasing trophic levels, and that organisms at lower trophic levels act as a sink to all the environmental MPs than the apex predators. Trophic transfer of MPs from the prey to the predator was demonstrated when faecal matter of penguins and northern fur seals were tested positive for the presence of MPs (Nelms et al., 2019; Donohue et al., 2019) with no reported toxicity. MPs were also reported to be present in the gut contents of both adult and calves of a coastal delphnid (*Sousa chinensis*), through unintentional consumption along with the prey (Zhu et al., 2019), posing an immense risk potential to these organisms which are already threatened with extinction, further cutting down their survival rates. Phagocytosis mediated entry of PS-MPs in a dinoflagellate species *Heterocapsa triquetra* (Long et al., 2017) implicated another potential pathway of MP transfer to higher trophic levels. In a study by Duncan et al., 2018, species of marine turtles *viz* Bystranded green (*Chelonia mydas*) and Loggerhead (*Caretta caretta*) from the Mediterranean basin, Kemp's ridley (*Lepidochelys kempii*) and leatherback (*Dermochelys coriacea*) turtles from Atlantic basin and flatback (*Natator depressus*), hawksbill (*Eretmochelys imbricata*) and olive ridley (*Lepidochelys olivacea*) turtles from the pacific basin were found to be enriched with MPs by either environmental exposure of the turtles to contaminated sea water and sediments, or the consumption of contaminated primary producers and sessile filter feeders.

EFFECTS ON NUTRIENT CYCLES

The detection of MPs in the surface, subsurface, and deep waters as well as the sediments of the watersheds have been greatly explored around the globe to report enormous amounts of plastics pitted in each of the locations. Accumulations of MPs on the surface of the water due to their buoyancy have been reported to cause eutrophication, leading to a reduced light penetration increased microbial assemblages, and decreased oxygen levels in the water bodies (Law, 2017). Weathering renders MPs rough-surfaced and biofouling makes it reactive due to the presence of additional functional groups and molecules. This leads to an increased density and decreased ability to float, promoting such MPs-contaminant aggregate's downward movement towards the pristine seafloor altering their biogeochemistry. Such particles rich in organic content are known to create oxygen-less zones (Arias-Andres et al., 2018). MPs from the surface reach the sediments which are reported to have an increased ammonia content (Seeley et al., 2020). This sinking of the surface MPs affects the carbon and nitrogen on the water surfaces, the dissolved organic matter breakdown causing disturbances in the oceanic biological pump, global greenhouse gases (Khalid et al., 2020; Katija et al., 2017; Rogers et al., 2020). The carbon pools of the environment are affected a great deal due to the presence of Dissolved Organic Carbon (DOCs) in the surface layer which in turn disturb the natural carbon pool of the ocean and affect microbial growth and nutrient cycling (Castillo et al., 2018). Eutrophication was also reported due to the disturbed nitrogen content (Cluzard et al., 2015) whereas Chen et al., (2020) reported the increase in the oceanic phosphorus content due to the formation of biofilms on MPs in his microcosm experiment simulating the natural settings. Scanty data on the hydrogeochemical cycle is available and is hence a potential gap of research with MPs looming large.

EFFECTS ON HUMANS

With MPs being detected in air, water, sediments, soils, and even the edible biota; humans are not an exception. Reports of MPs in the daily commodities and its subsequent ingestion by humans are eventually reflecting their presence in feces, colon, placenta, scalp hair, hand skin, facial skin, and saliva (Basri et al., 2021; Ragusa et al., 2021) etc. These particles are already invading human body through gastric, dermal (weakened skin barrier or a wound), or inhalation (due to its size and hydrophobicity) routes (Yee et al., 2021). MPs can cross the cellular barrier by phagocytosis, micropinocytosis, clathrin- and caveolae-mediated endocytosis and are known to exert cytotoxicity and get accumulated (Ding et al., 2021). *In vitro* studies with the human cell lines such as human hepatoma cell line HepG2 (toxicity of single and combine PE-MPs and Polychlorinated biphenyls (PCBs)) where PCBs were reported to be exerting a 'trojan horse' effect in presence of MPs (Pedriza et al., 2022). Shrinzi et al., (2017) reported oxidative stress mediated cytotoxicity in T98G (cerebral) and HeLa (epithelial human cells) when exposed to NPs. It has been noted that exposure of PS-NPs resulted in metabolic disorders of human cancer cell lines A549, HepG-2, and HCT116 through the formation of binucleated cells (Yee et al., 2021). Apart from cell lines approach, studies from mammalian models have also reported microplastics induced neurotoxicity (Deng et al., 2017), lesions and inflammations, decreased body weight, altered microbiota (Lu et al., 2018; Jin et al., 2021), and transgenerational toxicity (Luo et al., 2019).

DEGRADATION AND REMOVAL OF MPs

The irreversible breakdown of polymers by mechanisms such as biological, physical, and chemical such that their physico-chemical properties are altered into simpler product is commonly referred to as degradation phenomenon (Oliveira et al., 2020). The degradation mechanisms are generally classified based on the pathways such as abiotic (light, heat, UV, stress), chemical, biodegradation, photodegradation, thermo-oxidative, thermal degradation, and hydrolysis (Oliveira et al., 2020; Aljaradin et al., 2020; Liu et al., 2021).

Biodegradation

The action of biotic agents such as bacteria, fungi and their enzymes destroy plastic by their innate ability to decompose by the formation of biofilm on the MPs. Microorganisms such as *Ideonella sakaiensis, Fusarium oxysporum, Fusarium solani, Thermobifida fusca* are known to degrade PET; *Shewanella* sp., *Moritella* sp., *Psychtobactor* sp., *Pseudomonas* sp. *Clonostachys Rosea*, Trichoderma sp. Are known to degrade Polycaprolactone (PCL); *Vibrio Alginolyticus, Vibrio Parahemolyticus, Aspergillus Versicolor, Aspergillus sp* (PVA-LDPE); *Zalerion Maritimum, Aspergillus niger, A. versicolor, Penicillium pinophilum, P. frequentan, P. oxalicum, and P. chrysogenum, (*PE); *Alcanivorax* sp., Tenacibaculum sp., (Polybutylene PBS) (Aljaradin, 2020).

Photodegradation

The degradation of MPs in water by the sun's solar radiation cause plastics to become brittle, discolored, hard, and of decreased mechanical properties eventually degrading it, however the speed depends largely upon many factors such as the size of the particles, amount of light reaching the particles and other physicochemical properties of the water (Klein et al., 2018). Photo catalytic degradation of MPs have been reported to reduce the MP-particle volume by 65% in visible light irradiating Zinc oxide nanorods (Uheida et al., 2021)

Thermal and Thermo-Oxidative Degradation

The breakdown of MPs by the action of high temperatures than those bearable by their polymeric structures, inducing chemical changes in the polymers is an efficient method of MPs removal while oxidative degradation of MPs at moderate temperatures lead to formation of degradation products such as ketones, aldehydes, alcohols, carboxylic acids, and low molecular mass hydrocarbon waxes (Aljaradin et al., 2020).

Hydrolysis

The action of water at high temperature and pressure is an efficient and cost-effective method of MPs degradation. Acidic hydrolysis (H_2SO_4; for PET), Alkaline hydrolysis (NaOH), and neutral (Steam) are reported to degrade MPs with above 80% yield (Oliveira et al., 2020; Shirke et al., 2018; Sinha et al., 2018).

Removal of MPs

Membrane removal tool designed by Ward et al., (2015) and membrane bioreactors investigated by Talvite et al., (2017) efficiently removed MPs from synthetic water. Coagulations and agglomeration of MPs to form bigger particles using Iron and Aluminium salts and ultrafiltration and electrocoagulation techniques are also practiced (Ariza-Tarazona et al., 2019). Yang et al., (2019) designed a combination of activated sludge treatment plant and membrane bioreactors with a removal efficiency of 99.4%. MPs removal by green unicellular algae was mediated by Cole et al., (2011), Nolte et al., (2017) using seaweed *Fucus*

Figure 1. MPs Production, Release, and Transport in Aquatic Ecosystem

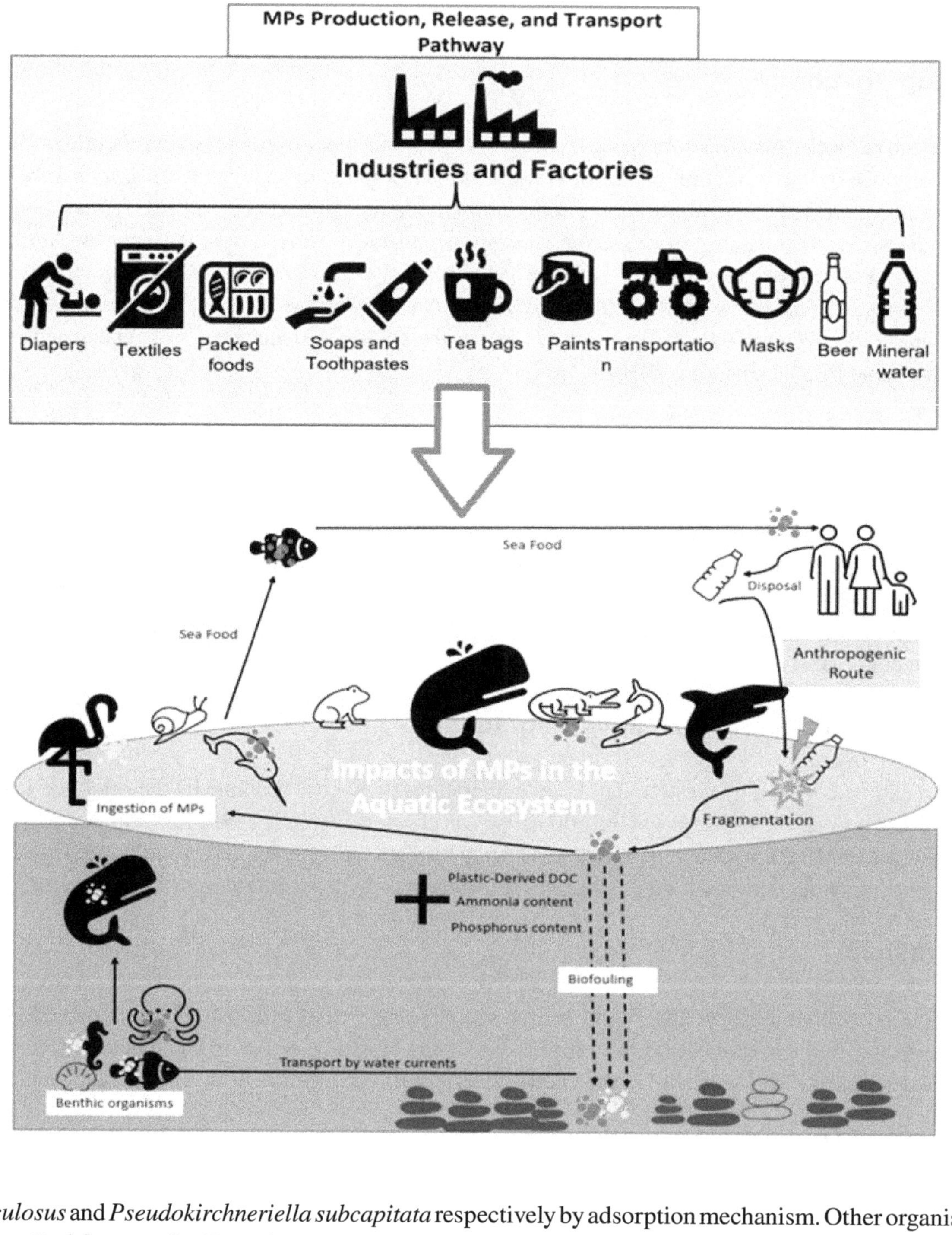

vesiculosus and *Pseudokirchneriella subcapitata* respectively by adsorption mechanism. Other organisms such as Red Sea coral's (*Danafungia scruposa*), crustacean Antarctic Krill *(Euphausia superba)* have been known to fragmentize and remove MPs (Corona et al., 2020; Padervand et al., 2020). However, their health status remains unclear under such circumstances. Alternatives such as starch (Ferreira et al.,

2016), polylactic acid (PLA) (Oi et al., 2017), Polyhydroxyalkanoates (PHA) (Perez et al. 2018) have been recommended as MPs removal agents from environmental matrices.

CONCLUSION

The chapter highlighted the occurrence of MPs and their detrimental effects on various organisms at different levels of biological organization. Besides, it also dealt with the available degradation approaches to minimize the impact on the biosphere. However, its omnipresence cannot be neglected as of now. Besides, the vector potential of the MPs with other hydrophobic organic contaminants threatens the relative pristine areas with significant impact on the ecosystem services. This eventually destroys the natural ambience of the waterways, compromising the organisms' health and perturbing the biogeochemical cycling of respective ecosystem by the depleting the essential nutrients. Among the organisms, planktonic species, filter-feeders, bivalves, large vertebrates including turtles, seals, sharks, whales, penguins, and seabirds etc., are found to be vulnerable to MPs uptake through feeding in polluted water resulting in several stress pathways from false satiation, mechanical injuries in the gut, reduced reproductive output, developmental toxicity, immunotoxicity, cytotoxicity, and neurotoxicity etc. This needs a thorough risk assessment strategy for ecosystem sustainability.

REFERENCES

Aljaradin, M. (n.d.). *Biodegradation of Microplastics in Drinking Water, A review*. Academic Press.

Allen, A. S., Seymour, A. C., & Rittschof, D. (2017). Chemoreception drives plastic consumption in a hard coral. *Marine Pollution Bulletin*, *124*(1), 198–205. doi:10.1016/j.marpolbul.2017.07.030 PMID:28743368

Ambrosini, R., Azzoni, R. S., Pittino, F., Diolaiuti, G., Franzetti, A., & Parolini, M. (2019). First evidence of microplastic contamination in the supraglacial debris of an alpine glacier. *Environmental Pollution*, *253*, 297–301. doi:10.1016/j.envpol.2019.07.005 PMID:31323612

Amrutha, K., & Warrier, A. K. (2020). The first report on the source-to-sink characterization of microplastic pollution from a riverine environment in tropical India. *The Science of the Total Environment*, *739*, 140377. doi:10.1016/j.scitotenv.2020.140377 PMID:32758976

Arias-Andres, M., Kettner, M. T., Miki, T., & Grossart, H. P. (2018). Microplastics: New substrates for heterotrophic activity contribute to altering organic matter cycles in aquatic ecosystems. *The Science of the Total Environment*, *635*, 1152–1159. doi:10.1016/j.scitotenv.2018.04.199 PMID:29710570

Barboza, L. G. A., Vieira, L. R., Branco, V., Figueiredo, N., Carvalho, F., Carvalho, C., & Guilhermino, L. (2018). Microplastics cause neurotoxicity, oxidative damage and energy-related changes and interact with the bioaccumulation of mercury in the European seabass, Dicentrarchus labrax (Linnaeus, 1758). *Aquatic Toxicology (Amsterdam, Netherlands)*, *195*, 49–57. doi:10.1016/j.aquatox.2017.12.008 PMID:29287173

Basri, K., Syaputra, E. M., & Handayani, S. (2021). Microplastic Pollution in Waters and its Impact on Health and Environment in Indonesia: A Review. *Journal of Public Health for Tropical and Coastal Region*, *4*(2), 63–77. doi:10.14710/jphtcr.v4i2.10809

Berber, A. A. (2019). *Polystyrene nanoplastics trigger toxicity on two different aquatic organisms (Brachionus plicatilis, Daphnia magna)*. Academic Press.

Bergami, E., Bocci, E., Vannuccini, M. L., Monopoli, M., Salvati, A., Dawson, K. A., & Corsi, I. (2016). Nano-sized polystyrene affects feeding, behavior and physiology of brine shrimp Artemia franciscana larvae. *Ecotoxicology and Environmental Safety*, *123*, 18–25. doi:10.1016/j.ecoenv.2015.09.021 PMID:26422775

Bergmann, M., Mützel, S., Primpke, S., Tekman, M. B., Trachsel, J., & Gerdts, G. (2019). White and wonderful? Microplastics prevail in snow from the Alps to the Arctic. *Science Advances*, *5*(8), eaax1157. doi:10.1126ciadv.aax1157 PMID:31453336

Boucher, J., & Friot, D. (2017). *Primary microplastics in the oceans: a global evaluation of sources* (Vol. 43). IUCN. doi:10.2305/IUCN.CH.2017.01.en

Burkhardt-Holm, P., & N'Guyen, A. (2019). Ingestion of microplastics by fish and other prey organisms of cetaceans, exemplified for two large baleen whale species. *Marine Pollution Bulletin*, *144*, 224–234. doi:10.1016/j.marpolbul.2019.04.068 PMID:31179992

Canniff, P. M., & Hoang, T. C. (2018). Microplastic ingestion by Daphnia magna and its enhancement on algal growth. *The Science of the Total Environment*, *633*, 500–507. doi:10.1016/j.scitotenv.2018.03.176 PMID:29579661

Carpenter, E. J., Anderson, S. J., Harvey, G. R., Miklas, H. P., & Peck, B. B. (1972). Polystyrene spherules in coastal waters. *Science*, *178*(4062), 749–750. doi:10.1126cience.178.4062.749 PMID:4628343

Carr, S. A., Liu, J., & Tesoro, A. G. (2016). Transport and fate of microplastic particles in wastewater treatment plants. *Water Research*, *91*, 174–182. doi:10.1016/j.watres.2016.01.002 PMID:26795302

Cedervall, T., Hansson, L. A., Lard, M., Frohm, B., & Linse, S. (2012). Food chain transport of nanoparticles affects behaviour and fat metabolism in fish. *PLoS One*, *7*(2), e32254. doi:10.1371/journal.pone.0032254 PMID:22384193

Chae, Y., Kim, D., & An, Y. J. (2019). Effects of micro-sized polyethylene spheres on the marine microalga Dunaliella salina: Focusing on the algal cell to plastic particle size ratio. *Aquatic Toxicology (Amsterdam, Netherlands)*, *216*, 105296. doi:10.1016/j.aquatox.2019.105296 PMID:31541944

Chahine, M. T. (1992). The hydrological cycle and its influence on climate. *Nature*, *359*(6394), 373–380. doi:10.1038/359373a0

Chan, C. K., Park, C., Chan, K. M., Mak, D. C., Fang, J. K., & Mitrano, D. M. (2021). Microplastic fibre releases from industrial wastewater effluent: A textile wet-processing mill in China. *Environmental Chemistry*, *18*(3), 93–100. doi:10.1071/EN20143

Chen, G., Li, Y., & Wang, J. (2021). Occurrence and ecological impact of microplastics in aquaculture ecosystems. *Chemosphere*, *274*, 129989. doi:10.1016/j.chemosphere.2021.129989 PMID:33979917

Chen, X., Chen, X., Zhao, Y., Zhou, H., Xiong, X., & Wu, C. (2020). Effects of microplastic biofilms on nutrient cycling in simulated freshwater systems. *The Science of the Total Environment, 719*, 137276. doi:10.1016/j.scitotenv.2020.137276 PMID:32114222

Cluzard, M., Kazmiruk, T. N., Kazmiruk, V. D., & Bendell, L. I. (2015). Intertidal concentrations of microplastics and their influence on ammonium cycling as related to the shellfish industry. *Archives of Environmental Contamination and Toxicology, 69*(3), 310–319. doi:10.100700244-015-0156-5 PMID:25916196

Coppock, R. L., Galloway, T. S., Cole, M., Fileman, E. S., Queirós, A. M., & Lindeque, P. K. (2019). Microplastics alter feeding selectivity and faecal density in the copepod, Calanus helgolandicus. *The Science of the Total Environment, 687*, 780–789. doi:10.1016/j.scitotenv.2019.06.009 PMID:31412481

Corona, E., Martin, C., Marasco, R., & Duarte, C. M. (2020). Passive and active removal of marine microplastics by a mushroom coral (Danafungia scruposa). *Frontiers in Marine Science, 7*, 128. doi:10.3389/fmars.2020.00128

Costa, E., Gambardella, C., Piazza, V., Vassalli, M., Sbrana, F., Lavorano, S., Garaventa, F., & Faimali, M. (2020). Microplastics ingestion in the ephyra stage of Aurelia sp. triggers acute and behavioral responses. *Ecotoxicology and Environmental Safety, 189*, 109983. doi:10.1016/j.ecoenv.2019.109983 PMID:31785944

Dantas, N. C., Duarte, O. S., Ferreira, W. C., Ayala, A. P., Rezende, C. F., & Feitosa, C. V. (2020). Plastic intake does not depend on fish eating habits: Identification of microplastics in the stomach contents of fish on an urban beach in Brazil. *Marine Pollution Bulletin, 153*, 110959. doi:10.1016/j.marpolbul.2020.110959 PMID:32275522

Deidda, I., Russo, R., Bonaventura, R., Costa, C., Zito, F., & Lampiasi, N. (2021). Neurotoxicity in marine invertebrates: An update. *Biology (Basel), 10*(2), 161. doi:10.3390/biology10020161 PMID:33670451

Deng, Y., Zhang, Y., Lemos, B., & Ren, H. (2017). Tissue accumulation of microplastics in mice and biomarker responses suggest widespread health risks of exposure. *Scientific Reports, 7*(1), 1–10. doi:10.1038rep46687 PMID:28436478

Diana, Z., Sawickij, N., Rivera, N. A. Jr, Hsu-Kim, H., & Rittschof, D. (2020). Plastic pellets trigger feeding responses in sea anemones. *Aquatic Toxicology (Amsterdam, Netherlands), 222*, 105447. doi:10.1016/j.aquatox.2020.105447 PMID:32145485

Ding, Y., Zhang, R., Li, B., Du, Y., Li, J., Tong, X., Wu, Y., Ji, X., & Zhang, Y. (2021). Tissue distribution of polystyrene nanoplastics in mice and their entry, transport, and cytotoxicity to GES-1 cells. *Environmental Pollution, 280*, 116974. doi:10.1016/j.envpol.2021.116974 PMID:33784569

Donohue, M. J., Masura, J., Gelatt, T., Ream, R., Baker, J. D., Faulhaber, K., & Lerner, D. T. (2019). Evaluating exposure of northern fur seals, Callorhinus ursinus, to microplastic pollution through fecal analysis. *Marine Pollution Bulletin, 138*, 213–221. doi:10.1016/j.marpolbul.2018.11.036 PMID:30660265

Duan, J., Bolan, N., Li, Y., Ding, S., Atugoda, T., Vithanage, M., Sarkar, B., Tsang, D. C. W., & Kirkham, M. B. (2021). Weathering of microplastics and interaction with other coexisting constituents in terrestrial and aquatic environments. *Water Research, 196*, 117011. doi:10.1016/j.watres.2021.117011 PMID:33743325

Espinosa, C., Beltrán, J. M. G., Esteban, M. A., & Cuesta, A. (2018). In vitro effects of virgin microplastics on fish head-kidney leucocyte activities. *Environmental Pollution, 235*, 30–38. doi:10.1016/j.envpol.2017.12.054 PMID:29274535

Europe, P. (2020). Plastics–the facts 2020. *PlasticEurope, 1*, 1–64.

Everaert, G., Van Cauwenberghe, L., De Rijcke, M., Koelmans, A. A., Mees, J., Vandegehuchte, M., & Janssen, C. R. (2018). Risk assessment of microplastics in the ocean: Modelling approach and first conclusions. *Environmental Pollution, 242*, 1930–1938. doi:10.1016/j.envpol.2018.07.069 PMID:30061084

Farrell, P., & Nelson, K. (2013). Trophic level transfer of microplastic: Mytilus edulis (L.) to Carcinus maenas (L.). *Environmental Pollution, 177*, 1–3. doi:10.1016/j.envpol.2013.01.046 PMID:23434827

Galgani, L., & Loiselle, S. A. (2021). Plastic pollution impacts on marine carbon biogeochemistry. *Environmental Pollution, 268*, 115598. doi:10.1016/j.envpol.2020.115598 PMID:33158618

Ge, J., Li, H., Liu, P., Zhang, Z., Ouyang, Z., & Guo, X. (2021). Review of the toxic effect of microplastics on terrestrial and aquatic plants. *The Science of the Total Environment, 791*, 148333. doi:10.1016/j.scitotenv.2021.148333 PMID:34412379

Geng, X., Wang, J., Zhang, Y., & Jiang, Y. (2021). How do microplastics affect the marine microbial loop? Predation of microplastics by microzooplankton. *The Science of the Total Environment, 758*, 144030. doi:10.1016/j.scitotenv.2020.144030 PMID:33340809

George, M., & Fabre, P. (2021). Floating plastics in oceans: A matter of size. *Current Opinion in Green and Sustainable Chemistry, 32*, 100543. doi:10.1016/j.cogsc.2021.100543

Gonçalves, H. C., Mercante, M. A., & Santos, E. T. (2011). Hydrological cycle. *Brazilian Journal of Biology, 71*(1), 241–253. doi:10.1590/S1519-69842011000200003 PMID:21537597

Goss, H., Jaskiel, J., & Rotjan, R. (2018). Thalassia testudinum as a potential vector for incorporating microplastics into benthic marine food webs. *Marine Pollution Bulletin, 135*, 1085–1089. doi:10.1016/j.marpolbul.2018.08.024 PMID:30301005

Gutow, L., Eckerlebe, A., Giménez, L., & Saborowski, R. (2016). Experimental evaluation of seaweeds as a vector for microplastics into marine food webs. *Environmental Science & Technology, 50*(2), 915–923. doi:10.1021/acs.est.5b02431 PMID:26654910

Hale, R. C., Seeley, M. E., La Guardia, M. J., Mai, L., & Zeng, E. Y. (2020). A global perspective on microplastics. *Journal of Geophysical Research: Oceans, 125*(1), e2018JC014719.

Hamed, M., Soliman, H. A., Osman, A. G., & Sayed, A. E. D. H. (2020). Antioxidants and molecular damage in Nile Tilapia (Oreochromis niloticus) after exposure to microplastics. *Environmental Science and Pollution Research International, 27*(13), 14581–14588. doi:10.100711356-020-07898-y PMID:32048193

Hartmann, N. B., Hüffer, T., Thompson, R. C., Hassellöv, M., Verschoor, A., Daugaard, A. E., Rist, S., Karlsson, T., Brennholt, N., Cole, M., Herrling, M. P., Hess, M. C., Ivleva, N. P., Lusher, A. L., & Wagner, M. (2019). Are We Speaking the Same Language? Recommendations for a Definition and Categorization Framework for Plastic Debris. *Environmental Science & Technology*, *53*(3), 1039–1047. doi:10.1021/acs.est.8b05297 PMID:30608663

Hintersteiner, I., Himmelsbach, M., & Buchberger, W. W. (2015). Characterization and quantitation of polyolefin microplastics in personal-care products using high-temperature gel-permeation chromatography. *Analytical and Bioanalytical Chemistry*, *407*(4), 1253–1259. doi:10.100700216-014-8318-2 PMID:25410643

Hossain, M. S., Rahman, M. S., Uddin, M. N., Sharifuzzaman, S. M., Chowdhury, S. R., Sarker, S., & Chowdhury, M. S. N. (2020). Microplastic contamination in Penaeid shrimp from the Northern Bay of Bengal. *Chemosphere*, *238*, 124688. doi:10.1016/j.chemosphere.2019.124688 PMID:31524623

Huang, W., Chen, M., Song, B., Deng, J., Shen, M., Chen, Q., Zeng, G., & Liang, J. (2021). Microplastics in the coral reefs and their potential impacts on corals: A mini-review. *The Science of the Total Environment*, *762*, 143112. doi:10.1016/j.scitotenv.2020.143112 PMID:33172634

Jeong, C. B., Won, E. J., Kang, H. M., Lee, M. C., Hwang, D. S., Hwang, U. K., Zhou, B., Souissi, S., Lee, S.-J., & Lee, J. S. (2016). Microplastic size-dependent toxicity, oxidative stress induction, and p-JNK and p-p38 activation in the monogonont rotifer (Brachionus koreanus). *Environmental Science & Technology*, *50*(16), 8849–8857. doi:10.1021/acs.est.6b01441 PMID:27438693

Jin, H., Ma, T., Sha, X., Liu, Z., Zhou, Y., Meng, X., Chen, Y., Han, X., & Ding, J. (2021). Polystyrene microplastics induced male reproductive toxicity in mice. *Journal of Hazardous Materials*, *401*, 123430. doi:10.1016/j.jhazmat.2020.123430 PMID:32659591

Jovanović, B., Gökdağ, K., Güven, O., Emre, Y., Whitley, E. M., & Kideys, A. E. (2018). Virgin microplastics are not causing imminent harm to fish after dietary exposure. *Marine Pollution Bulletin*, *130*, 123–131. doi:10.1016/j.marpolbul.2018.03.016 PMID:29866538

Kaiser, D., Kowalski, N., & Waniek, J. J. (2017). Effects of biofouling on the sinking behavior of microplastics. *Environmental Research Letters*, *12*(12), 124003. doi:10.1088/1748-9326/aa8e8b

Katija, K., Sherlock, R. E., Sherman, A. D., & Robison, B. H. (2017). New technology reveals the role of giant larvaceans in oceanic carbon cycling. *Science Advances*, *3*(5), e1602374. doi:10.1126ciadv.1602374 PMID:28508058

Khalid, N., Aqeel, M., Noman, A., Hashem, M., Mostafa, Y. S., Alhaithloul, H. A. S., & Alghanem, S. M. (2021). Linking effects of microplastics to ecological impacts in marine environments. *Chemosphere*, *264*, 128541. doi:10.1016/j.chemosphere.2020.128541 PMID:33059282

Klein, S., Dimzon, I. K., Eubeler, J., & Knepper, T. P. (2018). Analysis, occurrence, and degradation of microplastics in the aqueous environment. In *Freshwater microplastics* (pp. 51–67). Springer. doi:10.1007/978-3-319-61615-5_3

Krüger, L., Casado-Coy, N., Valle, C., Ramos, M., Sánchez-Jerez, P., Gago, J., Carretero, O., Beltran-Sanahuja, A., & Sanz-Lazaro, C. (2020). Plastic debris accumulation in the seabed derived from coastal fish farming. *Environmental Pollution, 257*, 113336. doi:10.1016/j.envpol.2019.113336 PMID:31753624

Lagarde, F., Olivier, O., Zanella, M., Daniel, P., Hiard, S., & Caruso, A. (2016). Microplastic interactions with freshwater microalgae: Hetero-aggregation and changes in plastic density appear strongly dependent on polymer type. *Environmental Pollution, 215*, 331–339. doi:10.1016/j.envpol.2016.05.006 PMID:27236494

Lahens, L., Strady, E., Kieu-Le, T. C., Dris, R., Boukerma, K., Rinnert, E., Gasperi, J., & Tassin, B. (2018). Macroplastic and microplastic contamination assessment of a tropical river (Saigon River, Vietnam) transversed by a developing megacity. *Environmental Pollution, 236*, 661–671. doi:10.1016/j.envpol.2018.02.005 PMID:29438952

Law, K. L. (2017). Plastics in the marine environment. *Annual Review of Marine Science, 9*(1), 205–229. doi:10.1146/annurev-marine-010816-060409 PMID:27620829

Lebreton, L., & Andrady, A. (2019). Future scenarios of global plastic waste generation and disposal. *Palgrave Communications, 5*(1), 1–11. doi:10.105741599-018-0212-7

Lechner, A., & Ramler, D. (2015). The discharge of certain amounts of industrial microplastic from a production plant into the River Danube is permitted by the Austrian legislation. *Environmental Pollution, 200*, 159–160. doi:10.1016/j.envpol.2015.02.019 PMID:25734504

Leslie, H. A. (2014). Review of microplastics in cosmetics. *IVM Institute for Environmental Studies, 476*, 1–33.

Li, J., Liu, H., & Chen, J. P. (2018). Microplastics in freshwater systems: A review on occurrence, environmental effects, and methods for microplastics detection. *Water Research, 137*, 362–374. doi:10.1016/j.watres.2017.12.056 PMID:29580559

Lim, X. (2021). *Microplastics are everywhere—but are they harmful?* Academic Press.

Liu, F., Olesen, K. B., Borregaard, A. R., & Vollertsen, J. (2019). Microplastics in urban and highway stormwater retention ponds. *The Science of the Total Environment, 671*, 992–1000. doi:10.1016/j.scitotenv.2019.03.416 PMID:31604201

Liu, X., Shi, H., Xie, B., Dionysiou, D. D., & Zhao, Y. (2019). Microplastics as both a sink and a source of bisphenol A in the marine environment. *Environmental Science & Technology, 53*(17), 10188–10196. doi:10.1021/acs.est.9b02834 PMID:31393116

Long, M., Paul-Pont, I., Hegaret, H., Moriceau, B., Lambert, C., Huvet, A., & Soudant, P. (2017). Interactions between polystyrene microplastics and marine phytoplankton lead to species-specific hetero-aggregation. *Environmental Pollution, 228*, 454–463. doi:10.1016/j.envpol.2017.05.047 PMID:28558286

Long, M., Paul-Pont, I., Hegaret, H., Moriceau, B., Lambert, C., Huvet, A., & Soudant, P. (2017). Interactions between polystyrene microplastics and marine phytoplankton lead to species-specific hetero-aggregation. *Environmental Pollution, 228*, 454–463. doi:10.1016/j.envpol.2017.05.047 PMID:28558286

Lu, L., Wan, Z., Luo, T., Fu, Z., & Jin, Y. (2018). Polystyrene microplastics induce gut microbiota dysbiosis and hepatic lipid metabolism disorder in mice. *The Science of the Total Environment*, *631*, 449–458. doi:10.1016/j.scitotenv.2018.03.051 PMID:29529433

Luo, H., Liu, C., He, D., Xu, J., Sun, J., Li, J., & Pan, X. (2022). Environmental behaviors of microplastics in aquatic systems: A systematic review on degradation, adsorption, toxicity and biofilm under aging conditions. *Journal of Hazardous Materials*, *423*, 126915. doi:10.1016/j.jhazmat.2021.126915 PMID:34461541

Luo, T., Zhang, Y., Wang, C., Wang, X., Zhou, J., Shen, M., Zhao, Y., Fu, Z., & Jin, Y. (2019). Maternal exposure to different sizes of polystyrene microplastics during gestation causes metabolic disorders in their offspring. *Environmental Pollution*, *255*, 113122. doi:10.1016/j.envpol.2019.113122 PMID:31520900

Mao, Y., Ai, H., Chen, Y., Zhang, Z., Zeng, P., Kang, L., Li, W., Gu, W., He, Q., & Li, H. (2018). Phytoplankton response to polystyrene microplastics: Perspective from an entire growth period. *Chemosphere*, *208*, 59–68. doi:10.1016/j.chemosphere.2018.05.170 PMID:29860145

Mendrik, F. M., Henry, T. B., Burdett, H., Hackney, C. R., Waller, C., Parsons, D. R., & Hennige, S. J. (2021). Species-specific impact of microplastics on coral physiology. *Environmental Pollution*, *269*, 116238. doi:10.1016/j.envpol.2020.116238 PMID:33321308

Menéndez-Pedriza, A., Jaumot, J., & Bedia, C. (2022). Lipidomic analysis of single and combined effects of polyethylene microplastics and polychlorinated biphenyls on human hepatoma cells. *Journal of Hazardous Materials*, *421*, 126777. doi:10.1016/j.jhazmat.2021.126777 PMID:34364209

Morgana, S., Ghigliotti, L., Estévez-Calvar, N., Stifanese, R., Wieckzorek, A., Doyle, T., Christiansen, J. S., Faimali, M., & Garaventa, F. (2018). Microplastics in the Arctic: A case study with sub-surface water and fish samples off Northeast Greenland. *Environmental Pollution*, *242*, 1078–1086. doi:10.1016/j.envpol.2018.08.001 PMID:30096546

Murphy, F., Ewins, C., Carbonnier, F., & Quinn, B. (2016). Wastewater treatment works (WwTW) as a source of microplastics in the aquatic environment. *Environmental Science & Technology*, *50*(11), 5800–5808. doi:10.1021/acs.est.5b05416 PMID:27191224

Napper, I. E., Davies, B. F., Clifford, H., Elvin, S., Koldewey, H. J., Mayewski, P. A., Miner, K. R., Potocki, M., Elmore, A. C., Gajurel, A. P., & Thompson, R. C. (2020). Reaching new heights in plastic pollution—Preliminary findings of microplastics on Mount Everest. *One Earth*, *3*(5), 621–630. doi:10.1016/j.oneear.2020.10.020

Nelms, S. E., Barnett, J., Brownlow, A., Davison, N. J., Deaville, R., Galloway, T. S., Lindeque, P. K., Santillo, D., & Godley, B. J. (2019). Microplastics in marine mammals stranded around the British coast: Ubiquitous but transitory? *Scientific Reports*, *9*(1), 1–8. doi:10.103841598-018-37428-3 PMID:30705316

Nelms, S. E., Galloway, T. S., Godley, B. J., Jarvis, D. S., & Lindeque, P. K. (2018). Investigating microplastic trophic transfer in marine top predators. *Environmental Pollution*, *238*, 999–1007. doi:10.1016/j.envpol.2018.02.016 PMID:29477242

Oliveira, J., Belchior, A., da Silva, V. D., Rotter, A., Petrovski, Ž., Almeida, P. L., Lourenço, N. D., & Gaudêncio, S. P. (2020). Marine environmental plastic pollution: Mitigation by microorganism degradation and recycling valorization. *Frontiers in Marine Science*, *7*, 1007. doi:10.3389/fmars.2020.567126

Padervand, M., Lichtfouse, E., Robert, D., & Wang, C. (2020). Removal of microplastics from the environment. A review. *Environmental Chemistry Letters*, *18*(3), 807–828. doi:10.100710311-020-00983-1

Pedersen, A. F., Gopalakrishnan, K., Boegehold, A. G., Peraino, N. J., Westrick, J. A., & Kashian, D. R. (2020). Microplastic ingestion by quagga mussels, Dreissena bugensis, and its effects on physiological processes. *Environmental Pollution*, *260*, 113964. doi:10.1016/j.envpol.2020.113964 PMID:31991349

Peng, X., Chen, M., Chen, S., Dasgupta, S., Xu, H., Ta, K., Du, M., Li, J., Guo, Z., & Bai, S. (2018). Microplastics contaminate the deepest part of the world's ocean. *Geochemical Perspectives Letters*, *9*, 1–5. doi:10.7185/geochemlet.1829

Petersen, F., & Hubbart, J. A. (2021). The occurrence and transport of microplastics: The state of the science. *The Science of the Total Environment*, *758*, 143936. doi:10.1016/j.scitotenv.2020.143936 PMID:33333307

Phuong, N. N., Zalouk-Vergnoux, A., Poirier, L., Kamari, A., Châtel, A., Mouneyrac, C., & Lagarde, F. (2016). Is there any consistency between the microplastics found in the field and those used in laboratory experiments? *Environmental Pollution*, *211*, 111–123. doi:10.1016/j.envpol.2015.12.035 PMID:26745396

Piarulli, S., & Airoldi, L. (2020). Mussels facilitate the sinking of microplastics to bottom sediments and their subsequent uptake by detritus-feeders. *Environmental Pollution*, *266*, 115151. doi:10.1016/j.envpol.2020.115151 PMID:32673992

Prata, J. C., da Costa, J. P., Lopes, I., Duarte, A. C., & Rocha-Santos, T. (2019). Effects of microplastics on microalgae populations: A critical review. *The Science of the Total Environment*, *665*, 400–405. doi:10.1016/j.scitotenv.2019.02.132 PMID:30772570

Praveena, S. M., Shaifuddin, S. N. M., & Akizuki, S. (2018). Exploration of microplastics from personal care and cosmetic products and its estimated emissions to marine environment: An evidence from Malaysia. *Marine Pollution Bulletin*, *136*, 135–140. doi:10.1016/j.marpolbul.2018.09.012 PMID:30509794

Ragusa, A., Svelato, A., Santacroce, C., Catalano, P., Notarstefano, V., Carnevali, O., Papa, F., Rongioletti, M. C. A., Baiocco, F., Draghi, S., D'Amore, E., Rinaldo, D., Matta, M., & Giorgini, E. (2021). Plasticenta: First evidence of microplastics in human placenta. *Environment International*, *146*, 106274. doi:10.1016/j.envint.2020.106274 PMID:33395930

Reichert, J., Schellenberg, J., Schubert, P., & Wilke, T. (2018). Responses of reef building corals to microplastic exposure. *Environmental Pollution*, *237*, 955–960. doi:10.1016/j.envpol.2017.11.006 PMID:29146203

Ribeiro, F., Garcia, A. R., Pereira, B. P., Fonseca, M., Mestre, N. C., Fonseca, T. G., Ilharco, L. M., & Bebianno, M. J. (2017). Microplastics effects in Scrobicularia plana. *Marine Pollution Bulletin*, *122*(1–2), 379–391. doi:10.1016/j.marpolbul.2017.06.078 PMID:28684108

Rillig, M. C., & Bonkowski, M. (2018). Microplastic and soil protists: A call for research. *Environmental Pollution, 241*, 1128–1131. doi:10.1016/j.envpol.2018.04.147 PMID:30029321

Rogers, K. L., Carreres-Calabuig, J. A., Gorokhova, E., & Posth, N. R. (2020). Micro-by-micro interactions: How microorganisms influence the fate of marine microplastics. *Limnology and Oceanography Letters, 5*(1), 18–36. doi:10.1002/lol2.10136

Romera-Castillo, C., Pinto, M., Langer, T. M., Álvarez-Salgado, X. A., & Herndl, G. J. (2018). Dissolved organic carbon leaching from plastics stimulates microbial activity in the ocean. *Nature Communications, 9*(1), 1–7. doi:10.103841467-018-03798-5 PMID:29651045

Rummel, C. D., Jahnke, A., Gorokhova, E., Kühnel, D., & Schmitt-Jansen, M. (2017). Impacts of biofilm formation on the fate and potential effects of microplastic in the aquatic environment. *Environmental Science & Technology Letters, 4*(7), 258–267. doi:10.1021/acs.estlett.7b00164

Sarasamma, S., Audira, G., Siregar, P., Malhotra, N., Lai, Y. H., Liang, S. T., Chen, J.-R., Chen, K. H.-C., & Hsiao, C. D. (2020). Nanoplastics cause neurobehavioral impairments, reproductive and oxidative damages, and biomarker responses in zebrafish: Throwing up alarms of wide spread health risk of exposure. *International Journal of Molecular Sciences, 21*(4), 1410. doi:10.3390/ijms21041410 PMID:32093039

Sarkar, D. J., Sarkar, S. D., Das, B. K., Manna, R. K., Behera, B. K., & Samanta, S. (2019). Spatial distribution of meso and microplastics in the sediments of river Ganga at eastern India. *The Science of the Total Environment, 694*, 133712. doi:10.1016/j.scitotenv.2019.133712 PMID:31400677

Savinelli, B., Fernández, T. V., Galasso, N. M., D'Anna, G., Pipitone, C., Prada, F., ... Musco, L. (2020). Microplastics impair the feeding performance of a Mediterranean habitat-forming coral. *Marine Environmental Research, 155*, 104887. doi:10.1016/j.marenvres.2020.104887 PMID:32072989

Scanes, E., Wood, H., & Ross, P. (2019). Microplastics detected in haemolymph of the Sydney rock oyster Saccostrea glomerata. *Marine Pollution Bulletin, 149*, 110537. doi:10.1016/j.marpolbul.2019.110537 PMID:31466014

Schirinzi, G. F., Pérez-Pomeda, I., Sanchís, J., Rossini, C., Farré, M., & Barceló, D. (2017). Cytotoxic effects of commonly used nanomaterials and microplastics on cerebral and epithelial human cells. *Environmental Research, 159*, 579–587. doi:10.1016/j.envres.2017.08.043 PMID:28898803

Seeley, M. E., Song, B., Passie, R., & Hale, R. C. (2020). Microplastics affect sedimentary microbial communities and nitrogen cycling. *Nature Communications, 11*(1), 1–10. doi:10.103841467-020-16235-3 PMID:32398678

Setälä, O., Fleming-Lehtinen, V., & Lehtiniemi, M. (2014). Ingestion and transfer of microplastics in the planktonic food web. *Environmental Pollution, 185*, 77–83. doi:10.1016/j.envpol.2013.10.013 PMID:24220023

Siegfried, M., Koelmans, A. A., Besseling, E., & Kroeze, C. (2017). Export of microplastics from land to sea. A modelling approach. *Water Research, 127*, 249–257. doi:10.1016/j.watres.2017.10.011 PMID:29059612

Sjollema, S. B., Redondo-Hasselerharm, P., Leslie, H. A., Kraak, M. H., & Vethaak, A. D. (2016). Do plastic particles affect microalgal photosynthesis and growth? *Aquatic Toxicology (Amsterdam, Netherlands)*, *170*, 259–261. doi:10.1016/j.aquatox.2015.12.002 PMID:26675372

Song, Y. K., Hong, S. H., Eo, S., Jang, M., Han, G. M., Isobe, A., & Shim, W. J. (2018). Horizontal and vertical distribution of microplastics in Korean coastal waters. *Environmental Science & Technology*, *52*(21), 12188–12197. doi:10.1021/acs.est.8b04032 PMID:30295469

Sun, Y., Yuan, J., Zhou, T., Zhao, Y., Yu, F., & Ma, J. (2020). Laboratory simulation of microplastics weathering and its adsorption behaviors in an aqueous environment: A systematic review. *Environmental Pollution*, *265*, 114864. doi:10.1016/j.envpol.2020.114864 PMID:32505960

Talvitie, J., Mikola, A., Koistinen, A., & Setälä, O. (2017). Solutions to microplastic pollution–Removal of microplastics from wastewater effluent with advanced wastewater treatment technologies. *Water Research*, *123*, 401–407. doi:10.1016/j.watres.2017.07.005 PMID:28686942

Tang, N., Liu, X., & Xing, W. (2020). Microplastics in wastewater treatment plants of Wuhan, Central China: Abundance, removal, and potential source in household wastewater. *The Science of the Total Environment*, *745*, 141026. doi:10.1016/j.scitotenv.2020.141026 PMID:32726699

Tang, Y., Liu, Y., Chen, Y., Zhang, W., Zhao, J., He, S., Yang, C., Zhang, T., Tang, C., Zhang, C., & Yang, Z. (2021). A review: Research progress on microplastic pollutants in aquatic environments. *The Science of the Total Environment*, *766*, 142572. doi:10.1016/j.scitotenv.2020.142572 PMID:33183825

Ter Halle, A., Ladirat, L., Martignac, M., Mingotaud, A. F., Boyron, O., & Perez, E. (2017). To what extent are microplastics from the open ocean weathered? *Environmental Pollution*, *227*, 167–174. doi:10.1016/j.envpol.2017.04.051 PMID:28460234

Trifuoggi, M., Pagano, G., Oral, R., Pavičić-Hamer, D., Burić, P., Kovačić, I., Siciliano, A., Toscanesi, M., Thomas, P. J., Paduano, L., Guida, M., & Lyons, D. M. (2019). Microplastic-induced damage in early embryonal development of sea urchin Sphaerechinus granularis. *Environmental Research*, *179*, 108815. doi:10.1016/j.envres.2019.108815 PMID:31629182

Uheida, A., Mejía, H. G., Abdel-Rehim, M., Hamd, W., & Dutta, J. (2021). Visible light photocatalytic degradation of polypropylene microplastics in a continuous water flow system. *Journal of Hazardous Materials*, *406*, 124299. doi:10.1016/j.jhazmat.2020.124299 PMID:33131945

Van Cauwenberghe, L., & Janssen, C. R. (2014). Microplastics in bivalves cultured for human consumption. *Environmental Pollution*, *193*, 65–70. doi:10.1016/j.envpol.2014.06.010 PMID:25005888

Van Colen, C., Vanhove, B., Diem, A., & Moens, T. (2020). Does microplastic ingestion by zooplankton affect predator-prey interactions? An experimental study on larviphagy. *Environmental Pollution*, *256*, 113479. doi:10.1016/j.envpol.2019.113479 PMID:31679869

Van Melkebeke, M., Janssen, C., & De Meester, S. (2020). Characteristics and sinking behavior of typical microplastics including the potential effect of biofouling: Implications for remediation. *Environmental Science & Technology*, *54*(14), 8668–8680. doi:10.1021/acs.est.9b07378 PMID:32551546

Van Sebille, E., Wilcox, C., Lebreton, L., Maximenko, N., Hardesty, B. D., Van Franeker, J. A., Eriksen, M., Siegel, D., Galgani, F., & Law, K. L. (2015). A global inventory of small floating plastic debris. *Environmental Research Letters*, *10*(12), 124006. doi:10.1088/1748-9326/10/12/124006

Vanapalli, K. R., Dubey, B. K., Sarmah, A. K., & Bhattacharya, J. (2021). Assessment of microplastic pollution in the aquatic ecosystems–An indian perspective. *Case Studies in Chemical and Environmental Engineering*, *3*, 100071. doi:10.1016/j.cscee.2020.100071

Vecchi, S., Bianchi, J., Scalici, M., Fabroni, F., & Tomassetti, P. (2021). Field evidence for microplastic interactions in marine benthic invertebrates. *Scientific Reports*, *11*(1), 1–12. doi:10.103841598-021-00292-9 PMID:34686714

Walkinshaw, C., Lindeque, P. K., Thompson, R., Tolhurst, T., & Cole, M. (2020). Microplastics and seafood: Lower trophic organisms at highest risk of contamination. *Ecotoxicology and Environmental Safety*, *190*, 110066. doi:10.1016/j.ecoenv.2019.110066 PMID:31846861

Wang, C., Zhao, J., & Xing, B. (2021). Environmental source, fate, and toxicity of microplastics. *Journal of Hazardous Materials*, *407*, 124357. doi:10.1016/j.jhazmat.2020.124357 PMID:33158648

Wang, J., Li, Y., Lu, L., Zheng, M., Zhang, X., Tian, H., Wang, W., & Ru, S. (2019). Polystyrene microplastics cause tissue damages, sex-specific reproductive disruption and transgenerational effects in marine medaka (Oryzias melastigma). *Environmental Pollution*, *254*, 113024. doi:10.1016/j.envpol.2019.113024 PMID:31454586

Wang, W., Ndungu, A. W., Li, Z., & Wang, J. (2017). Microplastics pollution in inland freshwaters of China: A case study in urban surface waters of Wuhan, China. *The Science of the Total Environment*, *575*, 1369–1374. doi:10.1016/j.scitotenv.2016.09.213 PMID:27693147

Weber, A., Jeckel, N., Weil, C., Umbach, S., Brennholt, N., Reifferscheid, G., & Wagner, M. (2021). Ingestion and toxicity of polystyrene microplastics in freshwater bivalves. *Environmental Toxicology and Chemistry*, *40*(8), 2247–2260. doi:10.1002/etc.5076 PMID:33928672

Xiong, X., Wu, C., Elser, J. J., Mei, Z., & Hao, Y. (2019). Occurrence and fate of microplastic debris in middle and lower reaches of the Yangtze River–from inland to the sea. *The Science of the Total Environment*, *659*, 66–73. doi:10.1016/j.scitotenv.2018.12.313 PMID:30597469

Yang, L., Li, K., Cui, S., Kang, Y., An, L., & Lei, K. (2019). Removal of microplastics in municipal sewage from China's largest water reclamation plant. *Water Research*, *155*, 175–181. doi:10.1016/j.watres.2019.02.046 PMID:30849731

Ye, S., & Andrady, A. L. (1991). Fouling of floating plastic debris under Biscayne Bay exposure conditions. *Marine Pollution Bulletin*, *22*(12), 608–613. doi:10.1016/0025-326X(91)90249-R

Yee, M. S. L., Hii, L. W., Looi, C. K., Lim, W. M., Wong, S. F., Kok, Y. Y., Tan, B.-K., Wong, C.-Y., & Leong, C. O. (2021). Impact of microplastics and nanoplastics on human health. *Nanomaterials (Basel, Switzerland)*, *11*(2), 496. doi:10.3390/nano11020496 PMID:33669327

Yurtsever, M. (2019). Glitters as a source of primary microplastics: An approach to environmental responsibility and ethics. *Journal of Agricultural & Environmental Ethics*, *32*(3), 459–478. doi:10.100710806-019-09785-0

Zhang, C., Chen, X., Wang, J., & Tan, L. (2017). Toxic effects of microplastic on marine microalgae Skeletonema costatum: Interactions between microplastic and algae. *Environmental Pollution*, *220*, 1282–1288. doi:10.1016/j.envpol.2016.11.005 PMID:27876228

Zhang, C., Zhou, H., Cui, Y., Wang, C., Li, Y., & Zhang, D. (2019). Microplastics in offshore sediment in the yellow Sea and east China Sea, China. *Environmental Pollution*, *244*, 827–833. doi:10.1016/j.envpol.2018.10.102 PMID:30390456

Zhang, Y., Wang, J., Geng, X., & Jiang, Y. (2021). Does microplastic ingestion dramatically decrease the biomass of protozoa grazers? A case study on the marine ciliate Uronema marinum. *Chemosphere*, *267*, 129308. doi:10.1016/j.chemosphere.2020.129308 PMID:33352364

Zhao, Y. B., Gao, P. P., & Ni, H. G. (2019). A chemical time bomb: Future risks of microplastics. *Water, Air, and Soil Pollution*, *230*(11), 1–5. doi:10.100711270-019-4320-9

Zheng, Y., Li, J., Cao, W., Liu, X., Jiang, F., Ding, J., Yin, X., & Sun, C. (2019). Distribution characteristics of microplastics in the seawater and sediment: A case study in Jiaozhou Bay, China. *The Science of the Total Environment*, *674*, 27–35. doi:10.1016/j.scitotenv.2019.04.008 PMID:31003085

Zhu, J., Yu, X., Zhang, Q., Li, Y., Tan, S., Li, D., Yang, Z., & Wang, J. (2019). Cetaceans and microplastics: First report of microplastic ingestion by a coastal delphinid, Sousa chinensis. *The Science of the Total Environment*, *659*, 649–654. doi:10.1016/j.scitotenv.2018.12.389 PMID:31096394

Chapter 11
Development of Bioplastic and Biodegradable Plastics

Nitai Charan Giri
https://orcid.org/0000-0002-0476-840X
Central Institute of Petrochemical Engineering and Technology, India

Vishal Verma
Central Institute of Petrochemical Engineering and Technology, India

Bhanja Prasad Patro
Central Institute of Petrochemical Engineering and Technology, India

ABSTRACT

Plastics are one of the essential materials due to their low cost and properties. Plastics are used almost everywhere including food packaging, home appliance, agriculture, automobile, electrical insulators, medical instruments, etc. However, due to the low biodegradability of conventional plastics, they remain in the environment for a very long time and thus pose a serious threat to our environment. Getting rid of these plastics is very difficult. The burning of plastics produces harmful chemicals that negatively impact the environment (e.g., global warming) and human health. Plastic management via recycling is an incomplete measure to address the environmental impacts of plastic. Therefore, there is a demand for developing alternative plastic materials that will be more environmentally friendly. Bioplastics have attracted much attention as a potential replacement for conventional plastics. This chapter will focus on the development, properties, and applications of various bioplastics. The biodegradability of the bioplastics will also be discussed.

INTRODUCTION

Plastics are ubiquitous in our society. It is estimated that 407 million tons of plastic were produced in 2018. (Sushmitha et al., 2016) Only 7% of this is recycled, and the rest is dumped into ocean and land-

DOI: 10.4018/978-1-7998-9723-1.ch011

Figure 1. Various bio-based and biodegradable plastics

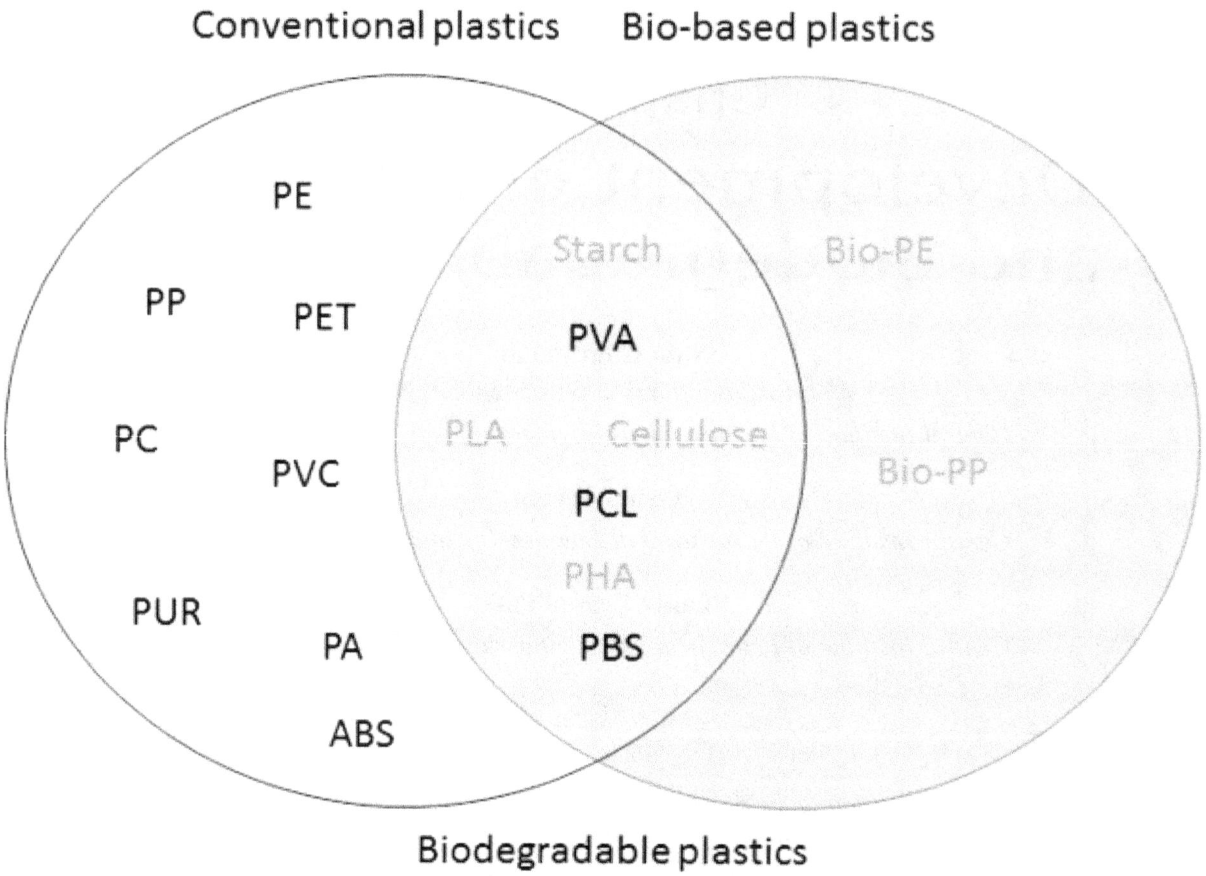

fills. Conventional plastics degrade very slowly, (DiGregorio, 2009) and remain in the environment for a very long time. Thus, these plastics pose a serious threat to

freshwater, natural terrestrial, and marine ecosystems. Bioplastic has attracted much attention as a potential replacement for conventional plastics. The increased interest is due to several advantages of bioplastic over conventional plastics. One advantage is their biodegradability. For example, bioplastic such as polyhydroxyalkanoate (PHA) has been shown to be completely biodegradable. (Eubeler et al., 2010) Other advantages include their adaptability to the human body, reduced reliance on fossil fuel, etc. Bioplastics can be bio-based and made from biomass and renewable resources such as corn starch, potato starch, rice straw, vegetable oil and fat, etc. However, all bio-based plastics are not biodegradable (Figure 1) such as bio-based-polyethylene (Bio-PE), bio-based-polypropylene (Bio-PP), etc. The rate of biodegradation depends on the bioplastics. Thus, bio-based and biodegradable plastics include polylactic acid (PLA), (Auras et al., 2004) PHA, (Liu et al., 2010) cellulose, (Privas et al., 2013) starch, etc. (Mostafa et al., 2014) It is worth mentioning that starch, cellulose, etc. are not plastics in their native form. However, they can be converted to plastic through innovative fermentation and polymer technology. Moreover, some protein-rich sources such as soy, (Alvarez-Castillo et al., 2018) wheat, (Jerez et al., 2005) pea (Perez-Puyana et al., 2016) have also been used for making bioplastic materials and films. Several bioplastic materials such as PHA, cellulose, starch, etc., have been used in food packaging. Bioplastics also have great potential application in the textile industry. However, there are some challenges to the growth of the bioplastic market. These include interference with food sources and high production costs. The issue with interference with food sources can be addressed by using non-food resources. Also, different biological alternatives such as bioplastic production from microalgae consortia has been reported. (López Rocha et al., 2020) Much research is being done to optimize the production and make bioplastic economically viable. This chapter will focus on the development, properties, and applications of various bioplastics. The biodegradability of the bioplastics will also be discussed.

BACKGROUND

Plant-based biodegradable plastics are often considered with zero or negative carbon footprint. (Filiciotto & Rothenberg, 2021) The global warming potential of biodegradable mulch films is 2-3 times lower than landfill and incineration. (Razza & Cerutti, 2017) Composting and anaerobic processing have a higher environmental impact than incineration with energy recovery. (Yates & Barlow, 2013) The variability of the results reflects the difficulty in determining the environmental impact of biodegradable plastics. However, a significant reduction of the carbon footprint is commonly recognized for bio-plastics compared to conventional plastics. Most of today's bio-based plastics are made from food crops. The feedstocks used for producing biodegradable plastics will impact the environment due to the use of water and land. According to European Bioplastics, the land required for biomaterials (also including materials other than plastic such as biofuel) is 2% of the overall land use. (Filiciotto & Rothenberg, 2021) The land use for plastic represent only 0.016% in 2019. (Filiciotto & Rothenberg, 2021) The land use for biofuel, on the other hand, is 60 times higher. One of the sustainable development goals (UN: SDG 15) is to have zero net lands taken by 2050 to favor natural habitats and improve agricultural practices. (United Nations, 2020) Thus, the use of waste products may provide an alternative that has zero impact land use. According to the UN FAO, one-third of all food resources were wasted worldwide. (Ishangulyyev et al., 2019) Converting waste into plastic creates product value from zero, which is economically very attractive. (Sanchez-Vazquez et al., 2013)

One of the major challenges in plastic is waste management. Especially, sorting different waste and the presence of hazardous materials are challenges in the present recycling effort. (Didier [2015)] ~45-75% of plastics are disposed of in landfills or natural environment. (Agamuthu, 2013) Most plastics in landfill are likely to leach into the environment and create microplastics. The high mobility of microplastic leads to water contamination, affecting human and animal health. (Prata et al., 2020) Thus, environmental analysis should consider the potential release of microplastic. Also, the molecules making the polymer have a significant impact on life and environment. For example, PVC was found to be more harmful than high-density polyethylene and PLA. This can be attributed to the toxicity of halogen-containing molecules. Therefore, plastics made from safer molecules will have a lower effect on life and environment. The degradation of biodegradable plastic was found to be much slower in turtles compared to the claimed biodegradability. 100% biodegradability resulted in the degradation of up to 8.5% in the turtle's digestive tract. (Filiciotto & Rothenberg, 2021) However, biodegradable plastics will still have an undeniably positive impact on uses where the material is prone to enter the environment.

The global bioplastic production was 2.11 million tons in 2019. (Jõgi & Bhat, 2020) Starch blends were the most common type of bioplastic (Table 1). Starch blends will continue to be the most common

Table 1. Global bioplastic production in 2019 and projection for 2024

Bioplastic type	2019 (%)	2024 (%)
Starch blends	21.3	18.5
PLA	13.9	13.1
PBAT	13.4	12.5
PE*	11.8	12
PA*	11.6	11.6
PET	9.8	8
PTT	9.2	6.6
PBS	4.3	6
Other (biodegradable)	1.4	5.3
PHA	1.2	3.8
Other (bio-based, non-biodegradable)*	1.1	1.3
PP*	0.9	0.9
PEF*	0	0.2
* indicates bio-based, but not biodegradable		

type of bioplastics in the coming years (Table 1). Plastic materials such as polyethylene furanoate (PEF) are expected to enter the bioplastic market soon. In 2019, biodegradable plastics accounted for 55.5% of bioplastics produced. In terms of bioplastic production, Asia led the way with 45% of bioplastics produced, followed by Europe (25%), North America (18%), and South America (12%). (Jõgi & Bhat, 2020)

The lack of consistent data on the biodegradability of different plastics hinders finding a clear correlation between physicochemical properties and biodegradation, hence the final fate of plastic materials. Often, literature studies focus on monitoring one change (e.g., change of structure by FTIR) or only report the evolution of CO_2, hindering the creation of a database. A complete database can predict the biodegradation of new plastic material or aid in designing biodegradable plastic materials. Future studies may correlate repeating unit, elemental analysis, physical properties (such as T_g and T_m) with biodegradability. Kinetic studies on biodegradability may also provide helpful information for comparing new plastic materials.

SOURCES OF BIOPLASTICS

1. **Plant sources:** Plant sources include starch-based sources such as wheat, corn, starch, rice, potato, barley, and cellulose derivatives which account for almost 80% of the bioplastic market. Pure starch can absorb humidity which makes it a suitable material for manufacturing drug capsules. Cane sugar is also used for the manufacture of bioplastic such as PLA. Genetic engineering is utilized in plants (e.g., genetically modified corn and potato) to produce bioplastic in plants. However, interference with food sources is one of the limitations in bioplastic production from plant sources. Recently, bioplastic films have been made from low-cost plant resources such as jackfruit waste flour and sago (low-cost starch source). (Krishnamurthy & Amritkumar, 2019) Using starch as a renewable source

Figure 2. Bacterial production of polyhydroxybutyrate (PHB)

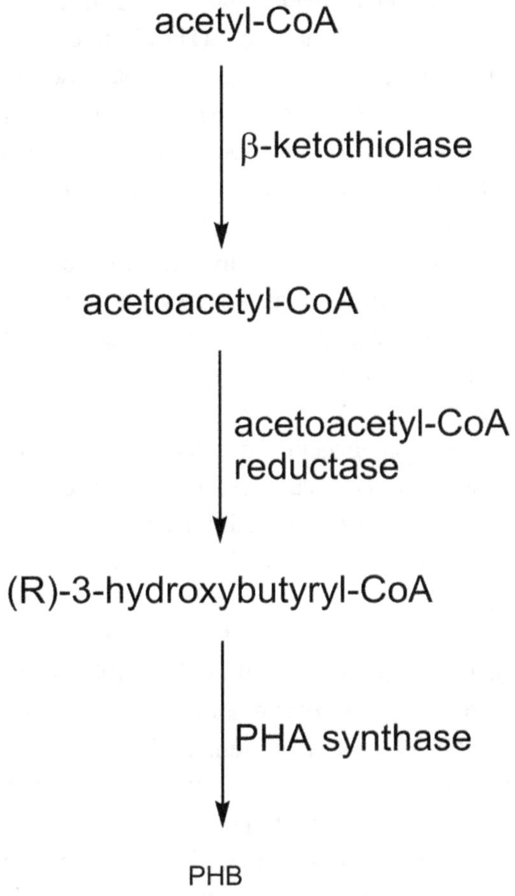

for bioplastic production has several advantages, such as low cost and abundance. However, starch in its native form has very limited application due to poor solubility, thermal decomposition, low shear stress resistance, brittleness, etc. (BeMiller & Whistler, 2009; Kalambur & Rizvi, 2006) Also, the mechanical property worsen upon exposure to environmental conditions (e.g., humidity leads to hydrolysis). However, some of these properties can be improved by using suitable plasticizers such as sugar glycerol, glycol, xylitol, and amides (e.g., urea, formamide, etc.). (Yang et al., 2006; Dai et al., 2009) Zinc nanofillers and glycerol have been added to starch-based bioplastic film to improve mechanical properties. (Harunsyah et al., 2017) Starch-based bioplastics were also reinforced by coconut husk fibers. (Babalola & Olorunnisola, 2019) Glass and carbon fibers are commonly used to reinforce bioplastics. However, these are not biodegradable. For this reason, these have been replaced by more environmentally friendly materials. (Yang et al., 2019) Apart from plasticizers and fillers, starch can also be blended with other synthetic polymers to improve mechanical properties and the rate of degradation. Other physical strengthening methods are mold temperature increase, dehydrothermal treatment, ultrasound, etc. (JIminez-Rosado et al., 2020) Thermal treatment of soy protein-based bioplastics enhanced mechanical properties. Its dehydrothermal treatment increased absorbent capacity, while ultrasound led to structure with smaller pores. Thus, differently treated bioplastics will have different applications. Fine smooth, flexible, and strong bioplastic was produced from tapioca starch. (Gokce, 2018) However, potato-based starch showed better properties in terms of ease of working (e.g., extraction, crying, etc.). (Hamidon et al., 2018) Ultrasound treatment of composite bioplastic from tapioca starch and sugarcane bagasse fiber improved properties such as tensile strength and a lower rate of moisture absorption. (Asrofi et al., 2020) Proteins (e.g., wheat gluten, soy, etc.) have been used to produce bioplastic. (Rasheed, 2011) Oil can also be used for the production of bioplastics. (Magar et al., 2015) Cottonseed oil, soybean oil, jatropha oil, palm oil, corn oil, coconut oil, etc., have been investigated. (Park and Kim, 2011; Wong et al., 2012) Ligninocellulosic biomass is another good resource for bioplastic production. (Brodin et al., 2017) This process avoids the utilization of food crops. However, it requires suitable, cost-effective pre-treatment for decomposition into sugar monomer. (Govil et al., 2020)

2. **Bacterial sources:** Some of the important bacterial species used for the production of PHA are B. Megaterium, (Mirtha et al., 1995) K. Aerogenes, (Eggink et al., 1995) and P. Aerogenosa. (Zhang et al., 1994) During metabolism, bacteria produce acetyl CoA, which is converted to PHB by three biosynthesis enzymes – 3-ketothiolase, acetoacetyl CoA reductase, and PHA synthase (Figure 2). Sugarcane has been used for bioplastic production by bacterial sugar assimilation. However, one limitation for bacterial production of bioplastic is that optimum bacterial growth requires specific conditions.
3. **Algal sources:** Algae are autotrophic organisms that can be unicellular or multicellular. Compared with bioplastics production from food staples, microalgae offer an advantage due to the high percentage of carbohydrates and proteins, fast growth, and no competition with food. (Wang et al., 2016) For example, spirulina has 46-63% protein content, and chlorella has 51-58% protein content (on a dry weight basis). (Ummanyma et al., 2020) Thus, these two are the most investigated microalgae. Microalgae can be used directly as biomass to produce bioplastics or indirectly by extracting PHB and starch within microalgae cells. (Coppola et al., 2021) Other approaches include the production of microalgae polymer blends through compression or hot molding, solvent casting, melt mixing, or twin-screw extrusion. (Cinnar et al., 2020) A bioplastic film was produced from salt-rich spirulina species residues with the addition of polyvinyl alcohol. (Zhang et al., 2020) Several microalgae were screened for starch production and starch-based bioplastic development. (Mathiot et al., 2019) C. reinhardtii was the most promising starch-producing strain. Composites were formed by combing microalgal biomass and petroleum. (Chia et al., 2020) Leftover biomass after biodiesel production can also be treated chemically to produce bioplastic. (Das et al., 2018) However, microalgae cannot be easily harvested. (Thurmund, 2010) Thus, macroalgae like seaweeds are better options for bioplastic production considering their high biomass, ability to grow in many different environments, and ease of harvesting. Seaweeds are photosynthetic algae that live in the bottom of the sea and are well known for natural polysaccharides. These polysaccharides can be extracted from seaweeds and used to produce bioplastic. The whole red macroalgae Kappaphycus alvarezzi was used to produce a bioplastic film adding polyethylene glycol as a plasticizer for food packaging applications. (Sudhakar et al., 2020) Since they are polymers made from sugars, they can be used to produce biodegradable plastics.

Figure 3. Polymer production via the fermentation of sugar

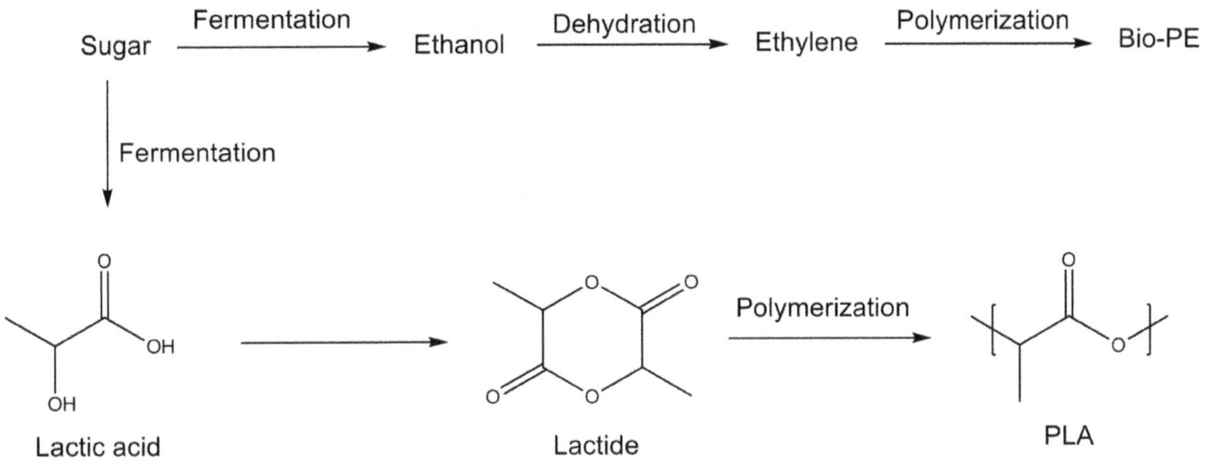

PRODUCTION OF BIOPLASTICS

1. **Bioplastic production from seaweed:** Polysaccharides such as starch, alginate, agar, carrageenan, floridean, etc., in seaweeds are used to produce bioplastic. (Rajendran et al., 2012) The seaweed is gathered, quickly dried, and then baled to maintain its quality. The dried seaweed is ground, sieved, and washed to eliminate impurities such as sand, salt, etc. Then, seaweed is subjected to a hot extraction process to separate the polysaccharides. This extraction process involves two steps. In the first step, the dissolved polysaccharide
mixture is centrifuged to eliminate the dense cellulosic particles. The smaller particles are removed by filtration. Then the solution is concentrated by evaporating water. In the second step, polysaccharides are recovered using one of the two methods. In one method, KCl is added to the concentrated solution of polysaccharide so that the filtrate will gel immediately. The gel is then frozen and compressed to remove excess water. In the second method, the concentrated solution is precipitated in isopropyl alcohol. The filtrate turns into a coagulum of polysaccharide alcohol and water. The coagulum is compressed to remove excess liquid and vacuum dried to remove the alcohol. Drying is completed in a belt drier and is blended to meet the specification of the finished product.
2. **Fermentation of sugar:** Polysaccharides can be converted to sugar (e.g., glucose, xylose, etc.) chemically or enzymatically. Fermentation of the sugar leads to lactic acid, ethanol, etc. This process can be carried out at room temperature and pressure using water as a solvent. However, sugars are derived from crops that compete with food sources. Thus, the development of lignocellulosic sugar processes will enhance the sustainability of this process. Lactic acid can be chemically converted to lactide(Figure 3).
PLA can be obtained by condensation polymerization of lactic acid or by the ring-opening polymerization of lactide. (Lim et al., 2008)
PLA is a thermoplastic and can be converted to end products using techniques such as injection moulding, blow moulding, film extrusion, etc. The processing temperature of PLA is low compared to conventional plastics. PLA can be used in a wide range of applications including, geotextile,

Figure 4. Different types of PHA

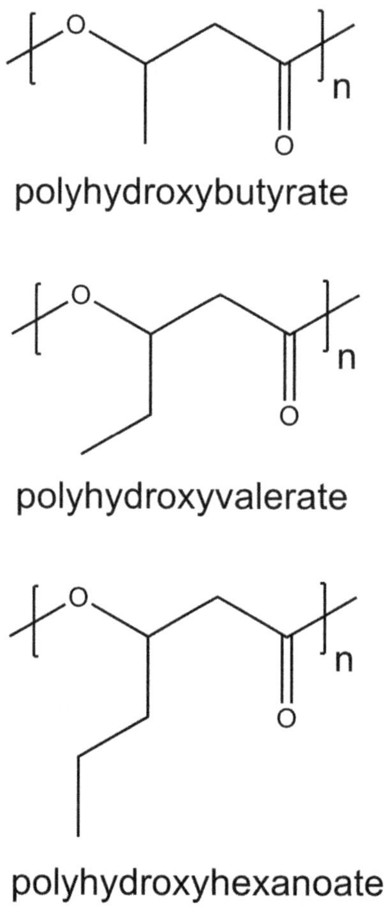

agricultural film, packaging, etc. Since it is compatible with the human body, it has been used in medical devices. (Lasprilla et al., 2012; Auras et al., 2004)

In this process, bio-PE can also be prepared. Bio-PE can be prepared from the polymerization of ethylene which can be prepared from ethanol (Figure 3). Ethanol represents a chemically identical alternative to ethylene production from petrochemical feedstocks. However, the production of ethylene from sugar-based ethanol needs further optimization. The most developed production routes of ethanol are the fermentation of sucrose and hydrolysis, followed by fermentation of starchy biomass. The dehydration of ethanol to ethylene is an established and commercial technology. It is based on dehydration of preheated blend of ethanol and water (1:1 M) at 350 °C and 5 bar. Further cooling and compression of the gas stream in a fractionating column lead to ethylene recovery. The final product contains 99.99% ethylene by weight. (Haro et al., 2013) Lignocellulosic biomass can also be used for Bio-PE production. However, the conversion of biomass to ethanol is more costly. This limits the use of lignocellulosic bio-ethanol for the production of bioplastic and emphasizes the need for more research and development in this area.

It is worth mentioning that bioethanol production decides the production cost of bioethylene. Thus, the origin of bioethanol is crucial. The cost of petrochemical ethylene is around $ 600-1300 per

Figure 5. Liquefaction of lignocellulosic biomass

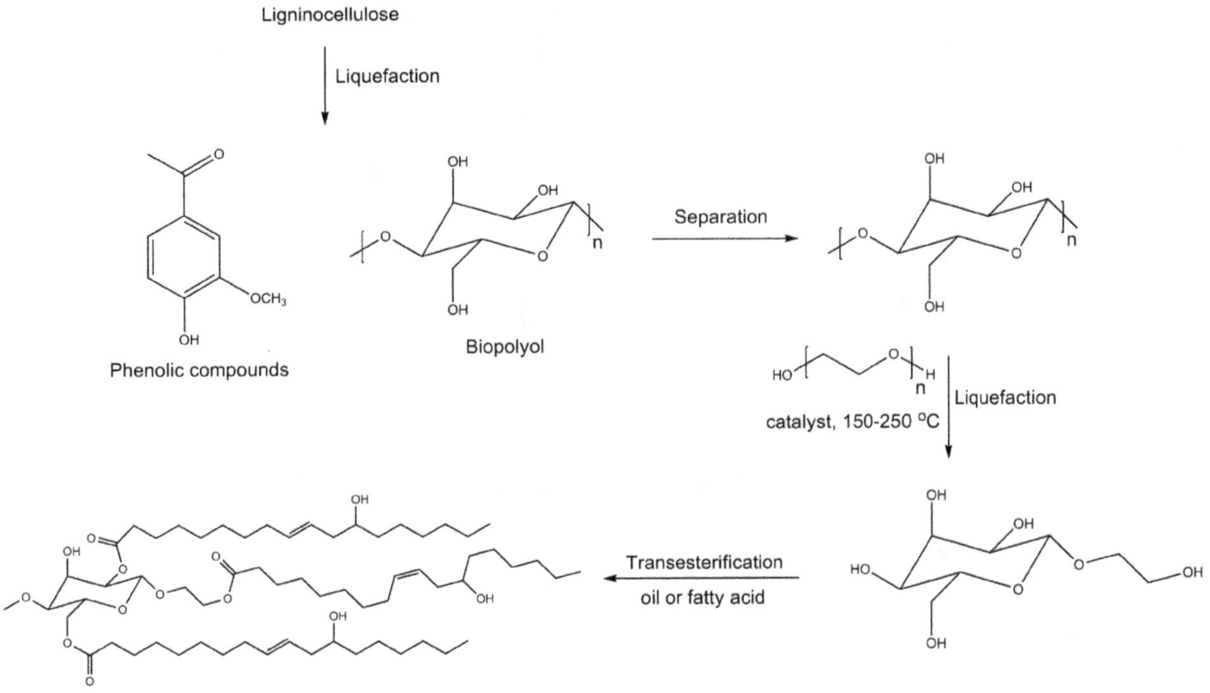

Figure 6. Oxyprolylation of lignocellulosic material

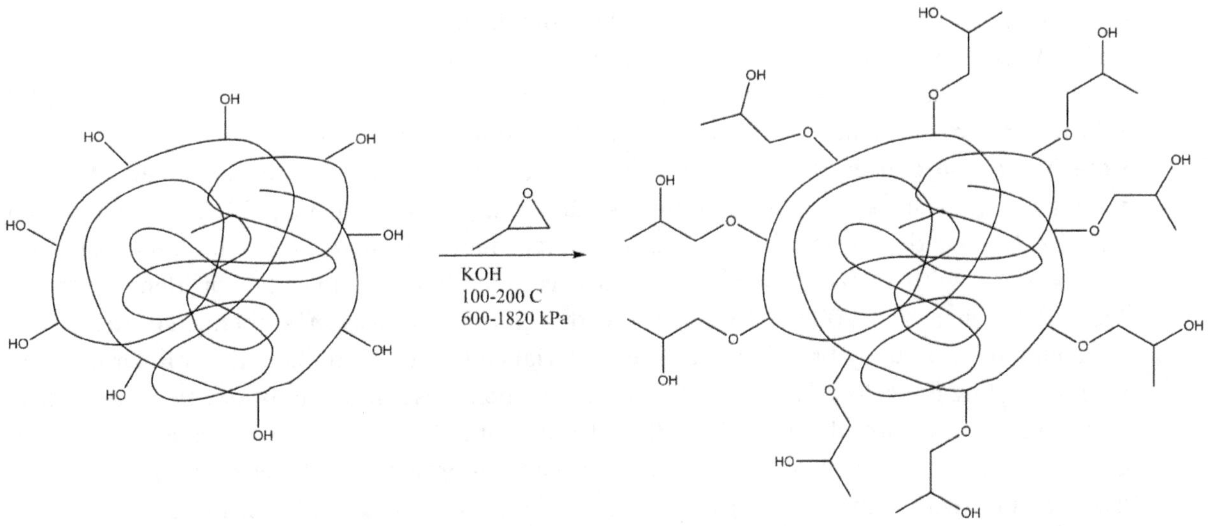

Figure 7. Synthesis of isocyanates for PUR production

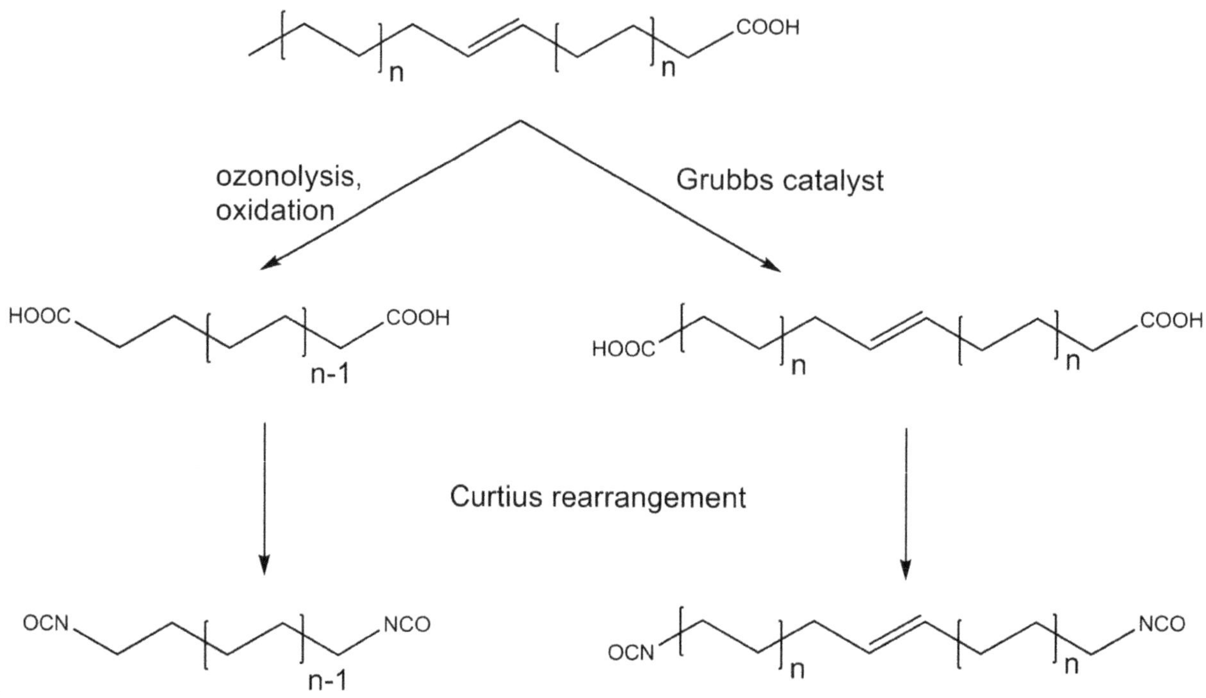

ton. The production cost of sugarcane ethylene in Brazil is about \$ 1200 per ton. (Brodin et al., 2017) Thus, Brazil can produce cost-competitive ethanol for ethylene production. This has been attributed to the cheap sugarcane feedstock, and their extensive experience in bioethanol production. (Broeren, 2013) According to a report by Nova-Institute, the production of 1Kg of Bio-PE and PLA requires 4 and 1.6 Kg of fermentable sugar, respectively. (Carus, 2016) From 1 ha of sugarcane, 2-3 and 6-7 tons of BIO-PE and PLA, respectively, can be produced. However, PLA and Bio-PE have different properties and, thus, have different applications.

3. **Biotechnological conversion:** In this way, bioplastics such as polyhydroxyalkanoate (PHA) is synthesized from sugar using different microorganisms. (Kawaguchi et al., 2016; Suriyamongkol et al., 2007) Depending on the choice of carbon source, microorganism, processing condition, additives, polymers with different characteristics such as crystallinity, chain length, brittleness, etc., are obtained. (Keenan et al., 2006) PHA granules with significant purity can be obtained from bacterial fermentation followed by breaking open the bacterial cells and solubilizing the cellular material. After separating the cells from the broth, the enzymatic digestion (using lysozyme, exonuclease, proteinases, etc.) is carried out to release the intracellular PHA granules. (Wang et al., 2014) High purity PHA can be obtained by solvent extraction using chloroform, methylene chloride, etc. 2006) PHA granules with significant purity can be obtained from bacterial fermentation followed by breaking open the bacterial cells and solubilizing the cellular material. After separating the cells from the broth, the enzymatic digestion (using lysozyme, exonuclease, proteinases, etc.) is carried out to release the intracellular PHA granules. (Wang et al., 2014) High purity PHA can be obtained by solvent extraction using chloroform, methylene chloride, etc.

Figure 8. Modification of cellulose

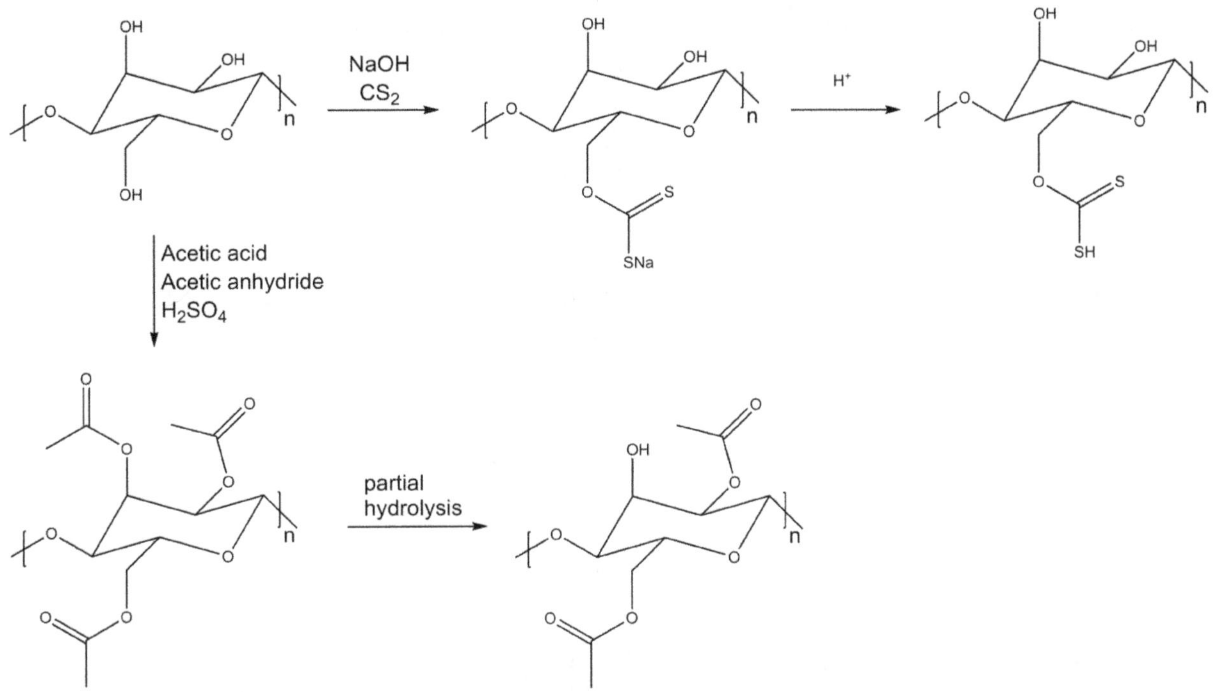

Like PLA, PHA can be thermoformed. Several companies are producing different types of PHA (Figure 4), including polyhydroxybutyrate (PHB), copolymer of the monomers R-3-hydroxyvalerate, and R-3-hydroxybutyrate. Applications of PHA include packaging, textile, and medical devices. However, PHA has not seen the wide application. (Chen, 2009) The main reason behind this is the high production cost of PHA. There is a possibility of using less costly feedstocks for PHA production. (Silva et al., 2007)

4. **Chemical conversion:** In this process, bioplastics like polyurethane (PUR) can be produced from lignin. Lignin is subjected to chemical modifications such as liquefaction (Kim et al., 2019; Wu et al., 2020) (Figure 5) and oxypropylation (Aniceto et al., 2012; Tenorio-Alfonso et al., 2020) (Figure 6) to produce polyols. Liquefaction is based on solvolysis of lignocellulosic biomass at 150-200 °C in the presence of polyhydric alcohols (e.g., ethylene or polyethylene glycol) as the liquefaction solvent and usually an acid catalyst. The resulting liquid is subjected to transesterification to produce natural polyester polyol. The solvolysis process increases both the functionality and sustainable nature of the starting polyols. Oxyproplynation can incorporate more readily available OH groups avoiding the utilization of any solvent while maintaining the biomass functionality. This process involves base-catalyzed grafting of propylene oxide onto lignocellulosic material under high pressure (650-1820 kPa) and temperature (100-200 °C). This process leads to the incorporation of the propylene oxide chain onto lignocellulosic biomass. Thus, the starting material is converted to a viscous polyol. Now polymerization can be carried out in the presence of isocyanate, catalyst (triethanol amine and dibutyltin dilaurate), blowing agent (water), and surfactant (polydimethyl siloxane). Much research has been done on developing bio-based PUR based on bio-based polyol and isocyanate, which come from petroleum resources. Recently isocyanates have been synthesized

Figure 9. Oxo-degradation of plastics

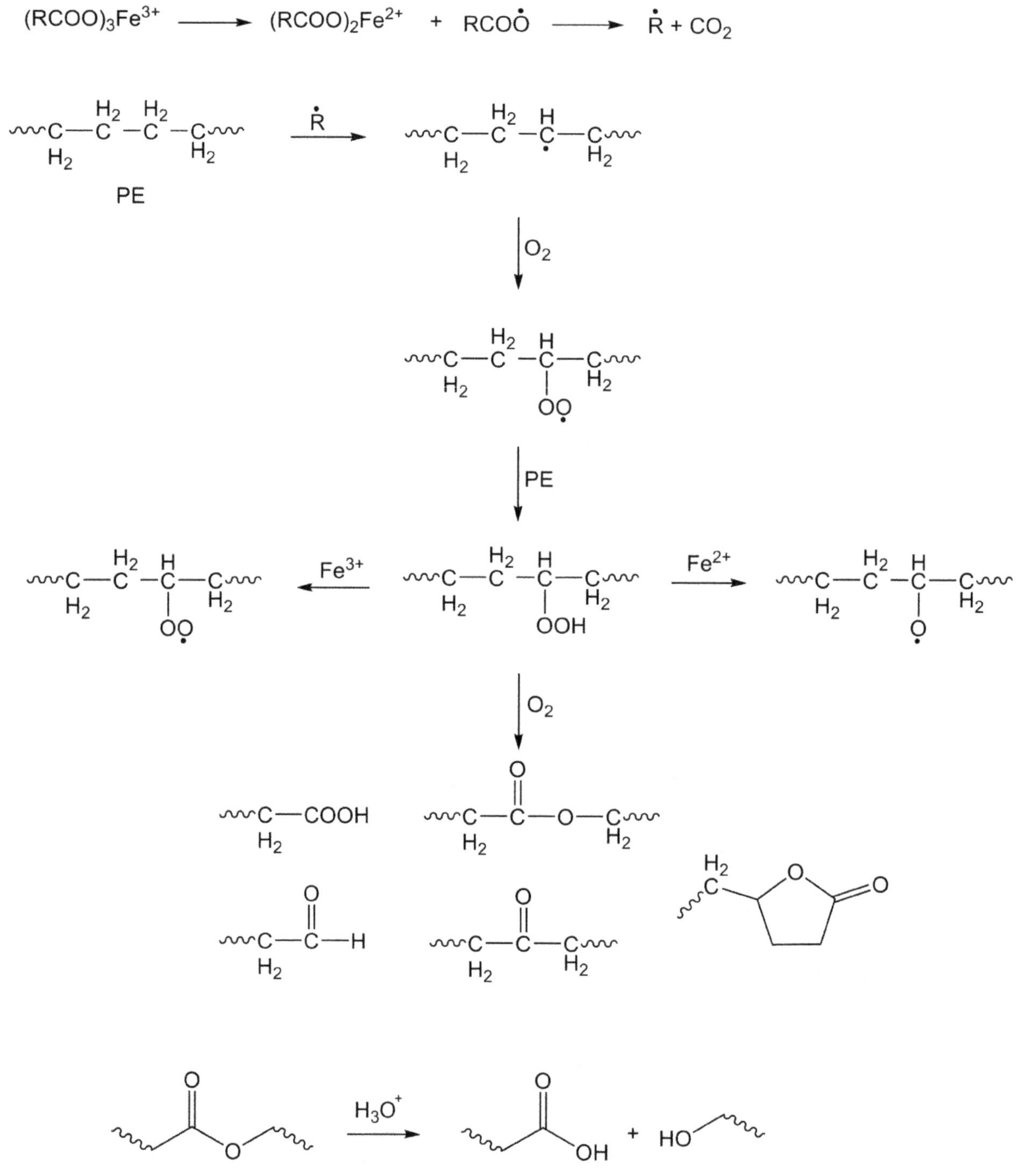

from natural feedstocks such as vegetable oil and fat. In one of these pathways, isocyanates have been obtained by treating diacids with sodium azide (Figure 7). (Hojabri et al., 2009) In another pathway, the bio-based isocyanate has been prepared using Grubbs catalyst (Figure 7). More recently, bio-based isocyanate has been produced from amino acids (L-lysine isocyanate) and fatty acids (dimeryldiisocyanate). (Morales-Cerrada et al., 2021) These bio-based polyurethanes do not show any cytotoxicity in vivo.

5. **Chemical modification:** In this process, bioplastics such as cellulose acetate can be prepared from polysaccharides. These polysaccharides can be shaped into films, for example, after dissolution. Cellulose films possess good strength, toughness, transparency, and surface gloss. (Yano et al., 2005) Also, cellulose is modified chemically during the dissolution process to ease the disintegration of the polymeric chain. For example, cellulose acetate is prepared by reacting with acetic anhydride in the presence of acetic acid (Figure 8). Cellulose acetate is optically transparent and is used as polarized films for liquid crystal displays, film base in photographic film, sunglass, etc. It is biodegradable since many microorganisms have acetyl esterase enzymes. (Puls et al., 2011) Cellulose Xanthate is produced by the reaction of cellulose with CS_2 in the presence of a base (Figure 8). (Paunonen, 2013) Films produced from cellulose xanthates are often used in food packaging.

PHYSICOCHEMICAL PROPERTIES AND BIODEGRADABILITY

Several physical and chemical properties influence biodegradability. The surface area of plastic material is proportional to its biodegradation. Hydrophilicity and hydrophobicity of plastic material also influence biodegradation. For example, biodegradation of petroleum-based plastics (e.g., PE) improves if the carboxylic acid group is introduced. (Gewert et al., 2015) Thus, biobased plastics containing heteroatoms will be more biodegradable. In fact, the presence of oxygen will improve the interaction with water and hence hydrolysis. (Okey & Stensel, 1996) Introduction of amine or amide group will also enhance biodegradability. (Ebbesen et al., 2016; Luo et al., 2011) However, the presence of halogen may decrease biodegradability due to their toxicity. (Boethling et al., 2007) Generally, the low reactivity of aliphatic groups is a barrier to biodegradability. However, UV light may lead to homolytic cleavage of the C-H bond, particularly in systems with conjugated bonds. However, the presence of conjugated alkene may lead to photo-initiated cross-linking rather than biodegradation. The presence of aromatic groups usually confers radical scavenging properties, which reduce biodegradability. The introduction of ester groups can improve the biodegradability of aromatic groups. (Shah et al., 2014) This is the case with PBAT. Other factors like crystallinity, molecular weight, etc., also influence biodegradability. For example, biodegradability decreases with increasing molecular weight. Some plastic materials, such as LDPE biodegrade faster due to their amorphous character. (Rudin & Choi, 2013) The crystalline/amorphous character is determined by branching. However, branching alone does not determine biodegradability.

BIODEGRADABILITY OF PLASTICS IN THE ENVIRONMENT

Plastics can end up in the environment with or without modification. (Horodytska et al., 2019) In 2013, 32% of the plastics produced (78 million tons) ended up in the environment. (Filiciotto & Rothenberg, 2021) The high amount of mismanaged plastic waste lead to the formation of microplastic that builds up in the environment. (Lebreton & Andrady, 2019) Major sources of microplastics are the wear and tear of automotive wheels, loss of plastic pellet during transport, washing of synthetic clothing, etc. However, the total weight of these microplastic is very small compared to global plastic production. Also,

Figure 10. Biodegradation of PET

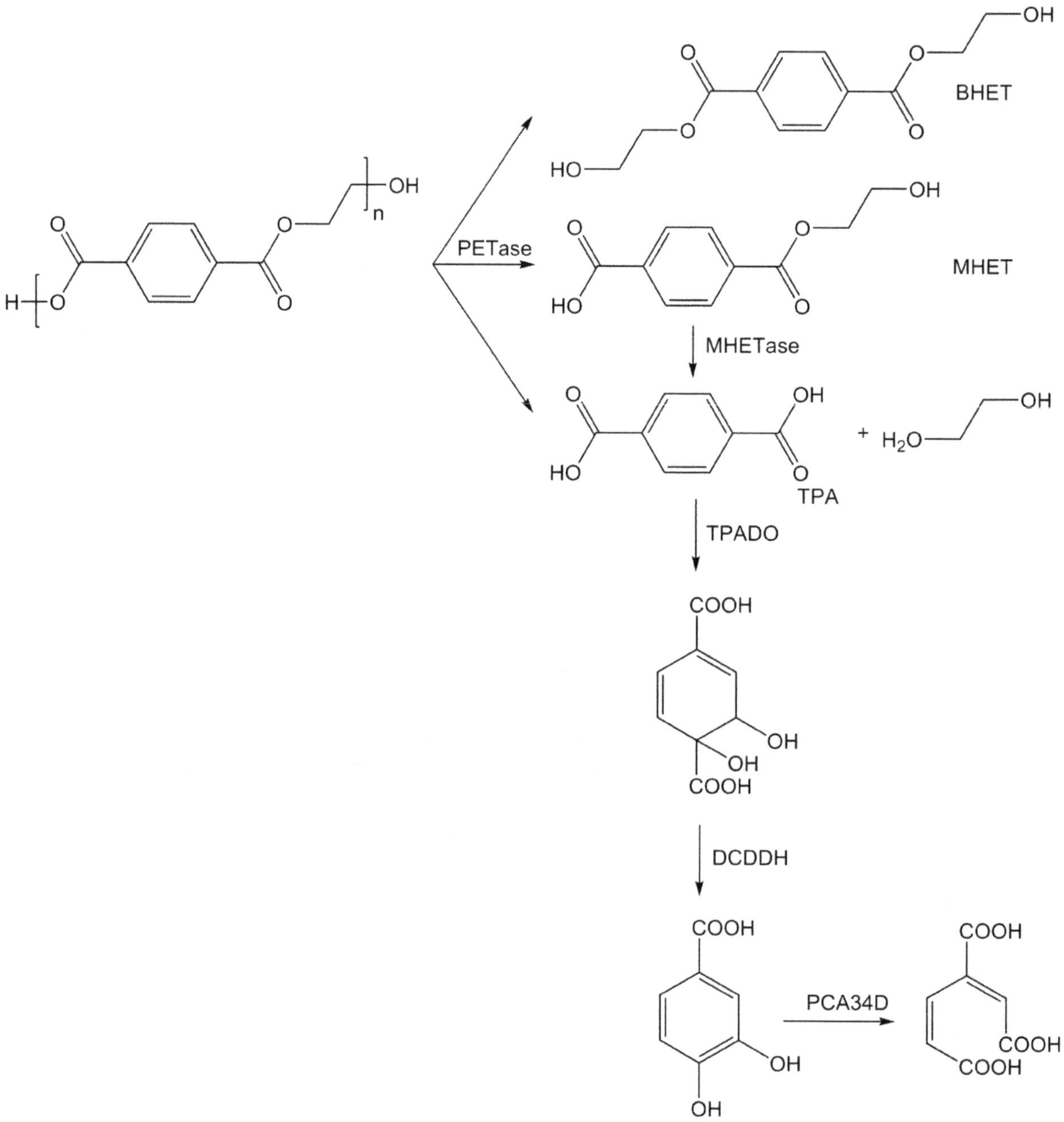

the dynamic nature of our environment causes various ecosystems to be contaminated with plastics and become part of the human/animal food chain. (Eerkes-Medrano et al., 2015; Law & Thompson, 2014) Thus, reducing microplastics will bring immense benefits to our society.

All plastics undergo some degradation. These degradation processes include physicochemical and/or biological. Physicochemical processes include hydrolysis, oxidation, weathering (degradation due to sunlight, wind, or waves). These processes affect all plastics and are the primary mechanism of microplastic

Figure 11. Biodegradation of PHA

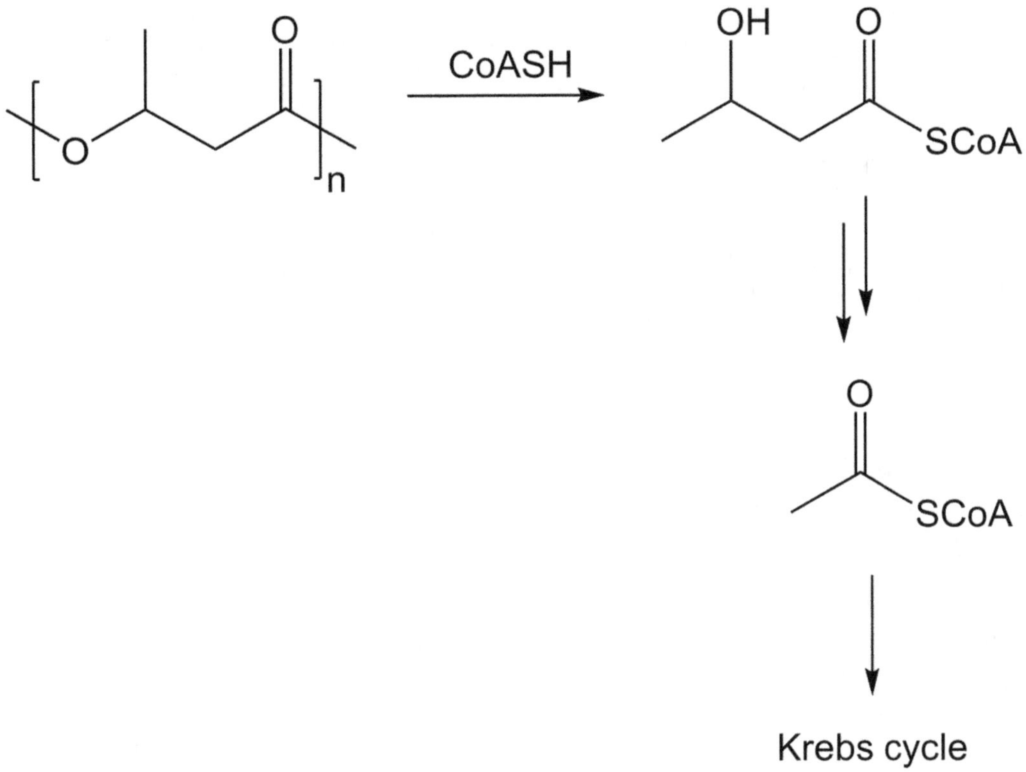

formation. (Kalogerakis et al., 2017) The plastics that are designed to undergo degradation by oxidation are called oxo-degradable plastics (Figure 9). (Scott, 2002) Similarly, the plastics that are designed to undergo degradation by hydrolysis is called hydro-degradable plastics. Both of these are usually non-biodegradable as-is and require modification. Oxo-degradable plastics are generally petroleum-derived plastics (e.g., polyethylene, polypropylene, etc.) with a mixture of additives. These additives are both pro- and anti-oxidant. The combination of these additives induces time-controlled oxidation. Pro-oxidants are often metal stearates (e.g., iron stearate)

and are balanced by phenolic or phosphite anti-oxidant. (Rahman,2012; Zbořilova & Pac, 2014) Photodegradable plastics are a sub-category of oxo-degradable plastics, where the oxidation is induced by UV light. (da Luz et al., 2014) Hydro-degradable plastics are often a blend of petro-based plastics and natural polymer (e.g., starch). (Lambert & Wagner, 2017) These plastics rely on the hydrophilic nature of the polymer for their decomposition into smaller oligomers.

Degradation of biodegradable plastics is carried out by microorganisms, such as bacteria, fungi, etc. (Greene, 2014) This

microbial degradation can be aerobic or anaerobic. It can go all the way to CO_2, methane, water, biomass/compost, etc. Most commercial biodegradable plastics are converted to compost rather than gaseous products. For a plastic material to be compostable, the organic matter resulting from the degradation should be harmless to animals and plants. However, there is a difference between biodegradable plastics and bio-based plastics/bioplastics. Bioplastics are made from biomass, generally involve the use

Figure 12. Proposed biodegradation of PVC

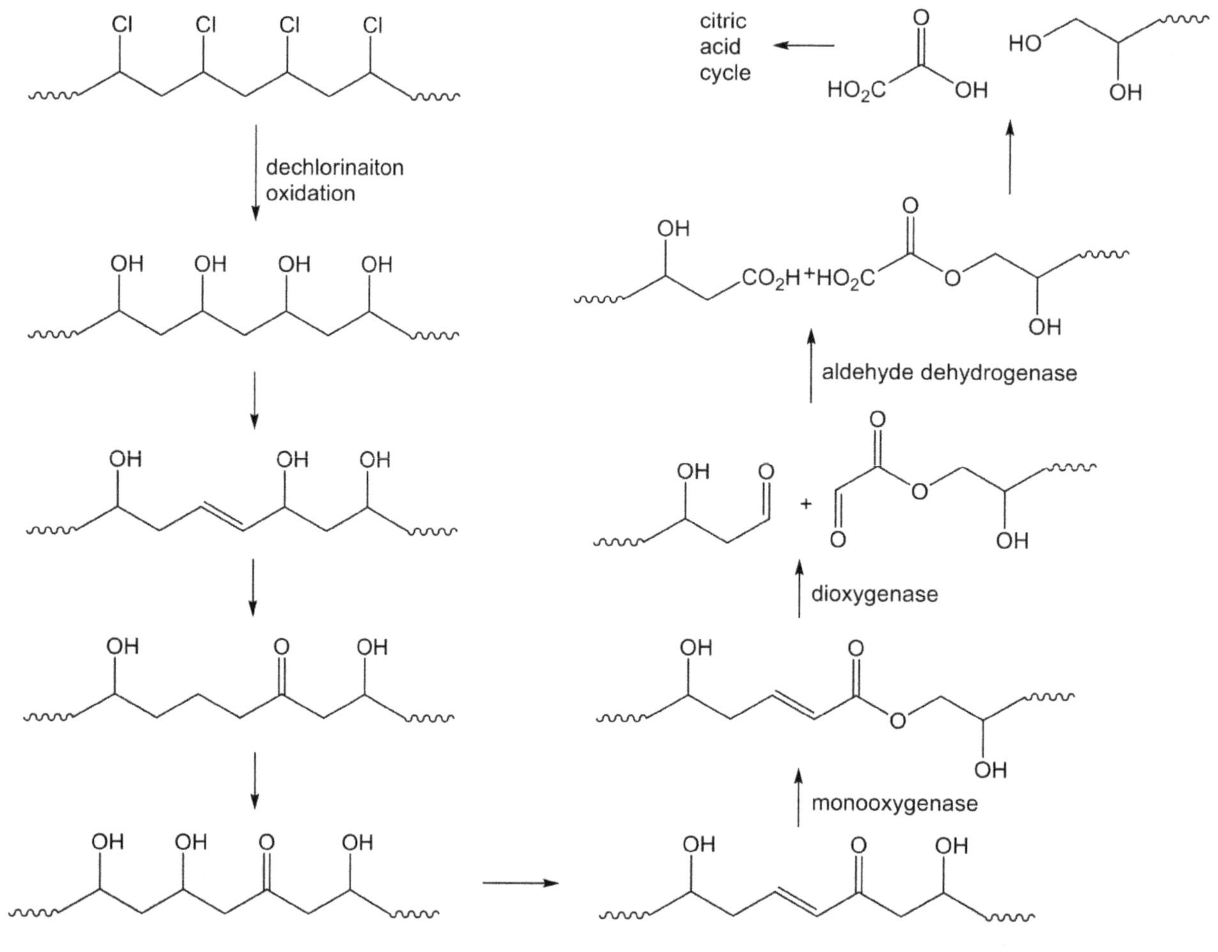

of the plant as feedstocks. Due to their origin, people sometimes erroneously assume all bioplastics are biodegradable. However,

biodegradability does not depend on the source but the chemical structure of the polymer. Thus, bio-based but not biodegradable plastics mimic petroleum-based plastics. Some examples include bio-polyethylene (Bio-PE), bio-polyethylene terephthalate (Bio-PET), bio-polyamides (Bio-PA or nylon). However, these plastics often have low feedstock efficiency and sometimes include petroleum-based monomers. (Hann et al., 2018) For example, current Bio-PET production includes 32% of bio-derived ethylene glycol, and the remaining 68% is petroleum-based terephthalic acid. The low feedstock efficiency has been attributed to the inherently different chemical structure of petroleum-based and plant-derived feedstocks. Also, the highly oxygenated nature of the biomass will hinder the synthesis of linear alkyl plastics, such as Bio-PE. The production of polyethylene furanoate (PEF) gives another approach for high-performance bioplastics. (de Jong et al., 2012) PEF is analogous to PET, with the aromatic ring substituted by a furan ring. Thus, less oxygen is removed from the original feedstock leading to better yield. The use of CO_2 as feedstock can also be seen as bio-based. However, the current production of CO_2 based plastics are based on petroleum-based copolymers. (Xu et al., 2018)

Figure 13. Biodegradation of bisphenol A polycarbonate

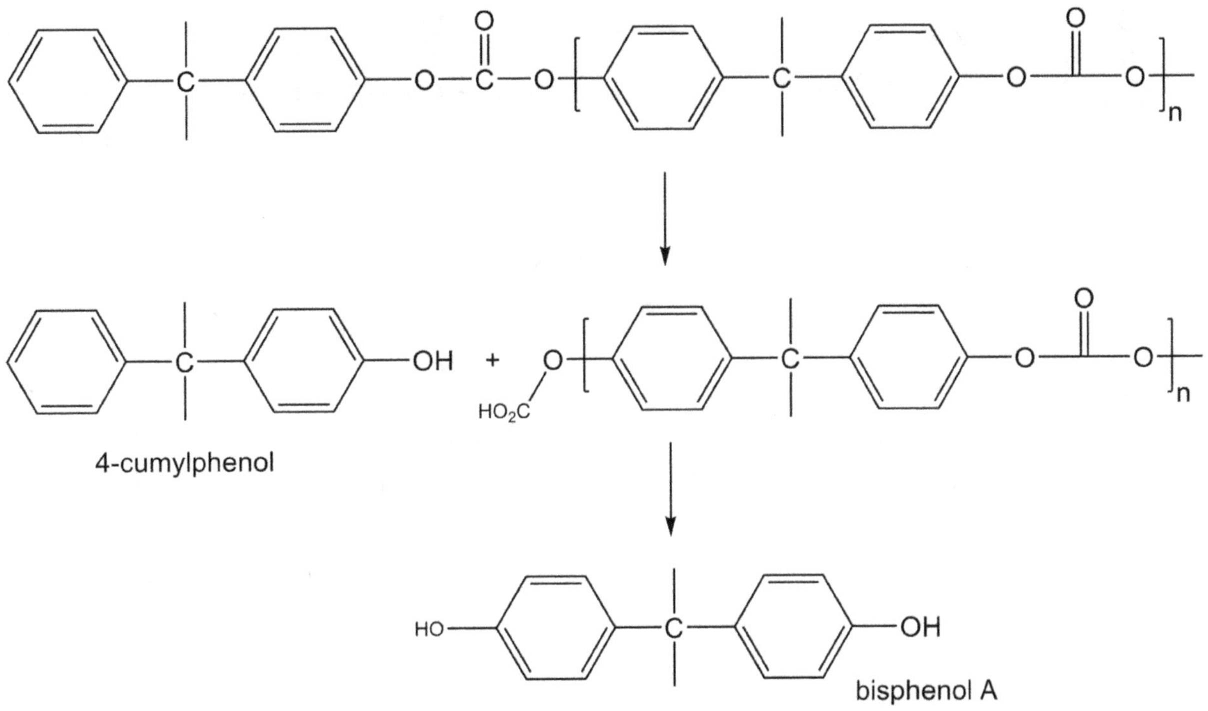

Some petroleum-based plastics are also biodegradable. These include polybutylene adipate terephthalate (PBAT), polyvinyl alcohol, etc. These plastics are used in mulch film or dishwasher tablet packaging. Given its high water solubility, Poly (vinyl alcohol), PVA can be regarded as a hydro-degradable plastic. Both of these plastics can be produced by bio-routes. For example, a fermentation route has been developed for 1,4-butanediol, which is a monomer of PBAT. (Ye et al., 2019)

Notable biobased and biodegradable plastics are PHAs and PLA. Out of PHAs, polyhydroxy valerate (PHV) and polyhydroxy butyrate (PHB) are most common (Figure 4). The hydrophilic nature of these polymers also enables hydro-degradation. PHAs and PLA are produced by the bacterial fermentation of sugar (discussed earlier). Biodegradation of some of the common polymers is discussed below.

1. **Biodegradation of PET:** PET is one of the most abundantly produced synthetic polymers, and its accumulation in the environment is of global concern. Since the ability to degrade PET has been thought to be limited to a few fungal species, it may last centuries in the environment. (Austin et al., 2018) Recently, it has been shown that a newly discovered bacterium uses PET as a major energy and carbon source. (Yoshida et al., 2016) When grown on PET, the strain produces two hydrolytic enzymes. Both enzymes are required to convert PET into its environmentally benign monomers – terephthalic acid (TPA) and ethylene glycol (Figure 10). TPA is incorporated into the cell via TPA transporter and catabolized by TPA 1,2-dioxygenase (TPADO), followed by dihydroxy-3,5-cyclohexadiene-1,4-dicarboxylate dehydrogenase (DCDDH) to produce protocatechuate. The benzene ring of protocatechuate will be cleaved by protocatechuate-3,4-dioxygenase (PCA34D).

Figure 14. Biodegradation of PU

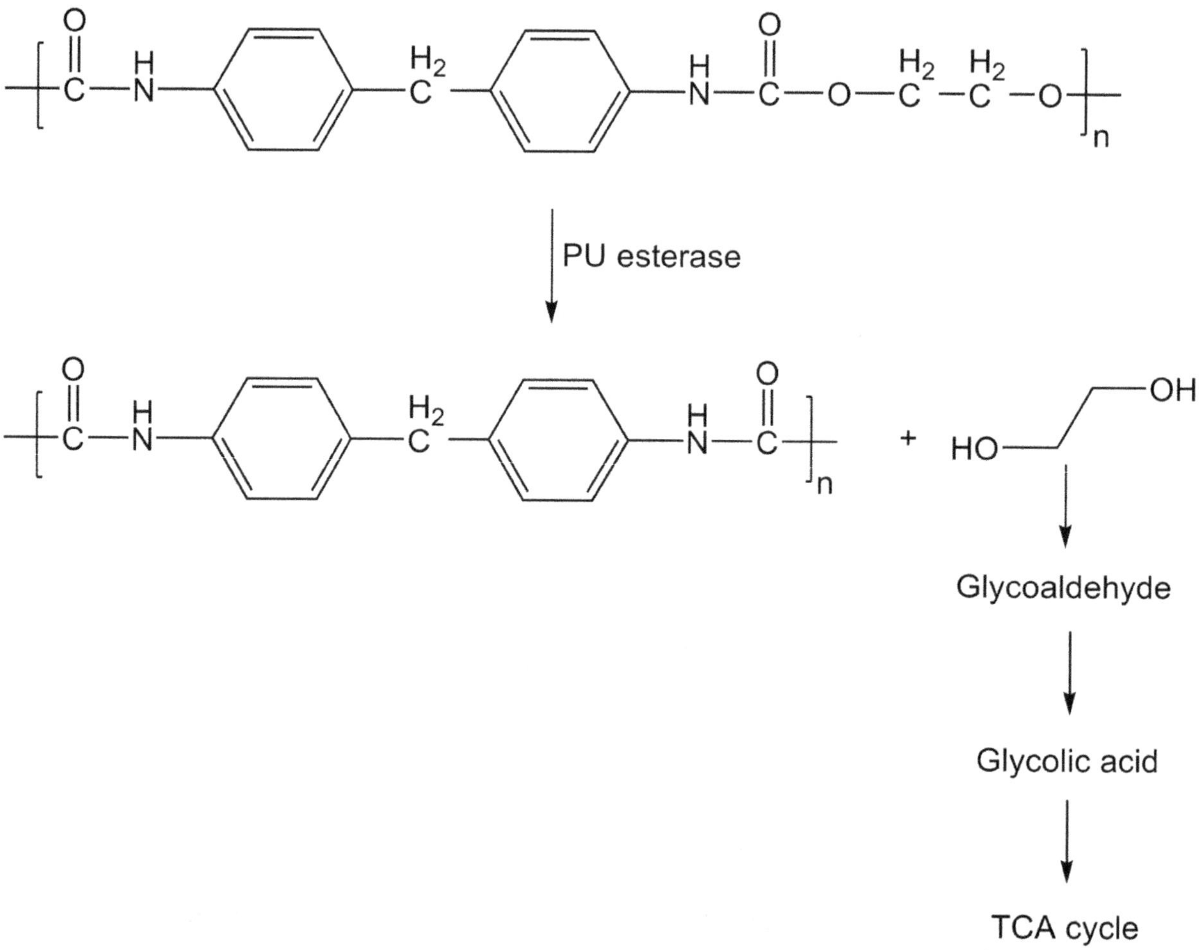

2. **Biodegradation of PHA:** Microorganisms produce and store PHA in their cells. (Muthukumar & Veerappapillai, 2015) PHA cannot pass through the semi-permeable membrane unless they are broken down to smaller oligomers or monomers. Thus, bacteria have evolved to produce hydrolases that convert PHA into hydroxyl acid monomers. Short and medium-chain PHAs are biodegraded by a number of bacteria (e.g., Variovorax, Stenotrophomonas, Acinetobacter, Pseudomonas, Bacillus, Burkholderia, Cupriavidus, Mycobacterium, and Streptomyces.). (Meereboer et al., 2020) Fungi such as Ascomycota, Basidiomycetes, Deuteromycetes, and Zygomycotina can also biodegrade PHAs. (Sang et al., 2002) In fact, they are more effective PHA degrader compared to bacteria. The biodegradation of PHA is mediated by lipases and hydrolases. The biodegradation process involves the breakdown of polymer into shorter chain polymers by hydrolytic depolymerases. These shorter chain polymers are further converted to trimer and dimer units, which are then processed by lipases and hydrolases. (Kobayashi et al., 2005) The hydrolysis process is not very specific and releases oligomers of various sizes into the surrounding medium. (Scherer et al., 1999; Slepecky & Law, 1961) The degradation product depends on the type of PHA. For example, biodegradation of PHB produces 3-hydroxybutyric acid (Figure 11). (Eldsäter et al., 1997) This acid is taken into

Figure 15. Biodegradation of nylon

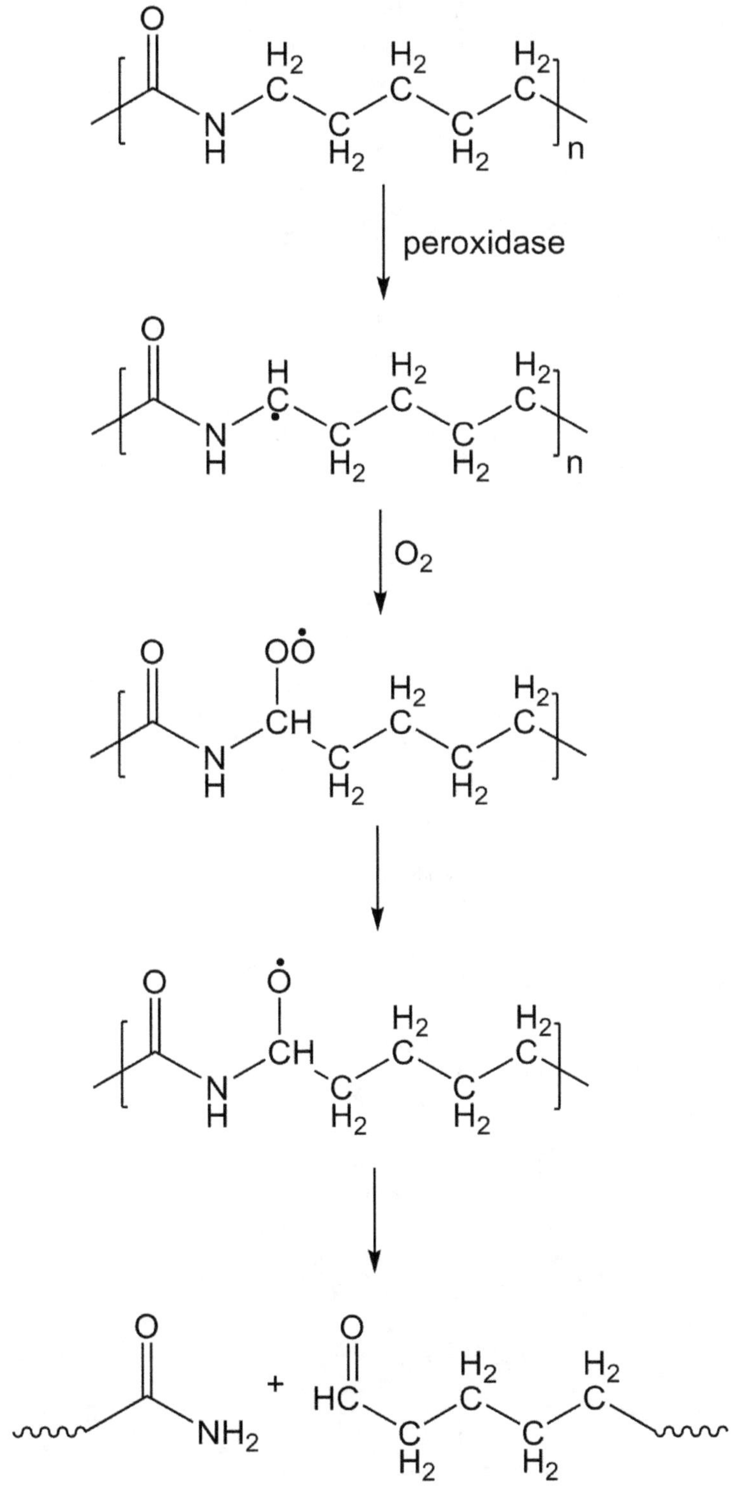

Figure 16. Biodegradation of PE

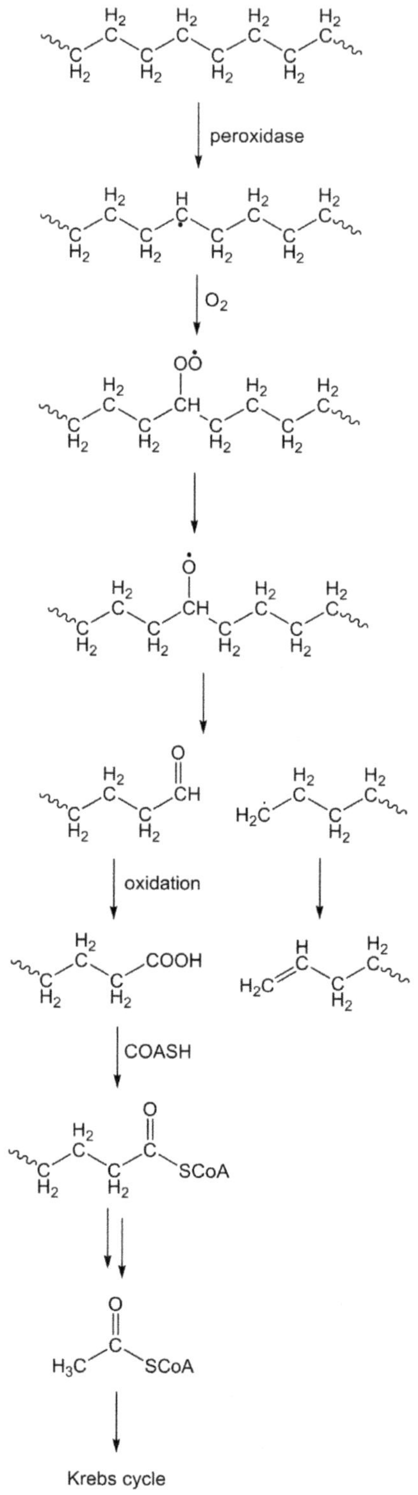

Figure 17. Biodegradation of PVA

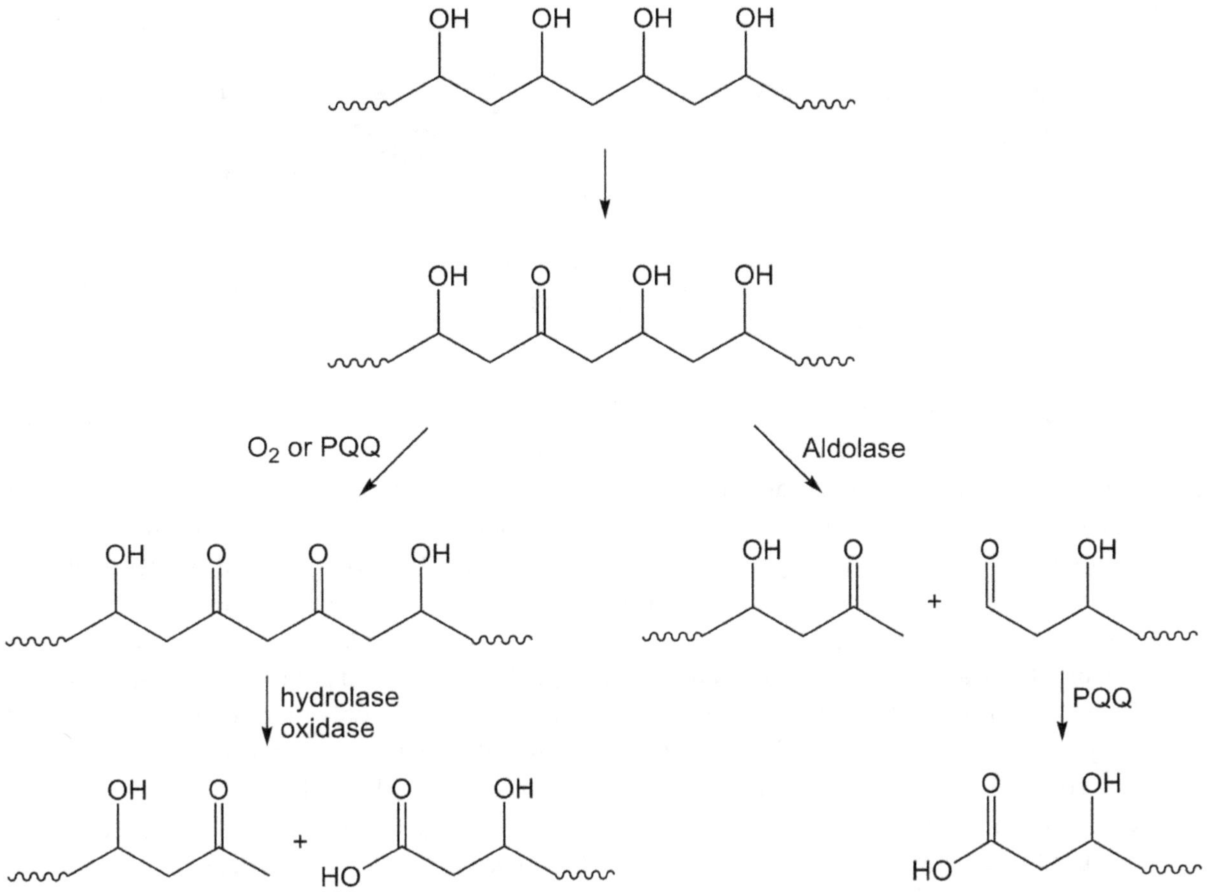

the cell for metabolism to produce CO_2 and H_2O. (Hakkarainen, 2002) It is worth mentioning that no harmful product is produced in this process.

3. **Biodegradation of polyvinyl chloride (PVC):** Microbial degradation of PVC is environmentally friendly and economically attractive. Recently a strain of Klebsiella that can actively degrade and utilize PVC has been discovered. (Zhang et al., 2021) Based on the metabolic products and the biodegradation genes, a biodegradation mechanism has been proposed for PVC (Figure 12). This process is initiated by dechlorination and oxidation. A monooxygenase has been proposed to produce ester compounds via Baeyer-Villiger oxidation. Further action of a dioxygenase has been proposed to produce aldehydes. These aldehydes can be converted to acids by dehydrogenases. Finally, these acid molecules will be utilized by the citric acid cycle.
4. **Biodegradation of bisphenol A (BPA) polycarbonate:** BPA polycarbonate (PC) is a widely used thermoplastic. However, its release into the environment cause damage to the ecosystem as well as human health. Thus, microbial degradation provides one way of reducing PC in our environment. Recently, a bacterial strain capable of degrading PC has been isolated. (Yue et al., 2021) Two degradation products (BPA and 4-cumylphenol) have also been isolated. Based on these results, a biodegradation pathway has been proposed (Figure 13). In this pathway, a hydrolase may cleave

Figure 18. Biodegradation of PLA

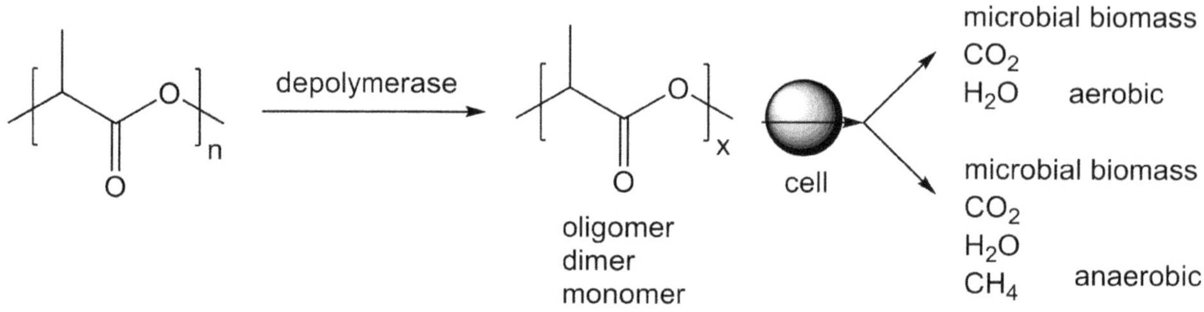

the carbonate bonds in PC. 4-cumylphenol may be initially produced by the chain-end scission. The carbonate bond will then be broken to release BPA.

5. **Biodegradation of polyurethane (PU):** Despite its xenobiotic origin, PU is susceptible to biodegradation (Filiciotto & Rothenberg, 2021). PU is not abundant in nature, and only a few microbial strains have been reported to degrade it. (Mohanan et al., 2020) PU is biodegraded through hydrolytic cleavage of urethane bonds (Figure 14). (Nakajima-Kambe et al., 1999) Few bacterial (P. aeruginosa, Corynebacterium sp., Comamonas acidovorans, Pseudomonas fluorescens, Acinetobacter calcoaceticus, and Bacillus subtilis) and fungal (e.g., Aureobasidium pullulans, Cladosporium sp., Curvularia senegalensis, and Fusarium solani) species degrade polyester-polyurethane through enzymatic hydrolysis of ester linkages. (Crabbe et al., 1994) These bacterial strains use polyester-polyethylene polymer as C, N, and energy sources for growth. (Howard, 2002)
6. **Biodegradation of nylon:** Marine bacteria were shown to degrade nylon 6 and 66. These bacteria can use the polymer as the sole carbon source. (Sudhakar et al., 2007) The degradation led to the formation of new functional groups such as NHCHO, CH_3, $CONH_2$, and COOH. Based on these functional groups, a mechanism has been proposed for the biodegradation of nylon (Figure 15). The formation of NHCHO and CH_3 groups may be due to the cleavage of the C-C bond in CH_2-CH_2 adjacent to the N-atom. The formation of $CONH_2$, CHO, and COOH may be due to the cleavage of the C-N bond in NH-CH_2. It is possible that the methylene group near the N-atom can be attacked by the peroxidase enzyme, and the subsequent reaction proceeds through auto-oxidation.
7. **Biodegradation of PE:** Previous studies have suggested biodegradation of polyethylene in the presence of microorganisms. (Ghatge et al., 2020) Polyethylene can be made susceptible to microbial degradation by adding starch and/or pro-oxidant (Muthukumar & Veerappapillai, 2015). Starch increases the hydrophilic nature of polyethylene so that microorganisms can easily degrade this part. In the presence of pro-oxidant, biodegradation is preceded by photo- and chemical-degradation. Biodegradation of high molecular weight polyethylene by lignin-degrading fungi has been reported. Both fungi were found to produce manganese peroxidase that may initiate the oxidation of PE (Figure 16). These oxidized products will eventually form fatty acids. These fatty acids will then be transported into the cell, where these will undergo β-oxidation and completely mineralized into CO_2, H_2O and biomass.
8. **Biodegradation of PVA:** Among the vinyl polymers produced industrially, PVA is the only one known to be mineralized by microorganisms. (Shimao, 2001) PVA degrading strains are not ubiquitous in the environment and only a few PVA degrading bacterial strains have been reported. PVA

is completely degraded and utilized by various pseudomonas strains. (Suzuki et al., 1973) Among the PVA degrading bacteria reported so far, a few strains showed the requirement of PQQ (pyrroloquinoline quinone) cofactor. (Shimao et al., 1984) However, other PVA degrading strains do not require PQQ cofactor. (Sakai et al., 1986) In the proposed PVA degrading mechanism (Figure 17), C-C bond is cleaved by a dehydrogenase or an oxidase. The resulting intermediate will then undergo further reaction in the presence of hydrolase or aldolase.

9. **Biodegradation of PLA:** Studies on PLA biodegrading microorganisms show that PLA degraders are not widely distributed. (Ghosh et al., 2013) Thus, PLA is less vulnerable to microbial attack. Biodegradation of PLA in the soil is slow and takes a long time to start. (Uruyama et al., [2002;] Ohkita & Lee, 2006) Microbial biodegradation of PLA was first reported using Amycolatopsis sp. (Pranamuda et al., 1997) Since then a number of microbial and enzymatic degradation of PLA has been reported. (Tokiwa & Calabia, 2006) Enzymatic degradation of PLA was investigated using proteinase K, bromelain and pronase. (Williams, 1981) Among these, proteinase K was most effective in for PLA degradation. It has been reported that the degradation of PLA was accelerated by several esterase type enzymes. (Fukuzaki et al., [1989)] During microbial degradation, the microorganism excrete extracellular depolymerase. (Qi et al., 2017) The depolymerase cleaves intramolecular ester bonds, resulting in the formation of oligomers, dimers, and monomers (Figure 18). These low molecular weight compounds cross the cell membrane and enter the cell. Finally, these compounds are converted to CO_2, H_2O (aerobic), or methane (anaerobic).
10. **Biodegradation of polystyrene (PS):** Mealworms were reported to rapidly degrade up to 50% of ingested Styrofoam (trade name of PS foam) in 24 hours. (Yang et al., 2015) Later it was shown that degradation of PS in mealworms is ubiquitous. (Yang et al., 2018; Peng et al., 2019) Among PS degrading enzymes, only hydroquinone peroxidase was able to depolymerize PS into low molecular weight products in dichloromethane. (Nakamiya et al., 1997) For the main chain cleavage, styrene and structures analogous to styrene can be processed through aromatic catabolism. (Ru et al., 2020) The products from aromatic catabolism may enter the microbial metabolism and ultimately be converted to CO_2 via the citric acid cycle (Figure 19). Another pathway involve the side chain oxidation (Figure 19). This pathway also ultimately leads to the formation of CO_2 via the citric acid cycle. Both of these pathways have been observed in several microorganisms. (Oelschlägel et al., 2018)

FUTURE PERSPECTIVES

Human reliance on plastic is unlikely to diminish, considering its superior property to many materials. High-priced petroleum products and concern about the environment and ecology have led scientists and industrialists to investigate renewable and biodegradable polymers. Biodegradability is dependent on the interaction of plastic material and microorganisms. Biodegradability is also affected by the physical and chemical properties of bioplastics. The biodegradation studies performed in labs often overestimate natural biodegradability rates. Therefore, studies will benefit from the development of standardized methodologies, adopting a clear definition of biodegradation, maximizing the number of techniques used to access biodegradation processes. The final point will differentiate between superficial surface deterioration and the more desirable bio-fragmentation and utilization of the plastic material necessary for substantial biodegradation. Thus, enhancing the efficiency of biodegradation is a big challenge. The

Figure 19. Biodegradation of PS

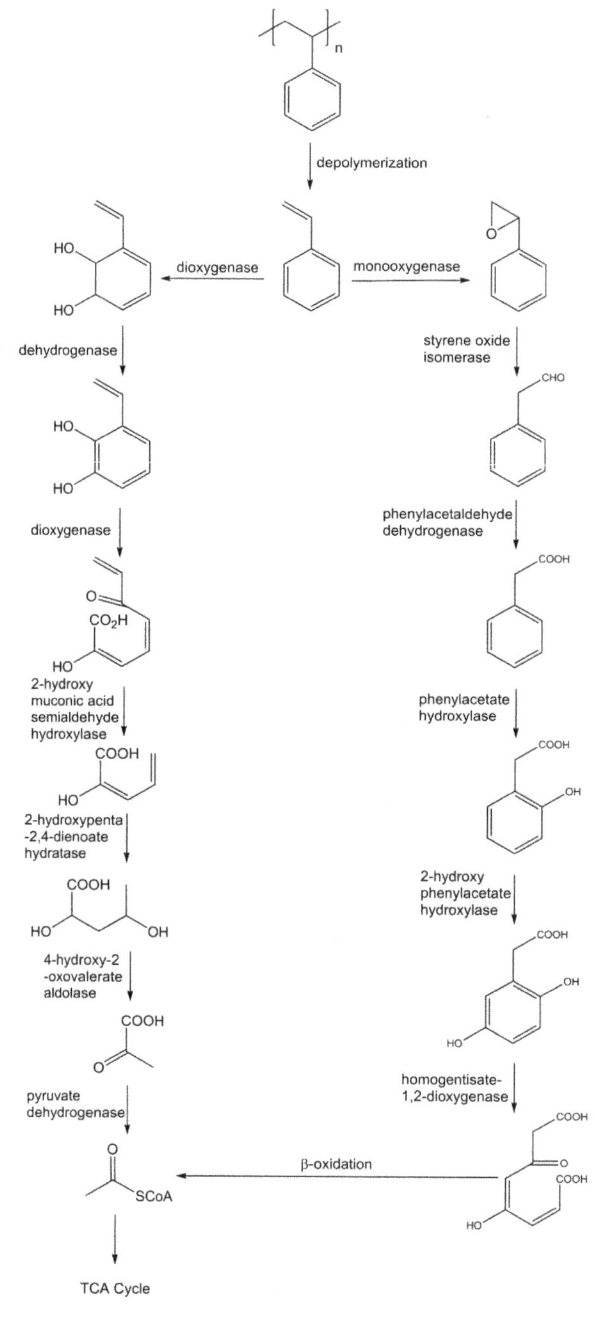

macromolecular structure of plastic materials impedes degradation. The use of physical pretreatments such as mechanical grinding, γ-radiations may improve enzymatic degradation. Rational protein design and directed evolution should improve the stability and activity of the enzymes, enhancing degradation efficiency. Colder environment, ecosystem dynamics, etc., can hinder biodegradation. Given the long life span of plastic materials, methods to use short-term experimental results to predict long-term degradation pathways and methods to simulate degradation should be used. The partial biodegradation will lead to the formation of microplastics. Very few enzymes (bacterial or fungal origin) have been demonstrated in polymer degradation. The function of these enzymes is mostly confined to the more susceptible, hydrolyzable backbones of PET and PUR. Thus, further investigation on the mechanism of enzymatic degradation will highlight the pathway for efficient biodegradation of polymers at the molecular level. (Ghatge et al., 2020) These investigations will allow the identification of the biomass structure generated due to the biodegradation of bioplastics. This understanding will help us produce next-generation bio-based biodegradable plastics by slight modification in structure to build a more sustainable society. These investigations may also lead to the development of microbes and enzymes that degrade plastics into high-value compounds. More research may also lead to a better technological solution to plastic waste and microplastic problems. Overall, biodegradation can partially make up for littering and waste management problems. Also, carbon emissions can be reduced if plants are used as feedstock. (Filiciotto & Rothenberg, 2021) Whether plastic materials are bio-based or not, biodegradable plastics give an environmental advantage.

CONCLUSION

The development of biodegradable plastic requires chemistry, chemical engineering, microbiology, and process engineering knowledge. Researchers in these areas should use their expertise and collaborate to make society more sustainable by developing eco-friendly plastics. Other vital factors in the development of biodegradable plastics are environmental conditions and socio-economic impacts. As already mentioned, biodegradable plastics are eco-friendly, made from plants (reduced reliance on fossil fuel), etc. However, biodegradable plastics have not been commercialized on a large scale. There are several reasons behind this. The main reason is the higher cost of production. Synthesis of polymers such as PHA in plants, which relies on CO_2 and light, may represent a cost-effective approach to produce this biopolymer in large quantities. Also, there remain some technical challenges in the large-scale production of bioplastics. However, developing robust strains capable of synthesizing polymers (e.g., PLA) from sugars derived from biomass in a one-step process could provide a commercially viable technology for bioplastic production. Thus, the future of biodegradable plastic is bright considering the environmental awareness throughout the world. Stricter government regulations and higher carbon taxes will provide further motivation for developing biodegradable plastics.

REFERENCES

Agamuthu, P. (2013). Landfilling in developing countries. *Waste Management & Research*, *31*(1), 1–2. doi:10.1177/0734242X12469169 PMID:23255612

Alvarez-Castillo, E., Del Toro, A., Aguilar, J. M., Bengoechea, C., & Guerrero, A. (2018). Optimization of a thermal process for the production of superabsorbent materials based on a soy protein isolate. *Industrial Crops and Products*, *125*, 573–581. doi:10.1016/j.indcrop.2018.09.051

Aniceto, J. P., Portugal, I., & Silva, C. M. (2012). Biomass-based polyols through oxypropylation reaction. *ChemSusChem*, *5*(8), 1358–1368. doi:10.1002/cssc.201200032 PMID:22807440

Asrofi, M., Sapuan, S. M., Ilyas, R. A., & Ramesh, M. (2020). Characteristic of composite bioplastics from tapioca starch and sugarcane bagasse fiber: Effect of time duration of ultrasonication (Bath-Type). *Materials Today: Proceedings*, *46*(4), 1626–1630.

Auras, R., Harte, B., & Selke, S. (2004). An overview of polylactides as packaging materials. *Macromolecular Bioscience*, *4*(9), 835–864. doi:10.1002/mabi.200400043 PMID:15468294

Auras, R., Harte, B., & Selke, S. (2004). An overview of polylactides as packaging materials. *Macromolecular Bioscience*, *4*(9), 835–864. doi:10.1002/mabi.200400043 PMID:15468294

Austin, H. P., Allen, M. D., Donohoe, B. S., Rorrer, N. A., Kearns, F. L., Silveira, R. L., Pollard, B. C., Dominick, G., Duman, R., El Omari, K., Mykhaylyk, V., Wagner, A., Michener, W. E., Amore, A., Skaf, M. S., Crowley, M. F., Thorne, A. W., Johnson, C. W., Woodcock, H. L., ... Beckham, G. T. (2018). Characterization and engineering of a plastic-degrading aromatic polyesterase. *Proceedings of the National Academy of Sciences of the United States of America*, *115*(19), E4350–E4357. doi:10.1073/pnas.1718804115 PMID:29666242

Babalola, O. A., & Olorunnisola, A. O. (2019). Evaluation of coconut (Cocos nucifera) husk fibre as a potential reinforcing material for bioplastic production. *Material Research Proceedings*, *11*, 195–200. doi:10.21741/9781644900178-14

BeMiller, J. N., & Whistler, R. L. (2009). Starch—chemistry and technology. In Food science and technology. Academic Press.

Boethling, R. S., Sommer, E., & DiFiore, D. (2007). Designing small molecules for biodegradability. *Chemical Reviews*, *107*(6), 2207–2227. doi:10.1021/cr050952t PMID:17530907

Brodin, M., Vallejos, M., Opedal, M. T., Area, M. C., & Chinga-Carrasco, G. (2017). Lignocellulosics as sustainable resources for production of Bioplastics – A Review. *Journal of Cleaner Production*, *162*, 646–664. doi:10.1016/j.jclepro.2017.05.209

Brodin, M., Vallejos, M., Opedal, M. T., Area, M. C., & Chinga-Carrasco, G. (2017). Lignocellulosics as sustainable resources for production of bioplastics—A review. *Journal of Cleaner Production*, *162*, 646–664. doi:10.1016/j.jclepro.2017.05.209

Broeren, M. (2013). *Production of Bio-ethylene. Technology Brief. Energy Technology Systems Analysis Programme (ETSAP)*. International Energy Agency (IEA). www.irena.org/Publications

Carus, M. (2016). Bio-based materials – Technical, Economic and Market Data on the Bio-based Economy. Technology and Polymerdagene, Gjøvik, Norway.

Chen, G.-Q. (2009). A microbial polyhydroxyalkanoates (PHA) based vio- and materials industry. *Chemical Society Reviews*, *38*(8), 2434–2446. doi:10.1039/b812677c PMID:19623359

Chia, W. Y., Ying Tang, D. Y., Khoo, K. S., Kay Lup, A. N., & Chew, K. W. (2020). Nature's fight against plastic pollution: Algae for plastic biodegradation and bioplastics production. *Environmental Science and Ecotechnology*, *4*, 100065. doi:10.1016/j.ese.2020.100065

Cinar, S. O., Chong, Z. K., Kucuker, M. A., Wieczorek, N., Cengiz, U., & Kuchta, K. (2020). Bioplastic production from microalgae: A review. *International Journal of Environmental Research and Public Health*, *17*(11), 3842. doi:10.3390/ijerph17113842 PMID:32481700

Coppola, G., Gaudio, M. T., Lopresto, C. G., Calabro, V., Curcio, S., & Chakraborty, S. (2021). Bioplastic from Renewable Biomass: A Facile Solution for a Greener Environment. *Earth Systems and Environment*, *5*(2), 231–251. doi:10.100741748-021-00208-7

Crabbe, J. R., Campbell, J. R., Thompson, L., Walz, S. L., & Schultz, W. W. (1994). Biodegradation of a colloidal ester-based polyurethane by soil fungi. *International Biodeterioration & Biodegradation*, *33*(2), 103–113. doi:10.1016/0964-8305(94)90030-2

da Luz, J. M. R., Paes, S. A., Bazzolli, D. M. S., Totola, M. R., Demuner, A. J., & Kasuya, M. C. M. (2014). Abiotic and biotic degradation of oxo-biodegradable plastic bags by Pleurotus ostreatus. *PLoS One*, *9*(11), e107438. doi:10.1371/journal.pone.0107438 PMID:25419675

Dai, H., Chang, P. R., Geng, F., Yu, J., & Ma, X. (2009). Preparation and properties of thermoplastic starch/montmorillonite nanocomposite using N-(2-Hydroxyethyl) formamide as a new additive. *Journal of Polymers and the Environment*, *17*(4), 225–232. doi:10.100710924-009-0142-y

Das, K. A., Sathish, A., & Stanley, J. (2018). Production of biofuel and bioplastic from Chlorella pyrenoidosa. *Proceedings: Material Today*, *5*(8), 16774-16781.

de Jong, E., Dam, M. A., Sipos, L., & Gruter, G.-J. M. (2012). *Biobased Monomers, Polymers, and Materials*. American Chemical Society.

Didier, B. (2015). *Briefing of the European Parliament*. https://www.europarl.europa.eu/RegData/etudes/BRIE/2015/559493/EPRS_BRI(2015)559493_EN.pdf

DiGregorio, B. E. (2009). Biobased performance bioplastic: Mirel. *Chemistry & Biology*, *16*(1), 1–2. doi:10.1016/j.chembiol.2009.01.001 PMID:19171300

Ebbesen, M. F., Gerke, C., Hartwig, P., & Hartmann, L. (2016). Biodegradable poly(amidoamine)s with uniform degradation fragments via sequence-controlled macromonomers. *Polymer Chemistry*, *7*(46), 7086–7093. doi:10.1039/C6PY01700B

Eerkes-Medrano, D., Thompson, R. C., & Aldridge, D. C. (2015). Microplastics in freshwater systems: A review of the emerging threats, identification of knowledge gaps and prioritization of research needs. *Water Research*, *2015*(75), 63–82. doi:10.1016/j.watres.2015.02.012 PMID:25746963

Eggink, G., deWaard, P., & Huijberts, G. N. (1995). Formation of novel poly(hydroxyalkanoates) from long-chain fatty acids. *Canadian Journal of Microbiology*, *41*(13), 14–21. doi:10.1139/m95-163 PMID:7606658

Eldsäter, C., Albertsson, A. C., & Karlsson, S. (1997). Impact of degradation mechanisms on poly(3-hydroxybutyrate-co-3-hydroxyvalerate) during composting. *Acta Polymerica*, *48*(11), 478–483. doi:10.1002/actp.1997.010481103

Eubeler, J. P., Bernhard, M., & Knepper, T. P. (2010). Environmental biodegradation of synthetic polymers II. Biodegradation of different polymer groups. Trends in Analytical Chemistry (Reference Ed.), 29, 84–100.

Filiciotto, L., & Rothenberg, G. (2021). Biodegradable plastics: Standards, policies, and impacts. *ChemSusChem, 14*(1), 56–72. doi:10.1002/cssc.202002044 PMID:33112051

Fukuzaki, H., Yoshida, M., Asano, M., & Kumakura, M. (1989). Synthesis of copoly(d, l-lactic acid) with relative low molecular weight and in vitro degradation. *European Polymer Journal, 25*(10), 1019–1026. doi:10.1016/0014-3057(89)90131-6

Gewert, B., Plassmann, M. M., & MacLeod, M. (2015). Pathways for degradation of plastic polymers floating in the marine environment. *Environmental Science. Processes & Impacts, 17*(9), 1513–1521. doi:10.1039/C5EM00207A PMID:26216708

Ghatge, S., Yang, Y., Ahn, J. H., & Hur, H.-G. (2020). Biodegradation of polyethylene: A brief review. *Applied Biological Chemistry, 63*(1), 27. doi:10.118613765-020-00511-3

Ghosh, S. K., Pal, S., & Ray, S. (2013). Study of microbes having potentiality for biodegradation of plastics. *Environmental Science and Pollution Research International, 20*(7), 4339–4355. doi:10.100711356-013-1706-x PMID:23613206

Gokce, E. (2018). Rethinking sustainability: A research on starch based bioplastic. *Journal of Sustainable Construction Materials and Technologies, 3*(3), 249–260. doi:10.29187/jscmt.2018.28

Govil, T., Wang, J., Samanta, D., David, A., Tripathi, A., Rauniyar, S., Salem, D. R., & Sani, R. K. (2020). Lignocellulosic feedstock: A review of a sustainable platform for cleaner production of nature's plastics. *Journal of Cleaner Production, 270*, 122521. doi:10.1016/j.jclepro.2020.122521

Greene, J. P. (2014). *Sustainable Plastics*. John Wiley & Sons, Ltd. doi:10.1002/9781118899595

Hakkarainen, M. (2002). Aliphatic polyesters: Abiotic and biotic degradation products. *Advances in Polymer Science, 157*, 113–138. doi:10.1007/3-540-45734-8_4

Hamidon, N. (2018). Potential of production bioplastic from potato starch. *Sustainable Environmental Technology, 1*, 115–123.

Hann, S., Scholes, R., Briedis, R., & Kirkevaag, K. (2018). *Bio-Based and Biodegradable Plastics: An Assessment of the Value Chain for Bio-Based and Biodegradable Plastics in Norway*. Eunomia For The Norwegian Environment Agency.

Haro, P., Ollero, P., & Trippe, F. (2013). Technoeconomic assessment of potential processes for bioethylene production. *Fuel Processing Technology, 114*, 35–48. doi:10.1016/j.fuproc.2013.03.024

Harunsyah, Y. M., & Fauzan, R. (2017). Mechanical properties of bioplastics cassava starch film with Zinc Oxide nanofiller as reinforcement. *IOP Conference Series. Materials Science and Engineering, 210*, 012015. doi:10.1088/1757-899X/210/1/012015

Hojabri, L., Kong, X., & Narine, S. S. (2009). Fatty Acid-Derived Diisocyanate and Biobased Polyurethane Produced from Vegetable Oil: Synthesis, Polymerization, and Characterization. *Biomacromolecules, 10*(4), 884–891. doi:10.1021/bm801411w PMID:19281152

Horodytska, O., Cabanes, A., & Fullana, A. (2019). *The Handbook of Environmental Chemistry*. Springer.

Howard, G. T. (2002). Biodegradation of polyurethane: A review. *International Biodeterioration & Biodegradation, 49*(4), 245–252. doi:10.1016/S0964-8305(02)00051-3

Ishangulyyev, R., Kim, S., & Lee, S. H. (2019). Understanding food loss and waste – why are we losing and wasting food? *Foods, 8*(8), 297. doi:10.3390/foods8080297 PMID:31362396

Jerez, A., Partal, P., Martínez, I., Gallegos, C., & Guerrero, A. (2005). Rheology and processing of gluten based bioplastics. *Biochemical Engineering Journal, 26*(2-3), 131–138. doi:10.1016/j.bej.2005.04.010

Jimenez-Rosado, M., Bouroudian, E., Perez-Puyana, V., Guerrero, A., & Romero, A. (2020). Evaluation of different strengthening methods in the mechanical and functional properties of soy proteinbased bioplastics. *Journal of Cleaner Production, 262*, 121517. doi:10.1016/j.jclepro.2020.121517

Jõgi, K., & Bhat, R. (2020). Valorization of food processing wastes and by-products for bioplastic production. *Sustainable Chemistry and Pharmacy, 18*, 100326. doi:10.1016/j.scp.2020.100326

Kalambur, S., & Rizvi, S. S. H. (2006). An overview of starch-based plastic blends from reactive extrusion. *Journal of Plastic Film & Sheeting, 22*(1), 39–58. doi:10.1177/8756087906062729

Kalogerakis, N., Karkanorachaki, K., Kalogerakis, G. C., Triantafyllidi, E. I., Gotsis, A. D., Partsinevelos, P., & Fava, F. (2017). Microplastics generation: Onset of fragmentation of polyethylene films in marine environment mesocosms. *Frontiers in Marine Science, 4*, 84. doi:10.3389/fmars.2017.00084

Kawaguchi, H., Hasunuma, T., Ogino, C., & Kondo, A. (2016). Bioprocessing of biobased chemicals produced from lignocellulosic feedstocks. *Current Opinion in Biotechnology, 42*, 30–39. doi:10.1016/j.copbio.2016.02.031 PMID:26970511

Keenan, T. M., Nakas, J. P., & Tanenbaum, S. W. (2006). Polyhydroxyalkanoate copolymers from forest biomass. *Journal of Industrial Microbiology & Biotechnology, 33*(7), 616–626. doi:10.100710295-006-0131-2 PMID:16761168

Kim, J.-Y., Lee, H. W., Lee, S. M., Jae, J., & Park, Y.-K. (2019). Overview of the recent advances in lignocellulose liquefaction for producing biofuels, bio-based materials and Chemicals. *Bioresource Technology, 279*, 373–384. doi:10.1016/j.biortech.2019.01.055 PMID:30685133

Kobayashi, T., Uchino, K., Abe, T., Yamazaki, Y., & Saito, T. (2005). Novel intracellular 3-hydroxybutyrate-oligomer hydrolase in Wautersia eutropha H16. *Journal of Bacteriology, 187*(15), 5129–5135. doi:10.1128/JB.187.15.5129-5135.2005 PMID:16030206

Krishnamurthy, A., & Amritkumar, P. (2019). Synthesis and characterization of eco-friendly bioplastic from low-cost plant resources. *SN Applied Sciences, 1*(11), 1432. doi:10.100742452-019-1460-x

Lambert, S., & Wagner, M. (2017). Environmental performance of bio-based and biodegradable plastics: The road ahead. *Chemical Society Reviews, 46*(22), 6855–6871. doi:10.1039/C7CS00149E PMID:28932844

Lasprilla, A. J. R., Martinez, G. A. R., Lunelli, B. H., Jardini, A. L., & Filho, R. M. (2012). Poly-lactic acid synthesis for application in biomedical devices – A review. *Biotechnology Advances*, *30*(1), 321–328. doi:10.1016/j.biotechadv.2011.06.019 PMID:21756992

Law, K. L., & Thompson, R. C. (2014). Oceans: Microplastics in the seas. *Science*, *345*(6193), 144–145. doi:10.1126cience.1254065 PMID:25013051

Lebreton, L., & Andrady, A. (2019). Future scenarios of global plastic waste generation and disposal. *Palgrave Communications*, *5*(1), 1–11. doi:10.105741599-018-0212-7

Lim, L.-T., Auras, R., & Rubino, M. (2008). Processing technologies for poly(lactic acid). *Progress in Polymer Science*, *33*(8), 820–852. doi:10.1016/j.progpolymsci.2008.05.004

Liu, B., Jiang, L., & Zhang, J. (2010). *Development of soy protein/poly (lacctic acid) bioplastics*. Society of Plastic Engineers.

López Rocha, C. J., Álvarez-Castillo, E., Estrada Yáñez, M. R., Bengoechea, C., Guerrero, A., & Orta Ledesma, M. T. (2020). Development of bioplastics from a microalgae consortium from wastewater. *Journal of Environmental Management*, *263*, 110353. doi:10.1016/j.jenvman.2020.110353 PMID:32883472

Luo, K., Yang, J., Kopečkova, P., & Kopeček, J. (2011). Biodegradable multiblock poly[N-(2-hydroxypropyl)methacrylamide] via reversible addition-fragmentation chain transfer polymerization and click chemistry. *Macromolecules*, *44*(8), 2481–2488. doi:10.1021/ma102574e PMID:21552355

Magar, S. P., Ingle, A. B., & Ganorkar, R. N. (2015). Production of bioplastic (PHA) from emulsified cotton seed oil medium by Ralstonia Spp. *International Journal of Engineering Research and General Science*, *3*(1), 436–441.

Mathiot, C., Ponge, P., Gallard, B., Sassi, J. F., Delrue, F., & Le Moigne, N. (2019). Microalgae starch-based bioplastics: Screening of ten strains and plasticization of unfractionated microalgae by extrusion. *Carbohydrate Polymers*, *208*, 142–151. doi:10.1016/j.carbpol.2018.12.057 PMID:30658785

Meereboer, K. W., Misra, M., & Mohanty, A. K. (2020). Review of recent advances in the biodegradability of polyhydroxyalkanoate (PHA) bioplastics and their composites. *Green Chemistry*, *22*(17), 5519–5558. doi:10.1039/D0GC01647K

Mirtha, E.F., & Lopez, N.I., Mendez, B.S., Furst, U.P., & Steinbuchel, A. (1995). Isolation and partial characterization of Bacillus megaterium mutants deficient in poly(3-hydroxybutyrate) synthesis. *Canadian Journal of Microbiology*, *41*(1), 77–79.

Mohanan, N., Montazer, Z., Sharma, P. K., & Levin, D. B. (2020). Microbial and Enzymatic Degradation of Synthetic Plastics. *Frontiers in Microbiology*, *11*, 580709. doi:10.3389/fmicb.2020.580709 PMID:33324366

Morales-Cerrada, R., Tavernier, R., & Caillol, S. (2021). Fully bio-based thermosetting polyurethanes from bio-based polyols and isocyanates. *Polymers*, *13*(8), 1255. doi:10.3390/polym13081255 PMID:33924399

Mostafa, N. A., Farag, A. A., Abo-dief, H. M., & Tayeb, A. M. (2014). Production of biodegradable plastic from agricultural wastes. *Arabian Journal of Chemistry*, 4–11.

Muthukumar, A., & Veerappapillai, S. (2015). Biodegradation of Plastics - A Brief Review. *International Journal of Pharmaceutical Sciences Review and Research*, *31*(2), 204–209.

Nakajima-Kambe, T., Shigeno-Akutsu, Y., Nomura, N., Onuma, F., & Nakahara, T. (1999). Microbial degradation of polyurethane, polyester polyurethanes and polyether polyurethanes. *Applied Microbiology and Biotechnology*, *51*(2), 134–140. doi:10.1007002530051373 PMID:10091317

Nakamiya, K., Ooi, T., & Kinoshita, S. (1997). Non-heme hydroquinone peroxidase from Azotobacter beijerinckii HM121. *Journal of Fermentation and Bioengineering*, *84*(1), 14–21. doi:10.1016/S0922-338X(97)82780-8

Oelschlägel, M., Zimmerling, J., & Tischler, D. (2018). A review: The Styrene metabolizing cascade of side-chain oxygenation as biotechnological basis to gain various valuable compounds. *Frontiers in Microbiology*, *9*, 9. doi:10.3389/fmicb.2018.00490 PMID:29623070

Ohkita, T., & Lee, S. H. (2006). Thermal degradation and biodegradability of poly (lactic acid)/corn starch biocomposites. *Journal of Applied Polymer Science*, *100*(4), 3009–3017. doi:10.1002/app.23425

Okey, R. W., & Stensel, H. D. (1996). A QSAR based biodegradability model – A QSBR. *Water Research*, *30*(9), 2206–2214. doi:10.1016/0043-1354(96)00098-X

Park, D. H., & Kim, B. S. (2011). Production of poly(3-hydroxybutyrate) and poly(3-hydroxybutyrate-co-4-hydroxybutyrate) by Ralstonia eutropha from soybean oil. *New Biotechnology*, *28*(6), 719–724. doi:10.1016/j.nbt.2011.01.007 PMID:21333767

Paunonen, S. (2013). Strength and barrier enhancement of cellophane and cellulose derivative films: A review. *BioResources*, *8*(2), 3098–3121. doi:10.15376/biores.8.2.3098-3121

Peng, B. Y., Su, Y., Chen, Z., Chen, J., Zhou, X., Benbow, M. E., Criddle, C. S., Wu, W.-M., & Zhang, Y. (2019). Biodegradation of Polystyrene by Dark (Tenebrio obscurus) and Yellow (Tenebrio molitor) Mealworms (Coleoptera: Tenebrionidae). *Environmental Science & Technology*, *53*(9), 5256–5265. doi:10.1021/acs.est.8b06963 PMID:30990998

Perez-Puyana, V., Felix, M., Romero, A., & Guerrero, A. (2016). Effect of the injection moulding processing conditions on the development of pea protein-based bioplastics. *Journal of Applied Polymer Science*, *133*(20), 43306. doi:10.1002/app.43306

Pranamuda, H., Tokiwa, Y., & Tanaka, H. (1997). Polylactide degradation by an Amycolatopsis sp. *Applied and Environmental Microbiology*, *63*(4), 1637–1640. doi:10.1128/aem.63.4.1637-1640.1997 PMID:16535586

Prata, J. C., da Costa, J. P., Lopes, I., Duarte, A. C., & Rocha-Santos, T. (2020). Environmental exposure to microplastics: An overview on possible human health effects. *The Science of the Total Environment*, *702*, 134455. doi:10.1016/j.scitotenv.2019.134455 PMID:31733547

Privas, E., Leroux, F., & Navard, P. (2013). Preparation and properties of blends composed of lignosulfonated layered double hydroxide/pasticized starch thermoplastics. *Carbohydrate Polymers*, *96*(1), 91–100. doi:10.1016/j.carbpol.2013.03.042 PMID:23688458

Puls, J., Wilson, S. A., & Hölter, D. (2011). Degradation of cellulose acetate-based materials: A review. *Journal of Polymers and the Environment*, *19*(1), 152–165. doi:10.100710924-010-0258-0

Qi, X., Ren, Y., & Wang, X. (2017). New advances in the biodegradation of poly(lactic) acid. *International Biodeterioration & Biodegradation*, *117*, 215–223. doi:10.1016/j.ibiod.2017.01.010

Rahman, A. U. (2012). *Oxo-Biodegradable Additives for Use in Fossil Fuel Polymer Films and Once-Used Packaging*. Academic Press.

Rajendran, N. N., Puppala, S., Raj, M. S., Angeeleena, B. R., & Venkata Rajam, Ch. (2012). Seaweeds can be a new source for bioplastics. *Journal of Pharmacy Research*, *5*, 1476–1479.

Rasheed, F. (2011). Production of Sustainable Bioplastic Materials from Wheat Gluten Proteins. The Swedish University of Agricultural Sciences, 4.

Razza, F., & Cerutti, A. K. (2017). *Soil Degradable Bioplastics for a Sustainable Modern Agriculture*. Springer. doi:10.1007/978-3-662-54130-2_7

Ru, J., Huo, Y., & Yang, Y. (2020). Microbial degradation and valorization of plastic wastes. *Frontiers in Microbiology*, *11*, 11. doi:10.3389/fmicb.2020.00442 PMID:32373075

Rudin, A., & Choi, P. (2013). *The Elements of Polymer Science & Engineering* (3rd ed.). Academic Press.

Sakai, K., Hamada, N., & Watanabe, Y. (1986). Degradation mechanism of poly(vinyl alcohol) by successive reactions of secondary alcohol oxidase and ®-diketone hydrolase from *Pseudomonas* sp. *Agricultural and Biological Chemistry*, *50*(4), 989–996. doi:10.1080/00021369.1986.10867494

Sanchez-Vazquez, S. A., Hailes, H. C., & Evans, J. R. G. (2013). Hydrophobic Polymers from Food Waste: Resources and Synthesis. *Polymer Reviews (Philadelphia, Pa.)*, *53*(4), 627–694. doi:10.1080/15583724.2013.834933

Sang, B. I., Hori, K., Tanji, Y., & Unno, H. (2002). Fungal contribution to in situ biodegradation of poly(3-hydroxybutyrate-co-3-hydroxyvalerate) film in soil. *Applied Microbiology and Biotechnology*, *58*, 241–247. doi:10.100700253-001-0884-5 PMID:11876418

Scherer, T. M., Fuller, R. C., Lenz, R. W., & Goodwin, S. (1999). Hydrolase activity of an extracellular depolymerase from Aspergillus fumigatus with bacterial and synthetic polyesters. *Polymer Degradation & Stability*, *64*(2), 267–275. doi:10.1016/S0141-3910(98)00201-8

Scott, G. (2002). *Degradable Polymers*. Springer. doi:10.1007/978-94-017-1217-0

Shah, A. A., Kato, S., Shintani, N., Kamini, N. R., & Nakajima-Kambe, T. (2014). Microbial degradation of aliphatic and aliphatic-aromatic co-polyesters. *Applied Microbiology and Biotechnology*, *98*(8), 3437–3447. doi:10.100700253-014-5558-1 PMID:24522729

Shimao, M. (2001). Biodegradation of plastics. *Current Opinion in Biotechnology*, *12*(3), 242–247. doi:10.1016/S0958-1669(00)00206-8 PMID:11404101

Shimao, M., Yamamoto, H., Ninomiya, K., Kato, N., Adachi, O., Ameyama, M., & Sakazawa, C. (1984). Pyrroloquinoline quinone as an essential growth factor for a poly(vinyl alcohol)-degrading symbiont, *Pseudomonas* sp. VM15C. *Agricultural and Biological Chemistry*, *48*(11), 2873–2876. doi:10.1271/bbb1961.48.2873

Silva, J. A., Tobella, L. M., Becerra, J., Godoy, F., & Matrínez, M. A. (2007). Biosynthesis of poly-β-hydroxyalkanoate by Brevundimonas vesicularis LMG P-23615 and Sphingopyxis macrogoltabida LMG 17324 using acid-hydrolyzed sawdust as carbon source. *Journal of Bioscience and Bioengineering*, *103*(6), 542–546. doi:10.1263/jbb.103.542 PMID:17630126

Slepecky, R. A., & Law, J. H. (1961). Synthesis and degradation of poly-b-hydroxybutyric acid in connection with sporulation of Bacillus megaterium. *Journal of Bacteriology*, *82*, 37–42. doi:10.1128/jb.82.1.37-42.1961 PMID:16561914

Sudhakar, M. P., Magesh, P. D., & Dharani, G. (2020). Studies on the development and characterization of bioplastic film from the red seaweed (Kappaphycus alvarezii). *Environmental Science and Pollution Research International*, *28*(26), 33899–33913. doi:10.100711356-020-10010-z PMID:32935218

Sudhakar, M., Priyadarshini, C., Doble, M., Sriyutha Murthy, P., & Venkatesan, R. (2007). Marine bacteria mediated degradation of nylon 66 and 6. *International Biodeterioration & Biodegradation*, *60*(3), 144–151. doi:10.1016/j.ibiod.2007.02.002

Suriyamongkol, P., Weselake, R., Narine, S., Moloney, M., & Shah, S. (2007). Biotechnological approaches for the production of polyhydroxyalkanoates in microorganisms and plants – a review. *Biotechnology Advances*, *25*(2), 148–175. doi:10.1016/j.biotechadv.2006.11.007 PMID:17222526

Sushmitha, B. S., Vanitha, K. P., & Rangaswamy, B. E. (2016). Bioplastics - A Review. *International Journal of Modern Trends in Engineering and Research*, *3*(4), 411–413.

Suzuki, T., Ichihara, Y., Yamada, M., & Tonomura, K. (1973). Some characteristics of *Pseudomonas* O-3 which utilizes polyvinyl alcohol. *Agricultural and Biological Chemistry*, *37*(4), 747–756. doi:10.1271/bbb1961.37.747

Tenorio-Alfonso, A., Sánchez, M. C., & Franco, J. M. (2020). A review of the sustainable approaches in the production of bio-based polyurethanes and their applications in the adhesive field. *Journal of Polymers and the Environment*, *28*(3), 749–774. doi:10.100710924-020-01659-1

Thurmund, W. (2010). *Seaweed: A new wave of investment in macroalgae*. Biofuels International.

Tokiwa, Y., & Calabia, B. P. (2006). Biodegradability and biodegradation of poly(lactide). *Applied Microbiology*, *72*, 244–251. PMID:16823551

Ummalyma, S. B., Sahoo, D., & Pandey, A. (2020). Microalgal Biorefineries for Industrial Products. In Microalgae Cultivation for Biofuels Production. Academic Press.

Uruyama, H., Kanamori, T., & Kimura, Y. (2002). Properties and biodegradability of polymer blends of poly(L-lactide)swith different optical purity of the lactate units. *Macromolecular Materials and Engineering*, *287*(2), 116–121. doi:10.1002/1439-2054(20020201)287:2<116::AID-MAME116>3.0.CO;2-Z

Wang, K., Mandal, A., Ayton, E., Hunt, R., Zeller, M.A., & Sharma, S. (2016). Modification of protein rich algal biomass to form bioplastics and odor removal. *Protein Byproduct*, 107-117.

Wang, Y., Yin, J., & Chen, G.-Q. (2014). Polyhydroxyalkanoates, challenges and opportunities. *Current Opinion in Biotechnology*, *30*, 59–65. doi:10.1016/j.copbio.2014.06.001 PMID:24976377

Williams, D. F. (1981). Enzymatic hydrolysis of polylactic acid. *Engineering in Medicine*, *10*(1), 5–7. doi:10.1243/EMED_JOUR_1981_010_004_02

Wong, Y.-M., Brigham, C. J., Rha, C. K., Sinskey, A. J., & Sudesh, K. (2012). Biosynthesis and characterization of polyhydroxyalkanoate containing high 3-hydroxyhexanoate monomer fraction from crude palm kernel oil by recombinant Cupriavidus necator. *Bioresource Technology*, *121*, 320–327. doi:10.1016/j.biortech.2012.07.015 PMID:22858502

Wu, Z., Wang, F., Hu, L., Jiang, Y., Wang, X., & Xu, J. (2020). Directional liquefaction of lignocellulose in 1, 4-dioxane–ethanol–formic acid co-solvents. *Journal of Chemical Technology and Biotechnology (Oxford, Oxfordshire)*, *96*(4), 971–979. doi:10.1002/jctb.6606

Xu, Y., Lin, L., Xiao, M., Wang, S., Smith, A. T., Sun, L., & Meng, Y. (2018). Synthesis and properties of CO2-based plastics: Environmentally-friendly, energy-saving and biomedical polymeric materials. *Progress in Polymer Science*, *80*, 163–182. doi:10.1016/j.progpolymsci.2018.01.006

Yang, J. H., Yu, J. G., & Ma, X. F. (2006). A novel plasticizer for the preparation of thermoplastic starch. *Chinese Chemical Letters*, *17*(1), 133–136.

Yang, J., Ching, Y. C., & Chuah, C. H. (2019). Applications of lignocellulosic fibers and lignin in bioplastics: A review. *Polymers*, *11*(5), 1–26. doi:10.3390/polym11050751 PMID:31035331

Yang, S. S., Wu, W. M., Brandon, A. M., Fan, H. Q., Receveur, J. P., Li, Y., Wang, Z.-Y., Fan, R., McClellan, R. L., Gao, S.-H., Ning, D., Phillips, D. H., Peng, B.-Y., Wang, H., Cai, S.-Y., Li, P., Cai, W.-W., Ding, L.-Y., Yang, J., ... Criddle, C. S. (2018). Ubiquity of polystyrene digestion and biodegradation within yellow mealworms, larvae of Tenebrio molitor Linnaeus (Coleoptera: Tenebrionidae). *Chemosphere*, *212*, 262–271. doi:10.1016/j.chemosphere.2018.08.078 PMID:30145418

Yang, Y., Yang, J., Wu, W. M., Zhao, J., Song, Y., Gao, L., Yang, R., & Jiang, L. (2015). Biodegradation and mineralization of polystyrene by plastic-eating mealworms. Part 1. Chemical and physical characterization and isotopic tests. *Environmental Science & Technology*, *49*(20), 12080–12086. doi:10.1021/acs.est.5b02661 PMID:26390034

Yano, H., Sugiyama, J., Nakagaito, A. N., Nogi, M., Matsuura, T., Hikita, M., & Handa, K. (2005). Optically transparent composites reinforced with networks of bacterial nanofibers. *Advanced Materials*, *17*(2), 153–155. doi:10.1002/adma.200400597

Yates, M. R., & Barlow, C. Y. (2013). Life Cycle assessment of biodegradable, commercial biopolymers – a critical review. *Resources, Conservation and Recycling*, *78*, 54–66. doi:10.1016/j.resconrec.2013.06.010

Ye, S., Wang, S., Lin, L., Xiao, M., & Meng, Y. (2019). CO2 derived biodegradable polycarbonates: Synthesis, modification and applications. *Advanced Industrial and Engineering Polymer Research*, *2*(4), 143–160. doi:10.1016/j.aiepr.2019.09.004

Yoshida, S., Hiraga, K., Takehana, T., Taniguchi, I., Yamaji, H., Maeda, Y., Toyohara, K., Miyamoto, K., Kimura, Y., & Oda, K. (2016). A bacterium that degrades and assimilates poly(ethylene terephthalate). *Science*, *351*(6278), 1196–1199. doi:10.1126cience.aad6359 PMID:26965627

Yue, W., Yin, C. F., Sun, L., Zhang, J., Xu, Y., & Zhou, N. Y. (2021). Biodegradation of bisphenol-A polycarbonate plastic by Pseudoxanthomonas sp. strain NyZ600. *Journal of Hazardous Materials, 15.*

Zbořilova, P., & Pac, J. (2014). *Oxo-Degradable Polyolefinic Material.* Academic Press.

Zhang, C., Wang, C., Cao, G., Wang, D., & Ho, S.-H. (2020). A sustainable solution to plastics pollution: An eco-friendly bioplastic film production from high-salt contained Spirulina sp. residues. *Journal of Hazardous Materials*, *388*, 121773. doi:10.1016/j.jhazmat.2019.121773 PMID:31836373

Zhang, H., Obias, V., Gonyer, K., & Dennis, D. (1994). Production of polyhydroxyalkanoates in sucrose-utilizing recombinant Escherichia coli and Klebsiella strains. *Applied and Environmental Microbiology*, *60*(4), 1198–1205. doi:10.1128/aem.60.4.1198-1205.1994 PMID:8017916

Zhang, Z., Peng, H., Yang, D., Zhang, J., & Ju, F. (2021). Polyvinyl Chloride Biodegradation Fuels Survival of Invasive Insect Larva and Intestinal Degrading Strain of Klebsiella. *bioRxiv*.

Chapter 12
Analysis of Microplastics

Namrata Pandey
Ecotoxicology Laboratory, Regulatory Toxicology Group, Academy of Scientific and Innovative Research (AcSIR), Ghaziabad, India

Kavita Krishna
Ecotoxicology Laboratory, Regulatory Toxicology Group, Academy of Scientific and Innovative Research (AcSIR), Ghaziabad, India

Alina Zehra
Ecotoxicology Laboratory, Regulatory Toxicology Group, Academy of Scientific and Innovative Research (AcSIR), Ghaziabad, India & CSIR-Indian Institute of Toxicology Research, Lucknow, India

S. Anbumani
Ecotoxicology Laboratory, Regulatory Toxicology Group, Academy of Scientific and Innovative Research (AcSIR), Ghaziabad, India & CSIR-Indian Institute of Toxicology Research, Lucknow, India

ABSTRACT

The ever-growing demand and consumption of plastic has created irrevocable havoc on earth. The exponential increase in the production of plastic is expected to create 2,134 million tons of waste by 2050, which surpasses the fish mass in the oceans. With no proper reuse or recycling policies and gruesome exploitation of this persistent pollutant, plastic has started accumulating and overflowing beyond control. The prevalence and the undefined harm from micro and nano plastic pollution calls for a vigilant screening and periodic upgradation of analytical methodology for efficient and standard reporting. This chapter aims to provide a summary of currently available extraction protocols and instrumental methodologies for microplastics analysis in various environmental samples to fully understand the implications it possesses.

INTRODUCTION

Plastic in the environment is exposed to various forces in nature. Weathering caused by water, air, sediment, wind or sun makes the plastic brittle and cause its degradation into smaller fragments, pellets and

DOI: 10.4018/978-1-7998-9723-1.ch012

fibres(Hernandez et al., 2019)(Chamas et al., 2020). These smaller versions, measuring < 5mm and <100 nm is termed as microplastics (MPs) and nano plastics (NPs), respectively. Owing to their virtue of extremely small size and complex physiochemical properties, micro- and nano-plastics have been dominating the world by polluting the most pristine ecosystems on earth ranging from darkest corners of deep sea like Mariana trench to white and wonderful snow of Swiss alps (Rhodes, 2018), creeping further into the wide array of organisms disrupting the habitat and functional ecology. This widespread global pollutant has unfortunately surpassed its presence beyond expectance in recent times. Micro and nano plastics have found its way into aqueous, terrestrial and aerial ecosystems (Sridharan et al., 2021). With no immunity to mankind, microplastics have found its way into human systems *via* trophic transfer through food consumption, a drizzle of honey (Diaz-Basantes et al., 2020), few shakes of table salt (Peixoto et al., 2019), or while opening plastic packaging (Sobhani et al., 2020), etc. Scientists are concerned that a human being is alarmingly consuming a credit card worth of plastic every year (Dalberg Advisors et al., 2019).

The fate of MPs/NPs, hence, can be deciphered by the knowledge of their abundance, characteristics, chemical composition, and surface morphology, as accurate and reliable investigations of MPs and NPs are an important source of explanation of their environmental health impacts.(Campanale et al., 2020) This chapter addresses the currently available analytical and methodological approaches for MPs, challenges within various environmental matrices and commercial products like salt(Lee et al., 2019), honey and beer,(Diaz-Basantes et al., 2020) canned food etc. Studies reporting the presence of MPs in both outdoor and indoor air along with the possibility of long distanced atmospheric transport of microplastic has spiked interest over the likelihood of inhalation exposure and its target organ toxicity (Dong et al., 2020). MPs are omnipresent and it came to no surprise when the pollutant was and kept getting detected in a wide range of concentrations in marine water, fresh water and bottled and tap drinking water (Nelms et al., 2019). Similarly, sediments play a regulating role in distribution of micro and nano plastics in benthic- pelagic layers of aquatic ecosystems. These watersheds act as both source and a sink for micro and nano plastic pollution while sparing no one, from biota inhabiting these bodies to humans consuming their produce. (Yao et al., 2019). Analysis and quantification of MPs/NPs from these environmental niches is the requisite towards measuring the plastic pollution, however, there is a need for optimisation of these analytical protocols so as to eliminate the incidences of false positives and false negatives.

For the ease of navigation and comprehension, the chapter is categorised into five major sections, *viz* sampling, sample preparation, visual identification, instrumental analysis and quantification, highlighting the majorly explored methodologies and instrumentation approaches. Sampling approaches depend upon the targeted ecosystem's location, sample volume and sample size. Retrieval methods include collection of samples using bottles, cans and pumps for water, shovels and scoops for soils and sediments, nets and fishing gears for aquatic and/or traps for terrestrial organisms. In the current chapter, a vital necessity of procedural blanks and contamination control to avoid overestimation of MPs is mentioned.

SAMPLING

One of the most crucial steps towards MPs analysis is the collection and process of samples. This should be done in a way that it represents the area it is collected from in its most natural way to avoid the over estimation of the pollution. The first and the foremost method in the sampling protocol is the appropriate selection of the site reflecting the best representation of the study area. The site for sampling should be done based on a thorough field analysis in terms of any accidental or unnatural contamination from a nearby source. The strategy for sediment sampling can be of three types (Adomat & Grischek, 2021), based on the research hypothesis as Deterministic, Stochastic, and Regular Grid systems where the sampling is done keeping in mind the previous literature survey information, statistical analysis as well as in a regular pattern at random locations respectively. Approaches of sampling as described (Möller et al., 2020) are judgemental sampling (biased; verifying a contamination site based on expert information), simple random sampling (unbiased, selecting point samples from a supposedly homogenous area), systematic and grid sampling (distribution of samples in patterns of triangles or squares defining the coordinate axis), transect sampling (samples collected in a single line equidistant from another in a one dimensional way), unaligned grid sampling (combination of random and grid sampling, points located randomly in a grid), and stratified sampling (samples collected from the sub areas of the total site, assuming each divided strata is having homogenous pollution). MPs have been reported to be present in soil (Rafique et al., 2020), air (Chen et al., 2020), water (Lv et al., 2021), sediments (Zhang et al., 2020) (Asadi et al., 2019)(Di Renzo et al., 2021), biota(Hermsen et al., 2018), and have been continuously analysed for their properties and quantities. The solid and sludge samples from WWTPs are collected by manual sieving, using tools such as steel quadrants, spades, spatulas, shovels, augers, corers (hand corers, piston corers, box corers and gravity corers, drill corers, freeze coring), extraction pump, buckets, glass jars, Van Veen Grab Sampler, dredges, or a combination of methods such as a Ruttner sampler (Magnusson & Norén, 2014), mobile pumping (Mintenig et al., 2017), and multiuse pump (Long et al., 2019). The water and its inhabitants are collected using a collecting unit such as a basin metallic pan, and anti-static wooden brush (Dehghani et al., 2017); a passive collector (Total deposition), and an active pump sampler are used to collect air samples. The biota samples are collected mostly through nets (water borne organisms), purchased from markets (commercially important organisms such as mussels, fishes, toads, and shrimps) or bell dived and collected. Bigger organisms such as the stranded whales, dolphins, turtles, and seal are samples too for MPs analysis (Dehghani et al., 2017; Nelms et al., 2019; Schirinzi et al., 2020). The most common method of sampling accumulated street dust is sweeping the surface with small natural fibre paint brush into a metal dust pan with a quadrate of 1 meter square (Patchaiyappan et al., 2021), (Kitahara & Nakata, 2020). Dry sweeping method efficiently captures bigger sized particles of >75-100µm whereas particles smaller than this are collected with lesser efficiency (O'Brien et al., 2021). An additional sampling methodology collect road dust from the respective sample quadrate using a vacuum cleaner. The dust is collected in a plastic bag and no filter is present in the machine before the collection bag to collect raw samples from the site (Yukioka et al., 2020).

SAMPLE PREPARATION

Soil and sediment are dried below 60°C to avoid plastic degradation and lose the moisture content. The dried soil is then sieved using a metallic mesh of sizes ranging from 5 µm to 5 mm to remove particles other than the particles of choice. Mesh sizes of various range of 0.2µm – 300 µm is preferred to filter water samples (Cutroneo et al., 2020). Biota samples are thoroughly washed, measured and weighed before dissection (in case of bigger vertebrate fishes) or processed as a whole.

CHEMICAL DIGESTION

Enumeration of plastic masked in complex environmental samples like biota tissue or organic built up requires action of strong reagents which will allow detection of the plastic and some recalcitrant type chemicals. Chemical digestion at high temperature should be carefully employed since these reactions can hamper the chemical and structural integrity of the particle and misidentification of particle. Lack or loss of particles during chemical treatments should also be considered to avoid false reporting.

Acid Digestion

Some of the most commonly used acids for digestion of organic matter for extraction of microplastic are H_2SO_4, HNO_3, HCl, $HClO_4$ in various concentrations and ratios. However, the polymer degradation and problems in polymer identification in field samples, have also been reported (Amy L. Lusher et al., 2020); (Joana C. Prata et al., 2019). Karami et al reported that HCl (37%) is known to have the recovery efficiency of the MPs of >95% but with little effect of the PET polymer (Karami et al., 2017). Adaptation of various concentrations, incubation temperature periods have been tried and tested with HNO_3. Proving to deliver highest digestion efficiency than other strong acids, nitric acid is often used to digest tissue samples in biota. If inefficient alone, HNO_3 is used in combination with perchloric acid in ratio of 4;1 v/v (Dehaut et al., 2016).

Alkaline Digestion

Some of the most common alkaline solutions used for digestion are 1 M and 10 M NaOH, 10% KOH. The sieved samples of different size categories are digested in 10% potassium hydroxide (KOH) at 60 °C for fourteen hours to remove organic matter (A. L. Lusher et al., 2017). KOH was found to be the most used alkali digestant at (KOH-10%) 60ºC overnight or for 24 hours. It was found to affect the polymers causing discoloration in nylon, PE, and uPVC (unplasticized PVC) (Joana Correia Prata et al., 2019). Sodium hydroxide has also been used to digest organic material, reported in zooplankton with 90% efficiency. Unlike acids, alkali digestion suggested polymer resistance to 10%KOH.

Oxidizing Digestion

Different samples of environmental matrices pose different challenges of extraction and analysis. Soil and sludge samples are particularly harder due to their higher organic content. MPs entering soil gets coated with organic matter and form soil aggregates. MP wrapped these soil particles are difficult to extract and need strong chemical treatments (Li et al., 2019).

Digestion with Hydrogen Peroxide

Peroxidation is currently being used and Oxidation through H_2O_2 has been employed in various studies to digest waste water samples. Various volume of H_2O_2 is subjected to temperature to digest the settled organically rich portion or filter membrane retentate of samples for clear visualisation and analysis of MPs (Ahmed et al., 2021) (Hamidian et al., 2021). Digestion with H_2O_2 requires large incubation time of days and temperature, endangering the polymeric characteristics of the plastic and restricting large sample analysis.

Digestion With Fenton's Reagent

also known as wet peroxide oxidation. Clearly, digestion of organically rich samples needs stronger digestion techniques without resulting into polymer degradation. Fenton reagents have been used in many studies as a promising alternative. Reaction involves an inorganic ferrous salt solution which activates peroxide, obtained from H_2O_2, leading to the formation of hydroxyl radicals which has a high oxidation potential. The high oxidation potential of hydroxyl radicals provides ambient temperature and oxidation conditions to the reactants. The pH of the reaction is maintained by sulphuric acid to 3. Not only Fenton's reaction requires shorter time and doesn't need any external application of energy, the reaction doesn't significantly change the chemical composition of polymers (Elkhatib & Oyanedel-Craver, 2020) (Jung et al., 2021).

Enzymatic Digestion

Enzymatic digestion is a non-aggressive extraction method. Studies have reported the use of various enzymes like Proteinase-K, trypsin, collagenase, Protease, Cellulase, Chitinase and papain individually or in combination. Sparing high temperature and polymer damage enzymatic digestion is not an economically viable option and requires large incubation periods, especially while processing large volume of organically rich data, as WWTPs samples (Bakaraki Turan et al., 2021). Enzymes presents a wide angle to the possibility of MP extraction from the organic matter in terms of minimal handling, inexpensiveness, safety, and efficiency (von Friesen et al., 2019). One such enzymatic digestion demonstration using pancreatic enzymes along with Tris, (isolated commercially) and bivalves. The method was proved to be a better alternative than KOH in terms of effectiveness and time. Other enzymes such as proteinase K (500 µg/mL) with CaCl2 at 50 °C and 60°C for 2 hours and 20 mins respectively in a sequence and moving on to 30% H_2O_2 (Karlsson et al., 2017); Trypsin, Collagenase and Papain (Courtene-Jones et al., 2017); Protease, Cellulase, Chitinase (Time of action: 15 days) with intermittent H_2O_2 treatments; Industrial enzyme blend (2.5%; at 45 °C) for 1 hour before the oxidation step (Crichton et al., 2017) (Joana Correia Prata et al., 2019).

DENSITY SEPERATION

Density separation is one of the advanced analytical methods which helps separate microplastics <500 µm from complex and organic rich sample material. As the research ventures sampling and extraction of microplastics from various matrices, samples with high content of organic material pose limitations. A sample with high organic content interfere with spectroscopic analysis and cause increased background noise in the spectra. MPs have been known to have densities around 0.8-1.8 g/cm^3 which are lighter and can be separated using solutions with higher density. (Rocha-Santos & Duarte, 2015). A super dense solution of salts and water causes the MPs to isolate to the surface whereas the heavier particles of the sand and organic noise, is settled at the bottom. Sodium chloride (NaCl) (1.15–1.3 g cm– 3) was found to be the most used salt in the density separation step and was employed by around 46.6% of the studies reported by (Cutroneo et al., 2021). NaCl is safe and inexpensive, however, the polymers such as polyester, PVC and PET (denser than NaCl; 1.23-1.38 g/cm^3) cannot be separated. Apart from this distilled water and Dichloromethane (1.3 g/cm^3; for low density MPs) is used for low density MPs. PET (polyethylene terephthalate), PVC (polyvinyl chloride), PBT (polybutylenes terephthalate), PLA (polylactic acid) whose density ranges from 1.32 to 1.58 g/cm^3. Other dense salts include Calcium chloride ($CaCl_2$) 1.3–1.35 g/cm^3, Zinc chloride ($ZnCl_2$; the second most used salt- 19.3%) 1.5–1.8 g/cm^3, Zinc bromide (ZnBr2) 1.7 g/cm^3, Sodium iodide (NaI; the third most used salt- 17.5%) 1.55–1.8 g/cm^3, Sodium bromide (NaBr) 1.37 g/cm^3, Sodium polytungstate (SPT; ($3Na_2WO_4{\cdot}9WO_3{\cdot}H_2O$)) 1.4–1.65 g/cm^3, Sodium tungstate dihydrate ($Na_2WO_4{\cdot}2H_2O$) 1.4 g/cm^3, Lithium meta tungstate (Li_2WO_4) 1.62 g/cm^3, Potassium iodide (KI) 1.7 g/cm^3, and Monosodium phosphate (MSP; NaH_2PO_4) 1.4–1.45 g/cm^3 have shown a promising recovery but have been in the harmful chemical category as per the US EPA and REACH Regulations, hence cannot be generally used for the analysis (Bellasi et al., 2021; Coppock et al., 2017). NaI is the costliest and cause environment harm. However, NaI having the maximum density is able to extract polymers of higher density which NaCl cannot. Examples are polyethylene (PE) (0.91– 0.92 g/cm3), polystyrene (PS) (1.04–1.1 g/cm3) and polypropylene (PP) (0.9–0.91 g/cm3). On the other hand, NaI or $ZnCl_2$ are applied for the extraction of MPs with high density polymers mainly polyethyleneterephtalate (PET) (1.37–1.45 g/cm3) and polyvinylchloride (PVC) (1.6–1.58 g/cm3) (Hidalgo-ruz et al., 2012; Wang et al., 2017). The mixture of density solution and processed sample are stirred, allowed to sit to settle and then the supernatant is filtered to extract MPs.

Oil Separation

The oil-based separation uses the oleophilic properties of the polymers such that the hydrophilic sediment particles are separated in the water layers while the polymeric content is trapped in the oil layer on the top (Huppertsberg & Knepper, 2018; He et al., 2020). Castor, Canola, Olive as well as mineral oil is efficiently used in separating MPs from the sediments and other environment matrix. The disadvantage of this technique involves washing off the oil layer before proceeding for the polymer identification procedures including FTIR or Raman which is time consuming.

Electrostatic Separation

The soil or sediments can be separated using the electrostatic discharge-based technique of where the conductive components (Sediments or soil) are distinguished from its non-conducting counter class (MPs/polymers) as done by Felsing et al., 2018 using a Korona-Walzen-Scheider (KWS) electrostatic bell separator (Felsing et al., 2018). The instrument charges the particles and discards the particles based on their charge into different sample holders where the least charged MPs fall into the holders different from that of the charged ones.

Magnetic Separation

The protocol to separate MPs from the environmental matrix such as soil or sediments or water, is based on the process of magnetizing the hydrophobic surface of the MPs with the iron particles rendering magnetic properties to the polymer particles which can be separated with an addition of a magnetic field. The recovery rate for the bigger particles is lesser than the particles which are smaller than 20 μm.

Pressurized Fluid Extraction (PFE)

A solvent based approach which utilizes the subcritical temperature and pressure to extract the hydrophobic organic compounds from soil, sediments, clay and wastes performed by Stephen and Gautam to extract MPs < 30 µm with a recovery rate of 100% from soil samples (Fuller & Gautam, 2016). Apart from the above listed methods of separation of MPs from unwanted particles in the sediment matrix, an eco-friendly alternative was used where NaCl was combined with sucrose to achieve the desired (Bellasi et al., 2021).

FILTRATION

Filtration is the final step of MP extraction. The technique is relatively simpler, cost effective and time efficient. The efficiency of filtration largely depends upon the efficient result of aforementioned steps, with the final aim of collecting the MPs from the strata with minimum organic debris. The processed sample solutions can be filtered using various types of filter membrane distinguished on the basis of pore size and type of membrane. Filter structure and pore size affect the abundance of microplastics of varying shapes (H. Cai et al., 2020). Glass fibre, PDFE, nitrocellulose and polycarbonate filters are cited in various studies (Bretas Alvim et al., 2020). Pore size of filtration membrane also plays an important role in filtration efficiency. A smaller pore size will filter less volume of sample solution, clog quickly and will need frequent change of filter with high debris content making identification of MP a gruesome task. A smaller pore size retentate a wide size range of MPs. However, a larger pore size will allow small particles to pass through and can result in underestimated reporting of MP. For instance, Whatman No. 42 filter paper (retention >8 µm) (Afrin et al., 2020), Whatman Anodisc filter (13 mm diameter, 0.2 µm pore size), glass fibre filter with pore size of 0.45 µm have been used to extract MPs from soil. In the case of sediments, various filters of pore size ranging from 0.2 µm to 5000 µm were used for filtering the solutions twice. It is important to choose the right type of membrane to avoid any damage or tear to filter membrane due to the usage of highly corrosive solutions and filtration under high pressure.

VISUAL IDENTIFICATION

Identification by eye is the first visual identification of MPs in extracted samples. However, this is restricted only to larger size microplastics. The preliminary observation is used to record information like size, surface texture, colour and shape. (Silva et al., 2018). Large sized MPs, corresponding to size range of 2-5 mm, can be sorted while inspection with forceps and a spatula. Visual sorting is easy, inexpensive and a fast method to see the contaminant (Shim et al., 2017).

While large particles can be observed through naked eyes, smaller particles of size <500 µm needs to be observed in dissecting or stereomicroscope (Hamidian et al., 2021). Stereomicroscope with or without a digital camera attached have been commonly used for the visual sorting and inspection (Piehl et al., 2018). The dried filter paper is inspected under a dissecting microscope at various magnification ranging from 10x-35x. Both the "break test" and the "hot needle test" are used to distinguish plastic and non-plastic particles to complete the primary MPs identification step (Egessa et al., 2020) (A. L. Lusher et al., 2017). The MPs were characterized based on their size, shape and colour after microscopic examination using a stereo microscope. The analysis and categorization of MPs can be well described in two ways that is the morphometrics or the physical and visible properties including the colour, shape, size, brittleness, weather-age, etc. and the chemical properties of the particles including the chemical nature of the MPs in terms of the polymer type. The visual characteristics have been described by the authors using an optical microscope in most of the literature (Barrett et al., 2020; Guerranti et al., 2020; Id et al., 2020). Earlier, large obvious sized microplastic was visually identified using simple microscopic techniques for presence and quantification (Dris et al., 2016). The techniques hinders accurate determination of plastic particulates of size <500 μm and limits quantification of the size fraction which can only be examined using microscope since the abundance of microplastic increase with decreasing size (Käppler et al., 2016) (Araujo, Nolasco, Ribeiro, & Ribeiro-claro, 2018). Visual identification coupled with confirmatory presence can overcome limitations imposed by human bias, microscope quality, magnification, sample matrix etc. and is recommended in recent studies. (Hendrickson et al., 2018) (Hidalgo-ruz et al., 2012). For particles <500 μm, it is recommended that non-visual, spectroscopy methods can ensure the determination of plastic.

Physical Characterization

Shapes

Microplastic is present is various shapes and forms in the environment. The most frequent terms to describe their morphology are fibres, fragments, films, foam, pellets, beads, sphere and flakes. A dominance of fragment shape was reported in atmospheric deposition of microplastic in snow sampled from remote areas of Swiss Alps (Bergmann et al., 2019), while in the street dust of the most abundant shapes are Iran, fibrous (33.5%) and granule (65.9%) (Abbasi & Turner, 2021). While reporting atmospheric abundance shape of microplastic is may affect its transport in the environment. Films are thin and flat plastic particles and so their deposition can happen longer distance and quantity. While shapes like pellets or fragments with sharp edges may harm the organism physically, smaller particles can pass the membrane barrier and cause disruption in physiological functions (Rochman et al., 2019). The influence of shape on atmospheric transport enquires further research.

Size

Microplastics encompass a broad range of sizes of plastic particles, typically between 1 μm to 5 mm in length. Various size of microplastic belonging to different shapes are reported in the environment. The length of plastic fibres in Pyrenees mountains was predominantly found to be less than 300 μm (~50%) with about 70% of the fragment size was less than 50 μm. In Hamburg, an urban city in Europe, the fragments were mostly of size less than 63 μm accounting for about 60%, followed by 63–300 μm accounting for about 30% of all the particles analysed. Fibre size were predominantly between 300 and 5000 μm in length (Klein & Fischer, 2019). Among the previous studies, the longest atmospheric microfibre identified is ~5000 μm (L. Cai et al., 2017) and the size can go as long as 5mm which can be visible through the naked eye. The snow in European and Arctic regions was sampled for detection of microplastic were 80% of microplastics were less than or equal to 25 μm (Bergmann et al., 2019).

Colour

As colourful and attractive plastic came to place in form of packaging, toys and other utility items microplastics have been reported in a range of various colours, including red, orange, yellow, brown, tan, off white, white, grey, blue, green, transparent etc. The list is endless and even more vibrant. Dark, white, transparent, or translucent particles may be under represented during visual inspection. Clear and transparent items have been ascribed to polypropylene, white to polyethylene and opaque colours to LDPE. However, the colour of a plastic particle cannot easily be used to deduce the type or origin. Importantly, colour information can be biased as brighter colours are spotted more easily during visual inspection (Rochman et al., 2019).

INSTRUMENTAL ANALYSIS

Polymer based identification of plastic pollutants extracted from various environmental matrices give assured answers to the speculation of visually identified plastic particles. Particles analysed give spectral analysis of the polymer type which is then compared with the reference spectral library values of the instrument and give suitable match results. Confirming MPs with their polymers characteristics eradicates the problem of false positives but perpetuates the issue of false negatives. A sound knowledge of type of MP polymer contamination in environment gives insight about their interaction in various natural conditions in addition to evaluating source of plastic pollution in the first place.

Fourier Transform Infrared (FTIR) Spectroscopy

The working principle of FTIR involves obtaining a vibration spectrum when an IR wavelength range of 400–4000 cm^{-1} acts on the given substance, the atoms of the material fall from an excited state to ground state along with a decrease in energy. This decrease in energy is characteristic of a particular molecular structure and gives unique peaks in the vibration spectra (Lenz et al., 2015). This spectra obtained is screened for the presence and absence of characteristic frequency bands and matched with references of spectral libraries (Araujo, Nolasco, Ribeiro, & Ribeiro-Claro, 2018).

FT-IR can be employed to detect MPs through two measurement mode, reflectance and transmittance (Huppertsberg & Knepper, 2018). A special mode of reflectance called Attenuated total reflectance (ATR)- FTIR measures vibrational spectrum of microplastic through contact analysis. The pressure probed by the ATR probe can damage highly-weathered or fragile microplastics. There is a chance of losing MP as particles can be pulled from the filter paper by adhesion to or electrostatic interaction with the probe tip. A hard particle can easily damage the ATR probe made of germanium. The samples and crystal surfaces are prone to contamination during analysis. Measurement of particles with ATR-FTIR is laborious since each particle to be analysed is kept on the crystal manually and size restricted up to 500 µm, due to contact analysis. Another mode of spectral measurement is transmission mode. During analysis, transmission spectra is recorded directly on filter. Suitable filter materials like, silica or aluminium oxide are used as these filters are IR transparent. It is critical to investigate the effects of chemical degradation on vibrational spectral bands of plastics before MP identification (Xu et al., 2019).

FTIR analysis spectra is impeded by oxidative damage of polymer in natural conditions, which then hampers the polymer identification due to lack of reference data on weathered plastics. It is important to investigate, the characteristic vibrational spectra of chemically weathered plastics. Small microplastics with of size of 10 μm can be analysed by micro-FTIR (μ-FTIR), which performs microscopic observation on plastic particles prior to spectroscopic confirmation on a single platform by switching between the object lens and IR probe. Hence, μ-FTIR gives morphological and chemical characteristic of particles analysed. The technique provides an advantage of analysing plastic particles on the filter paper, sparing energy and time to handle particles individually.

Raman Spectroscopy

Based on the principle of irradiation of sample with monochromatic radiation, Raman spectroscopy is a vibrational spectroscopy technique which provides information on molecular vibration of the system excited by the incident monochromatic radiation. The Raman spectral corresponds to the characteristic vibrations of the molecules and give confirmatory analysis for the microplastic observed (Araujo, Nolasco, Ribeiro, & Ribeiro-claro, 2018) (Halfar et al., 2021). Often coupled with a microscope, the coupled spectroscopic method is able to collect spectra from different points and generate images of morphological properties (Huppertsberg & Knepper, 2018).

The smallest sample analysed from Raman in practical application is 10 μm due to surface weathering, however with improved techniques this size can go as low up to 2 μm. The samples analysed by Raman are not destroyed, need minimal sample preparation and quantity. High sensitivity to non-polar functional groups, lower interference of water on spectra and narrower spectral bands are some of the advantages of Raman spectroscopy. Some critical limitations of Raman are fluorescence and sample degradation. In addition, biofouling and surface alterations due to surface oxidation introduce numerous various alterations which impede polymer detection. The use of laser as a light source might cause sample heating which leads to background emission and polymer degradation (Silva et al., 2018).

SEM/EDS Analysis

To further determine the chemical composition of both plastic and non-plastic particles, scanning electron microscopy (SEM) can be used on plastic particles. SEM provides clear and high magnification images which gives information on surface structure of the particle. This helps in discrimination of MP from organic particles. After imaging at high magnification all samples undergo electron dispersive x-ray spectroscopy (EDS) which analyse the elemental composition of the polymer and distinguish carbon-dominant plastics from organic impurities. Fairly inexpensive, SEM/EDS requires extensive sample preparation and direct handling (Shim et al., 2017).

Thermochemical Methods

Pyrolysis coupled with mass spectrometry is one of the confirmatory non-visual methods to determine microplastic in a sample. Py-GC/MS can identify the type (e.g., PET, PVC, PE) and the concentration of this plastic (ppb) through thermo-analytical methods. The size of plastic particles necessary within the sample to obtain a clear result has been suggested as 100 μm (Fries et al., 2013; Gillibert et al., 2019; Käppler et al., 2016). While analysing one particle at a time, Py-GC/MS can analyse both polymer type and organic additive in the MP by analysing thermal degradation products (Reichert et al., 2019). Some impactful advantages, provided by high sensitivity of GC/MS, are minimum sample quantity requirement and minimal to no need to sample preparation as samples is thermally degraded. Although small quantity is an advantage, this compromises the representativeness of sample composition. There are some limitations of instrumental analysis using Py-GC/MS like,it is not possible to quantify particles and define their shapes. The thermo analytical methods are by nature destructive. Hence, the technique can only be employed for verification of the composition of suspected microplastics.

With pyrolysis of weathered environmental plastic samples, the m/z signals of samples are impeded with various disturbances caused by additives on plastic particles, known as co-elution of pyrolysis products. To solve this, (Matsui et al., 2020) suggests to define a library containing characteristic pyrolysis products for any given polymer and isolating their characteristic m/z ion profiles from the total ion pyrograms. On selection of correct m/z signals this strategy can dissolve the problem of co-elution, as the extracted ion pyrograms will only show the peaks of the compounds of interest. Although time consuming, the automation of data processing can improve the efficiency of Py-GC/MS.

There have been recent advancements in pyrolysis methods coupled with spectrometry techniques which are being used toidentify smaller quantities of particles in environmental and laboratory experiment samples (Shim et al., 2017). These advancements, including the use of thermal desorption (TDS-GC/MS) coupled with thermogravimetric analysis (TGA) and solid phase extraction can provide enhanced analysis of very small plastic particles sampled from complex environmental matrices. Another variation called differential scanning calorimetry (DSC) is yet another thermogravimetric method which studies the thermal properties of polymeric materials. TGA-DSC is based on the change in heat capacities of polymer during solid-liquid phase transition, at elevated temperature. Every plastic product has a characteristic DSC value and so the samples in question can be matched to the standards and polymer types of the unknown samples can be identified. DSC can be useful for identifying specific primary microplastics, such as polyethylene microbeads, for which reference materials are available. One of the major drawbacks of TGA-DSC is ambiguous identification of polymer due to overlapping in transition temperatures. Dominique explained the working and standardisation of polymers in GC/MS very in elaborated forms (*Dominique Remy.Pdf*, n.d.).

QUANTIFICATION

Quantification of microplastics is an essential part of data reporting as it works towards unifying the representation of environmental concentration of the pollutant in different strata. The concentration units of microplastics in surface water are reported in items/particles per m^2 and items/particles per m^3. The latter represents the concentration of MP in surface area whereas the former represents it in volume of water. In case of sediment samples, it is represented in items/particles per m^2 or grams/mg per m^2. Items/particles per kilogram dry/wet weight and items/particles per m^2 sampling area are also used for sediment samples. The concentration unit can be converted from m^2 to m^3 if the sampling is done in standard methods at specific are and at specific depth. In case of biota, the concentrations are reported in particles/gram where gram can represent either the weight of the organ or the whole individual. This unit representation helps in deciphering the amount of MP directly or indirectly being consumed by humans. Studies also report MP concentration in biota in particles/individual to discuss the intensity of the contamination.

Usually, Microplastics are counted manually by technicians with or without using microscope. The task demanded skill and time with a risk of inaccurate results. Wang et. al developed a method to directly quantify PC and PET microplastic in environment by depolymerizing plastic particles and identifying emerging structural unit compounds (Wang et al., 2017). The method has successfully quantified MP particles in marine sediments, sludge, indoor dust, biota samples of mussel and earthworm, sea salt and rock salt samples. Although being truly transformative in quantifying MP, the method only works for 2 polymers PC and PET.

Staining with Nile Red can also aid in easy quantification of MP. Lv et al. has successfully applied this technique of fluorescence staining to quantify MP in biological samples (Lv et al., 2019). Erni-Cassola et al. used a more automated version of MP quantification with Nile Red. Fluorescence microscopy, and image analysis software for high-throughput detection can quantify MP of size range 20 µm to 1000 µm.

The abundance of MPs varies with sampling sites and cannot be considered a strict representative of the entire environmental matrices. The choice of pore size for sampling tools and during filtration. For instance, Desforges et al. (Desforges et al., 2014) observed more MP abundance while using filtration pore size of 0.062 mm whereas Doyle et al. obtained much less while using a trawl size of 0.5 mm, sampling site of both the studies is North East Pacific Ocean (Stifanese et al., 2018).

CONTAMINATION CONTROL AND QUALITY ANALYSIS

A very important aspect of microplastic research is data accuracy. The pouring in of alarming data should not lack representation and have credibility. While Gwinette et al state that its inevitable to avoid contamination during field samples, stating genuine data and addressing contamination control increase the reliability on the work (Rivers et al., n.d.). Quality control is essential in every step of the study. Procedural blanks containing pure water and spiked blanks, containing pure water with a certain number of MPs of known composition and abundance, should be employed at the time of field sampling. Non-plastic sampling tools, latex gloves, and cotton coat should be used during sampling.

During handling of samples in laboratory for extraction and preparation, recovery rate of standards, should be provided (Stolte et al., 2015). To refrain from over estimation of microfibers, environmental fallout of fibres should always be considered. Thus, procedural blanks and inter-laboratory testing can be used for quality control. Performing laboratory extraction in closed spaces with minimal human interference and covering everything can reduce microfibre contamination. Zobkov and Esiukova suggested internal standards and periodic empty runs can ensure contamination free processing of sediment samples (Zobkov & Esiukova, 2017). Regular monitoring of atmospheric fallout can be practiced by keeping filter paper blanks in various positions and observing them under microscope.

Polymeric identification of environmentally extracted microplastics should be compared with data of standard MPs. While it is hard to analyse every particle extracted due to size, shape and quantity limitations, pooling of samples is a practical approach to analyse MPs and give a representative data in place of accurate data.

CONCLUSION

The extensive research on microplastic contamination brings undoubtedly numerous data and knots to be rectified for effective risk assessment. In this chapter, various extraction protocols for different environmental samples were discussed in-depth besides the instrumentation approaches for MPs visualization

Figure 1. Overview of sampling for extraction and analysis of plastic

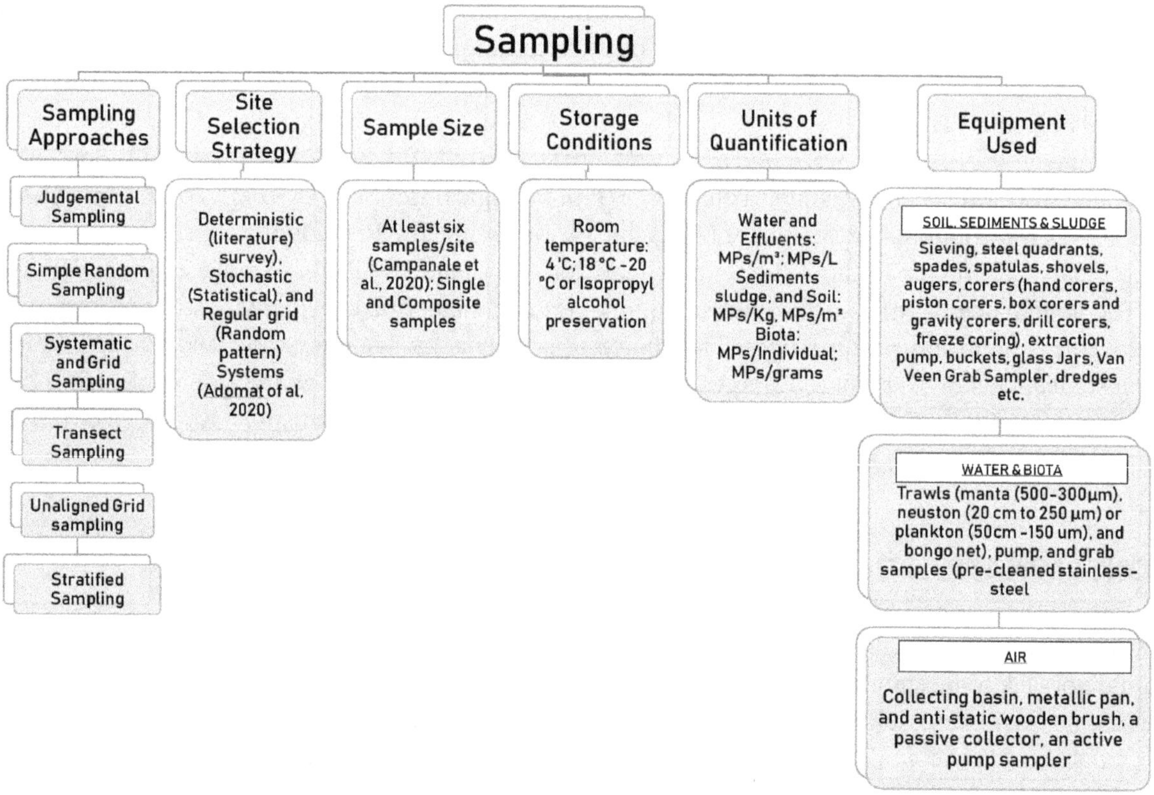

and polymeric characterization. Available methods like filtration, dissection, depurination, homogenization and digestion are widely employed in accordance to the size to be retracted. Characterization of the isolated MPs particles undergo very primitive to advance identification techniques to answer the most preliminary questionnaire of size, morphology, shape, colour etc. Among this, visual identification using stereomicroscopy, fluorescence staining *via* Nile Red is a widely accepted quick approach to produce cursory details. Further to this, instrumental analysis of particles is recommended to identify the polymeric composition of the detected MPs. Advanced microscopy and spectroscopy techniques such as SEM, FTIR, μ-FTIR, Raman, thermal analysis through py-GCMS etc. are endorsed at present. Lastly, the analytically identified particles are recorded, extrapolated and reported in standardised units. Quantification of data obtained is more important in order to keep a periodic check on the spread and consequence of MPs. Thus, each category in the chapter addressed most basic and important aspects regarding the analytical approaches of this emerging environmental contaminant.

Figure 2. Extraction and identification of microplastics

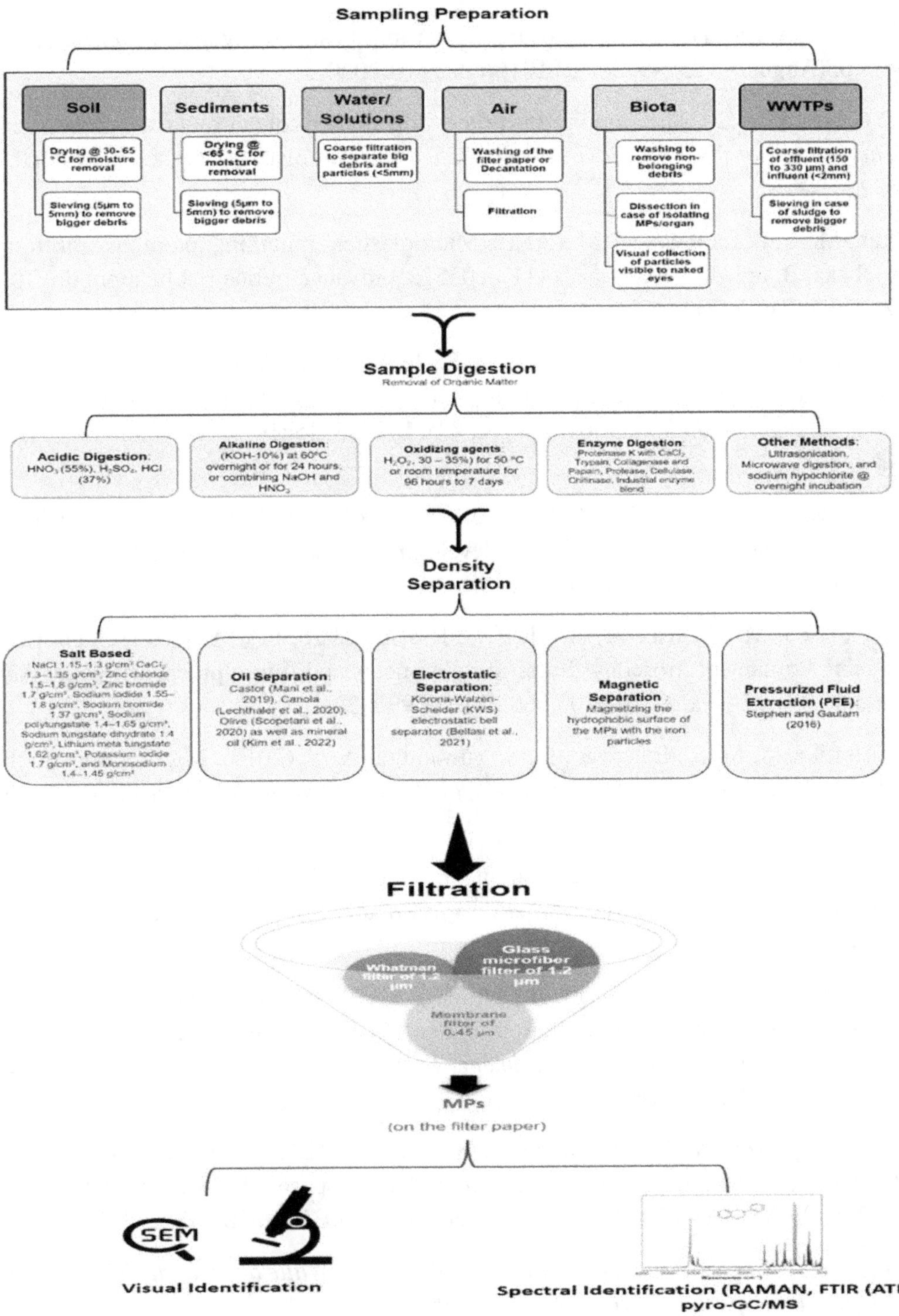

REFERENCES

Abbasi, S., & Turner, A. (2021). Human exposure to microplastics: A study in Iran. *Journal of Hazardous Materials, 403*(August), 123799. doi:10.1016/j.jhazmat.2020.123799

Adomat, Y., & Grischek, T. (2021). Sampling and processing methods of microplastics in river sediments - A review. *The Science of the Total Environment, 758*, 143691. doi:10.1016/j.scitotenv.2020.143691 PMID:33298323

Afrin, S., Uddin, M. K., & Rahman, M. M. (2020). Microplastics contamination in the soil from Urban Landfill site, Dhaka, Bangladesh. *Heliyon, 6*(11), e05572. Advance online publication. doi:10.1016/j.heliyon.2020.e05572 PMID:33294704

Ahmed, M. B., Rahman, M. S., Alom, J., Hasan, M. S., Johir, M. A. H., Mondal, M. I. H., Lee, D. Y., Park, J., Zhou, J. L., & Yoon, M. H. (2021). Microplastic particles in the aquatic environment: A systematic review. *The Science of the Total Environment, 775*, 145793. doi:10.1016/j.scitotenv.2021.145793 PMID:33631597

Araujo, C. F., Nolasco, M. M., Ribeiro, A. M. P., & Ribeiro-claro, P. J. A. (2018). Identi fi cation of microplastics using Raman spectroscopy : Latest developments and future prospects. *Water Research, 142*, 426–440. doi:10.1016/j.watres.2018.05.060 PMID:29909221

Araujo, C. F., Nolasco, M. M., Ribeiro, A. M. P., & Ribeiro-Claro, P. J. A. (2018). Identification of microplastics using Raman spectroscopy: Latest developments and future prospects. *Water Research, 142*, 426–440. doi:10.1016/j.watres.2018.05.060 PMID:29909221

Asadi, M. A., Hertika, A. M. S., Iranawati, F., & Yuwandita, A. Y. (2019). Microplastics in the sediment of intertidal areas of Lamongan, Indonesia. *Aquaculture, Aquarium, Conservation & Legislation, 12*(4), 1065–1073.

Bakaraki Turan, N., Sari Erkan, H., & Onkal Engin, G. (2021). Microplastics in wastewater treatment plants: Occurrence, fate and identification. *Process Safety and Environmental Protection, 146*, 77–84. doi:10.1016/j.psep.2020.08.039

Barrett, J., Chase, Z., Zhang, J., Holl, M. M. B., Willis, K., Williams, A., Hardesty, B. D., Wilcox, C., & Pennino, M. G. (2020). Microplastic Pollution in Deep-Sea Sediments From the Great Australian Bight. *Microplastic Pollution in Deep-Sea Sediments From the Great Australian Bight., 7*(October), 1–10. doi:10.3389/fmars.2020.576170

Bellasi, A., Binda, G., Pozzi, A., Boldrocchi, G., & Bettinetti, R. (2021). The extraction of microplastics from sediments: An overview of existing methods and the proposal of a new and green alternative. *Chemosphere, 278*, 130357. doi:10.1016/j.chemosphere.2021.130357 PMID:33823347

Bergmann, M., Mützel, S., Primpke, S., & Tekman, M. B. (2019). *White and wonderful ? Microplastics prevail in snow from the Alps to the Arctic*. Academic Press.

Bretas Alvim, C., Mendoza-Roca, J. A., & Bes-Piá, A. (2020). Wastewater treatment plant as microplastics release source – Quantification and identification techniques. *Journal of Environmental Management, 255*(June). doi:10.1016/j.jenvman.2019.109739

Cai, H., Chen, M., Chen, Q., Du, F., Liu, J., & Shi, H. (2020). Microplastic quantification affected by structure and pore size of filters. *Chemosphere*, *257*, 127198. doi:10.1016/j.chemosphere.2020.127198 PMID:32512329

Cai, L., Wang, J., Peng, J., Tan, Z., Zhan, Z., Tan, X., & Chen, Q. (2017). *Characteristic of microplastics in the atmospheric fallout from Dongguan city, China : Preliminary research and first evidence.* doi:10.1007/s11356-017-0116-x

Campanale, C., Massarelli, C., Savino, I., Locaputo, V., & Uricchio, V. F. (2020). A detailed review study on potential effects of microplastics and additives of concern on human health. *International Journal of Environmental Research and Public Health*, *17*(4), 1212. Advance online publication. doi:10.3390/ijerph17041212 PMID:32069998

Chamas, A., Moon, H., Zheng, J., Qiu, Y., Tabassum, T., Jang, J. H., Abu-Omar, M., Scott, S. L., & Suh, S. (2020). Degradation Rates of Plastics in the Environment. *ACS Sustainable Chemistry & Engineering*, *8*(9), 3494–3511. doi:10.1021/acssuschemeng.9b06635

Chen, G., Feng, Q., & Wang, J. (2020). Mini-review of microplastics in the atmosphere and their risks to humans. *The Science of the Total Environment*, *703*, 135504. doi:10.1016/j.scitotenv.2019.135504 PMID:31753503

Coppock, R. L., Cole, M., Lindeque, P. K., Queirós, A. M., & Galloway, T. S. (2017). A small-scale, portable method for extracting microplastics from marine sediments. *Environmental Pollution*, *230*, 829–837. doi:10.1016/j.envpol.2017.07.017 PMID:28734264

Courtene-Jones, W., Quinn, B., Murphy, F., Gary, S. F., & Narayanaswamy, B. E. (2017). Optimisation of enzymatic digestion and validation of specimen preservation methods for the analysis of ingested microplastics. *Analytical Methods*, *9*(9), 1437–1445. doi:10.1039/C6AY02343F

Crichton, E. M., Noël, M., Gies, E. A., & Ross, P. S. (2017). A novel, density-independent and FTIR-compatible approach for the rapid extraction of microplastics from aquatic sediments. *Analytical Methods*, *9*(9), 1419–1428. doi:10.1039/C6AY02733D

Cutroneo, L., Reboa, A., Besio, G., Borgogno, F., Canesi, L., Canuto, S., Dara, M., Enrile, F., Forioso, I., Greco, G., Lenoble, V., Malatesta, A., Mounier, S., Petrillo, M., Rovetta, R., Stocchino, A., Tesan, J., Vagge, G., & Capello, M. (2020). Microplastics in seawater: Sampling strategies, laboratory methodologies, and identification techniques applied to port environment. *Environmental Science and Pollution Research International*, *27*(9), 8938–8952. doi:10.100711356-020-07783-8 PMID:32026372

Cutroneo, L., Reboa, A., Geneselli, I., & Capello, M. (2021). Considerations on salts used for density separation in the extraction of microplastics from sediments. *Marine Pollution Bulletin*, *166*(March), 112216. doi:10.1016/j.marpolbul.2021.112216 PMID:33684703

de Wit, W., & Bigaud, N. (2019). No Plastic In Nature: Assessing plastic ingestion from nature to people (AN ANALYSIS for WWF). *World Wide Fund For Nature*, 7.

Dehaut, A., Cassone, A. L., Frère, L., Hermabessiere, L., Himber, C., Rinnert, E., Rivière, G., Lambert, C., Soudant, P., Huvet, A., Duflos, G., & Paul-Pont, I. (2016). Microplastics in seafood: Benchmark protocol for their extraction and characterization. *Environmental Pollution*, *215*(August), 223–233. doi:10.1016/j.envpol.2016.05.018 PMID:27209243

Dehghani, S., Moore, F., & Akhbarizadeh, R. (2017). Microplastic pollution in deposited urban dust, Tehran metropolis, Iran. *Environmental Science and Pollution Research International*, *24*(25), 20360–20371. doi:10.100711356-017-9674-1 PMID:28707239

Desforges, J. W., Galbraith, M., Dangerfield, N., & Ross, P. S. (2014). Widespread distribution of microplastics in subsurface seawater in the NE Pacific Ocean. *Marine Pollution Bulletin*, *79*(1-2), 94–99. Advance online publication. doi:10.1016/j.marpolbul.2013.12.035 PMID:24398418

Di Dong, C., Chen, C. W., Chen, Y. C., Chen, H. H., Lee, J. S., & Lin, C. H. (2020). Polystyrene microplastic particles: In vitro pulmonary toxicity assessment. *Journal of Hazardous Materials*, *385*, 121575. doi:10.1016/j.jhazmat.2019.121575 PMID:31727530

Di Renzo, L., Mascilongo, G., Berti, M., Bogdanović, T., Listeš, E., Brkljača, M., Notarstefano, V., Gioacchini, G., Giorgini, E., Olivieri, V., Silvestri, C., Matiddi, M., D'Alterio, N., Ferri, N., & Di Giacinto, F. (2021). Potential Impact of Microplastics and Additives on the Health Status of Loggerhead Turtles (Caretta caretta) Stranded Along the Central Adriatic Coast. *Water, Air, and Soil Pollution*, *232*(3), 98. Advance online publication. doi:10.100711270-021-04994-8

Diaz-Basantes, M. F., Conesa, J. A., & Fullana, A. (2020). Microplastics in honey, beer, milk and refreshments in Ecuador as emerging contaminants. *Sustainability (Switzerland)*, *12*(12), 5514. Advance online publication. doi:10.3390u12145514

Dris, R., Gasperi, J., Saad, M., Mirande, C., & Tassin, B. (2016). Synthetic fi bers in atmospheric fallout : A source of microplastics in the environment? *MPB*, *4–7*(1-2), 290–293. Advance online publication. doi:10.1016/j.marpolbul.2016.01.006 PMID:26787549

Egessa, R., Nankabirwa, A., Ocaya, H., & Pabire, W. G. (2020). Microplastic pollution in surface water of Lake Victoria. *The Science of the Total Environment*, *741*, 140201. doi:10.1016/j.scitotenv.2020.140201 PMID:32603936

Elkhatib, D., & Oyanedel-Craver, V. (2020). A Critical Review of Extraction and Identification Methods of Microplastics in Wastewater and Drinking Water. *Environmental Science & Technology*, *54*(12), 7037–7049. doi:10.1021/acs.est.9b06672 PMID:32432459

Felsing, S., Kochleus, C., Buchinger, S., Brennholt, N., Stock, F., & Reifferscheid, G. (2018). A new approach in separating microplastics from environmental samples based on their electrostatic behavior. *Environmental Pollution*, *234*, 20–28. doi:10.1016/j.envpol.2017.11.013 PMID:29154206

Fries, E., Deki, H., Willmeyer, J., Nuelle, M., & Remy, D. (2013). *Environmental Science Processes & Impacts scanning electron microscopy*. doi:10.1039/c3em00214d

Fuller, S. G., & Gautam, A. (2016). *A Procedure for Measuring Microplastics using Pressurized Fluid Extraction*. doi:10.1021/acs.est.6b00816

Gillibert, R., Balakrishnan, G., Deshoules, Q., Tardivel, M., Magazzu, A., Donato, M. G., Marago, O. M., Lamy, M., Chapelle, D. La, Colas, F., Lagarde, F., & Gucciardi, P. G. (2019). *Raman Tweezers for Small Microplastics and Nanoplastics Identi fi cation in Seawater*. doi:10.1021/acs.est.9b03105

Guerranti, C., Perra, G., Martellini, T., Giari, L., & Cincinelli, A. (2020). Knowledge about microplastic in mediterranean tributary river ecosystems: Lack of data and research needs on such a crucial marine pollution source. *Journal of Marine Science and Engineering*, *8*(3), 216. Advance online publication. doi:10.3390/jmse8030216

Halfar, J., Cabanov, K., Hevi, S., & Kašp, A. (2021). *Disparities in Methods Used to Determine Microplastics in the Aquatic Environment : A Review of Legislation*. Sampling Process and Instrumental Analysis.

Hamidian, A. H., Ozumchelouei, E. J., Feizi, F., Wu, C., Zhang, Y., & Yang, M. (2021). A review on the characteristics of microplastics in wastewater treatment plants: A source for toxic chemicals. *Journal of Cleaner Production*, *295*, 126480. doi:10.1016/j.jclepro.2021.126480

He, D., Zhang, X., & Hu, J. (2020). Jo u rn a l P of. *Journal of Hazardous Materials*, *124640*. Advance online publication. doi:10.1016/j.jhazmat.2020.124640 PMID:33246814

Hendrickson, E., Minor, E. C., & Schreiner, K. (2018). *Microplastic Abundance and Composition in Western Lake Superior As Determined via Microscopy*. Pyr-GC/MS, and FTIR. doi:10.1021/acs.est.7b05829

Hermsen, E., Mintenig, S. M., Besseling, E., & Koelmans, A. A. (2018). Quality Criteria for the Analysis of Microplastic in Biota Samples. *Critical Reviews in Environmental Science and Technology*, *52*(18), 10230–10240. doi:10.1021/acs.est.8b01611 PMID:30137965

HernandezL. M.XuE. G.LarssonH. C. E.TaharaR.MaisuriaV. B.TufenkjiN. (2019). *into Tea*. doi:10.1021/acs.est.9b02540

Hidalgo-ruz, V., Gutow, L., Thompson, R. C., & Thiel, M. (2012). *Microplastics in the Marine Environment: A Review of the Methods Used for Identification and Quantification*. doi:10.1021/es2031505

Huppertsberg, S., & Knepper, T. P. (2018). *Instrumental analysis of microplastics — benefits and challenges*. Academic Press.

Id, A. K. B., Spanjer, A. R., Id, M. R. R., & Thom, T. (2020). *Microplastics in Lake Mead National Recreation Area, USA : Occurrence and biological uptake*. doi:10.1371/journal.pone.0228896

Jung, S., Cho, S. H., Kim, K. H., & Kwon, E. E. (2021). Progress in quantitative analysis of microplastics in the environment: A review. *Chemical Engineering Journal*, *422*(April), 130154. doi:10.1016/j.cej.2021.130154

Käppler, A., Fischer, D., Oberbeckmann, S., Schernewski, G., Labrenz, M., Eichhorn, K., & Voit, B. (2016). Analysis of environmental microplastics by vibrational microspectroscopy : FTIR, Raman or both? *Analytical and Bioanalytical Chemistry*, *408*(29), 8377–8391. doi:10.100700216-016-9956-3 PMID:27722940

Karami, A., Golieskardi, A., Choo, C. K., Romano, N., Ho, Y., & Salamatinia, B. (2017). A high-performance protocol for extraction of microplastics in fish. *The Science of the Total Environment*, *578*, 485–494. doi:10.1016/j.scitotenv.2016.10.213 PMID:27836345

Karlsson, T. M., Vethaak, A. D., Almroth, B. C., Ariese, F., van Velzen, M., Hassellöv, M., & Leslie, H. A. (2017). Screening for microplastics in sediment, water, marine invertebrates and fish: Method development and microplastic accumulation. *Marine Pollution Bulletin, 122*(1–2), 403–408. doi:10.1016/j.marpolbul.2017.06.081 PMID:28689849

Kitahara, K. I., & Nakata, H. (2020). Plastic additives as tracers of microplastic sources in Japanese road dusts. *The Science of the Total Environment, 736*, 139694. doi:10.1016/j.scitotenv.2020.139694 PMID:32502788

Klein, M., & Fischer, E. K. (2019). Microplastic abundance in atmospheric deposition within the Metropolitan area of Hamburg, Germany. *The Science of the Total Environment, 685*, 96–103. doi:10.1016/j.scitotenv.2019.05.405 PMID:31174127

Lee, H., Kunz, A., Shim, W. J., & Walther, B. A. (2019). Microplastic contamination of table salts from Taiwan, including a global review. *Scientific Reports, 9*(1), 1–9. doi:10.103841598-019-46417-z PMID:31300670

Lenz, R., Enders, K., Stedmon, C. A., MacKenzie, D. M. A., & Nielsen, T. G. (2015). A critical assessment of visual identification of marine microplastic using Raman spectroscopy for analysis improvement. *Marine Pollution Bulletin, 100*(1), 82–91. doi:10.1016/j.marpolbul.2015.09.026 PMID:26455785

Li, Q., Wu, J., Zhao, X., Gu, X., & Ji, R. (2019). Separation and identification of microplastics from soil and sewage sludge. *Environmental Pollution, 254*, 113076. doi:10.1016/j.envpol.2019.113076 PMID:31472456

Long, Z., Pan, Z., Wang, W., Ren, J., Yu, X., Lin, L., Lin, H., Chen, H., & Jin, X. (2019). Microplastic abundance, characteristics, and removal in wastewater treatment plants in a coastal city of China. *Water Research, 155*, 255–265. doi:10.1016/j.watres.2019.02.028 PMID:30852313

Lusher, A. L., Munno, K., Hermabessiere, L., & Carr, S. (2020). Isolation and Extraction of Microplastics from Environmental Samples: An Evaluation of Practical Approaches and Recommendations for Further Harmonization. In Applied Spectroscopy (Vol. 74, Issue 9). doi:10.1177/0003702820938993

Lusher, A. L., Welden, N. A., Sobral, P., & Cole, M. (2017). Sampling, isolating and identifying microplastics ingested by fish and invertebrates. *Analytical Methods, 9*(9), 1346–1360. doi:10.1039/C6AY02415G

Lv, L., Qu, J., Yu, Z., Chen, D., Zhou, C., Hong, P., Sun, S., & Li, C. (2019). A simple method for detecting and quantifying microplastics utilizing fluorescent dyes - Safranine T, fluorescein isophosphate, Nile red based on thermal expansion and contraction property. *Environmental Pollution, 255*, 113283. doi:10.1016/j.envpol.2019.113283 PMID:31580990

Lv, L., Yan, X., Feng, L., Jiang, S., Lu, Z., Xie, H., Sun, S., Chen, J., & Li, C. (2021). Challenge for the detection of microplastics in the environment. *Water Environment Research, 93*(1), 5–15. doi:10.1002/wer.1281 PMID:31799785

Magnusson, K., & Norén, F. (2014). Screening of microplastic particles in and down-stream a wastewater treatment plant. *IVL Swedish Environmental Research Institute, 55*(C), 22.

Matsui, K., Ishimura, T., Mattonai, M., Iwai, I., Watanabe, A., Teramae, N., Ohtani, H., & Watanabe, C. (2020). Journal of Analytical and Applied Pyrolysis Identification algorithm for polymer mixtures based on Py-GC / MS and its application for microplastic analysis in environmental samples. *Journal of Analytical and Applied Pyrolysis*, *149*(April), 104834. doi:10.1016/j.jaap.2020.104834

Mintenig, S. M., Int-Veen, I., Löder, M. G. J., Primpke, S., & Gerdts, G. (2017). Identification of microplastic in effluents of waste water treatment plants using focal plane array-based micro-Fourier-transform infrared imaging. *Water Research*, *108*, 365–372. doi:10.1016/j.watres.2016.11.015 PMID:27838027

Möller, J. N., Löder, M. G. J., & Laforsch, C. (2020). Finding Microplastics in Soils: A Review of Analytical Methods. *Environmental Science & Technology*, *54*(4), 2078–2090. doi:10.1021/acs.est.9b04618 PMID:31999440

Nelms, S. E., Barnett, J., Brownlow, A., Davison, N. J., Deaville, R., Galloway, T. S., Lindeque, P. K., Santillo, D., & Godley, B. J. (2019). Microplastics in marine mammals stranded around the British coast: Ubiquitous but transitory? *Scientific Reports*, *9*(1), 1–8. doi:10.103841598-018-37428-3 PMID:30705316

O'Brien, S., Okoffo, E. D., Rauert, C., O'Brien, J. W., Ribeiro, F., Burrows, S. D., Toapanta, T., Wang, X., & Thomas, K. V. (2021). Quantification of selected microplastics in Australian urban road dust. *Journal of Hazardous Materials*, *416*(March), 125811. doi:10.1016/j.jhazmat.2021.125811 PMID:33892382

Patchaiyappan, A., Dowarah, K., Zaki Ahmed, S., Prabakaran, M., Jayakumar, S., Thirunavukkarasu, C., & Devipriya, S. P. (2021). Prevalence and characteristics of microplastics present in the street dust collected from Chennai metropolitan city, India. *Chemosphere*, *269*, 128757. doi:10.1016/j.chemosphere.2020.128757 PMID:33183789

Peixoto, D., Pinheiro, C., Amorim, J., Oliva-Teles, L., Guilhermino, L., & Vieira, M. N. (2019). Microplastic pollution in commercial salt for human consumption: A review. *Estuarine, Coastal and Shelf Science*, *219*(February), 161–168. doi:10.1016/j.ecss.2019.02.018

Piehl, S., Leibner, A., Löder, M. G. J., Dris, R., Bogner, C., & Laforsch, C. (2018). Identification and quantification of macro- and microplastics on an agricultural farmland. *Scientific Reports*, *8*(1), 1–9. doi:10.103841598-018-36172-y PMID:30560873

Prata, J. C., da Costa, J. P., Duarte, A. C., & Rocha-Santos, T. (2019). Methods for sampling and detection of microplastics in water and sediment: A critical review. *Trends in Analytical Chemistry*, *110*, 150–159. doi:10.1016/j.trac.2018.10.029

Prata, J. C., da Costa, J. P., Girão, A. V., Lopes, I., Duarte, A. C., & Rocha-Santos, T. (2019). Identifying a quick and efficient method of removing organic matter without damaging microplastic samples. *The Science of the Total Environment*, *686*, 131–139. doi:10.1016/j.scitotenv.2019.05.456 PMID:31176812

Rafique, A., Irfan, M., Mumtaz, M., & Qadir, A. (2020). Spatial distribution of microplastics in soil with context to human activities: A case study from the urban center. *Environmental Monitoring and Assessment*, *192*(11), 671. Advance online publication. doi:10.100710661-020-08641-3 PMID:33009943

Reichert, J., Arnold, A. L., Hoogenboom, M. O., Schubert, P., & Wilke, T. (2019). Impacts of microplastics on growth and health of hermatypic corals are species-specific. *Environmental Pollution*, *254*, 113074. doi:10.1016/j.envpol.2019.113074 PMID:31473388

Rhodes, C. J. (2018). Plastic pollution and potential solutions. *Science Progress, 101*(3), 207–260. doi:10.3184/003685018X15294876706211 PMID:30025551

Rivers, M., & Gwinnett, C. (n.d.). *Quantification is more than counting: Actions required to accurately quantify and report isolated marine microplastics.* Elsevier. Retrieved December 17, 2021, from https://www.sciencedirect.com/science/article/pii/S0025326X18308750

Rocha-Santos, T., & Duarte, A. C. (2015). A critical overview of the analytical approaches to the occurrence, the fate and the behavior of microplastics in the environment. *Trends in Analytical Chemistry, 65*, 47–53. doi:10.1016/j.trac.2014.10.011

Rochman, C. M., Brookson, C., Bikker, J., Djuric, N., Earn, A., Bucci, K., Athey, S., Huntington, A., McIlwraith, H., Munno, K., De Frond, H., Kolomijeca, A., Erdle, L., Grbic, J., Bayoumi, M., Borrelle, S. B., Wu, T., Santoro, S., Werbowski, L. M., ... Hung, C. (2019). Rethinking microplastics as a diverse contaminant suite. *Environmental Toxicology and Chemistry, 38*(4), 703–711. doi:10.1002/etc.4371 PMID:30909321

Schirinzi, G. F., Pedà, C., Battaglia, P., Laface, F., Galli, M., Baini, M., Consoli, P., Scotti, G., Esposito, V., Faggio, C., Farré, M., Barceló, D., Fossi, M. C., Andaloro, F., & Romeo, T. (2020). A new digestion approach for the extraction of microplastics from gastrointestinal tracts (GITs) of the common dolphinfish (Coryphaena hippurus) from the western Mediterranean Sea. *Journal of Hazardous Materials, 397*(February), 122794. doi:10.1016/j.jhazmat.2020.122794 PMID:32387826

Shim, W. J., Hong, S. H., & Eo, S. E. (2017). Identification methods in microplastic analysis: A review. *Analytical Methods, 9*(9), 1384–1391. doi:10.1039/C6AY02558G

Silva, A. B., Bastos, A. S., Justino, C. I. L., Duarte, A. C., & Rocha-santos, T. A. P. (2018). Analytica Chimica Acta Microplastics in the environment : Challenges in analytical chemistry -. *RE:view, 1017*. Advance online publication. doi:10.1016/j.aca.2018.02.043 PMID:29534790

Sobhani, Z., Lei, Y., Tang, Y., Wu, L., Zhang, X., Naidu, R., Megharaj, M., & Fang, C. (2020). Microplastics generated when opening plastic packaging. *Scientific Reports, 10*(1), 1–7. doi:10.103841598-020-61146-4 PMID:32193409

Sridharan, S., Kumar, M., Singh, L., Bolan, N. S., & Saha, M. (2021). Microplastics as an emerging source of particulate air pollution: A critical review. *Journal of Hazardous Materials, 418*(March), 126245. doi:10.1016/j.jhazmat.2021.126245 PMID:34111744

Stifanese, R., Morgana, S., Ghigliotti, L., Est, N., Wieckzorek, A., Doyle, T., Christiansen, J. S., Faimali, M., & Garaventa, F. (2018). *Microplastics in the Arctic : A case study with sub-surface water and fi sh samples off Northeast Greenland.* doi:10.1016/j.envpol.2018.08.001

Stolte, A., Forster, S., Gerdts, G., & Schubert, H. (2015). Microplastic concentrations in beach sediments along the German Baltic coast. *Marine Pollution Bulletin, 99*(1–2), 216–229. doi:10.1016/j.marpolbul.2015.07.022 PMID:26198261

von Friesen, L. W., Granberg, M. E., Hassellöv, M., Gabrielsen, G. W., & Magnusson, K. (2019). An efficient and gentle enzymatic digestion protocol for the extraction of microplastics from bivalve tissue. *Marine Pollution Bulletin, 142*(March), 129–134. doi:10.1016/j.marpolbul.2019.03.016 PMID:31232285

Vroom, R., Halsband, C., Besseling, E., & Koelmans, A. A. (2016). *Effects of microplastics on zooplankton*. https://library.wur.nl/WebQuery/wurpubs/510036

Wang, L., Zhang, J., Hou, S., & Sun, H. (2017). A Simple Method for Quantifying Polycarbonate and Polyethylene Terephthalate Microplastics in Environmental Samples by Liquid Chromatography-Tandem Mass Spectrometry. *Environmental Science & Technology Letters*, *4*(12), 530–534. doi:10.1021/acs.estlett.7b00454

Xu, J. L., Thomas, K. V., Luo, Z., & Gowen, A. A. (2019). FTIR and Raman imaging for microplastics analysis: State of the art, challenges and prospects. *Trends in Analytical Chemistry*, *119*, 115629. doi:10.1016/j.trac.2019.115629

Yao, P., Zhou, B., Lu, Y. H., Yin, Y., Zong, Y. Q., Chen, M. Te, & O'Donnell, Z. (2019). A review of microplastics in sediments: Spatial and temporal occurrences, biological effects, and analytic methods. *Quaternary International, 519*(October), 274–281. doi:10.1016/j.quaint.2019.03.028

Yukioka, S., Tanaka, S., Nabetani, Y., Suzuki, Y., Ushijima, T., Fujii, S., Takada, H., Van Tran, Q., & Singh, S. (2020). Occurrence and characteristics of microplastics in surface road dust in Kusatsu (Japan), Da Nang (Vietnam), and Kathmandu (Nepal). *Environmental Pollution*, *256*, 113447. doi:10.1016/j.envpol.2019.113447 PMID:31679875

Zhang, S., Liu, X., Hao, X., Wang, J., & Zhang, Y. (2020). Distribution of low-density microplastics in the mollisol farmlands of northeast China. *Science of the Total Environment, 708*, 135091. doi:10.1016/j.scitotenv.2019.135091

Zobkov, M., & Esiukova, E. (2017). Microplastics in Baltic bottom sediments: Quantification procedures and first results. *Marine Pollution Bulletin*, *114*(2), 724–732. doi:10.1016/j.marpolbul.2016.10.060 PMID:27810093

Chapter 13
Microplastics Analytical Techniques in Water, Sediments, and Biota

Erangi Imasha Hewawasam Udullege
Sirindhorn International Institute of Technology, Thammasat University, Thailand

Sandhya Babel
https://orcid.org/0000-0003-2378-4891
Sirindhorn International Institute of Technology, Thammasat University, Thailand

ABSTRACT

Identification and quantification of microplastics (MPs) pollution levels in all the environmental compartments including water, sediments, and biota are an hourly need. MPs analytical techniques in water, sediments, and biota consist of several laborious steps including sampling, sample handling, and analytical techniques for identification and quantification. Studies have employed a wide variety of techniques resulting in variation in MPs abundance and characteristics. MPs reporting techniques also vary between different studies. The sampling techniques, digestion reagents, the temperature applied, density separation reagents, and the techniques utilized cause significant impacts on the recovery rate of the MPs particles from samples. 20-10 μm has become the lower reliable, practical limit for MPs due to the limitations in identification methods. Since there is many more MPs research to be done, there is an urgency of establishing reliable and efficient standard methodologies for MPs monitoring enabling comparison of studies from different parts of the world.

INTRODUCTION

Plastics have become an essential material in product manufacturing in almost all sectors since the initial commercial application in the 1950s to 2020 with 359 million tonnes of global plastic manufacturing (Plastic Europe, 2020). Characteristics like durability, cheapness, and being easily discardable have made plastics more attractive. Covid 19 pandemic has dramatically increased the usage of plastics due

DOI: 10.4018/978-1-7998-9723-1.ch013

to safety reasons just within a short period. Plastic waste in the world's oceans was first reported in the 1970s and extensive studies have been started since 2005 (Rios Mendoza & Balcer, 2019). Environmental degradation turned larger plastics into smaller plastics called microplastics (MPs) when released into the environment (Peng et al., 2020) while specifically designed micrometer size primary MPs are introduce in to the environment by the industrial products such as personal care products, sand blasting media and synthetic fibers (Horton et al., 2017a). According to Frias and Nash (2019) MPs are defined as "any synthetic solid particle or polymeric matrix, with regular or irregular shape and with size ranging from 1 µm to 5 mm, of either primary or secondary manufacturing origin, which are insoluble in water" (p.146). MPs are a ubiquitous contaminant found in all most all environments including water, sediments, beaches, soil, air, biota and remote places like polar regions (Karbalaei et al., 2018; Lusher et al., 2015). Recently, there is an emerging trend of investigation of MPs in freshwater and aquatic organisms as it is a major source of transport of MPs into higher levels of food chains (Lusher et al., 2017).

Analysis of quantity and the characteristics of MPs in the environment is very important as it provides the regional and global MPs pollution status, distribution of MPs in various environmental matrices, varying trends of MP concentrations, possible sources of MPs generation, adhered pollutants and possibility of exposure of MPs to the biota. Several field experiments has been carried out to analyze the MPs in all the environmental compartments, land, water, and air. Increasing number of field and laboratory studies have been carried out to analyze the concentrations of MPs in biota and the responses of biota to the MPs. These studies have employed a wide variety of techniques for the quantification and characterization of MPs. The difference in the methodologies adopted makes it difficult to compare the results among the studies and under or overestimation of MP pollution. This urges the need of standardization of analytical methods and sampling procedures among researchers (Liu et al., 2020).

The sampling and analytical techniques varies based on the environmental matrices, but all have similar procedures such as sampling, quality assurance and quality control, processing of samples, digestion of organic matter, density separation, filtration and purification and the last step identification and quantification. Nets, sieves, or pumps are commonly used for water sampling while trowels, spoons/tablespoons, shovels, spatula, grabber (e.g. Ekman or Van Veen), and box corer used for sediment sampling (Prata et al., 2019a; Stock et al., 2019). The biota sampling procedure for analysis of MPs varies based on the target organisms (Zhu & Wang, 2020). After sample collection, sample processing which includes preparation, organic matter digestion, MP extraction, and filtration is required prior to identification and quantification of MPs.

Environmental samples need to be digested to remove the organic matter to prevent overestimation of concentrations and a higher number of particles selecting for further analysis (Prata et al., 2019b). Hydrogen peroxide (H_2O_2) and an iron (II) catalyst, Fenton's reagent, and potassium hydroxide, are some common reagents used for digestion of samples (Karami et al., 2017). The residual solution can be filtered and recovered directly after digestion. But sometimes inorganic particles dominate after digestion which arise the necessity of further exposure to a density separation (Bessa et al., 2019). Sodium chloride (NaCl), zinc chloride ($ZnCl_2$), and sodium iodide (NaI) are the most used density separation solutions (Zhu & Wang, 2020). Following these preparation steps, samples are clean to identify the MPs. Visual identification followed by analytical techniques to identify polymers is widely used (Lusher et al., 2017).

Several studies recently are focusing on analysis of negative effects of MPs to the environment, food chain, human and other biota. Research studies have shown that the ingestion of MPs causes physical damages to the organisms such as invade and harm the digestive organs, cause for illusion of satiety, lower ingestion, substitute nutrition and energy and may cause death sometimes (Zhang et al., 2019).

These ingested MPs particles can also cause various cellular and molecular level toxic effects. Smaller MPs particles are accumulating inside the organisms. This creates the path for MPs to accumulate in the food chain and reach to higher trophic levels creating chronic effects (Farrell & Nelson, 2013). Human intake of MPs via drinking water, seafood consumption and inhalation (Kankanige & Babel, 2020; Cho et al., 2019; Cox et al., 2019) has been reported. Accuracy of MPs concentrations in all the environmental matrices is important to determine the negative effects of MPs on biota, human and the environment. However, researchers believe that the present knowledge on concentration and adverse effects of MPs to the human is underestimated due to the limitation in data and analysis techniques (Cox et al., 2019). Hence, reviewing the existing MPs analytical methods is of greater importance to understand the pros and cons of the techniques employed currently.

This book chapter discusses the sampling methods for MPs, quality assurance and quality control procedures, sample processing techniques, and identification methods of MPs in water, sediments, and biota samples based on literature. It also highlights the limitation of each process employed for analysis and detection.

Sampling of MPs

MPs are present in the water (surface layer, water column, and benthic sediments) beaches, and a variety of aquatic organisms. The sampling technique is mainly based on the matrices and the limitations of sizes of MPs to be targeted. Selective, bulk and volume-reduced sampling are the major technique used to collect samples of MPs in the aquatic areas. Selective sampling is a simple and straightforward method usually applied in beach where plastics are large enough for detection using the naked eye and hence can be extracted directly. However, there is a great risk as the higher limitations of detectable sizes of MPs, and less obvious particles are easily ignored especially when they are combined with other surrounding debris (Shim et al., 2017). Bulk sampling is known as the collection of the whole sample without decreasing the water volume. This method is largely used for sediment collection and occasionally for water samples. The representativeness of the sample collected by this method is problematic. In the volume-reduced sampling, the volume of the sample is decreased by filtration while sampling and preserve only a little portion of the sample for further analysis. This method is the most popular approach for water sampling as it covers larger amounts or areas of samples while sampling (Wang & Wang, 2018).

Water Sampling

The distribution of MPs in the water column is mainly dependent on the characteristics of MPs (size, shape, density, biofouling, and adsorption of chemicals) and environmental conditions (water density, wind, currents, and waves). Hence, the quantity and quality of MPs recovered are largely reliant on sampling place and depth (Picó & Barceló, 2019). Sampling, as well as processing techniques, are the same for both fresh water and saltwater MPs samples. However, MPs in the freshwater systems appear deeper in the water column due to the density difference between fresh and saltwater. Therefore, depth and location need to be changed depending on the sampling place and salinity. Nets, sieves, or pumps are commonly used for sampling (Prata et al., 2019a). Figure 1 shows the general procedure for identification of microplastics in water, sediments, and biota.

Surface Water

Most often nets have been used for surface water sampling as it can filter high volumes of water and particles are directly concentrated during sampling (Hidalgo-Ruz et al., 2012). Nets with a mesh sizes of 50-3000 μm have been used (Klein S. et al., 2018). Dris et al. (2015) reported that the MPs abundance is much greater in the net which has a smaller mesh size. However, researchers tend to use nets with larger mesh sizes rather than the smaller mesh sizes nets which clog more easily. Filtered water volume is measured by using a flow meter mounted on the net opening and hence the concentration of MPs can be calculated (Klein S. et al., 2018). Water surface up to a depth of 0.5 m can be sampled by using manta trawls, plankton or neuston nets (Stock et al., 2019). Neuston catamarans are utilized in marine environments with higher waves while a manta trawl works best in calm waters which prevents destruction to the device. Manta net once deployed off a boat, should be towed linearly at a low speed of 3- 5 knots for a set distance or time (30-15 minutes) depending on the flow rate. Net opening is submerged while towing. Neuston networks in the same manner but while towing, the neuston net opening is partly submerged in water (Löder & Gerdts, 2015). European Commission (2013) along with other monitoring programs recommends MPs sampling from seawater preferably using nets with 333 mm mesh size, 6 m length for 30 minutes. González et al. (2016) recommended to perform sampling over time (over the seasons) and under different environmental conditions (during floods or high/low discharges for lakes). Mai et al. (2018) recommended to perform large-scale surface water sampling in lakes or seas using manta trawls or nets, as they can filter a huge quantity of water to collect floating MPs. In addition to common methods, other approaches such as the surface microlayer method, acoustic doppler current profilers, hand-net collection, 3D hydrodynamic-numerical modeling, and bulk water sampling have been used. In bulk water sampling, volume varies among the studies. Klein. et al. (2018) have used a bulk sampling method with 3 liters of water samples collected utilizing glass bottles to estimate the MPs pollution levels in aquaculture fishponds water in The Pearl River estuary of China. In rivers and lakes, bulk water samples can be collected by using buckets, pumps, or steel or polycarbonate sampling tubes from surface or depths up to 18 cm (Rios Mendoza & Balcer, 2019).

Water Column

Still, there are no specific sampling depths for samples taken below the water surface. Therefore, sampling depth varies according to the research focus. Water column sampling has been carried out by direct filtration of the water with submersible Teflon pumps, acquisition of batch samples, or plankton or bongo nets (Picó & Barceló, 2019).

Nylon nets and pumping systems can be a source of MPs contamination while sampling. It is important that plastic-free materials such as metal sieves and glass bottles should be used during sampling to avoid contamination (Prata et al., 2019a).

Sediment Sampling

MPs sampling techniques for sediments in both marine and freshwater environments are similar. The sampling procedure depends on the goal of the research and varies in terms of sampling volume, area, size, and depth. In general, it is advantageous to collect as many samples as possible for getting more understandings of the distribution and number of MPs particles in sediments (Frias et al., 2018). Sampling locations in marine environments differ in terms of the tideline, intertidal, supralittoral, and flot-

Figure 1.

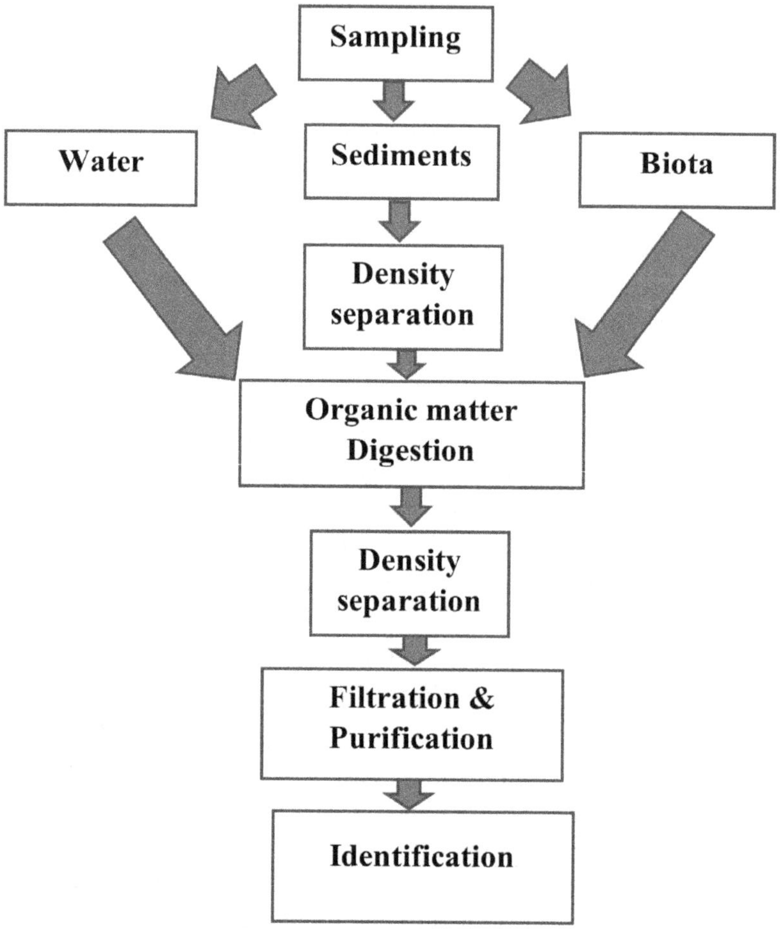

sam deposits (Mai et al., 2018). Up to 500 g to 10 kg size of sediment samples have been analyzed by researchers (Hidalgo-Ruz et al., 2012). Sampling of sediments in the beach environments is conducted with trowels, spoons/tablespoons, shovels, or spatula. Plastic tools should be avoided due to contamination. In sublittoral zone, in the sea, or freshwater environments sediments can be sampled with a grabber (e.g., Ekman or Van Veen) or a box corer for superficial sediments. The sampling depth varies from the upper 5 cm of the surface layer up to 32 cm. Some studies do not mention the depth. Bottom sediments in the water can be sampled by using a corer with a closed tube can (Stock et al., 2019). Frias et al. (2018) suggested a standardized protocol for monitoring intertidal and subtidal sediments. They propose observing intertidal sediments on beaches once per season in at least three random squares of 30 cm edge length 100 m parallel to the water line. Then collect the sediments in the top 5 cm (4.5 l) with a metal shovel and kept in glass jars in order to prevent contamination. For subtidal sediments, a Van Veen grabber or box corer (e.g. Reineck box corer) or drill corer or a Pürckhauer is recommended. Frias et al. (2018) recommended to take 6 samples per site in different depths and of different matrixes and directly freeze the sediments at -20 °C, if not analyzed soon after sampling.

Biota Sampling

Investigations on the ingestion of MPs by various marine vertebrates and invertebrates have been very commonly reported in the literature. Recently, there is an emerging trend of investigation of MPs in freshwater and aquaculture organisms as it is a major source of transport of MPs into higher levels of food chains. The biota sampling method is determined by the research question, available resources, habitat, and target organism (Lusher et al., 2017). The most frequently monitored biota in aquaculture environments is fish (Karami et al., 2017), clams, mussels (Li et al., 2021), and oysters (Phuong et al., 2018), etc. Fish species in marine environments are generally collected depending on their habitats using surface, midwater, and benthic trawls. Fish species in riverine systems usually have been collected using gill nets. Benthic invertebrate species such as Norway lobsters (*Nephrops norvegicus*) may be collected in grabs, traps, and creels, or by bottom trawling. Planktonic and nektonic invertebrates recovered by way of manta and bongo nets. Bivalves, crustaceans, and annelids are usually collected by hand from the field (Lusher et al., 2017). Another method is a direct collection from commercial fish markets, where the capture method is unknown (Li et al., 2018; Sparks et al., 2021)

Bessa et al. (2019) have developed a harmonized protocol for monitoring MPs in biota. They recommended choosing species with high abundance and wide geographic distribution, that are easy to sample and process in the laboratory, species that are already used as bioindicators, and species with ecological and socio-economic relevance for investigations. It is recommended to take a sample size of at least 50 specimens of similar size per research unit (species, food web, feeding type, etc.) for representativeness of the sample. Researchers have also used less than 50 samples depending on the objectives of the research and the environment of sampling with appropriate justifications. Bessa et al. (2019) also suggests record the data such as date and time, sampling site or location data, mesh size, polymer typology, material used for sampling, gear used for collection of specimens, analyzed/processed tissues, length and weight of the individuals', and additional observations during/after sampling.

Collection of representative biota sample is a challenge as aquatic environmental factors alter periodically at different times, for instance, seasons and climate, or along ecological gradients at various spatial scales like basin and water depths. Thus, special care should be given when selecting sampling sites and times. Furthermore, biota is dissected to collect MPs from various tissues and organs, and this also affects the assessment of MPs. The stomach, liver, gastrointestinal tract, and whole organism have been used as biological samples for analysis of different species by different researchers (Zhu & Wang, 2020).

Special care should be taken to avoid contamination and mitigation during sampling and sample analysis.

Microplastic Losses during Sampling of Biota

During sampling, there is a possibility of a loss of MPs due to handling stress, physical movement, and the physiological and behavioral specificities of the sampled biota. Gut evacuation times for organisms are diverse. For example, gut evacuation time is 30 minutes for decapod crustaceans while over 150 hours for larger lobsters. Thus, there is a possibility to egest MPs debris prior to analysis. Therefore, keeping a short gap between the collection and preservation of organisms is important. Handling stress can cause regurgitation (Lusher et al., 2017). Bromley 1994 reported regurgitating stomach contents by fish species. Regurgitation may bias the gut content estimation, changing consumption estimates, and the existence of MPs. Thus, care should be taken to minimize handling stress when sampling biota in order to reduce the MPs regurgitating.

Microplastic Accumulation during Sampling of Biota

Biota can be feeding on MPs during capture in nets as the mesh size of the net can collect MPs (ex; manta nets, mesh size 0.33 mm). Laboratory studies have confirmed that nano- and micro-plastics can stick to external appendages of aquatic organisms. Therefore, research studying external adherence of MPs should be careful when sampling. This can be prevented by exposing biota only for a short period to such situations (Lusher et al., 2017).

Biota Sample Storage

Biota samples should be stored just after sampling until examine in the laboratory. Biological samples conserved on board using aluminum foil for freezing at −20 °C or preservation in ethanol in glass containers have been recommended by the ICES (2015). In some studies, specimens were kept in a closed container instead of wrapping each individual using aluminum foil (Hermsen et al., 2018). Instead of 70% ethanol, 4% formaldehyde is also used as a common fixative. At higher concentrations, these fixatives might damage some polymers (Lusher et al., 2017). Desiccation also has been used to store organisms in some studies (Cole et al., 2014).

Quality Assurance and Quality Control

MPs samples are highly sensitive to external contamination which can be air-borne, water-borne, or contamination by uncleansed equipment. Thus, conducting quality assurance and quality control procedures are vital and of great importance for the accuracy of the data during the whole sampling process (Mai et al., 2018). Quality assurance and quality control procedures cover four mains aspects;

I. **Operators' cloth protection**- wearing latex gloves and pure cotton clothes
II. **Appropriate cleaning of the material**- clean workplace, use ultra-pure water for analytical steps, use steel or glass devices, replace plastic materials with non-plastics materials, clean glassware with sodium dodecyl sulfate solution (a detergent) in an ultrasonic bath, and then rinsing with 50% ethanol followed by ultra-pure water in a laminar flow box, rinsing with Milli-Q water prior to every step or rinse all the equipment three times using filtered deionized water prior to use
III. **Protect samples for the air**- filtering the laboratory air over the filter paper for a certain period under vacuum condition, covering glassware with watch glasses when not in use (90% reduction of contamination), sample handling under a clean laminar flow cabinet (50% reduction of contamination)
IV. **Perform sampling and laboratory blanks**- conduct daily controls with a glass microfiber filter, use procedural blanks and spiked blanks in field sampling, provide recovery rates of standard MPs by applied extraction method (Hermsen et al., 2018; Mai et al., 2018; Stock et al., 2019; Wang & Wang, 2018; Picó & Barceló, 2019; Prata et al., 2021; Miller et al., 2021).

Processing of Biota Samples

A large number of studies focus on the investigation of the MPs in the digestive tract including the intestines and stomach (Cole et al., 2011). This is especially applied to larger animals like fish. For smaller species like bivalves, zooplankton, worms, and shrimps, whole specimen were analyzed (Hermsen et al., 2018). To ensure that only the MPs in the intestinal tracts are investigated, around three days depuration for clearing the gut must be done for live biota (Van Cauwenberghe & Janssen, 2014). Depurations make sure only MPs remained within tissues or trapped in the intestinal tract are considered. Depuration also allows fecal analysis to investigate MPs consumption (Lusher et al., 2017). Frozen samples should be unfrozen, or preserved samples must be extracted from the fixative (Lusher et al., 2013). If the objective of the study is to investigate the ingestion of the MPs, biota samples must be washed using water, saline water, or forceps to prevent contamination with externally adhered plastics. European Commission (2013) proposes to use a dissecting microscope to extract the gut or the entire digestive tract.

Processing of Sediment Samples

Munich Plastic Sediment Separator (MPSS) and the electrostatic separator have commonly used for sediment sample processing. Munich Plastic Sediment Separator, a density separator that can analyze larger sample volumes up to 6 L can be used to optimize sediment extraction procedure. This method also can be used to reduce the sample volume of sediments containing a higher amount of organic materials. This method better separates the smaller MPs particles (<1 mm) from sediments. It achieved 95.5-100% of MPs recovery rate. This method allows larger sediment samples to process easily allowing only filtration afterward (Imhof et al., 2012). Imhof et al. 2012 have used a smaller scale MPSS for very small sample volumes like less than 250 mL.

The electrostatic separator can also be used to reduce the non-polymer substance up to 90% of larger sediment samples (Felsing et al., 2018). This method is based on the common property of most polymers, non-conductors. Dry particles are separately transported via a vibrating conveyer onto a rotating metal drum where particles are subjected to an electric field of up to 30 kV. Then the particles get charged and when the drum rotates particles discharge based on their electrostatic properties. This method has the advantages such as low cost, less time consumption, no chemicals required for the first separation step of large samples. However, organic digestion and density separation are still required for the remaining sample portion of sediment and plastics.

Digestion of Organic Matter

Environmental samples collected from aquaculture systems contain organic materials which disrupt the accurate identification and characterization of MPs. Plastic materials will result in overestimation of concentrations and a higher number of particles selecting to further analysis (Prata et al., 2019b). Therefore, samples are mainly pre-treated with chemical or enzymatic digestion to remove the organic matter. Sediments processed with the MPSS does not require digestion. Only clean water samples can be directly filtered for polymer identification (Stock et al., 2019). Acid, oxidation, alkali, and enzyme treatments are the most common chemical digestion methods (Zhu & Wang, 2020).

Digestion of Water Samples

Water samples are mostly digested using (30%) H_2O_2 and an iron (II) catalyst to remove the organic matter (Masura et al., 2015).

Digestion of Sediment Samples

Hydrogen peroxide with different concentrations has been commonly used for sediment sample digestion. Frias et al. (2018) recommended using hydrogen peroxide (H_2O_2) 6-10% solution for sediment sample digestion. Hurley et al. (2018) found that soil and sludge samples can be effectively digested by using Fenton's reagent (consisted of 30% (v/v) H_2O_2 and a mixture of 20 g iron (II) sulfate heptahydrate and 1 L filtered RO water catalyst) at temperatures below 40 °C at pH 3 for 2 h. This method has minor negative effects on the size and mass of MPs.

Digestion of Biota Samples

Several chemical digestion methods have been used to digest biota samples. Acid digestion (mixture of acids or HNO_3 alone) of biota tissues for MPs analysis is a very common practice adopted by researcher's. ICES (2015) recommended using a mixture of HNO_3:$HClO_4$ (4:1) to digest animal tissue with the aim of standardizing the digestion practices. However, Enders et al. (2017) have proved this ICES recommended procedure as detrimental to many of the common plastic polymers. They have proved that 30% KOH: NaClO mixture is a more effective digester agent than ICES recommended digester agent. These findings are also in line with the findings of Catarino et al. (2017) which strongly discourage further use of acid digestion. Dehaut et al. (2016) reported the degradation of polyamide when using HNO_3 to digest biological tissues. Polyamide represents a significant volume of worldwide plastic production, and thus care should be taken. Thiele et al. (2019) mentioned 10% KOH at a temperature less than 40 °C as the most economical and fast method for digestion of bivalve's tissues. This method has shown a digestion efficacy of more than 95% for oysters. They do not recommend using KOH at 60 °C which will destroy rayon. They suggest using this method as the standard method for degradation of all the biota tissue to extract MPs. This is also in line with the findings of Prata et al. (2019b), and Karami et al. (2017). However, Bessa et al. (2019) reported that this method (10% KOH at 40 °C) is not suitable for fatty tissues. They recommended using KOH 10% combined with a detergent (e.g. Tween 20) to faster digestion of fatty tissues.

Catarino et al. (2017) have compared the recovery rate and efficiency of three different digestive agents: 1M NaOH, 35% HNO_3, and 0.1 UHb/mL protease. This paper recommended using industrial enzymes which have a higher recovery rate and least destruction compared to other methods as the standard procedure for mussel's digestion.

H_2O_2 is widely using to digest organic matter from biota tissues (Qu et al., 2018; Li et al., 2015; Wu et al., 2020; Bom & Sá, 2021). Nuelle et al. (2014) have identified 30% H_2O_2 as an effective oxidizing agent to digest organic matter though it slightly changes the polymers. Frias et al. (2018) recommended using 10% H_2O_2 as plastics react with high concentrations of H_2O_2 solutions. However, Zhang et al. (2019) reporting that digestion with 2-7% of H_2O_2 results in underestimation of MPs weight and number. Table 1 summarize the digestion reagents widely used in water, sediments, and biota. A recent study by

Fraissinet et al. (2021) has revealed that a mixture of 2.5% KOH, 5% H_2O_2 and 2.7% methanol at 60 °C for 3h allows a 99% digestion of mussel tissues.

Efficacy of Reagents in Organic Matter Reduction and Recovery Rate

The organic matter removal rate is varying among different digestion agents. Digestion efficacy can be calculated by comparing the relative organic material removing rate using Equation 1. Digestion efficacy should be ³95.0% to select as a suitable digestion agent. The existence of undigested organic substances on the filter paper could disturb the optical analysis of MPs (Karami et al., 2017).

$$\text{Efficacy}(\%)100 = \frac{\text{Wet weight entire organism's tissue}(g) - \text{Dry weight on filter paper}(g)}{\text{Wet weight entire organism's tissue}(g)} * 100$$

Equation 1

After digestion, the solution is filtered through a membrane. The recovery rate (equation 2) can be calculated by using the weight of the MPs remaining on the membrane (Karami et al., 2017).

$$\text{Recovery } \% = \frac{\text{Dry weight on filter paper}(g)}{\text{Wet weight entire organism's tissue}(g)} * 100 \text{ Equation 2}$$

Effects of Digestion Methods on MPs

The reagents used, the temperature applied, and the heat generated from the exothermic oxidation reactions utilized in the chemical digestion methods cause significant impacts on polymers such as visual damage, partial destruction of polymers, etc. It eventually affects the recovery rate of the MPs particles from samples. Chemical reagents cause both physical and spectral changes on polymeric particles. Digestions at high temperatures should be avoided. Thus, care should be given to select a digestion reagent that has lower effects on MPs particles (Hurley et al., 2018; Karami et al., 2017).

Density Separation

The residual solution can be filtered and recovered directly after digestion. But sometimes inorganic particles dominate after digestion which arise the necessity of further exposure to a density separation (Bessa et al., 2019). Plastic particles have lighter densities than sand or other sediments. This density difference is used to extract the lighter plastic fragments from the denser sediment grains (Hidalgo-Ruz et al., 2012). Different high-density solutions are mixed with the sample and shaken for a certain period and allow to settle down for several hours. Then the supernatant can be separated through filtration. NaCl (1.0-1.2 g/cm^3) is the most widely used solution due to its low cost and non-hazardous nature (Stock et al., 2019). EU Marine Strategy Framework Directive (MSFD) Technical Subgroup of Marine Litter and Frias et al. (2018) recommended using NaCl or sodium tungstate dihydrate ($Na_2WO_4 \cdot 2H_2O$) to digest sediment samples. It can separate polymers that have a lower density like polypropylene or polyamide, but it cannot separate PVC or PET which have high densities. This results in underestimation of polymer types and the total particle count as PVC and PET account for 17% of the world's plastic manufacturing (Plastics Europe, 2017). Liebezeit & Dubaish (2012) reported that $ZnCl_2$ can be utilized to recover all kinds of plastics. Coppock et al. (2017) compared the costs and efficiency of NaCl, NaI, and $ZnCl_2$ and decided that $ZnCl_2$ is the most efficient and cheap method for density separation. NaI is an expensive solution and Nuelle et al. (2014) suggest using NaCl solution to reduce the initial sample size and then use $ZnCl_2$ for further separation. Both $ZnCl_2$ and NaI can separate PVC polymers. Potassium formate (K(HCOO)) is another high-density solution use for the extraction of MPs that is reusable (Corcoran et al., 2009). Table 1 summarize the widely used solution for density separation.

Filtration and Purification

Filtration is used for extracting MPs from digested solutions. The appropriate selection of filter membranes is crucial for the filtration as well as for the post-identification of MPs. Cellulose nitrate membrane filter, nylon membrane filter, glass fiber filter, cellulose acetate membrane filter, and polycarbonate membrane filter have been used in literature widely. Features like smooth filter surface and not easily rolling up makes cellulose nitrate membrane filter, cellulose acetate membrane filter and nylon membrane filter beneficial for the quantitation and identification of MPs. The selection of membrane filter varies and is based on the applied digestion reagent. Cellulose nitrate membrane filter and cellulose acetate membrane filter cannot be used for filtration of alkali digested solution as alkali solution (NaOH/KOH) can react with the membrane. Alkali digested solutions are recommended to be filtered by using nylon membrane filters. Cellulose nitrate membrane, cellulose acetate membrane, and nylon membrane filters are appropriate for filtration of oxidative digested solutions (Zhu & Wang, 2020). The pore size of the filters should be decided in line with the spatial resolution of the identification technique going to be applied. The common pore size of cellulose nitrate membrane filters is 0.45 (Hu et al., 2016) 0.8 (Mathalon & Hill, 2014), and 5 μm (Li et al., 2018). Five μm is the common pore size of cellulose acetate membrane filters and nylon membrane filters used in literature (Hermsen et al., 2018; Horton et al., 2017b). Glass fiber filters are also used for filtration (Davidson & Dudas, 2016) and it is not recommended for the identification of MPs as the rough surface interferes during the experiment. The polycarbonate filter membrane is also not recommended as it has a powerful infrared signal which can disrupt identification. Filtration is also affected by the temperature of digested solutions (Zhu & Wang, 2020).

Identification Methods

After the preparation, the quantity and types of MPs should be found. Visual identification followed by analytical techniques for polymer identification is widely used (Lusher et al., 2017). Analysis of MPs generally comprises of two steps: physical characterization of possible plastics (e.g., microscopy) subsequently chemical characterization (e.g., spectroscopy) for verification of plastics (Shim et al., 2017). Even though the worldwide accepted lower value for small MPs is 1 μm, present chemical characterization equipment like micro- FTIR and micro-Raman spectroscopy only can reliably identify MPs up to 20-10 μm. Thus, 20-10 μm has become the lower reliable, practical limit for MPs (Bessa et al., 2019). Table 2 summarize the advantages and limitations of each identification technique.

Table 1. Summary of the different reagents used for digestion and density separation

Purpose	Reagent	Remarks
Digestion of organic matter	(30%) H_2O_2	Widely used Long reaction time slightly changes the polymers
	Fenton's reagent (Consisted of 30% (v/v) H_2O_2 and a mixture of 20 g iron (II) sulfate heptahydrate and 1 L filtered RO water catalyst)	Effective digestion method. Has minor negative effects on the size and mass of MPs.
	Acid digestion (HNO_3 alone or mixture of acids; mixture of HNO_3:$HClO_4$ (4:1))	Detrimental to many of the common plastic polymers
	10% KOH	Economical and faster method for digestion of bivalve's tissues and other fatty tissues in biota
Density separation	NaCl	Most widely used solution low cost Non-hazardous Cannot separate higher density particles like PVC or PET
	$ZnCl_2$	High recovery rate Cheap Environmentally hazardous
	NaI	Expensive

Optical Techniques

Visual sorting by the naked eye or with the help of an optical microscope (usually a stereomicroscope) is the most common and simplest technique used when there are many samples to analyze. The observer can directly identify the MPs in the size range of 1-5 mm by the naked eye. (Wang & Wang, 2018). This technique is based on the physical characteristics of MPs like size, color, and shape. The quality of visual analysis is affected by the observer, the quality and magnification of the used microscope, and the sample type (Löder & Gerdts, 2015). Following criteria are recommended to follow in optical analysis.

- fibers must have consistent color and thickness all along the entire length
- particles should be uniformly colored and clear
- white particles must be further analyzed (Wang & Wang, 2018)

Many studies have proved that MPs recognized by the visual method were confirmed as non-plastic in following infrared spectroscopy analysis (Zhu & Wang, 2020). Many studies only have used a smaller subset of sorted particles for further analysis. Therefore, care should be given to select a representative subset of sorted particles for further analysis. It is recommended to further analyze all the particles if the presorted particles are less than 100 to reduce the uncertainty. If the pre-sorted particles are larger than 100, more than fifty percent of the particles should be included in the subset for future analysis (Hermsen et al., 2018). Because of the limitations, this method is not recommended as an independent analysis technique (Löder & Gerdts, 2015).

Scanning Electron Microscope (SEM)

Scanning electron microscope (SEM) can provide extremely clear and high-resolution (<0.5 nm resolution) images of plastic-like particles by providing pictures of the surface texture of the particles. Furthermore, by examining the images of the surface textures, like pits and cracks, weathering progress of recovered MPs from natural matrices can be identified. Further analysis of SEM and energy-dispersive X-ray spectroscopy (SEM-EDS) provides the elemental composition and inorganic additives of the particles. The application of SEM-EDS helps in further distinguishing between natural materials and MPs through imaging and elemental analysis, thus reduces the number of particles necessary for the spectroscopic examination. However, this method is time-consuming and requires extra effort for sample preparation (gold or carbon surface coat) hence, not appropriate for the analysis of a large number of samples (Wang & Wang, 2018; Shim et al., 2017; Zarfl, 2019).

Fourier Transform Infrared (FTIR) Spectroscopy

FTIR is a simple, non-destructive, and highly accurate method which mostly used for the identification of MPs recovered from environmental matrices (Zarfl, 2019). Bond composition of materials differs from each other making it feasible to identify spectra of an unknown substance by comparing with the standard spectra of a material in the spectral library (Löder M.G.J., 2015). FTIR can not only identify the MPs but also verify specific polymer types, giving clues for the sources of the sample analyzed. Furthermore, FTIR provides information about the physiochemical weathering of MPs by examining their oxidation intensity. However, FTIR is time-consuming, requires an experienced operator, requires manual sorting of sample particles and small size particles cannot analyze (only capable of analyzing particles greater than 10–20 μm) (Zhu & Wang, 2020).

FTIR micro spectroscopy (micro-FTIR), attenuated total reflectance-FTIR (ATR-FTIR), and focal plane array (FPA)-FTIR spectroscopy are optimized techniques of FTIR which is highly utilized for MPs research at present (Wang & Wang, 2018).

FTIR Micro Spectroscopy (Micro-FTIR)

This technology combines both microscopy and FTIR spectroscopy on a single platform and enables the identification of smaller MPs. This method does not require a sample preparation step. But samples should be completely dried before analysis. Transmission mode, reflection mode, and attenuated total reflection mode are three major modes utilized in the analysis and identification of MPs. Mode is selected based on the application. Transmission mode delivers high-resolution spectra of thin and transparent plastic film due to penetration of infrared rays through the plastics. Opaque and thick MPs can be analyzed using the reflection mode. Unevenly thick MPs and MPs larger than 300 μm can be identified by using the attenuated total reflection mode. Currently, Micro-FTIR cannot identify smaller MPs of sub-20-μm-range (Zhu & Wang, 2020).

Focal Plane Array (FPA) Based Micro-FTIR Imaging

Conventional Micro-FTIR cannot examine the multi-point spectral curves of MPs samples, thus limit the detection of smaller size MPs. But this would be possible with the development of Micro-FTIR based on focal plane array technology. This method occupies two techniques to evaluate the acquired spectra; artificial interpretation of appropriate vibration bands based on reference tables and database retrieval function matched with reference spectrum library (Klein S. et al., 2018; Shim et al., 2017; Löder & Gerdts, 2015).

Raman Spectroscopy

This technology is also widely applicable in MPs research. This also provides the polymer composition of the MPs sample. Raman spectroscopy and FTIR are complementary techniques. FTIR can identify some molecular vibrations, which are Raman spectroscopy inactive, and vice versa (Qiu et al., 2016). Unlike FTIR this method allows detection of thicker or strongly absorbing MPs as it is not relying on the transmission of the exciting light across the sample material (Zarfl, 2019). This technique irradiated samples with a laser light which results in different frequencies of backscattered light (Löder & Gerdts, 2015). These techniques allow identifying MPs particles down to 1 µm. Microscopy combined with Raman spectroscopy (Micro- Raman spectroscopy) can even successfully identify MPs less than 1 µm. This method allows quick and accurate identification of samples by matching the sample Raman spectra with the standard spectral library. However, this technique is disturbed by the presence of additives, color, and adhered contaminants MPs (Qiu et al., 2016).

Thermal Analysis

This method is also used to identify MPs in literature studies, but not so frequently. This method measures changes in the physical and chemical properties of polymers based on the thermal stability of the sample (Shim et al., 2017). Thermal analysis methods are destructive techniques hence further analysis of the samples is impossible. This method only provides the total mass fraction of polymers and does not provide the quantity, shape, and size range of the MPs in the sample. However, it provides data about the polymer type along with the organic or inorganic additives present in the samples. These limitations urge to put more effort to explore more about the practicability of this method (Shim et al., 2017). It is recommended to use thermal analysis methods only as complementary methods to the spectroscopic methods (Wang & Wang, 2018).

Pyrolysis – Gas Chromatography-Mass Spectrometry (Pyr-GC-MS)

This method decides the polymer type of MPs by examining the pyrolysis products of the MPs sample. Polymer composition is identified by comparing the obtained thermal spectra of the sample thermal spectra of known polymer samples in the reference library (Fischer & Scholz-Böttcher, 2017). This method avoids background contamination as it does not require any solvents when analyzing. Pyrolysis products of the different polymers can be the same, thus misjudgment of types of MPs is possible. Also, permit only 0.5 mg of samples to be analyzed making it inappropriate to use for biological samples. In addition, it has disadvantages like time-consuming and unsuitable to analyze large-scale samples (Dümichen et al., 2015).

Thermal Extraction and Desorption – Gas Chromatography-Mass Spectrometry (TED-GC-MS)

TED-GC-MS is a novel technique that develops to evade the problems with Pyr-GC-MS. TED-GC-MS is a combination of two techniques: thermal extraction with thermogravimetric analysis (TGA) and thermal desorption gas chromatography-mass spectrometry (TD-GC-MS). The advantages of TGA is that it allows analysis of large samples and fast analysis (Wang & Wang, 2018).

Fluorescent Staining Methods

The development of fast, less expensive, easy and most specially accurate quantification of MPs particles as small as a single micron has long been a crucial necessity in MPs research studies (Shruti et al., 2022). These issues were addressed by the introduction of fluorescence-led identification technique using staining dyes such as Rose Bengal or Nile Red (NR). The dye adsorbs into MPs surfaces and when observed under a fluorescence microscope, it can easily be distinguished from mineral and other organic substances in the sample. NR staining method is widely employed for MPs quantification around the world recently (Imasha & Babel, 2021; Dowarah et al., 2020). However, various staining protocols for MPs in water samples identification have been used in the literature. But still, there is not any harmonized protocols (Prata, et al., 2019c; Shruti et al., 2022). Wang et al. (2021) have proved that addition of H_2O_2 or combined addition of H_2O_2 and NaCl help to reduce the false positive of MPs when stained with Nile red. Moreover, this technique is mainly introduced to increase the accuracy of MPs counts by visual identification. This method is only recommended to use as a complementary technique for a fast and inexpensive estimation of plastic particles in a sample along with a chemical identification technique (Zarfl, 2019).

CONCLUSION

Identification and quantification of MPs are very important to understand the contamination level and potential impacts on the environment of this emerging pollutant. A wide variety of analytical methods have been applied to identify MPs in water, sediments, and biota. The variation in analytical methods has made it difficult to compare the studies. Also, these identification methods involve several time-consuming steps.

Quality assurance and quality control procedures should be followed throughout the analysis procedures to prevent external MPs contamination. Sampling procedures always depend on the goal of the research, and it varies in terms of sampling volume, area, size, and depth. Special care should be given to prevent accumulation and losses of MPs during sampling of biota. The selection of a proper digestion reagent is important to remove the organic matter from the environmental samples which have lower effects on MPs particles. Usage of efficient density separation reagent can recover a wide range of MPs polymer types. Filter papers selection should be done considering the identification techniques employed and the digestion reagent applied. The combination of the microscopic method followed by chemical identification has improved the efficiency and reliability of MPs identification. Micro FTIR and micro- Raman spectroscopy appear to be promising techniques in MPs identification.

Table 2. Advantages and limitations of microplastics identification techniques

Identification techniques	Advantages	Limitations
Optical method	Quick identification Low cost	Polymer composition cannot be identified Further confirmation of particles needed
Scanning electron microscope and energy-dispersive X-ray spectroscopy	High resolution pictures provide surface texture of the particles along with the understanding of the weathering process	Time-consuming Requires extra effort for sample preparation
Fourier Transform Infrared (FTIR) spectroscopy	Nondestructive method High accuracy Can be identified MPs along with the polymer type	Time-consuming Requires an experienced operator Underestimation (particles <20μm cannot be identified)
Raman spectroscopy	Micro- Raman spectroscopy can be used to identify smaller MPs >1 μm Nondestructive method	Disturbed by the presence of additives, color, and adhered contaminants to MPs Time consuming
Pyrolysis – gas chromatography-mass spectrometry (Pyr-GC-MS)	Better sensitivity Organic and inorganic impurities attached to MPS can also be identified	Time-consuming Unsuitable to analyze large-scale samples

There is an urgency of standardizing the analytical methods considering the following aspects. Sampling protocols should be standardized with regards to the number of sampling locations, amount of samples, sample volume sizes, sampling depths and sampling frequency for each environmental matrices, water, sediments, and biota. Different studies have analyzed MPs in different size ranges. Hence there should be a uniformity in analyzing MPs size ranges in different studies to make them comparable. Quality assurance and quality control procedures also need to be strict. Current analytical methods are time consuming and expensive. Hence simple, easy, and less expensive analytical methods should be developed. Consideration should be given to develop automated procedures for MPs analysis instead of current manual handling process. Results reporting, especially the MPs in biota, should be standardized.

Still, there are much research to be carried out in the analysis of MPs in water, sediments, and biota. Hence, future research should be focused on establishing reliable and efficient standard methodologies for MPs monitoring enabling comparison of studies from different parts of the world. Moreover, more emphasis should be given to develop reliable methodologies to identify MPs down to few micrometers.

REFERENCES

Bessa, F., Kogel, T., Frias, J., & Lusher, A. (2019). Harmonized protocol for monitoring microplastics in biota. *Micropoll-Multilevel Assessment of Microplastics and Associated Pollutants in the Baltic Sea View Project*, (March), 1–30. doi:10.13140/RG.2.2.28588.72321/1

Bom, F. C., & Sá, F. (2021). Concentration of microplastics in bivalves of the environment: A systematic review. *Environmental Monitoring and Assessment*, *193*(12), 846. Advance online publication. doi:10.100710661-021-09639-1 PMID:34839390

Bromley, P. J. (1994). The role of gastric evacuation experiments in quantifying the feeding rates of predatory fish. *Reviews in Fish Biology and Fisheries*, *4*(1), 36–66. doi:10.1007/BF00043260

Catarino, A. I., Thompson, R., Sanderson, W., & Henry, T. B. (2017). Development and optimization of a standard method for extraction of microplastics in mussels by enzyme digestion of soft tissues. *Environmental Toxicology and Chemistry*, *36*(4), 947–951. doi:10.1002/etc.3608 PMID:27583696

Cole, M., Lindeque, P., Halsband, C., & Galloway, T. S. (2011). Microplastics as contaminants in the marine environment: A review. *Marine Pollution Bulletin*, *62*(12), 2588–2597. doi:10.1016/j.marpolbul.2011.09.025 PMID:22001295

Cole, M., Webb, H., Lindeque, P. K., Fileman, E. S., Halsband, C., & Galloway, T. S. (2014). Isolation of microplastics in biota-rich seawater samples and marine organisms. *Scientific Reports*, *4*(1), 1–8. doi:10.1038rep04528 PMID:24681661

Coppock, R. L., Cole, M., Lindeque, P. K., Queirós, A. M., & Galloway, T. S. (2017). A small-scale, portable method for extracting microplastics from marine sediments. *Environmental Pollution*, *230*, 829–837. doi:10.1016/j.envpol.2017.07.017 PMID:28734264

Corcoran, P. L., Biesinger, M. C., & Grifi, M. (2009). Plastics and beaches: A degrading relationship. *Marine Pollution Bulletin*, *58*(1), 80–84. doi:10.1016/j.marpolbul.2008.08.022 PMID:18834997

Cox, K. D., Covernton, G. A., Davies, H. L., Dower, J. F., Juanes, F., & Dudas, S. E. (2019). Human Consumption of Microplastics. *Environmental Science & Technology*, *53*(12), 7068–7074. doi:10.1021/acs.est.9b01517 PMID:31184127

Davidson, K., & Dudas, S. E. (2016). Microplastic Ingestion by Wild and Cultured Manila Clams (Venerupis philippinarum) from Baynes Sound, British Columbia. *Archives of Environmental Contamination and Toxicology*, *71*(2), 147–156. doi:10.100700244-016-0286-4 PMID:27259879

Dehaut, A., Cassone, A. L., Frère, L., Hermabessiere, L., Himber, C., Rinnert, E., Rivière, G., Lambert, C., Soudant, P., Huvet, A., Duflos, G., & Paul-Pont, I. (2016). Microplastics in seafood: Benchmark protocol for their extraction and characterization. *Environmental Pollution*, *215*, 223–233. doi:10.1016/j.envpol.2016.05.018 PMID:27209243

Dowarah, K., Patchaiyappan, A., Thirunavukkarasu, C., Jayakumar, S., & Devipriya, S. P. (2020). Quantification of microplastics using Nile Red in two bivalve species Perna viridis and Meretrix meretrix from three estuaries in Pondicherry, India and microplastic uptake by local communities through bivalve diet. *Marine Pollution Bulletin*, *153*(February), 110982. doi:10.1016/j.marpolbul.2020.110982 PMID:32275539

Dris, R., Gasperi, J., Rocher, V., Saad, M., Renault, N., & Tassin, B. (2015). Microplastic contamination in an urban area: A case study in Greater Paris. *Environmental Chemistry*, *12*(5), 592–599. doi:10.1071/EN14167

Dümichen, E., Barthel, A. K., Braun, U., Bannick, C. G., Brand, K., Jekel, M., & Senz, R. (2015). Analysis of polyethylene microplastics in environmental samples, using a thermal decomposition method. *Water Research*, *85*, 451–457. doi:10.1016/j.watres.2015.09.002 PMID:26376022

Enders, K., Lenz, R., Beer, S., & Stedmon, C. A. (2017). Extraction of microplastic from biota: Recommended acidic digestion destroys common plastic polymers. *ICES Journal of Marine Science*, *74*(1), 326–331. doi:10.1093/icesjms/fsw173

Plastics Europe. (2017). *Plastics – the Facts 2017*. doi:10.1016/j.marpolbul.2013.01.015

Plastics Europe. (2020). Plastics – the Facts 2020. In *PlasticEurope*. https://www.plasticseurope.org/en/resources/publications/4312-plastics-facts-2020

European Commission. (2013). *MSDF Guidance on Monitoring Marine Litter*. doi:10.2788/99475

Felsing, S., Kochleus, C., Buchinger, S., Brennholt, N., Stock, F., & Reifferscheid, G. (2018). A new approach in separating microplastics from environmental samples based on their electrostatic behavior. *Environmental Pollution, 234*, 20–28. doi:10.1016/j.envpol.2017.11.013 PMID:29154206

Fischer, M., & Scholz-Böttcher, B. M. (2017). Simultaneous Trace Identification and Quantification of Common Types of Microplastics in Environmental Samples by Pyrolysis-Gas Chromatography-Mass Spectrometry. *Environmental Science & Technology, 51*(9), 5052–5060. doi:10.1021/acs.est.6b06362 PMID:28391690

Fraissinet, S., Pennetta, A., Rossi, S., De Benedetto, G. E., & Malitesta, C. (2021). Optimization of a new multi-reagent procedure for quantitative mussel digestion in microplastic analysis. *Marine Pollution Bulletin, 173*(PA), 112931. doi:10.1016/j.marpolbul.2021.112931

Frias, J., Pagter, E., Nash, R., O'Connor, I., Carretero, O., Filgueiras, A., Viñas, L., Gago, J., Antunes, J., Bessa, F., Sobral, P., Goruppi, A., Tirelli, V., Pedrotti, M. L., Suaria, G., Aliani, S., Lopes, C., Raimundo, J., Caetano, M., … Gerdts, G. (2018). Standardised protocol for monitoring microplastics in sediments. *JPI-Oceans BASEMAN Project,* 33. doi:10.13140/RG.2.2.36256.89601/1

Frias, J. P. G. L., & Nash, R. (2019). Microplastics: Finding a consensus on the definition. *Marine Pollution Bulletin, 138*(November), 145–147. doi:10.1016/j.marpolbul.2018.11.022

González, D., Hanke, G., Tweehuysen, G., Bellert, B., Holzhauer, M., Palatinus, A., Hohenblum, P., & Oosterbaan, L. (2016). Riverine Litter Monitoring - Options and Recommendations - Thematic Report. In *JRC Scientific and Technical Reports*. doi:10.2788/461233

Hermsen, E., Mintenig, S. M., Besseling, E., & Koelmans, A. A. (2018). Quality Criteria for the Analysis of Microplastic in Biota Samples. *Critical Reviews in Environmental Science and Technology, 52*(18), 10230–10240. doi:10.1021/acs.est.8b01611 PMID:30137965

Hidalgo-Ruz, V., Gutow, L., Thompson, R. C., & Thiel, M. (2012). Microplastics in the marine environment: A review of the methods used for identification and quantification. *Environmental Science & Technology, 46*(6), 3060–3075. doi:10.1021/es2031505 PMID:22321064

Horton, A. A., Spurgeon, D. J., Lahive, E., & Svendsen, C. (2017a). Microplastics in freshwater and terrestrial environments: Evaluating the current understanding to identify the knowledge gaps and future research priorities. *The Science of the Total Environment, 586*(February), 127–141. doi:10.1016/j.scitotenv.2017.01.190 PMID:28169032

Horton, A. A., Svendsen, C., Williams, R. J., Spurgeon, D. J., & Lahive, E. (2017b). Large microplastic particles in sediments of tributaries of the River Thames, UK – Abundance, sources and methods for effective quantification. *Marine Pollution Bulletin, 114*(1), 218–226. doi:10.1016/j.marpolbul.2016.09.004 PMID:27692488

Hu, L., Su, L., Xue, Y., Mu, J., Zhu, J., Xu, J., & Shi, H. (2016). Uptake, accumulation and elimination of polystyrene microspheres in tadpoles of Xenopus tropicalis. *Chemosphere, 164*, 611–617. doi:10.1016/j.chemosphere.2016.09.002 PMID:27635643

Hurley, R. R., Lusher, A. L., Olsen, M., & Nizzetto, L. (2018). Validation of a Method for Extracting Microplastics from Complex, Organic-Rich, Environmental Matrices. *Environmental Science & Technology, 52*(13), 7409–7417. doi:10.1021/acs.est.8b01517 PMID:29886731

ICES. (2015). OSPAR request on development of a common monitoring protocol for plastic particles in fish stomachs and selected shellfish on the basis of existing fish disease surveys. *IICES Advice,* 1–6.

Imasha, H. U. E., & Babel, S. (2021). Microplastics Contamination in Commercial Green Mussels from Selected Wet Markets in Thailand. *Archives of Environmental Contamination and Toxicology*, (3), 449–459. Advance online publication. doi:10.100700244-021-00886-4 PMID:34508277

Imhof, H. K., Schmid, J., Niessner, R., Ivleva, N. P., & Laforsch, C. (2012). A novel, highly efficient method for the separation and quantification of plastic particles in sediments of aquatic environments. *Limnology and Oceanography, Methods, 10*(July), 524–537. doi:10.4319/lom.2012.10.524

Kankanige, D., & Babel, S. (2020). Smaller-sized micro-plastics (MPs) contamination in single-use PET-bottled water in Thailand. *The Science of the Total Environment, 717*, 137232. doi:10.1016/j.scitotenv.2020.137232 PMID:32062244

Karami, A., Golieskardi, A., Choo, C. K., Romano, N., Ho, Y., & Salamatinia, B. (2017). A high-performance protocol for extraction of microplastics in fish. *The Science of the Total Environment, 578*, 485–494. doi:10.1016/j.scitotenv.2016.10.213 PMID:27836345

Karbalaei, S., Hanachi, P., Walker, T. R., & Cole, M. (2018). Occurrence, sources, human health impacts and mitigation of microplastic pollution. *Environmental Science and Pollution Research International, 25*(36), 36046–36063. doi:10.100711356-018-3508-7 PMID:30382517

Klein, S., D. I. K., J., E., & T.P., K. (2018). Analysis, Occurrence, and Degradation of Microplastics in the Aqueous Environment. In Freshwater Microplastics. The Handbook of Environmental Chemistry (p. 302). Springer. doi:10.1007/978-3-319-61615-5

Li, J., Green, C., Reynolds, A., Shi, H., & Rotchell, J. M. (2018). Microplastics in mussels sampled from coastal waters and supermarkets in the United Kingdom. *Environmental Pollution, 241*, 35–44. doi:10.1016/j.envpol.2018.05.038 PMID:29793106

Li, J., Wang, Z., Rotchell, J. M., Shen, X., Li, Q., & Zhu, J. (2021). Where are we? Towards an understanding of the selective accumulation of microplastics in mussels. *Environmental Pollution, 286*(June), 117543. doi:10.1016/j.envpol.2021.117543 PMID:34119866

Li, J., Yang, D., Li, L., Jabeen, K., & Shi, H. (2015). Microplastics in commercial bivalves from China. *Environmental Pollution, 207*, 190–195. doi:10.1016/j.envpol.2015.09.018 PMID:26386204

Liebezeit, G., & Dubaish, F. (2012). Microplastics in beaches of the East Frisian Islands Spiekeroog and Kachelotplate. *Bulletin of Environmental Contamination and Toxicology, 89*(1), 213–217. doi:10.100700128-012-0642-7 PMID:22526995

Liu, M., Lu, S., Chen, Y., Cao, C., Bigalke, M., & He, D. (2020). Analytical Methods for Microplastics in Environments: Current Advances and Challenges. In Handbook of Environmental Chemistry (Vol. 95, pp. 3–24). doi:10.1007/698_2019_436

Löder, M. G. J. G. G. (2015). Methodology Used for the Detection and Identification of Microplastics—A Critical Appraisal. In Marine Anthropogenic Litter. doi:10.1007/978-3-319-16510-3

Lusher, A. L., McHugh, M., & Thompson, R. C. (2013). Occurrence of microplastics in the gastrointestinal tract of pelagic and demersal fish from the English Channel. *Marine Pollution Bulletin*, *67*(1–2), 94–99. doi:10.1016/j.marpolbul.2012.11.028 PMID:23273934

Lusher, A. L., Tirelli, V., O'Connor, I., & Officer, R. (2015). Microplastics in Arctic polar waters: The first reported values of particles in surface and sub-surface samples. *Scientific Reports*, *5*(September), 1–9. doi:10.1038rep14947 PMID:26446348

Lusher, A. L., Welden, N. A., Sobral, P., & Cole, M. (2017). Sampling, isolating and identifying microplastics ingested by fish and invertebrates. *Analytical Methods*, *9*(9), 1346–1360. doi:10.1039/C6AY02415G

Mai, L., Bao, L. J., Shi, L., Wong, C. S., & Zeng, E. Y. (2018). A review of methods for measuring microplastics in aquatic environments. *Environmental Science and Pollution Research International*, *25*(12), 11319–11332. doi:10.100711356-018-1692-0 PMID:29536421

Masura, J., Baker, J., Foster, G., & Arthur, C. (2015). Laboratory Methods for the Analysis of Microplastics in the Marine Environment. *NOAA Marine Debris Program National*, (July), 1–39. doi:10.1016/j.jjcc.2016.11.011

Mathalon, A., & Hill, P. (2014). Microplastic fibers in the intertidal ecosystem surrounding Halifax Harbor, Nova Scotia. *Marine Pollution Bulletin*, *81*(1), 69–79. doi:10.1016/j.marpolbul.2014.02.018 PMID:24650540

Miller, E., Sedlak, M., Lin, D., Box, C., Holleman, C., Rochman, C. M., & Sutton, R. (2021). Recommended best practices for collecting, analyzing, and reporting microplastics in environmental media: Lessons learned from comprehensive monitoring of San Francisco Bay. *Journal of Hazardous Materials*, *409*(November), 124770. doi:10.1016/j.jhazmat.2020.124770

Nuelle, M. T., Dekiff, J. H., Remy, D., & Fries, E. (2014). A new analytical approach for monitoring microplastics in marine sediments. *Environmental Pollution*, *184*, 161–169. doi:10.1016/j.envpol.2013.07.027 PMID:24051349

Peng, L., Fu, D., Qi, H., Lan, C. Q., Yu, H., & Ge, C. (2020). Micro- and nano-plastics in marine environment: Source, distribution and threats — A review. *The Science of the Total Environment*, *698*, 134254. doi:10.1016/j.scitotenv.2019.134254 PMID:31514025

Phuong, N. N., Poirier, L., Pham, Q. T., Lagarde, F., & Zalouk-Vergnoux, A. (2018). Factors influencing the microplastic contamination of bivalves from the French Atlantic coast: Location, season and/or mode of life? *Marine Pollution Bulletin*, *129*(2), 664–674. doi:10.1016/j.marpolbul.2017.10.054 PMID:29106937

Picó, Y., & Barceló, D. (2019). Analysis and prevention of microplastics pollution in water: Current perspectives and future directions. *ACS Omega*, *4*(4), 6709–6719. doi:10.1021/acsomega.9b00222 PMID:31459797

Prata, J. C., da Costa, J. P., Duarte, A. C., & Rocha-Santos, T. (2019a). Methods for sampling and detection of microplastics in water and sediment: A critical review. *Trends in Analytical Chemistry*, *110*, 150–159. doi:10.1016/j.trac.2018.10.029

Prata, J. C., da Costa, J. P., Girão, A. V., Lopes, I., Duarte, A. C., & Rocha-Santos, T. (2019b). Identifying a quick and efficient method of removing organic matter without damaging microplastic samples. *The Science of the Total Environment*, *686*, 131–139. doi:10.1016/j.scitotenv.2019.05.456 PMID:31176812

Prata, J. C., Reis, V., da Costa, J. P., Mouneyrac, C., Duarte, A. C., & Rocha-Santos, T. (2021). Contamination issues as a challenge in quality control and quality assurance in microplastics analytics. *Journal of Hazardous Materials*, *403*(August), 123660. Advance online publication. doi:10.1016/j.jhazmat.2020.123660 PMID:33264868

Prata, J. C., Reis, V., Matos, J. T. V., da Costa, J. P., Duarte, A. C., & Rocha-Santos, T. (2019c). A new approach for routine quantification of microplastics using Nile Red and automated software (MP-VAT). *The Science of the Total Environment*, *690*, 1277–1283. doi:10.1016/j.scitotenv.2019.07.060 PMID:31470490

Qiu, Q., Tan, Z., Wang, J., Peng, J., Li, M., & Zhan, Z. (2016). Extraction, enumeration and identification methods for monitoring microplastics in the environment. *Estuarine, Coastal and Shelf Science*, *176*, 102–109. doi:10.1016/j.ecss.2016.04.012

Qu, X., Su, L., Li, H., Liang, M., & Shi, H. (2018). Assessing the relationship between the abundance and properties of microplastics in water and in mussels. *Science of the Total Environment, 621*(February), 679–686. doi:10.1016/j.scitotenv.2017.11.284

Rios Mendoza, L. M., & Balcer, M. (2019). Microplastics in freshwater environments: A review of quantification assessment. *Trends in Analytical Chemistry*, *113*, 402–408. doi:10.1016/j.trac.2018.10.020

Shim, W. J., Hong, S. H., & Eo, S. E. (2017). Identification methods in microplastic analysis: A review. *Analytical Methods*, *9*(9), 1384–1391. doi:10.1039/C6AY02558G

Shruti, V. C., Pérez-Guevara, F., Roy, P. D., & Kutralam-Muniasamy, G. (2022). Analyzing microplastics with Nile Red: Emerging trends, challenges, and prospects. *Journal of Hazardous Materials, 423*(August). doi:10.1016/j.jhazmat.2021.127171

Sparks, C., Awe, A., & Maneveld, J. (2021). Abundance and characteristics of microplastics in retail mussels from Cape Town, South Africa. *Marine Pollution Bulletin*, *166*(February), 112186. doi:10.1016/j.marpolbul.2021.112186 PMID:33676106

Stock, F., Kochleus, C., Bänsch-Baltruschat, B., Brennholt, N., & Reifferscheid, G. (2019). Sampling techniques and preparation methods for microplastic analyses in the aquatic environment – A review. *Trends in Analytical Chemistry*, *113*, 84–92. doi:10.1016/j.trac.2019.01.014

Thiele, C. J., Hudson, M. D., & Russell, A. E. (2019). Evaluation of existing methods to extract microplastics from bivalve tissue: Adapted KOH digestion protocol improves filtration at single-digit pore size. *Marine Pollution Bulletin, 142*(March), 384–393. doi:10.1016/j.marpolbul.2019.03.003 PMID:31232316

Torre, M., Digka, N., Anastasopoulou, A., Tsangaris, C., & Mytilineou, C. (2016). Anthropogenic microfibres pollution in marine biota. A new and simple methodology to minimize airborne contamination. *Marine Pollution Bulletin, 113*(1–2), 55–61. doi:10.1016/j.marpolbul.2016.07.050 PMID:27491365

Van Cauwenberghe, L., & Janssen, C. R. (2014). Microplastics in bivalves cultured for human consumption. *Environmental Pollution, 193*, 65–70. doi:10.1016/j.envpol.2014.06.010 PMID:25005888

Wang, C., Jiang, L., Liu, R., He, M., Cui, X., & Wang, C. (2021). Comprehensive assessment of factors influencing Nile red staining: Eliciting solutions for efficient microplastics analysis. *Marine Pollution Bulletin, 171*(July), 112698. doi:10.1016/j.marpolbul.2021.112698 PMID:34245991

Wang, W., & Wang, J. (2018). Investigation of microplastics in aquatic environments: An overview of the methods used, from field sampling to laboratory analysis. *Trends in Analytical Chemistry, 108*, 195–202. doi:10.1016/j.trac.2018.08.026

Wu, F., Wang, Y., Leung, J. Y. S., Huang, W., Zeng, J., Tang, Y., Chen, J., Shi, A., Yu, X., Xu, X., Zhang, H., & Cao, L. (2020). Accumulation of microplastics in typical commercial aquatic species: A case study at a productive aquaculture site in China. *The Science of the Total Environment, 708*, 135432. doi:10.1016/j.scitotenv.2019.135432 PMID:31806295

Zarfl, C. (2019). Promising techniques and open challenges for microplastic identification and quantification in environmental matrices. *Analytical and Bioanalytical Chemistry, 411*(17), 3743–3756. doi:10.100700216-019-01763-9 PMID:30919016

Zhang, S., Wang, J., Liu, X., Qu, F., Wang, X., Wang, X., Li, Y., & Sun, Y. (2019). Microplastics in the environment: A review of analytical methods, distribution, and biological effects. *Trends in Analytical Chemistry, 111*, 62–72. doi:10.1016/j.trac.2018.12.002

Zhu, J., & Wang, C. (2020). Recent advances in the analysis methodologies for microplastics in aquatic organisms: Current knowledge and research challenges. *Analytical Methods, 12*(23), 2944–2957. doi:10.1039/D0AY00143K PMID:32930155

Chapter 14
Environmental Effect of Plastics During the Anthropocene and the Great Acceleration

Elhoucine Essefi
University of Gabes, Tunisia

Soumaya Hajji
https://orcid.org/0000-0002-6371-7223
Faculty of Sciences of Sfax, Tunisia

ABSTRACT

The aim of this chapter is to investigate the environmental effect of plastics (macroplastic and microplastic) during the Anthropocene and the Great Acceleration. Plastic production has worldwide increased since 1950. For instance, many Tunisian regions such as Bizerte, Kerkennah, and Gabes witness a proliferation of plastic and microplastic. The manifestation of the plastic invasion is obviously dispersed within continental and marine environments. The detection of microplastic needs an extraction protocol and the use of the infrared spectroscopy. Added to their esthetic pollution, effect of plastics on environment and human health remains controversial. On the other hand, microplastic fragments obtained after the partial destruction of plastic represent more serious dangers. These fragments are integrated within the pedosphere, hydrosphere, and biosphere. They may be eaten by animals, including humans. Plastics are also good and safe niches for pathogenic viruses. They are considered as motivators of the Anthropocene virology.

INTRODUCTION

Small quantities of plastic could be accepted since they may be recycled (Joseph et al., 2021). But big quantities represent a real threat since they are defragmented to microplastic, which are in terns fragmented to nanoplastic (Kwak & An, 2021). In doing so, the plastic pollution becomes dispersed and lost within the atmosphere, hydrosphere, pedosphere and biosphere. To investigate the environmental pollution of

DOI: 10.4018/978-1-7998-9723-1.ch014

plastic, methods of extraction and detection as well as the remedial solutions are of great importance (Patil et al., 2022). The Anthropocene and Great Acceleration are marked by environmental changes recorded within the atmosphere (Albertsen et al., 2021; Lee & Lee, 2021), hydrosphere (Ahlström et al., 2020), bedosphere (Rossiter, 2021) and biosphere (Folke, 2021; Brauch, 2021). Great Acceleration may be identified as the set of human-driven major social, environmental and technological modifications taking place since 1950 (Shoshitaishvili, 2021). This transition is mainly driven by increasing energy consumption (Essefi, 2021a) leading to the setting of a new Anthropocene geochemistry and mineralogy (Essefi, 2020, 2021b) representing a serious threat of an apocalyptic scenario (Essefi, 2021c). As a geological layer, plastic becomes a "vibrant" memory of the nexus between capitalism and humanism, revealing its full political potential. Then, it enters a symbiotic relationship with all biotic and abiotic bodies, becoming endo-plastic. Plastic is a witness, by-product and determinant of the Anthropocene (Clinci, 2021). In terms of origin, plastic is a by-product of the main source of energy: the petrol. As a matter of fact, petroleum derivatives feed with many kinds of plastic (Palos et al., 2021). This may give an explanation of the parallel evolution of the Anthropocene setting and energy consumption (Essefi, 2021a). The environmental issue of plastic pollution is more severe than fragments of plastics damaging the esthetic side of a region. Instead, these big fragments are candidate to form smaller particles of less than 5 mm: microplastic. These products have been progressively integrated within terrestrial and marine ecosystems (Stubbins et al., 2021). Recent studies (Gkoutselis et al., 2021; Mincer, 2021) argued that plastic enhanced the pathogenic effect of some viruses including COVID-19; it is the Anthropocene virology. This chapter aims to investigate the detection of the environmental pollution by plastic and microplastic and their effect on human health. In this work, we dealt on a concrete example from Tunisia: the Gulf of Gabes.

GULF OF GABES: SOUTHEASTERN TUNISIA: AN EXAMPLE OF A PLASTIC POLLUTED REGION

The Gulf of Gabes (GG) or "small Sirte, located in the eastern Mediterranean in south eastern Tunisia; it is characterized by a high marine productivity, for this is considered as one of the most important fishing zones in Tunisia. In fact, it is the seat of a major fishery and industrial activity that is highly developed given the favourable climatic, topographic, geomorphologic and oceanographic conditions. But since 1972, this gulf is generally influenced by industrial waste. Mainly "chemical group Ghannouch-Gabes" located near the commercial port 3 km north of the city of Gabes. The chemical group rejects waste rich in organic and inorganic pollutants such as trace metals (cadmium, zinc, lead, mercury ...) and aromatic hydrocarbons, which are caused a very important modification of the biotic and abiotic parameters of this environment and consequently a variability of coastal marine biodiversity. The Gulf of Gabes has a very large continental shelf, which is marked by a relatively gentle slope, a low decline and a missing terrain with a network of channels and wadis more important to less important. The particle size characterizes by heterogeneity in the spatial distribution of the percentages of the fine and coarse fraction, Indeed, their percentages vary respectively between 1 and 40% and between 60 and 99%. In the Gulf of Gabes, the tide is among the major and particular hydrological parameters in the Mediterranean (Ben Rouina, 2016), they are semi-diurnal with significant amplitudes whose maximum is in the south of the gulf and decreases on the edges. Its amplitude is the highest in the Mediterranean Sea, with a height of 1.7 m. In addition, and according to studies carried out by the LCHF in 1958-1959, in the worst conditions the maximum level of tide is between 2.3 and 2.4 m and at the time of the open water high water, it is getting the maximum rating at 2.6 m. (Béjaoui et al., 2019). Regarding currents, golf is characterized by the presence of three main types of ocean currents, such as low-amplitude coastal currents, surface currents and tidal currents determined by wind regimes. The latter are represented by two south-westerly dynamics north of the Kerkennah Islands and a current directed towards the southern part of the Gulf of wind-generated speeds near the coast are the most intense, generally understood between 0.15 m / s and 0.30 m/s. The tidal currents measured during the flow vary between 0.1 and 0.15 m / s, and during the ebb tide are of the order of 0.05 m/s. During the 20th century, anthropogenic activities generated an increase of 1 mm / year in the level of the oceans. The tide gauge data studied over the period from 1901 to 2010 show that the average rate of sea level rise is about 1.7 ± 0.2 mm / year. Thus the altimetry data studied over the period 1993-2014 shows a sea level rise of 3.2 ± 0.mm / year. More particularly, the Gulf of Gabes is among the areas most affected by this rise, even though faster than the world average, it is estimated locally at 5.7 mm / year. From a climatic point of view, the Gulf of Gabes is characterized by an arid to semi-arid climate, with a low rainfall, with an annual average of 200 mm and a low annual average temperature with daily maximum peaks of (41 to 48 °C). The Mediterranean climatic regime is due to the displacement in latitude of the great centers of action of the atmosphere related to the cosmic mechanism of the seasons bringing during the summer and during the winter Among the factors responsible for climate change, the variations of the orbital and solar parameters (insolation and solar activity) as well as the volcanism can have a significant influence on the climatic conditions but for approximately 200 years the anthropic activities influence the climatic changes by various parameters.

METHODS OF MICROPLASTIC DETECTION

A core was collected throughout the Gulf of Gabes; one at the mouth of wadi in the coastal area of Gabes, the study in this area focused on a core 40 cm deep. It was collected in the coastal region of the city of Gabes (the mouth of wadi) on July 4th, 2017. Calcimetric analysis of sediments is an analytical approach not only to enhance the quality of a sample, but also a means to trace eustatic and environmental changes in sedimentary basins. There are two methods of calcimetry, used by several researchers: calcimetry by titration and calcimetry of Bernard. The principle of the method used consists of an attack of the rocks by hydrochloric acid (HCl) of relatively high concentration. The pH is a complex parameter whose value depends on many factors. The measurement of pH (or hydrogen potential) of a solution is done using a pH-meter and is done with a glass electrode. A pH equal to 7 corresponds to a neutral pH, between 0 and 7 at an acidic pH and between 7 and 14 a basic pH. Conductivity is the measure of the ability of the water to conduct an electrical current. Conductivity varies with temperature. It is related to the concentration and nature of the dissolved substances. The conductivity of a soil or sediment is a measure of the amount of ions present and could dissolve in the presence of water. The mineral salts are good drivers as opposed to the organic matter that drives little, in the case of wastewater heavily loaded with organic matter, the conductivity will not necessarily give an immediate idea of the environmental load. On the other hand, in other cases, it allows to quickly assess the degree of mineralization of water. The infrared radiation was discovered in 1800 by Frederick Wilhelm Hershel, it is a class of spectroscopy that deals with the infrared region of electromagnetic spectrum, between the region of the visible spectrum and radio waves. Infrared radiation invisible to the naked eye and located in a wavelength ranges greater than 800 nm. As early as

Figure 1. Geographical location of governorate of Gabes
(Chaabouni et al., 2012)

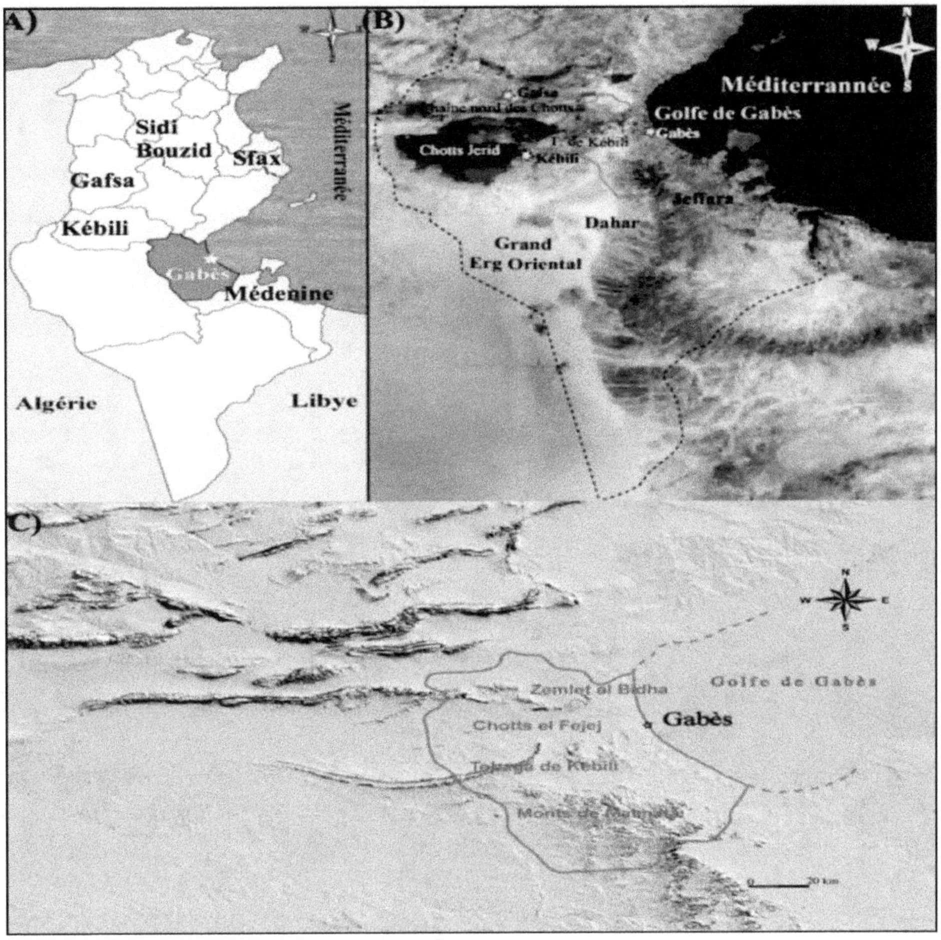

1924 it was found that the energy of the medium infrared radiation coincided with that of the internal movement of the molecule, also the relation between the absorption of IR radiation by a molecule and its molecular structure is highlighted. Infrared Absorption Spectrometry was proven to be a valuable tool for the diagnosis of microplastics in Golf of Gabes (Chouchene et al., 2021) (Fig.1). Polyethelene is detected along the bands 2970 cm-1, 2030 cm-1, 1730 cm-1, 1450 cm-1, 1000 cm-1 and 740 cm-1. Nylon is detected along the bands 3300 cm-1, 2950 cm-1, 1850 cm-1, 1625 cm-1, 1540 cm-1, 675 cm-1, and 560 cm-1. Polypropylene is detected along the bands 2950 cm-1, 2920 cm-1, 2875 cm-1, 2840 cm-1, 2840 cm-1, 1750 cm-1, 1650 cm-1, 1460 cm-1, 1375 cm-1, 1170 cm-1, 1000 cm-1, 970 cm-1, 850 cm-1 and 800 cm-1. Polysterene is detected along the bands 3050 cm-1, 3025 cm-1, 2920 cm-1, 2850 cm-1, 2360 cm-1, 1600 cm-1, 1490 cm-1, 1450 cm-1, 1370 cm-1, 1060 cm-1, 1025 cm-1, 900 cm-1, 750 cm-1, 700 cm-1, and 550 cm-1.

Figure 2. Detection of microplastics based on FTIR spectrum within the Golf of Gabes (Chouchene et al., 2021)

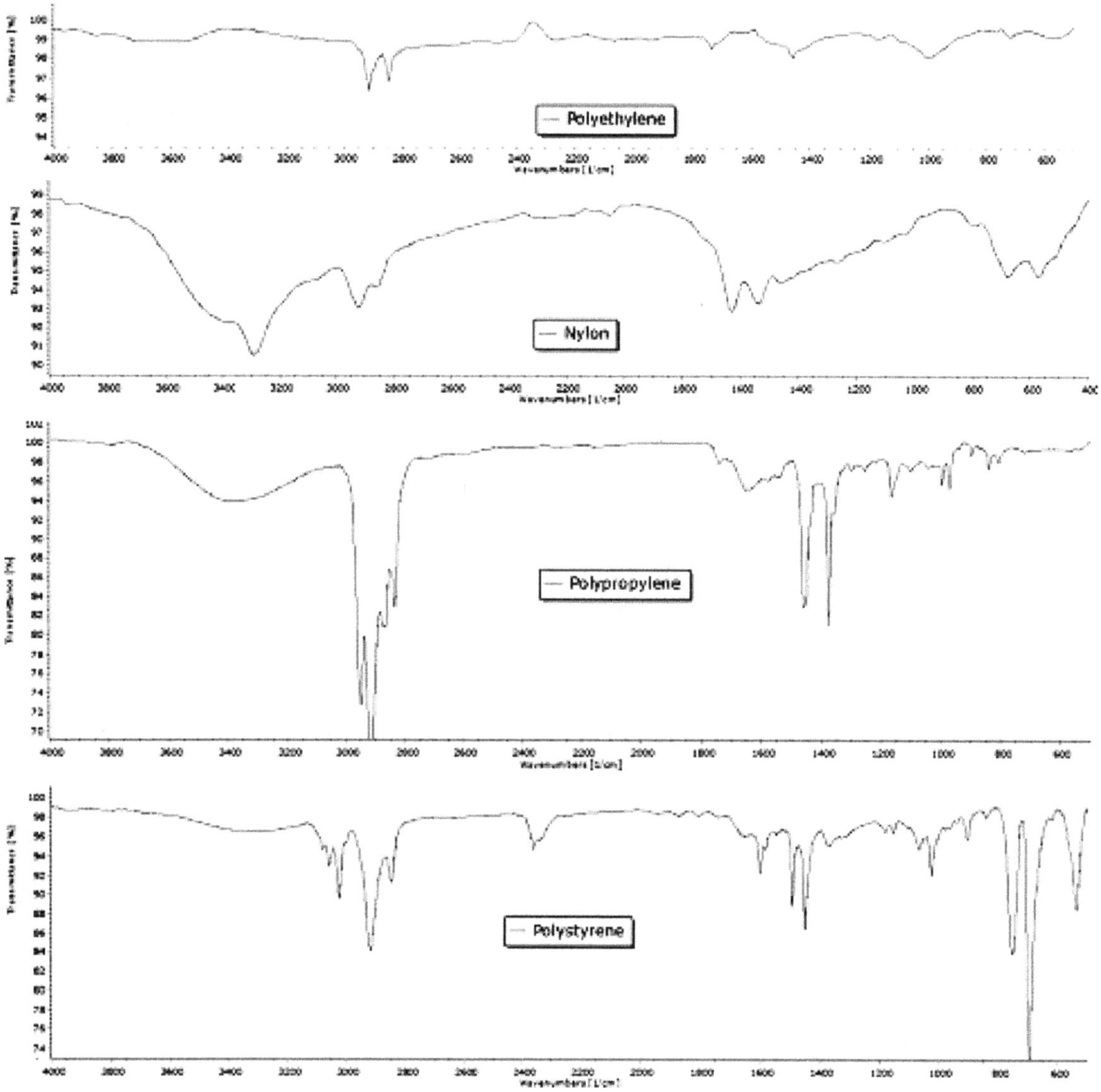

RESULTS

Manifestation of Plastic Evasion during the Anthropocene and Great Acceleration

Undoubtedly, the Anthropocene is the era of plastic; productions as well as consumptions have dramatically increased from 1950 onwards (Fig.3). The great acceleration of plastic production had started since 1950 but it has flourished since 1980. Recently, the coronavirus disease (COVID-19) pandemic has led to massive fossil fuel-derived plastic production (Gorrasi et al., 2021; Silva et al., 2021).

Figure 3. Great acceleration of plastic production

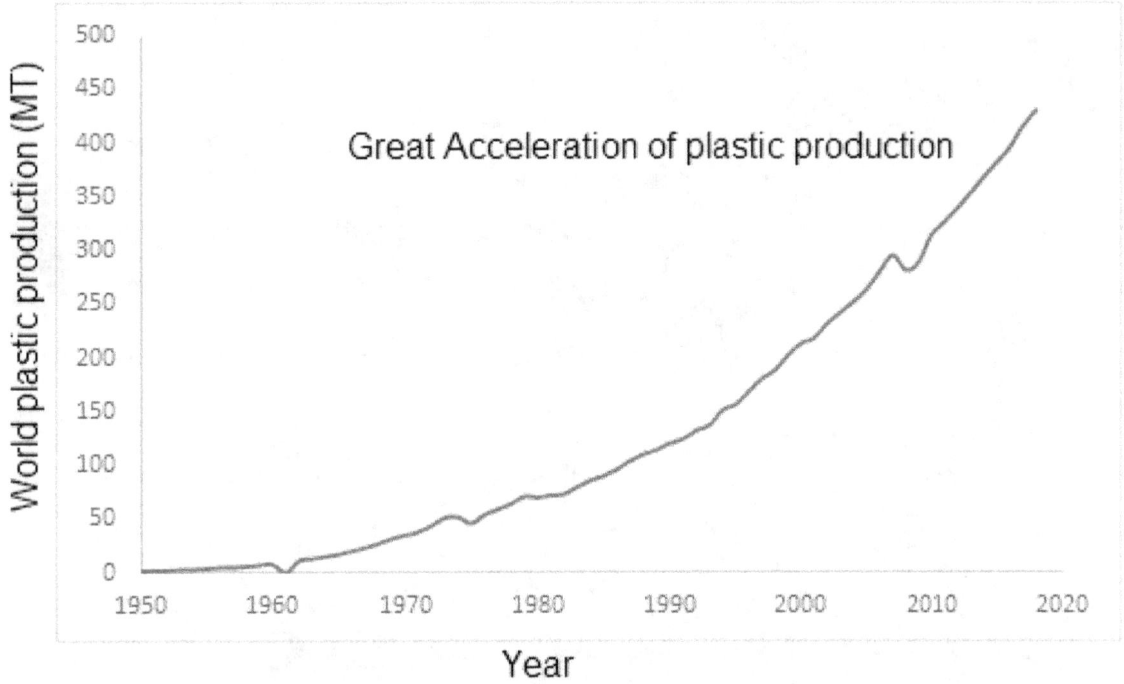

As concrete manifestation of plastic production and consumption were noticed in many regions around the world. As example of these regions, the coastal town of Gabes is evaded by mountains of plastic waste dispersed along continental as well as marine systems. As it is indicated (Fig.4), plastic wastes are collected within the natural outlet of the region: the sea. Hydrodynamics of this coastal zone makes these wastes crowded at the level of the harbor.

Record of the Anthropocene and Great Acceleration

Along the 40 cm core of Golf of Gabes, the Anthropocene and Great Acceleration are marked by a radical change in the geochemical record (Fig.5). The pH shows an upward decrease related to a global acidification taking place during the Anthropocene (300 yr) and Great Acceleration (70 yr) within water bodies in the world. This acidification resulted in calcite dissolution with the depositional environment. This dissolution is shown by an upward noticeable decrease of calcite percentage along the core. The setting of the Great Acceleration and Anthropocene was detected along some core of Tunisian wetlands (Essefi, 2021b,c; Essefi and Hajji, 2021a,b).

Microplastics as Marker of the Anthropocene and Great Acceleration

Infrared Absorption Spectrometry has been proven to be a valuable tool for the diagnosis chemical components at the level of core taken from the mouth of the wadi. The diffractograms of the infrared spectrum of the samples 1, 3, 6 and 9 respectively at 1cm, 3cm, 6cm and 9cm depth of the core G1

Figure 4. Accumulation of the plastic wastes at the level of Gabes harbor

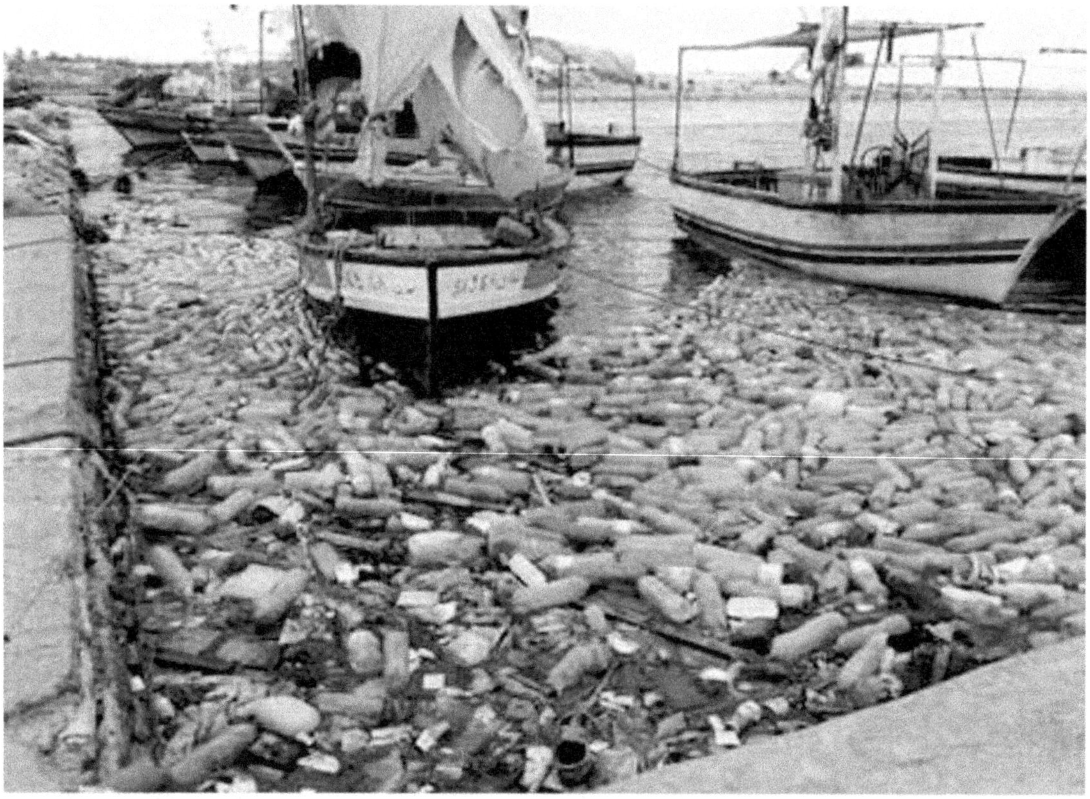

Figure 5. Setting of the Anthropocene and Great Acceleration conditions in the coast of Gabes, south-eastern Tunisia

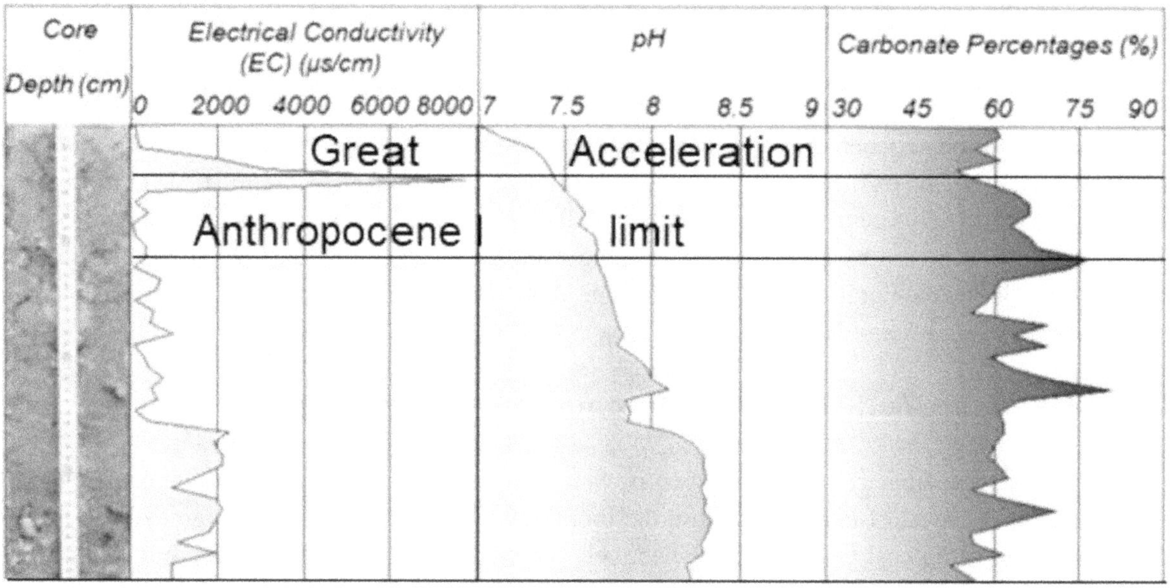

Figure 6. Diffractogram infrared spectrum of samples 1, 3, 6 and 9 of core G1 of Gabes

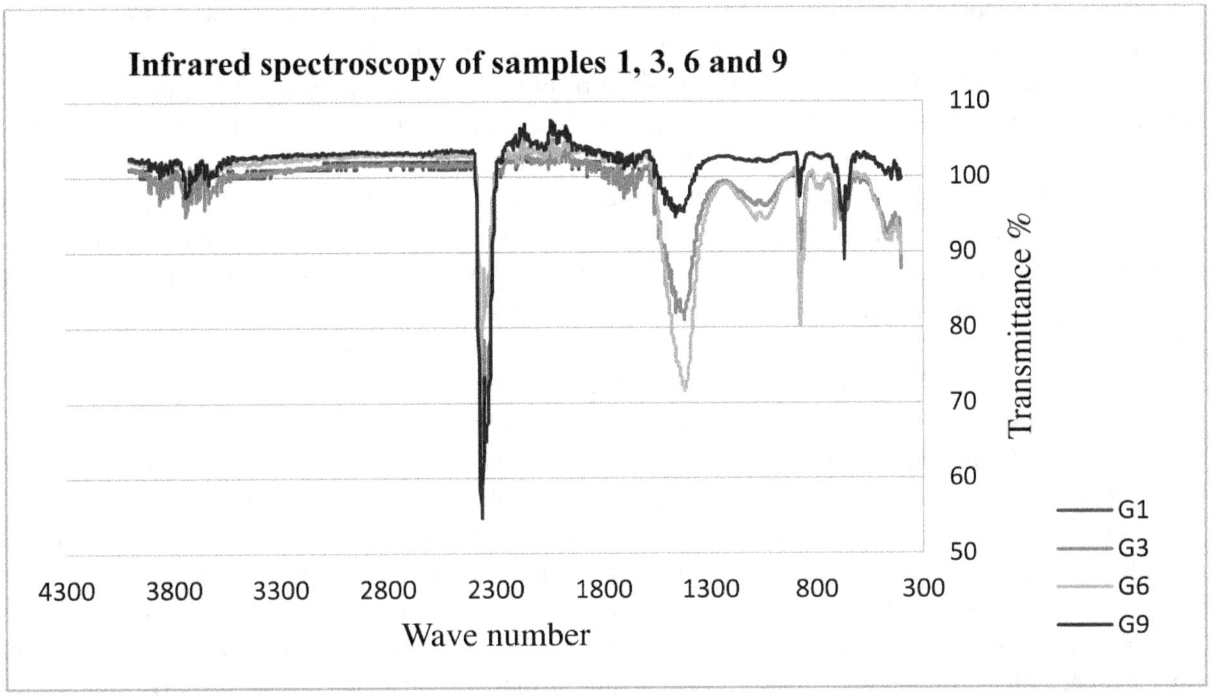

of the coastal area of Gabes clearly shows bands of remarkable absorbance (Fig.2) Wide and intense absorption bands centered around the wave number 1460 cm^{-1} and 670 cm^{-1} related to polypropylene. Thin and intense bands centered on the wave number 2360 1060 also a thin and a weak band at related to polysterene. Other minor harmonic are present at the bands 1750, 3650, and 3737 cm^{-1}. From the results obtained we can identify the different constituents of the first 9 cm of our core. Indeed the identification of calcium or calcium carbonate ($CaCO_3$) is verified by the C-O elongation of the carbonate group (1460 and 875 cm^{-1}). Gypsum ($CaSO_4.2\ H_2O$) is verified on the one hand by the modes of SO sulphate SO_4^{2-} (670 cm^{-1}) elongation vibrations and on the other hand by the characteristic bands of constitutive water (3650 and 3737 cm^{-1}). In practice, carbon dioxide also has absorption at 2349 cm^{-1}, which is often observed on spectra using air as a reference medium due to poor compensation.

Based on the carbonate percentage, pH and the infrared spectroscopy, we have been able to set the Holocene-Anthropocene limit. The values of carbonate percentage show an upward increase to an increasing sedimentary flux during the Anthropocene.

DISCUSSION: ENVIRONMENTAL AND HEALTH IMPACT

Big plastic fragments are obviously worldwide dispersed within marine as well as continental environments. The degradation of these particles takes long period of time; they persist within terrestrial ecosystems. In addition, they are subdivided into small (less than 5 mm) particles: microplastic. These microplastics are integrated within terrestrial ecosystems. In terms on analytical procedure, they may be extracted according to the protocol. Recently Abidli et al. (2021) investigated microplastic contamination within in the gastrointestinal tract of two commercial fish species from two lagoons in northern Tunisia: the lagoon of Bizerte and the lagoon of Ghar El Melh. Isolated microplastics appeared in a variety of coloured types, such as fibres> fragments> films and were identified as Polypropylene and Polyethylene polymers by FTIR-ATR analysis. The obtained results indicate the growing threat that affects the two sampling sites. On the other hand, southeastern Tunisia, the pollution level, the type, occurrence, and distribution of MPs in sediments from the southwestern Kerkennah archipelago, were investigated (Chouchene et al., 2021). This study showed that plastics and microplastics were, which emphasized that their extensive distribution throughout three lines by an average abundance of "MPs" was 611 items/m2. Microplastic (MP) is a pervasive pollutant colonised by diverse groups of microbes, including potentially pathogenic species. However, despite their impact as pathogens and affinity for plastics, fungi have been largely neglected. Recently, to unravel the role of MP as a carrier of fungal pathogens in terrestrial ecosystems and the immediate human environment, epiplastic mycobiomes from municipal plastic waste from Kenya were deciphered. It was proven that the terrestrial plastisphere is a suitable ecological niche for a variety of fungal organisms, including important animal and plant pathogens, which formed the plastisphere core mycobiome. MPs serve as selective artificial microhabitats that not only attract distinct fungal communities, but also accumulate certain opportunistic human pathogens, such as cryptococcal and Phoma-like species. Therefore, MP must be regarded a persistent reservoir and potential vector for fungal pathogens in soil environments. In face of the worldwide increasing amount of plastic waste in marine and continental ecosystems, a special care should be given to this interrelation with severe consequences of the fungal epidemiology appearing during the Anthropocene and flourishing during the Great Acceleration on a global scale.

From environmental viewpoint, the increased population during the Anthropocene and Great Acceleration leading to further plastic consumption resulted in an obvious environment pollution, which is evident in the decline of the natural environment (Singh et al., 2021), mortality of aquatic organisms (Lehtiniemi et al., 2021; Vazquez, & Rahman, 2021). In third world countries such as Tunisia, plastic waste causes the blockage of sewage systems (Hussein et al., 2021); such phenomena resulted in breeding grounds for mosquitoes and other disease-causing vectors as well as foul odours (Banu, 2021), reduced aeration and water percolation (Busman et al., 2021), causing reduced productivity in agricultural lands (Sarıdaş et al., 2021; Amare, & Desta, 2021). In terms of health impact, plastic polymers are considered harmless to human health with little risk (Halden et al., 2021). Most of the plastic additives have been proven as endocrine disruptors Chakraborty et al., 2022) and carcinogens (Alimba et al., 2021). Linked to dermatitis, these chemicals harm humans primarily through skin contact, ingestion and inhalation (Ahrensbøll-Friis et al., 2021). Microplastics are vital toxins that can form complexes in the food chain after being consumed by a variety of marine and freshwater life, resulting in a variety of health problems (Lehel & Murphy, 2021; Ahmad & Wankhade, 2022). Biomonitoring investigations on human tissues have indicated that plastic elements are found in the human species (Bousoumah et al., 2021). Some plastic particles circulate from the stomach to the lymphatic and circulatory systems (Davis, Rubin, 2021), leading hence to so-called plastic bronchitis which is affecting even children (Pałyga-Bysiecka et al., 2022). Other particles pass through cell tissues, the blood-brain barrier and the placenta (Braun et al., 2021).

CONCLUSION

Plastic and microplastic are considered as real threat for the environment and human health. Recent statistics showed an increase of plastic production and consumption. This increase is obviously noticed in many sites and they are hardly degradable. The danger of these products becomes certain with their fragmentation towards microplastic, which are progressively integrated within terrestrial ecosystems. They may be detected within sediment based on infrared spectroscopy. Within animal species, microplastics are found in their gastrointestinal tracts. In terms of environmental damage, plastic consumption resulted in obvious environment pollution, which is recorded in some features including mortality of aquatic organisms. In addition, plastic waste causes the blockage of sewage systems leading to the breeding grounds for mosquitoes and foul odours. Plastic additives have been proven as endocrine disruptors and carcinogens. Linked to dermatitis, these chemicals harm humans primarily through skin contact, ingestion and inhalation.

REFERENCES

Abidli, S., Akkari, N., Lahbib, Y., & El Menif, N. T. (2021). First evaluation of microplastics in two commercial fish species from the lagoons of Bizerte and Ghar El Melh (Northern Tunisia). *Regional Studies in Marine Science*, *41*, 101581. doi:10.1016/j.rsma.2020.101581

Ahlström, H., Hileman, J., Wang-Erlandsson, L., García, M. M., Moore, M. L., Jonas, K., Pranindita, A., Kuiper, J. J., Fetzer, I., Jaramillo, F., & Svedin, U. (2021). An Earth system law perspective on governing social-hydrological systems in the Anthropocene. *Earth System Governance*, *10*, 100120. doi:10.1016/j.esg.2021.100120

Ahmad, S. A., & Wankhade, V. (2022). Entry of Macro, Micro, and Nanoplastic in the Food Chain and Their Impact on Marine Life (from Source to Sink). In *Impact of Plastic Waste on the Marine Biota* (pp. 211–222). Springer. doi:10.1007/978-981-16-5403-9_11

Ahrensbøll-Friis, U., Simonsen, A. B., Dahlin, J., Isaksson, M., Zachariae, C., & Johansen, J. D. (2022). Allergic contact dermatitis from dyes used in the temple of spectacles. *Contact Dermatitis*, *86*(1), 25–28. doi:10.1111/cod.13989 PMID:34655078

Alimba, C. G., Faggio, C., Sivanesan, S., Ogunkanmi, A. L., & Krishnamurthi, K. (2021). Micro (nano)-plastics in the environment and risk of carcinogenesis: Insight into possible mechanisms. *Journal of Hazardous Materials*, *416*, 126143. doi:10.1016/j.jhazmat.2021.126143

Amare, G., & Desta, B. (2021). Coloured plastic mulches: Impact on soil properties and crop productivity. *Chemical and Biological Technologies in Agriculture*, *8*(1), 1–9. doi:10.118640538-020-00201-8

Banu, S. A. (2021). Reduction of solid waste dumps in religious places during pandemic outbreak in Bengaluru. *International Journal of Applied Research*, *7*(10).

Béjaoui, B., Ismail, S. B., Othmani, A., Hamida, O. B. A. B. H., Chevalier, C., Feki-Sahnoun, W., ... Hassen, M. B. (2019). Synthesis review of the Gulf of Gabes (eastern Mediterranean Sea, Tunisia): Morphological, climatic, physical oceanographic, biogeochemical and fisheries features. *Estuarine, Coastal and Shelf Science*, *219*, 395–408. doi:10.1016/j.ecss.2019.01.006

Ben Rouina, S. (2016). *Reconstitution des paléoenvironnements et des évènements extrêmes au cours du Quaternaire à l'oued El Akarit (Golfe de Gabès, Sud de la Tunisie)* (Doctoral dissertation). Perpignan.

Bousoumah, R., Leso, V., Iavicoli, I., Huuskonen, P., Viegas, S., Porras, S. P., Santonen, T., Frery, N., Robert, A., & Ndaw, S. (2021). Biomonitoring of occupational exposure to bisphenol A, bisphenol S and bisphenol F: A systematic review. *The Science of the Total Environment*, *783*, 146905. doi:10.1016/j.scitotenv.2021.146905 PMID:33865140

Brauch, H. G. (2021). Peace Ecology in the Anthropocene. In *Decolonising Conflicts, Security, Peace, Gender, Environment and Development in the Anthropocene* (pp. 51–185). Springer. doi:10.1007/978-3-030-62316-6_2

Braun, T., Ehrlich, L., Henrich, W., Koeppel, S., Lomako, I., Schwabl, P., & Liebmann, B. (2021). Detection of microplastic in human placenta and meconium in a clinical setting. *Pharmaceutics*, *13*(7), 921. doi:10.3390/pharmaceutics13070921 PMID:34206212

Busman, N. A., Maie, N., Ishak, C. F., Sulaiman, M. F., & Melling, L. (2021). Effect of compaction on soil CO2 and CH4 fluxes from tropical peatland in Sarawak, Malaysia. *Environment, Development and Sustainability*, *23*(8), 11646–11659. doi:10.100710668-020-01132-y

Chaabouni, R., Bouaziz, S., Peresson, H., & Wolfgang, J. (2012). Lineament analysis of South Jenein Area (Southern Tunisia) using remote sensing data and geographic information system. *The Egyptian Journal of Remote Sensing and Space Sciences*, *15*(2), 197–206. doi:10.1016/j.ejrs.2012.11.001

Chakraborty, P., Bharat, G. K., Gaonkar, O., Mukhopadhyay, M., Chandra, S., Steindal, E. H., & Nizzetto, L. (2022). Endocrine-disrupting chemicals used as common plastic additives: Levels, profiles, and human dietary exposure from the Indian food basket. *The Science of the Total Environment*, *810*, 152200. doi:10.1016/j.scitotenv.2021.152200 PMID:34890663

Chouchene, K., Rocha-Santos, T., & Ksibi, M. (2021). Types, occurrence, and distribution of microplastics and metals contamination in sediments from south west of Kerkennah archipelago, Tunisia. *Environmental Science and Pollution Research International*, *28*(34), 46477–46487. doi:10.100711356-020-09938-z PMID:32632691

Clinci, D. (2021). Plastic Memories of the Anthropocene. *Metacritic Journal for Comparative Studies and Theory*, *7*(1), 83–97. doi:10.24193/mjcst.2021.11.05

Davis, M. D., & Rubin, B. K. (2021). Plastic Bronchitis. In *Diagnostic and Interventional Bronchoscopy in Children* (pp. 289–293). Humana. doi:10.1007/978-3-030-54924-4_23

De-la-Torre, G. E., Dioses-Salinas, D. C., Pizarro-Ortega, C. I., & Santillán, L. (2021). New plastic formations in the Anthropocene. *The Science of the Total Environment*, *754*, 142216. doi:10.1016/j.scitotenv.2020.142216 PMID:33254855

Essefi, E. (2020). On the Geochemistry and Mineralogy of the Anthropocene. *Int J Water Wastewater Treat*, *6*(2).

Essefi, E. (2021a). Parallel evolution of energy consumption and environmental pollution during the Anthropocene. *Journal of Global Ecology and Environment*, 36-42.

Essefi, E. (2021b). Record of the Anthropocene-Great Acceleration along a core from the coast of Sfax, southeastern Tunisia. *Turkish Journal of Earth Science*, 1-16.

Essefi, E. (2021c). Homo Sapiens Sapiens Progressive Defaunation During The Great Acceleration: The Cli-Fi Apocalypse Hypothesis. *International Journal of Toxicology and Toxicity Assessment*, *1*(1), 1–6.

Essefi, E. (2022b). Millennial to Centennial Cyclicity Within the Exoreic Saline System of Boujmel, Southern Tunisia. In Handbook of Research on Monitoring and Evaluating the Ecological Health of Wetlands (pp. 230-251). IGI Global.

Essefi, E., & Hajji, S. (2022a). Response of Erosion to Environmental and Climate Changes During the Anthropocene Within the Endorheic System of Mhabeul, Southeastern Tunisia. In Prevention and Management of Soil Erosion and Torrential Floods (pp. 217-234). IGI Global.

Folke, C., Polasky, S., Rockström, J., Galaz, V., Westley, F., Lamont, M., ... Walker, B. H. (2021). Our future in the Anthropocene biosphere. *Ambio*, 1–36. PMID:33715097

Furukuma, S. (2021). A study of 'new plastic formations' found in the Seto Inland Sea, Japan. *Int. J. Sci. Res. Publ.*, *11*(6), 185–188. doi:10.29322/IJSRP.11.06.2021.p11427

Gkoutselis, G., Rohrbach, S., Harjes, J., Obst, M., Brachmann, A., Horn, M. A., & Rambold, G. (2021). Microplastics accumulate fungal pathogens in terrestrial ecosystems. *Scientific Reports*, *11*(1), 1–13. doi:10.103841598-021-92405-7 PMID:34267241

Gorrasi, G., Sorrentino, A., & Lichtfouse, E. (2021). Back to plastic pollution in COVID times. *Environmental Chemistry Letters*, *19*(1), 1–4. doi:10.100710311-020-01129-z PMID:33192208

Halden, R. U., Rolsky, C., & Khan, F. R. (2021). Time: A Key Driver of Uncertainty When Assessing the Risk of Environmental Plastics to Human Health. *Environmental Science & Technology*, *55*(19), 12766–12769. doi:10.1021/acs.est.1c02580 PMID:34520666

Hussein, B. A., Tsegaye, A. A., & Abdulahi, A. (2021). Assessment of the environmental and health impacts of disposal plastics in Gode town, Somali regional state, Eastern Ethiopia. *J Mater Environ Sci*, *12*(3), 455–471.

Joseph, B., James, J., Kalarikkal, N., & Thomas, S. (2021). Recycling of medical plastics. *Advanced Industrial and Engineering Polymer Research*, *4*(3), 199–208. doi:10.1016/j.aiepr.2021.06.003

Kwak, J. I., & An, Y. J. (2021). Microplastic digestion generates fragmented nanoplastics in soils and damages earthworm spermatogenesis and coelomocyte viability. *Journal of Hazardous Materials*, *402*, 124034. doi:10.1016/j.jhazmat.2020.124034 PMID:33254833

Lee, G. E., & Lee, J. H. (2021). Spatial correlation analysis using the indicators of the anthropocene focusing on atmospheric pollution: A case study of Seoul. *Ecological Indicators, 125*, 107535. doi:10.1016/j.ecolind.2021.107535

Lehel, J., & Murphy, S. (2021). Microplastics in the Food Chain: Food Safety and Environmental Aspects. *Reviews of Environmental Contamination and Toxicology, 259*, 1–49. PMID:34611754

Lehtiniemi, M., Hartikainen, S., Turja, R., Lehtonen, K. K., Vepsäläinen, J., Peräniemi, S., Leskinen, J., & Setälä, O. (2021). Exposure to leachates from post-consumer plastic and recycled rubber causes stress responses and mortality in a copepod Limnocalanus macrurus. *Marine Pollution Bulletin, 173*, 113103. doi:10.1016/j.marpolbul.2021.113103 PMID:34741928

Martin, J., Lusher, A. L., & Nixon, F. C. (2022). A review of the use of microplastics in reconstructing dated sedimentary archives. *The Science of the Total Environment, 806*, 150818. doi:10.1016/j.scitotenv.2021.150818 PMID:34637878

Mincer, J. (2021). *Aftershocks of SARS-CoV-2: A plastic pandemic*. Canadian Family Physician.

Palos, R., Gutiérrez, A., Vela, F. J., Olazar, M., Arandes, J. M., & Bilbao, J. (2021). Waste Refinery: The Valorization of Waste Plastics and End-of-Life Tires in Refinery Units. A Review. *Energy & Fuels, 35*(5), 3529–3557. doi:10.1021/acs.energyfuels.0c03918 PMID:35310012

Pałyga-Bysiecka, I., Polewczyk, A. M., Polewczyk, M., Kołodziej, E., Mazurek, H., & Pogorzelski, A. (2022). Plastic Bronchitis—A Serious Rare Complication Affecting Children Only after Fontan Procedure? *Journal of Clinical Medicine, 11*(1), 44. doi:10.3390/jcm11010044 PMID:35011785

Patil, S. M., Rane, N. R., Bankole, P. O., Krishnaiah, P., Ahn, Y., Park, Y. K., Yadav, K. K., Amin, M. A., & Jeon, B. H. (2022). An assessment of micro-and nanoplastics in the biosphere: A review of detection, monitoring, and remediation technology. *Chemical Engineering Journal, 430*, 132913. doi:10.1016/j.cej.2021.132913

Porta, R. (2021). Anthropocene, the plastic age and future perspectives. *FEBS Open Bio, 11*(4), 948–953. doi:10.1002/2211-5463.13122 PMID:33794071

Rossiter, D. G. (2021). Are soil phenoforms the new normal? Soil classification and soil mapping in the Anthropocene. *Soil Security, 5*, 100017. doi:10.1016/j.soisec.2021.100017

Sarıdaş, M. A., Kapur, B., Çeliktopuz, E., Şahiner, Y., & Kargı, S. P. (2021). Land productivity, irrigation water use efficiency and fruit quality under various plastic mulch colors and irrigation regimes of strawberry in the eastern Mediterranean region of Turkey. *Agricultural Water Management, 245*, 106568. doi:10.1016/j.agwat.2020.106568

Shoshitaishvili, B. (2021). From Anthropocene to Noosphere: The Great Acceleration. *Earth's Future, 9*(2).

Silva, A. L. P., Prata, J. C., Walker, T. R., Duarte, A. C., Ouyang, W., Barcelò, D., & Rocha-Santos, T. (2021). Increased plastic pollution due to COVID-19 pandemic: Challenges and recommendations. *Chemical Engineering Journal, 405*, 126683. doi:10.1016/j.cej.2020.126683 PMID:32834764

Singh, S., Naik, T. S. K., Anil, A. G., Dhiman, J., Kumar, V., Dhanjal, D. S., ... Ramamurthy, P. C. (2021). Micro (nano) plastics in wastewater: A critical review on toxicity risk assessment, behaviour, environmental impact and challenges. *Chemosphere*, 133169. PMID:34890615

Stubbins, A., Law, K. L., Muñoz, S. E., Bianchi, T. S., & Zhu, L. (2021). Plastics in the Earth system. *Science*, *373*(6550), 51–55. doi:10.1126cience.abb0354 PMID:34210876

Torres, F. G., & De-la-Torre, G. E. (2021). Historical microplastic records in marine sediments: Current progress and methodological evaluation. *Regional Studies in Marine Science*, *46*, 101868. doi:10.1016/j.rsma.2021.101868

Vazquez, O. A., & Rahman, M. S. (2021). An ecotoxicological approach to microplastics on terrestrial and aquatic organisms: A systematic review in assessment, monitoring and biological impact. *Environmental Toxicology and Pharmacology*, *84*, 103615. doi:10.1016/j.etap.2021.103615 PMID:33607259

Weber, C. J., & Lechthaler, S. (2021). Plastics as a stratigraphic marker in fluvial deposits. *Anthropocene*, *36*, 100314. doi:10.1016/j.ancene.2021.100314

Compilation of References

¨ohr, A., Savelli, H., Beunen, R., Kalz, M., Ragas, A., & Van Belleghem, F. (2017). Solutions for global marine litter pollution. *Current Opinion in Environmental Sustainability, 28*, 90–99. doi:10.1016/j.cosust.2017.08.009

Abbasi, S., & Turner, A. (2021). Human exposure to microplastics: A study in Iran. *Journal of Hazardous Materials, 403*(August), 123799. doi:10.1016/j.jhazmat.2020.123799

Abbasi, S., Keshavarzi, B., Moore, F., Delshab, H., Soltani, N., & Sorooshian, A. (2017). Investigation of microrubbers, microplastics and heavy metals in street dust: A study in Bushehr city, Iran. In Environmental Earth Sciences (Vol. 76, Issue 23). Springer. doi:10.100712665-017-7137-0

Abbasi, S., Keshavarzi, B., Moore, F., Turner, A., Kelly, F. J., Dominguez, A. O., & Jaafarzadeh, N. (2019). Distribution and potential health impacts of microplastics and microrubbers in air and street dusts from Asaluyeh County, Iran. *Environmental Pollution, 244*, 153–164. doi:10.1016/j.envpol.2018.10.039 PMID:30326387

Abeynayaka, A., Kojima, F., Miwa, Y., Ito, N., Nihei, Y., Fukunaga, Y., Yashima, Y., & Itsubo, N. (2020). Rapid Sampling of Suspended and Floating Microplastics in Challenging Riverine and Coastal Water Environments in Japan. In Water (Vol. 12, Issue 7). MDPI. doi:10.3390/w12071903

Abidli, S., Toumi, H., Lahbib, Y., & El Menif, N. T. (2017). The First Evaluation of Microplastics in Sediments from the Complex Lagoon-Channel of Bizerte (Northern Tunisia). In Water Air and Soil Pollution (Vol. 228, Issue 7). Springer International Publishing AG. doi:10.100711270-017-3439-9

Abidli, S., Akkari, N., Lahbib, Y., & El Menif, N. T. (2021). First evaluation of microplastics in two commercial fish species from the lagoons of Bizerte and Ghar El Melh (Northern Tunisia). *Regional Studies in Marine Science, 41*, 101581. doi:10.1016/j.rsma.2020.101581

Abidli, S., Pinheiro, M., Lahbib, Y., Neuparth, T., Santos, M. M., & Trigui El Menif, N. (2021). Effects of environmentally relevant levels of polyethylene microplastic on *Mytilus galloprovincialis* (Mollusca: Bivalvia): filtration rate and oxidative stress. *Environmental Science and Pollution Research International, 28*(21), 26643–26652. doi:10.100711356-021-12506-8 PMID:33495949

Abu-Hilal, A. H., & Al-Najjar, T. H. (2009). Plastic pellets on the beaches of the northern Gulf of Aqaba, Red Sea. *Aquatic Ecosystem Health & Management, 12*(4), 461–47. doi:10.1080/14634980903361200

Achari, G. A., & Kowshik, M. (2018). Recent developments on nanotechnology in agriculture: Plant mineral nutrition, health, and interactions with soil microflora. *Journal of Agricultural and Food Chemistry, 66*(33), 8647–8661. doi:10.1021/acs.jafc.8b00691 PMID:30036480

Adomat, Y., & Grischek, T. (2021). Sampling and processing methods of microplastics in river sediments - A review. *The Science of the Total Environment, 758*, 143691. doi:10.1016/j.scitotenv.2020.143691 PMID:33298323

Adu-Boahen, K., Dadson, I. Y., Mensah, D. K. D., & Kyeremeh, S. (2020). Mapping ecological impact of microplastics on freshwater habitat in the central region of Ghana: A case study of River Akora. *GeoJournal*, •••, 1–19. doi:10.100710708-020-10273-6

Afrin, S., Uddin, M. K., & Rahman, M. M. (2020). Microplastics contamination in the soil from Urban Landfill site, Dhaka, Bangladesh. *Heliyon*, *6*(11), e05572. Advance online publication. doi:10.1016/j.heliyon.2020.e05572 PMID:33294704

Agamuthu, P. (2013). Landfilling in developing countries. *Waste Management & Research*, *31*(1), 1–2. doi:10.1177/0734242X12469169 PMID:23255612

Ahlström, H., Hileman, J., Wang-Erlandsson, L., García, M. M., Moore, M. L., Jonas, K., Pranindita, A., Kuiper, J. J., Fetzer, I., Jaramillo, F., & Svedin, U. (2021). An Earth system law perspective on governing social-hydrological systems in the Anthropocene. *Earth System Governance*, *10*, 100120. doi:10.1016/j.esg.2021.100120

Ahmad, S. A., & Wankhade, V. (2022). Entry of Macro, Micro, and Nanoplastic in the Food Chain and Their Impact on Marine Life (from Source to Sink). In *Impact of Plastic Waste on the Marine Biota* (pp. 211–222). Springer. doi:10.1007/978-981-16-5403-9_11

Ahmed, M. B., Rahman, M. S., Alom, J., Hasan, M. S., Johir, M. A. H., Mondal, M. I. H., Lee, D. Y., Park, J., Zhou, J. L., & Yoon, M. H. (2021). Microplastic particles in the aquatic environment: A systematic review. *The Science of the Total Environment*, *775*, 145793. doi:10.1016/j.scitotenv.2021.145793 PMID:33631597

Ahrendt, C., Perez-Venegas, D. J., Urbina, M., Gonzalez, C., Echeveste, P., Aldana, M., Pulgar, J., & Galbán-Malagón, C. (2020). Microplastic ingestion cause intestinal lesions in the intertidal fish *Girella laevifrons*. *Marine Pollution Bulletin, 151*(November), 110795. doi:10.1016/j.marpolbul.2019.110795

Ahrensbøll-Friis, U., Simonsen, A. B., Dahlin, J., Isaksson, M., Zachariae, C., & Johansen, J. D. (2022). Allergic contact dermatitis from dyes used in the temple of spectacles. *Contact Dermatitis*, *86*(1), 25–28. doi:10.1111/cod.13989 PMID:34655078

Ajith, N., Arumugam, S., Parthasarathy, S., Manupoori, S., & Janakiraman, S. (2020). Global distribution of microplastics and its impact on marine environment—a review. In Environmental Science and Pollution Research (Vol. 27, Issue 21, pp. 25970–25986). doi:10.100711356-020-09015-5

Akbay, İ. K., & Özdemir, T. (2016). Monomer migration and degradation of polycarbonate via UV-C irradiation within aquatic and atmospheric environments. Journal of Macromolecular Science. *Part A*, *53*(6), 340–345.

Alice, P., Maud, G., Dominique, B., & Julien, G. (n.d.). Micro- and nanoplastic transfer in freezing saltwater: Implications for their fate in polar waters. In *Environmental Science-Processes & Impacts*. Royal Soc Chemistry. doi:10.1039/D1EM00280E

Alimba, C. G., Faggio, C., Sivanesan, S., Ogunkanmi, A. L., & Krishnamurthi, K. (2021). Micro (nano)-plastics in the environment and risk of carcinogenesis: Insight into possible mechanisms. *Journal of Hazardous Materials*, *416*, 126143. doi:10.1016/j.jhazmat.2021.126143

Alimi, O. S., Farner Budarz, J., Hernandez, L. M., & Tufenkji, N. (2018). Microplastics and nanoplastics in aquatic environments: Aggregation, deposition, and enhanced contaminant transport. *Environmental Science & Technology*, *52*(4), 1704–1724. doi:10.1021/acs.est.7b05559 PMID:29265806

Aljaradin, M. (n.d.). *Biodegradation of Microplastics in Drinking Water, A review*. Academic Press.

Allen, A. S., Seymour, A. C., & Rittschof, D. (2017). Chemoreception drives plastic consumption in a hard coral. *Marine Pollution Bulletin*, *124*(1), 198–205. doi:10.1016/j.marpolbul.2017.07.030 PMID:28743368

Allen, S., Allen, D., Phoenix, V. R., Le Roux, G., Durántez Jiménez, P., Simonneau, A., Binet, S., & Galop, D. (2019). Atmospheric transport and deposition of microplastics in a remote mountain catchment. *Nature Geoscience*, *12*(5), 339–344. doi:10.103841561-019-0335-5

Ally, B., Ismail, S. N. S., & Rasdi, I. (2014). Municipal solid waste management of Zanzibar: Current practice, the challenges and the future. *International Journal of Current Research and Academic Review*, *1*, 5-19. http://www.ijcrar.com/special/1/Biubwa%20Ally,%20et%20al.pdf

Alnajar, N., Jha, A. N., & Turner, A. (2020). Impacts of microplastic fibres on the marine mussel, *Mytilus galloprovinciallis. Chemosphere*, *128290*. Advance online publication. doi:10.1016/j.chemosphere.2020.128290 PMID:33182139

Alprol, A. E., Gaballah, M. S., & Hassaan, M. A. (2021). Micro and Nanoplastics analysis: Focus on their classification, sources, and impacts in marine environment. *Regional Studies in Marine Science*, *42*, 101625. doi:10.1016/j.rsma.2021.101625

Alvarez-Castillo, E., Del Toro, A., Aguilar, J. M., Bengoechea, C., & Guerrero, A. (2018). Optimization of a thermal process for the production of superabsorbent materials based on a soy protein isolate. *Industrial Crops and Products*, *125*, 573–581. doi:10.1016/j.indcrop.2018.09.051

Amare, G., & Desta, B. (2021). Coloured plastic mulches: Impact on soil properties and crop productivity. *Chemical and Biological Technologies in Agriculture*, *8*(1), 1–9. doi:10.118640538-020-00201-8

Ambrosini, R., Azzoni, R. S., Pittino, F., Diolaiuti, G., Franzetti, A., & Parolini, M. (2019). First evidence of microplastic contamination in the supraglacial debris of an alpine glacier. *Environmental Pollution*, *253*, 297–301. doi:10.1016/j.envpol.2019.07.005 PMID:31323612

Amrutha, K., & Warrier, A. K. (2020). The first report on the source-to-sink characterization of microplastic pollution from a riverine environment in tropical India. In *Science of the Total Environment* (Vol. 739). Elsevier. doi:10.1016/j.scitotenv.2020.140377

Anastasopoulou, A., Kovač Viršek, M., Bojanić Varezić, D., Digka, N., Fortibuoni, T., Koren, Š., Mandić, M., Mytilineou, C., Pešić, A., Ronchi, F., Šiljić, J., Torre, M., Tsangaris, C., & Tutman, P. (2018). Assessment on marine litter ingested by fish in the Adriatic and NE Ionian Sea macro-region (Mediterranean). *Marine Pollution Bulletin*, *133*(May), 841–851. doi:10.1016/j.marpolbul.2018.06.050 PMID:30041385

Anderson, J. C., Park, B. J., & Palace, V. P. (2016). Microplastics in aquatic environments: Implications for Canadian ecosystems. *Environmental Pollution*, *218*(Supplement C), 269–280. doi:10.1016/j.envpol.2016.06.074 PMID:27431693

Andrades, R., dos Santos, R. A., Martins, A. S., Teles, D., & Santos, R. G. (2019). Scavenging as a pathway for plastic ingestion by marine animals. *Environmental Pollution*, *248*, 159–165. Advance online publication. doi:10.1016/j.envpol.2019.02.010 PMID:30784834

Andrady, A. L. (2011). Microplastics in the marine environment. *Marine Pollution Bulletin*, *62*(8), 1596–1605. doi:10.1016/j.marpolbul.2011.05.030 PMID:21742351

Andrady, A. L., & Neal, M. A. (2009). Applications and societal benefits of plastics. *Philosophical Transactions of the Royal Society of London. Series B, Biological Sciences*, *364*(1526), 1977–1984. doi:10.1098/rstb.2008.0304 PMID:19528050

Angiolillo, M., Gerigny, O., Valente, T., Fabri, M.-C., Tambute, E., Rouanet, E., Claro, F., Tunesi, L., Vissio, A., Daniel, B., & Galgani, F. (2021). Distribution of seafloor litter and its interaction with benthic organisms in deep waters of the Ligurian Sea (Northwestern Mediterranean). In Science of the Total Environment (Vol. 788). Elsevier. doi:10.1016/j.scitotenv.2021.147745

Aniceto, J. P., Portugal, I., & Silva, C. M. (2012). Biomass-based polyols through oxypropylation reaction. *ChemSusChem, 5*(8), 1358–1368. doi:10.1002/cssc.201200032 PMID:22807440

Araujo, C. F., Nolasco, M. M., Ribeiro, A. M. P., & Ribeiro-claro, P. J. A. (2018). Identi fi cation of microplastics using Raman spectroscopy : Latest developments and future prospects. *Water Research, 142*, 426–440. doi:10.1016/j.watres.2018.05.060 PMID:29909221

ARCADIS. (2012). *Case study on the plastic cycle and its loopholes in the four European regional seas areas*. European Commission DG Environment Framework contract. ENV.D.2./ETU/2011/0041

Aretoulaki, E., Ponis, S., Plakas, G., & Agalianos, K. (2020). A systematic meta-review analysis of review papers in the marine plastic pollution literature. *Marine Pollution Bulletin, 161*, 111690. doi:10.1016/j.marpolbul.2020.111690 PMID:33039791

Arias-Andres, M., Kettner, M. T., Miki, T., & Grossart, H. P. (2018). Microplastics: New substrates for heterotrophic activity contribute to altering organic matter cycles in aquatic ecosystems. *The Science of the Total Environment, 635*, 1152–1159. doi:10.1016/j.scitotenv.2018.04.199 PMID:29710570

Asadi, M. A., Hertika, A. M. S., Iranawati, F., & Yuwandita, A. Y. (2019). Microplastics in the sediment of intertidal areas of Lamongan, Indonesia. *Aquaculture, Aquarium, Conservation & Legislation, 12*(4), 1065–1073.

Aslam, H., Ali, T., Mortula, M. M., & Attaelmanan, A. G. (2020). Evaluation of microplastics in beach sediments along the coast of Dubai, UAE. *Marine Pollution Bulletin, 150*(November), 110739. doi:10.1016/j.marpolbul.2019.110739

Asrofi, M., Sapuan, S. M., Ilyas, R. A., & Ramesh, M. (2020). Characteristic of composite bioplastics from tapioca starch and sugarcane bagasse fiber: Effect of time duration of ultrasonication (Bath-Type). *Materials Today: Proceedings, 46*(4), 1626–1630.

Auras, R., Harte, B., & Selke, S. (2004). An overview of polylactides as packaging materials. *Macromolecular Bioscience, 4*(9), 835–864. doi:10.1002/mabi.200400043 PMID:15468294

Au, S. Y., Bruce, T. F., Bridges, W. C., & Klaine, S. J. (2015). Responses of Hyalella azteca to acute and chronic microplastic exposures. *Environmental Toxicology and Chemistry, 34*(11), 2564–2572. doi:10.1002/etc.3093 PMID:26042578

Au, S. Y., Lee, C. M., Weinstein, J. E., van den Hurk, P., & Klaine, S. J. (2017). Trophic transfer of microplastics in aquatic ecosystems: Identifying critical research needs. *Integrated Environmental Assessment and Management, 13*(3), 505–509. doi:10.1002/ieam.1907 PMID:28440939

Austin, H. P., Allen, M. D., Donohoe, B. S., Rorrer, N. A., Kearns, F. L., Silveira, R. L., Pollard, B. C., Dominick, G., Duman, R., El Omari, K., Mykhaylyk, V., Wagner, A., Michener, W. E., Amore, A., Skaf, M. S., Crowley, M. F., Thorne, A. W., Johnson, C. W., Woodcock, H. L., ... Beckham, G. T. (2018). Characterization and engineering of a plastic-degrading aromatic polyesterase. *Proceedings of the National Academy of Sciences of the United States of America, 115*(19), E4350–E4357. doi:10.1073/pnas.1718804115 PMID:29666242

Auta, H. S., Emenike, C. U., & Fauziah, S. H. (2017). Screening of Bacillus strains isolated from mangrove ecosystems in Peninsular Malaysia for microplastic degradation. *Environmental Pollution, 231*, 1552–1559. doi:10.1016/j.envpol.2017.09.043 PMID:28964604

Auta, H. S., Emenike, C. U., Jayanthi, B., & Fauziah, S. H. (2018). Growth kinetics and biodeterioration of polypropylene microplastics by Bacillus sp. and Rhodococcus sp. isolated from mangrove sediment. *Marine Pollution Bulletin, 127*, 15–21. doi:10.1016/j.marpolbul.2017.11.036 PMID:29475646

Avio, C. G., Gorbi, S., Milan, M., Benedetti, M., Fattorini, D., d'Errico, G., Pauletto, M., Bargelloni, L., & Regoli, F. (2015). Pollutants bioavailability and toxicological risk from microplastics to marine mussels. *Environmental Pollution, 198*, 211–222. doi:10.1016/j.envpol.2014.12.021 PMID:25637744

Avio, C. G., Gorbi, S., & Regoli, F. (2017). Plastics and microplastics in the oceans: From emerging pollutants to emerged threat. *Marine Environmental Research, 128*, 2–11. doi:10.1016/j.marenvres.2016.05.012 PMID:27233985

Axworthy, J. B., & Padilla-Gamiño, J. L. (2019). Microplastics ingestion and heterotrophy in thermally stressed corals. *Scientific Reports, 9*(1), 18193. Advance online publication. doi:10.103841598-019-54698-7 PMID:31796829

Azzarello, M., & Van Vleet, E. (1987). Marine birds and plastic pollution. *Marine Ecology Progress Series, 37*, 295–303. doi:10.3354/meps037295

Babalola, O. A., & Olorunnisola, A. O. (2019). Evaluation of coconut (Cocos nucifera) husk fibre as a potential reinforcing material for bioplastic production. *Material Research Proceedings, 11*, 195–200. doi:10.21741/9781644900178-14

Bai, Z., Wang, N., & Wang, M. (2021). Effects of microplastics on marine copepods. *Ecotoxicology and Environmental Safety, 217*, 112243. doi:10.1016/j.ecoenv.2021.112243 PMID:33915449

Bakaraki Turan, N., Sari Erkan, H., & Onkal Engin, G. (2021). Microplastics in wastewater treatment plants: Occurrence, fate and identification. *Process Safety and Environmental Protection, 146*, 77–84. doi:10.1016/j.psep.2020.08.039

Bakir, A., O'Connor, I. A., Rowland, S. J., Hendriks, A. J., & Thompson, R. C. (2016). Relative importance of microplastics as a pathway for the transfer of hydrophobic organic chemicals to marine life. *Environmental Pollution, 219*, 56–65. doi:10.1016/j.envpol.2016.09.046 PMID:27661728

Balbi, T., Camisassi, G., Montagna, M., Fabbri, R., Franzellitti, S., Carbone, C., Dawson, K., & Canesi, L. (2017). Impact of cationic polystyrene nanoparticles (PS-NH2) on early embryo development of *Mytilus galloprovincialis*: Effects on shell formation. *Chemosphere, 186*, 1–9. doi:10.1016/j.chemosphere.2017.07.120 PMID:28759811

Baldwin, A. K., Corsi, S. R., & Mason, S. A. (2016). Plastic Debris in 29 Great Lakes Tributaries: Relations to Watershed Attributes and Hydrology. In Environmental Science & Technology (Vol. 50, Issue 19, pp. 10377–10385). Amer Chemical Soc. doi:10.1021/acs.est.6b02917

Banu, S. A. (2021). Reduction of solid waste dumps in religious places during pandemic outbreak in Bengaluru. *International Journal of Applied Research, 7*(10).

Barboza, L. G. A., Lopes, C., Oliveira, P., Bessa, F., Otero, V., Henriques, B., Raimundo, J., Caetano, M., Vale, C., & Guilhermino, L. (2020). Microplastics in wild fish from North East Atlantic Ocean and its potential for causing neurotoxic effects, lipid oxidative damage, and human health risks associated with ingestion exposure. *The Science of the Total Environment, 717*, 134625. doi:10.1016/j.scitotenv.2019.134625 PMID:31836230

Barboza, L. G. A., Vieira, L. R., Branco, V., Figueiredo, N., Carvalho, F., Carvalho, C., & Guilhermino, L. (2018). Microplastics cause neurotoxicity, oxidative damage and energy-related changes and interact with the bioaccumulation of mercury in the European seabass, *Dicentrarchus labrax* (Linnaeus, 1758). *Aquatic Toxicology (Amsterdam, Netherlands), 195*, 49–57. doi:10.1016/j.aquatox.2017.12.008 PMID:29287173

Barboza, L. G. A., Vieira, L. R., & Guilhermino, L. (2018). Single and combined effects of microplastics and mercury on juveniles of the European seabass (Dicentrarchus labrax): Changes in behavioural responses and reduction of swimming velocity and resistance time. *Environmental Pollution, 236*, 1014–1019. doi:10.1016/j.envpol.2017.12.082 PMID:29449115

Barboza, L., Dick Vethaak, A., Lavorante, B., Lundebye, A. K., & Guilhermino, L. (2018). Marine microplastic debris: An emerging issue for food security, food safety and human health. *Marine Pollution Bulletin*, *133*, 336–348. doi:10.1016/j.marpolbul.2018.05.047 PMID:30041323

Barnardo, T., & Ribbink, A. J. (2020). *African Marine Litter Monitoring Manual*. African Marine Waste Network. Sustainable Seas Trust, Port Elizabeth. https://sst.org.za/wp-content/uploads/2020/07/Barnardo-Ribbink-2020_African-Marine-Litter-Monitoring-Manual.pdf

Barnes, D. K., Galgani, F., Thompson, R. C., & Barlaz, M. (2009). Accumulation and fragmentation of plastic debris in global environments. *Philos. Trans. R. Soc. Lond. Ser. B Biol. Sci.*, *364*(1526), 1985–1998. PMID:19528051

Barnes, D. K., Galgani, F., Thompson, R. C., & Barlaz, M. (2009). Accumulation and fragmentation of plastic debris in global environments. *Philosophical Transactions of the Royal Society of London. Series B, Biological Sciences*, *364*(1526), 1985–1998. doi:10.1098/rstb.2008.0205 PMID:19528051

Barrett, J., Chase, Z., Zhang, J., Holl, M. M. B., Willis, K., Williams, A., Hardesty, B. D., & Wilcox, C. (2020). Microplastic Pollution in Deep-Sea Sediments From the Great Australian Bight. *Frontiers in Marine Science*, *7*(October), 1–10. doi:10.3389/fmars.2020.576170

Basri, K., Syaputra, E. M., & Handayani, S. (2021). Microplastic Pollution in Waters and its Impact on Health and Environment in Indonesia: A Review. *Journal of Public Health for Tropical and Coastal Region*, *4*(2), 63–77. doi:10.14710/jphtcr.v4i2.10809

Battulga, B., Kawahigashi, M., & Oyuntsetseg, B. (2019). Distribution and composition of plastic debris along the river shore in the Selenga River basin in Mongolia. *Environmental Science and Pollution Research International*, *26*(14), 14059–14072. doi:10.100711356-019-04632-1 PMID:30852749

Battulga, B., Kawahigashi, M., & Oyuntsetseg, B. (2020). Behavior and distribution of polystyrene foams on the shore of Tuul River in Mongolia. In *Environmental Pollution* (Vol. 260). ELSEVIER SCI LTD., doi:10.1016/j.envpol.2020.113979

Bayo, J., Martinez, A., Guillen, M., Olmos, S., Roca, M.-J., & Alcolea, A. (2017). Microbeads in Commercial Facial Cleansers: Threatening the Environment. In Clean-Soil Air Water (Vol. 45, Issue 7). Wiley. doi:10.1002/clen.201600683

Beiras, R., & Tato, T. (2019). Microplastics do not increase toxicity of a hydrophobic organic chemical to marine plankton. *Marine Pollution Bulletin*, *138*, 58–62. doi:10.1016/j.marpolbul.2018.11.029 PMID:30660309

Béjaoui, B., Ismail, S. B., Othmani, A., Hamida, O. B. A. B. H., Chevalier, C., Feki-Sahnoun, W., ... Hassen, M. B. (2019). Synthesis review of the Gulf of Gabes (eastern Mediterranean Sea, Tunisia): Morphological, climatic, physical oceanographic, biogeochemical and fisheries features. *Estuarine, Coastal and Shelf Science*, *219*, 395–408. doi:10.1016/j.ecss.2019.01.006

Bejgarn, S., MacLeod, M., Bogdal, C., & Breitholtz, M. (2015). Toxicity of leachate from weathering plastics: An exploratory screening study with *Nitocra spinipes. Chemosphere*, *132*, 114–119. doi:10.1016/j.chemosphere.2015.03.010 PMID:25828916

Bellasi, A., Binda, G., Pozzi, A., Boldrocchi, G., & Bettinetti, R. (2021). The extraction of microplastics from sediments: An overview of existing methods and the proposal of a new and green alternative. *Chemosphere*, *278*, 130357. doi:10.1016/j.chemosphere.2021.130357 PMID:33823347

Bell, M. L., Belanger, K., Ebisu, K., Gent, J. F., & Leaderer, B. P. (2012). Relationship between birth weight and exposure to airborne fine particulate potassium and titanium during gestation. *Environmental Research*, *117*, 83–89. doi:10.1016/j.envres.2012.05.004 PMID:22705336

BeMiller, J. N., & Whistler, R. L. (2009). Starch—chemistry and technology. In Food science and technology. Academic Press.

Ben Rouina, S. (2016). *Reconstitution des paléoenvironnements et des évènements extrêmes au cours du Quaternaire à l'oued El Akarit (Golfe de Gabès, Sud de la Tunisie)* (Doctoral dissertation). Perpignan.

Benkendorff, K. (2010). Molluscan biological and chemical diversity: Secondary metabolites and medicinal resources produced by marine molluscs. *Biological Reviews of the Cambridge Philosophical Society*, *85*(4), 757–775. doi:10.1111/j.1469-185X.2010.00124.x PMID:20105155

Berber, A. A. (2019). *Polystyrene nanoplastics trigger toxicity on two different aquatic organisms (Brachionus plicatilis, Daphnia magna)*. Academic Press.

Bergami, E., Bocci, E., Vannuccini, M. L., Monopoli, M., Salvati, A., Dawson, K. A., & Corsi, I. (2016). Nano-sized polystyrene affects feeding, behavior and physiology of brine shrimp Artemia franciscana larvae. *Ecotoxicology and Environmental Safety*, *123*, 18–25. doi:10.1016/j.ecoenv.2015.09.021 PMID:26422775

Bergami, E., Krupinski Emerenciano, A., González-Aravena, M., Cárdenas, C. A., Hernández, P., Silva, J. R. M. C., & Corsi, I. (2019). Polystyrene nanoparticles affect the innate immune system of the Antarctic sea urchin *Sterechinus neumayeri*. *Polar Biology*, *42*(4), 743–757. doi:10.100700300-019-02468-6

Bergami, E., Manno, C., Cappello, S., Vannuccini, M. L., & Corsi, I. (2020). Nanoplastics affect moulting and faecal pellet sinking in Antarctic krill (*Euphausia superba*) juveniles. *Environment International*, *143*(July), 105999. doi:10.1016/j.envint.2020.105999 PMID:32763632

Bergami, E., Pugnalini, S., Vannuccini, M. L., Manfra, L., Faleri, C., Savorelli, F., Dawson, K. A., & Corsi, I. (2017). Long-term toxicity of surface-charged polystyrene nanoplastics to marine planktonic species *Dunaliella tertiolecta* and *Artemia franciscana*. *Aquatic Toxicology (Amsterdam, Netherlands)*, *189*, 159–169. doi:10.1016/j.aquatox.2017.06.008 PMID:28644993

Berglund, E., Fogelberg, V., Nilsson, P. A., & Hollander, J. (2019). Microplastics in a freshwater mussel (Anodonta anatina. In N. Europe (Ed.), *Science of the Total Environment* (Vol. 697). Elsevier. doi:10.1016/j.scitotenv.2019.134192

Bergmann, M., Mützel, S., Primpke, S., & Tekman, M. B. (2019). *White and wonderful ? Microplastics prevail in snow from the Alps to the Arctic*. Academic Press.

Bergmann, M., Gutow, L., & Klages, M. (2015). Marine anthropogenic litter. In M. B. L. Gutow & M. Klages (Eds.), *Marine Anthropogenic Litter*. Springer., doi:10.1007/978-3-319-16510-3

Bergmann, M., Mützel, S., Primpke, S., Tekman, M. B., Trachsel, J., & Gerdts, G. (2019). White and wonderful? Microplastics prevail in snow from the Alps to the Arctic. *Science Advances*, *5*(8), eaax1157. Advance online publication. doi:10.1126ciadv.aax1157 PMID:31453336

Bergmann, M., Sandhop, N., Schewe, I., & D'Hert, D. (2016). Observations of floating anthropogenic litter in the Barents Sea and Fram Strait, Arctic. *Polar Biology*, *39*(3), 553–560. doi:10.100700300-015-1795-8

Berry, K. L. E., Epstein, H. E., Lewis, P. J., Hall, N. M., & Negri, A. P. (2019). Microplastic Contamination Has Limited Effects on Coral Fertilisation and Larvae. *Diversity (Basel)*, *11*(12), 228. doi:10.3390/d11120228

Bessa, F., Barría, P., Neto, J. M., Frias, J. P. G. L., Otero, V., Sobral, P., & Marques, J. C. (2018). Occurrence of microplastics in commercial fish from a natural estuarine environment. *Marine Pollution Bulletin*, *128*, 575–584. doi:10.1016/j.marpolbul.2018.01.044 PMID:29571409

Bessa, F., Kogel, T., Frias, J., & Lusher, A. (2019). Harmonized protocol for monitoring microplastics in biota. *Micropoll-Multilevel Assessment of Microplastics and Associated Pollutants in the Baltic Sea View Project*, (March), 1–30. doi:10.13140/RG.2.2.28588.72321/1

Besseling, E., Foekema, E. M., Van Franeker, J. A., Leopold, M. F., Kühn, S., Rebolledo, E. L. B., Heße, E., Mielke, L., IJzer, J., & Kamminga, P. (2015). Microplastic in a macro filter feeder: Humpback whale Megaptera novaeangliae. *Marine Pollution Bulletin*, *95*(1), 248–252. doi:10.1016/j.marpolbul.2015.04.007 PMID:25916197

Besseling, E., Wang, B., Lürling, M., & Koelmans, A. A. (2014). Nanoplastic affects growth of S. obliquus and reproduction of D. magna. *Environmental Science & Technology*, *48*(20), 12336–12343. doi:10.1021/es503001d PMID:25268330

Bettas, A. G., Tosin, M., Barbale, M., & Degli-Innocenti, F. (2014). Biodegradation of plastics in soil and efects on nitrifcation activity. A laboratory approach. *Frontiers in Microbiology*, *5*, 710–723. PMID:25566223

Betts, K. (2008). Why small plastic particles may pose a big problem in the oceans. *Environmental Science & Technology*, *42*(24), 8995. doi:10.1021/es802970v PMID:19174862

Bhadra, J., Al-Thani, N., & Abdulkareem, A. (2017). Recycling of polymer-polymer composites. In *Micro and nano fibrillar composites (MFCs and NFCs) from polymer blends* (pp. 263–277). Woodhead Publishing. doi:10.1016/B978-0-08-101991-7.00011-X

Bhargava, S., Chen Lee, S. S., Min Ying, L. S., Neo, M. L., Lay-Ming Teo, S., & Valiyaveettil, S. (2018). Fate of Nanoplastics in Marine Larvae: A Case Study Using Barnacles, *Amphibalanus amphitrite. ACS Sustainable Chemistry & Engineering*, *6*(5), 6932–6940. doi:10.1021/acssuschemeng.8b00766

Bhattacharya, P., Lin, S., Turner, J. P., & Ke, P. C. (2010). Physical adsorption of charged plastic nanoparticles affects algal photosynthesis. *The Journal of Physical Chemistry C*, *114*(39), 16556–16561. doi:10.1021/jp1054759

Biermann, L., Clewley, D., Martinez-Vicente, V., & Topouzelis, K. (2020). Finding plastic patches in coastal waters using optical satellite data. *Scientific Reports*, *10*(1), 1–10. doi:10.103841598-020-62298-z PMID:31913322

Bing, X., Bloemhof-Ruwaard, J., & van der Vorst, J. (2014). Sustainable reverse logistics network design for household plastic waste. *Flexible Services and Manufacturing Journal*, *26*(1-2), 119–142. doi:10.100710696-012-9149-0

Blair, R. M., Waldron, S., Phoenix, V. R., & Gauchotte-Lindsay, C. (2019). Microscopy and elemental analysis characterisation of microplastics in sediment of a freshwater urban river in Scotland, UK. *Environmental Science and Pollution Research International*, *26*(12), 12491–12504. doi:10.100711356-019-04678-1 PMID:30848429

Blöcker, L., Watson, C., & Wichern, F. (2020). Living in the plastic age - different short-term microbial response to microplastics addition to arable soils with contrasting soil organic matter content and farm management legacy. *Environmental Pollution*, *267*, 115468. doi:10.1016/j.envpol.2020.115468 PMID:32891047

Blomstrand, E., & Silander Hagström, T. (2014). *Waste management and production systems; The case of Zanzibar.* https://www.diva-portal.org/smash/get/diva2:853136/FULLTEXT01.pdf

Boerger, C. M., Lattin, G. L., Moore, S. L., & Moore, C. J. (2010). Plastic ingestion by planktivorous fishes in the North Pacific Central Gyre. *Marine Pollution Bulletin*, *60*(12), 2275–2278. doi:10.1016/j.marpolbul.2010.08.007 PMID:21067782

Boethling, R. S., Sommer, E., & DiFiore, D. (2007). Designing small molecules for biodegradability. *Chemical Reviews*, *107*(6), 2207–2227. doi:10.1021/cr050952t PMID:17530907

Bolan, N. S., Hedley, M. J., & White, R. E. (1991). Processes of soil acidification during nitrogen cycling with emphasis on legume based pastures. *Plant and Soil*, *134*(1), 53–63. doi:10.1007/BF00010717

Bölscher, T., Paterson, E., Freitag, T., Thornton, B., & Herrmann, A. M. (2017). Temperature sensitivity of substrate-use efficiency can result from altered microbial physiology without change to community composition. *Soil Biology & Biochemistry, 109*, 59–69. doi:10.1016/j.soilbio.2017.02.005

Bom, F. C., & Sá, F. (2021). Concentration of microplastics in bivalves of the environment: A systematic review. *Environmental Monitoring and Assessment, 193*(12), 846. Advance online publication. doi:10.100710661-021-09639-1 PMID:34839390

Bondelind, M., Sokolova, E., Nguyen, A., Karlsson, D., Karlsson, A., & Bjorklund, K. (2020). Hydrodynamic modelling of traffic-related microplastics discharged with stormwater into the Gota River in Sweden. In Environmental Science and Pollution Research (Vol. 27, Issues 19, SI, pp. 24218–24230). Springer Heidelberg. doi:10.100711356-020-08637-z

Boots, B., Russell, C. W., & Green, D. S. (2019). Effects of microplastics in soil ecosystems: Above and below ground. *Environmental Science & Technology, 53*(19), 11496–11506. doi:10.1021/acs.est.9b03304 PMID:31509704

Bordós, G., Urbányi, B., Micsinai, A., Kriszt, B., Palotai, Z., Szabó, I., Hantosi, Z., & Szoboszlay, S. (2019). Identification of microplastics in fish ponds and natural freshwater environments of the Carpathian basin, Europe. *Chemosphere, 216*, 110–116. doi:10.1016/j.chemosphere.2018.10.110 PMID:30359912

Born, M. P., & Brüll, C. (2021). From model to nature— A review on the transferability of marine (micro-) plastic fragmentation studies. *The Science of the Total Environment*. Advance online publication. doi:10.1016/j.scitotenv.2021.151389 PMID:34808157

Bosker, T., Bouwman, L. J., Brun, N. R., Behrens, P., & Vijver, M. G. (2019). Microplastics accumulate on pores in seed capsule and delay germination and root growth of the terrestrial vascular plant Lepidium sativum. *Chemosphere, 226*, 774–781. doi:10.1016/j.chemosphere.2019.03.163 PMID:30965248

Boucher, J., & Friot, D. (2017). *Primary microplastics in the oceans: A global evaluation of sources* (Vol. 10). Gland, Switzerland: IUCN. https://holdnorgerent.no/wp-content/uploads/2020/03/IUCN-report-Primary-microplastics-in-the-oceans.pdf

Boucher, J., & Friot, D. (2017). Primary microplastics in the oceans: A global evaluation of sources. In Primary microplastics in the oceans: A global evaluation of sources. doi:10.2305/IUCN.CH.2017.01.en

Boucher, C., Morin, M., & Bendell, L. I. (2016). The influence of cosmetic microbeads on the sorptive behavior of cadmium and lead within intertidal sediments: A laboratory study. In *Regional Studies in Marine Science* (Vol. 3, pp. 1–7). Elsevier Science BV. doi:10.1016/j.rsma.2015.11.009

Bousoumah, R., Leso, V., Iavicoli, I., Huuskonen, P., Viegas, S., Porras, S. P., Santonen, T., Frery, N., Robert, A., & Ndaw, S. (2021). Biomonitoring of occupational exposure to bisphenol A, bisphenol S and bisphenol F: A systematic review. *The Science of the Total Environment, 783*, 146905. doi:10.1016/j.scitotenv.2021.146905 PMID:33865140

Bouwmeester, H., Dekkers, S., Noordam, M. Y., Hagens, W. I., Bulder, A. S., de Heer, C., ten Voorde, S. E. C. G., Wijnhoven, S. W. P., Marvin, H. J. P., & Sips, A. J. A. M. (2009). Review of health safety aspects of nanotechnologies in food production. *Regulatory Toxicology and Pharmacology, 53*(1), 52–62. doi:10.1016/j.yrtph.2008.10.008 PMID:19027049

Bouwmeester, H., Hollman, P. C., & Peters, R. J. (2015). Potential Health Impact of Environmentally Released Micro- and Nanoplastics in the Human Food Production Chain: Experiences from Nanotoxicology. *Environmental Science & Technology, 49*(15), 8932–8947. doi:10.1021/acs.est.5b01090 PMID:26130306

Bouwstra, J., Pilgram, G., Gooris, G., Koerten, H., & Ponec, M. (2001). New aspects of the skin barrier organization. *Skin Pharmacology and Physiology, 14*(Suppl. 1), 52–62. doi:10.1159/000056391 PMID:11509908

Bradney, L., Wijesekara, H., Palansooriya, K. N., Obadamudalige, N., Bolan, N. S., Ok, Y. S., Rinklebe, J., Kim, K. H., & Kirkham, M. B. (2019). Particulate plastics as a vector for toxic trace-element uptake by aquatic and terrestrial organisms and human health risk. *Environment International, 131*, 104937. doi:10.1016/j.envint.2019.104937 PMID:31284110

Brandts, I., Barría, C., Martins, M. A., Franco-Martínez, L., Barreto, A., Tvarijonaviciute, A., Tort, L., Oliveira, M., & Teles, M. (2021). Waterborne exposure of gilthead seabream (*Sparus aurata*) to polymethylmethacrylate nanoplastics causes effects at cellular and molecular levels. *Journal of Hazardous Materials, 403*(July), 123590. doi:10.1016/j.jhazmat.2020.123590

Brandts, I., Teles, M., Tvarijonaviciute, A., Pereira, M. L., Martins, M. A., Tort, L., & Oliveira, M. (2018). Effects of polymethylmethacrylate nanoplastics on *Dicentrarchus labrax*. *Genomics, 110*(6), 435–441. doi:10.1016/j.ygeno.2018.10.006 PMID:30316739

Bråte, I. L. N., Blázquez, M., Brooks, S. J., & Thomas, K. V. (2018). Weathering impacts the uptake of polyethylene microparticles from toothpaste in Mediterranean mussels (*M. galloprovincialis*). *The Science of the Total Environment, 626*, 1310–1318. doi:10.1016/j.scitotenv.2018.01.141 PMID:29898538

Brauch, H. G. (2021). Peace Ecology in the Anthropocene. In *Decolonising Conflicts, Security, Peace, Gender, Environment and Development in the Anthropocene* (pp. 51–185). Springer. doi:10.1007/978-3-030-62316-6_2

Braun, T., Ehrlich, L., Henrich, W., Koeppel, S., Lomako, I., Schwabl, P., & Liebmann, B. (2021). Detection of microplastic in human placenta and meconium in a clinical setting. *Pharmaceutics, 13*(7), 921. doi:10.3390/pharmaceutics13070921 PMID:34206212

Brennecke, D., Ferreira, E. C., Costa, T. M. M., Appel, D., da Gama, B. A. P., & Lenz, M. (2015). Ingested microplastics (>100μm) are translocated to organs of the tropical fiddler crab *Uca rapax*. *Marine Pollution Bulletin, 96*(1–2), 491–495. doi:10.1016/j.marpolbul.2015.05.001 PMID:26013589

Bretas Alvim, C., Mendoza-Roca, J. A., & Bes-Piá, A. (2020). Wastewater treatment plant as microplastics release source – Quantification and identification techniques. *Journal of Environmental Management, 255*(June). doi:10.1016/j.jenvman.2019.109739

Bringer, A., Thomas, H., Dubillot, E., Le Floch, S., Receveur, J., Cachot, J., & Tran, D. (2021). Subchronic exposure to high-density polyethylene microplastics alone or in combination with chlortoluron significantly affected valve activity and daily growth of the Pacific oyster, *Crassostrea gigas*. *Aquatic Toxicology (Amsterdam, Netherlands), 237*, 105880. doi:10.1016/j.aquatox.2021.105880 PMID:34126365

Brodin, M., Vallejos, M., Opedal, M. T., Area, M. C., & Chinga-Carrasco, G. (2017). Lignocellulosics as sustainable resources for production of Bioplastics – A Review. *Journal of Cleaner Production, 162*, 646–664. doi:10.1016/j.jclepro.2017.05.209

Broeren, M. (2013). *Production of Bio-ethylene. Technology Brief. Energy Technology Systems Analysis Programme (ETSAP)*. International Energy Agency (IEA). www.irena.org/Publications

Bromley, P. J. (1994). The role of gastric evacuation experiments in quantifying the feeding rates of predatory fish. *Reviews in Fish Biology and Fisheries, 4*(1), 36–66. doi:10.1007/BF00043260

Brown, D. M., Wilson, M. R., MacNee, W., Stone, V., & Donaldson, K. (2001). Size dependent proinflammatory effects of ultrafine polystyrene particles: A role for surface area and oxidative stress in the enhanced activity of ultrafines. *Toxicology and Applied Pharmacology, 175*(3), 191–199. doi:10.1006/taap.2001.9240 PMID:11559017

Browne, M. A., Crump, P., Niven, S. J., Teuten, E., Tonkin, A., Galloway, T., & Thompson, R. (2011). Accumulation of microplastic on shorelines woldwide: Sources and sinks. *Environmental Science & Technology, 45*(21), 9175–9179. doi:10.1021/es201811s PMID:21894925

Browne, M. A., Dissanayake, A., Galloway, T. S., Lowe, D. M., & Thompson, R. C. (2008). Ingested microscopic plastic translocates to the circulatory system of the mussel, Mytilus edulis (L.). *Environmental Science & Technology, 42*(13), 5026–5031. doi:10.1021/es800249a PMID:18678044

Browne, M. A., Galloway, T. S., & Thompson, R. C. (2010). Spatial patterns of plastic debris along estuarine shorelines. *Environmental Science & Technology, 44*(9), 3404–3409. doi:10.1021/es903784e PMID:20377170

Budimir, S., Setälä, O., & Lehtiniemi, M. (2018). Effective and easy to use extraction method shows low numbers of microplastics in offshore planktivorous fish from the northern Baltic Sea. *Marine Pollution Bulletin, 127*(December), 586–592. doi:10.1016/j.marpolbul.2017.12.054

Buerki-Thurnherr, T., von Mandach, U., & Wick, P. (2012). Knocking at the door of the unborn child: Engineered nanoparticles at the human placental barrier. *Swiss Medical Weekly, 142*, w13559. doi:10.4414mw.2012.13559 PMID:22481566

Büks, F., Schaik, N. L. V., & Kaupenjohann, M. (2020). What do we know about how the terrestrial multicellular soil fauna reacts to microplastic? *Soil (Göttingen), 6*(2), 245–267. doi:10.5194oil-6-245-2020

Burke, L., Reytar, K., Spalding, M., & Perry, A. (2011). *Reefs at Risk: Revisted.* In World Resources Institute.

Burkhardt-Holm, P., & N'Guyen, A. (2019). Ingestion of microplastics by fish and other prey organisms of cetaceans, exemplified for two large baleen whale species. *Marine Pollution Bulletin, 144*, 224–234. doi:10.1016/j.marpolbul.2019.04.068 PMID:31179992

Busman, N. A., Maie, N., Ishak, C. F., Sulaiman, M. F., & Melling, L. (2021). Effect of compaction on soil CO2 and CH4 fluxes from tropical peatland in Sarawak, Malaysia. *Environment, Development and Sustainability, 23*(8), 11646–11659. doi:10.100710668-020-01132-y

Cai, H., Chen, M., Chen, Q., Du, F., Liu, J., & Shi, H. (2020). Microplastic quantification affected by structure and pore size of filters. *Chemosphere, 257*, 127198. doi:10.1016/j.chemosphere.2020.127198 PMID:32512329

Cai, L., Wang, J., Peng, J., Tan, Z., Zhan, Z., Tan, X., & Chen, Q. (2017). Characteristic of microplastics in the atmospheric fallout from Dongguan city, China: Preliminary research and first evidence. *Environmental Science and Pollution Research International, 24*(32), 24928–24935. doi:10.100711356-017-0116-x PMID:28918553

Cai, L., Wang, J., Peng, J., Wu, Z., & Tan, X. (2018). Observation of the degradation of three types of plastic pellets exposed to UV irradiation in three different environments. *The Science of the Total Environment, 628–629*, 740–747. doi:10.1016/j.scitotenv.2018.02.079 PMID:29454214

Calafat, A. M., Ye, X., Wong, L.-Y., Reidy, J. A., & Needham, L. L. (2008). Exposure of the U.S. Population to Bisphenol A and 4- tertiary-Octylphenol: 2003–2004. *Environmental Health Perspectives, 116*(1), 39–44. doi:10.1289/ehp.10753 PMID:18197297

Campanale, C., Massarelli, C., Savino, I., Locaputo, V., & Uricchio, V. F. (2020). A Detailed Review Study on Potential Effects of Microplastics and Additives of Concern on Human Health. *International Journal of Environmental Research and Public Health, 17*(4), 1212. doi:10.3390/ijerph17041212 PMID:32069998

Campanale, C., Stock, F., Massarelli, C., Kochleus, C., Bagnuolo, G., Reifferscheid, G., & Uricchio, V. F. (2020). Microplastics and their possible sources: The example of Ofanto river in southeast Italy. In *Environmental Pollution* (Vol. 258). Elsevier Sci Ltd. doi:10.1016/j.envpol.2019.113284

Canesi, L., Ciacci, C., Bergami, E., Monopoli, M. P., Dawson, K. A., Papa, S., Canonico, B., & Corsi, I. (2015). Evidence for immunomodulation and apoptotic processes induced by cationic polystyrene nanoparticles in the haemocytes of the marine bivalve *Mytilus*. *Marine Environmental Research, 111*, 34–40. doi:10.1016/j.marenvres.2015.06.008 PMID:26115607

Canniff, P. M., & Hoang, T. C. (2018). Microplastic ingestion by Daphnia magna and its enhancement on algal growth. *The Science of the Total Environment, 633*, 500–507. doi:10.1016/j.scitotenv.2018.03.176 PMID:29579661

Cao, D., Wang, X., Luo, X., Liu, G., & Zheng, H. (2017). Effects of polystyrene microplastics on the fitness of earthworms in an agricultural soil. *IOP C Ser. Earth Env., 61*, 012148.

Capolupo, M., Franzellitti, S., Valbonesi, P., Lanzas, C. S., & Fabbri, E. (2018). Uptake and transcriptional effects of polystyrene microplastics in larval stages of the Mediterranean mussel *Mytilus galloprovincialis*. *Environmental Pollution, 241*, 1038–1047. doi:10.1016/j.envpol.2018.06.035 PMID:30029311

Capolupo, M., Sørensen, L., Jayasena, K. D. R., Booth, A. M., & Fabbri, E. (2020). Chemical composition and ecotoxicity of plastic and car tire rubber leachates to aquatic organisms. *Water Research, 169*, 115270. doi:10.1016/j.watres.2019.115270 PMID:31731243

Capolupo, M., Valbonesi, P., & Fabbri, E. (2021). A Comparative Assessment of the Chronic Effects of Micro- and Nano-Plastics on the Physiology of the Mediterranean Mussel *Mytilus galloprovincialis*. *Nanomaterials (Basel, Switzerland), 11*(3), 649. doi:10.3390/nano11030649 PMID:33800064

Carbery, M., O'Connor, W., & Palanisami, T. (2018). Trophic transfer of microplastics and mixed contaminants in the marine food web and implications for human health. *Environment International, 115*, 400–409. doi:10.1016/j.envint.2018.03.007 PMID:29653694

Carpenter, E. J., Anderson, S. J., Harvey, G. R., Miklas, H. P., & Peck, B. B. (1972). Polystyrene spherules in coastal waters. *Science, 178*(4062), 749–750. doi:10.1126cience.178.4062.749 PMID:4628343

Carrasco, A., Pulgar, J., Quintanilla-Ahumada, D., Perez-Venegas, D., Quijón, P. A., & Duarte, C. (2019). The influence of microplastics pollution on the feeding behavior of a prominent sandy beach amphipod, *Orchestoidea tuberculata* (Nicolet, 1849). *Marine Pollution Bulletin, 145*(December), 23–27. doi:10.1016/j.marpolbul.2019.05.018

Carreras-Colom, E., Constenla, M., Soler-Membrives, A., Cartes, J. E., Baeza, M., Padros, F., & Carrasson, M. (2018). Spatial occurrence and effects of microplastic ingestion on the deep-water shrimp Aristeus antennatus. In *Marine Pollution Bulletin* (Vol. 133, pp. 44–52). Pergamon-Elsevier Science Ltd. doi:10.1016/j.marpolbul.2018.05.012

Carr, S. A., Liu, J., & Tesoro, A. G. (2016). Transport and fate of microplastic particles in wastewater treatment plants. *Water Research, 91*, 174–182. doi:10.1016/j.watres.2016.01.002 PMID:26795302

Carus, M. (2016). Bio-based materials – Technical, Economic and Market Data on the Bio-based Economy. Technology and Polymerdagene, Gjøvik, Norway.

Caruso, G. (2019). Microplastics as vectors of contaminants. *Marine Pollution Bulletin, 146*, 921–924. doi:10.1016/j.marpolbul.2019.07.052 PMID:31426238

Castro-Jiménez, J., González-Fernández, D., Fornier, M., Schmidt, N., & Sempéré, R. (2019). Macro-litter in surface waters from the Rhone River: Plastic pollution and loading to the NW Mediterranean Sea. *Marine Pollution Bulletin, 146*, 60–66. doi:10.1016/j.marpolbul.2019.05.067 PMID:31426199

Catarino, A. I., Macchia, V., Sanderson, W. G., Thompson, R. C., & Henry, T. B. (2018). Low levels of microplastics (MP) in wild mussels indicate that MP ingestion by humans is minimal compared to exposure via household fibres fallout during a meal. *Environmental Pollution, 237*, 675–684.

Catarino, A. I., Macchia, V., Sanderson, W. G., Thompson, R. C., & Henry, T. B. (2018). Low levels of microplastics (MP) in wild mussels indicate that MP ingestion by humans is minimal compared to exposure via household fibres fallout during a meal. *Environmental Pollution, 237*, 675–684. doi:10.1016/j.envpol.2018.02.069 PMID:29604577

Catarino, A. I., Thompson, R., Sanderson, W., & Henry, T. B. (2017). Development and optimization of a standard method for extraction of microplastics in mussels by enzyme digestion of soft tissues. *Environmental Toxicology and Chemistry, 36*(4), 947–951. doi:10.1002/etc.3608 PMID:27583696

Cedervall, T., Hansson, L.-A., Lard, M., Frohm, B., & Linse, S. (2012). Food chain transport of nanoparticles affects behaviour and fat metabolism in fish. *PLoS One, 7*(2), e32254. doi:10.1371/journal.pone.0032254 PMID:22384193

Chaabouni, R., Bouaziz, S., Peresson, H., & Wolfgang, J. (2012). Lineament analysis of South Jenein Area (Southern Tunisia) using remote sensing data and geographic information system. *The Egyptian Journal of Remote Sensing and Space Sciences, 15*(2), 197–206. doi:10.1016/j.ejrs.2012.11.001

Chae, Y., & An, Y. J. (2017). Effects of micro- and nanoplastics on aquatic ecosystems: Current research trends and perspectives. *Marine Pollution Bulletin, 124*(2), 624–632. doi:10.1016/j.marpolbul.2017.01.070 PMID:28222864

Chae, Y., & An, Y. J. (2018). Current research trends on plastic pollution and ecological impacts on the soil ecosystem: A review. *Environmental Pollution, 240*, 387–395. doi:10.1016/j.envpol.2018.05.008 PMID:29753246

Chae, Y., Kim, D., & An, Y. J. (2019). Effects of micro-sized polyethylene spheres on the marine microalga Dunaliella salina: Focusing on the algal cell to plastic particle size ratio. *Aquatic Toxicology (Amsterdam, Netherlands), 216*, 105296. doi:10.1016/j.aquatox.2019.105296 PMID:31541944

Chagnon, C., Thiel, M., Antunes, J., Ferreira, J. L., Sobral, P., & Ory, N. C. (2018). Plastic ingestion and trophic transfer between Easter Island flying fish (*Cheilopogon rapanouiensis*) and yellowfin tuna (*Thunnus albacares*) from Rapa Nui (Easter Island). *Environmental Pollution, 243*, 127–133. doi:10.1016/j.envpol.2018.08.042 PMID:30172118

Chahine, M. T. (1992). The hydrological cycle and its influence on climate. *Nature, 359*(6394), 373–380. doi:10.1038/359373a0

Chakraborty, P., Bharat, G. K., Gaonkar, O., Mukhopadhyay, M., Chandra, S., Steindal, E. H., & Nizzetto, L. (2022). Endocrine-disrupting chemicals used as common plastic additives: Levels, profiles, and human dietary exposure from the Indian food basket. *The Science of the Total Environment, 810*, 152200. doi:10.1016/j.scitotenv.2021.152200 PMID:34890663

Chamas, A., Moon, H., Zheng, J., Qiu, Y., Tabassum, T., Jang, J. H., Abu-Omar, M., Scott, S. L., & Suh, S. (2020). Degradation Rates of Plastics in the Environment. *ACS Sustainable Chemistry & Engineering, 8*(9), 3494–3511. doi:10.1021/acssuschemeng.9b06635

Chan, C. K., Park, C., Chan, K. M., Mak, D. C., Fang, J. K., & Mitrano, D. M. (2021). Microplastic fibre releases from industrial wastewater effluent: A textile wet-processing mill in China. *Environmental Chemistry, 18*(3), 93–100. doi:10.1071/EN20143

Chapman, P. M. (2007). Microplastic an emerging contaminant of potential concern. *Integrated Environmental Assessment and Management, 3*(2008), 1. doi:10.1897/IEAM_2008-022.1

Chapron, L., Peru, E., Engler, A., Ghiglione, J. F., Meistertzheim, A. L., Pruski, A. M., Purser, A., Vétion, G., Galand, P. E., & Lartaud, F. (2018). Macro- and microplastics affect cold-water corals growth, feeding and behaviour. *Scientific Reports*, *8*(1), 15299. Advance online publication. doi:10.103841598-018-33683-6 PMID:30333567

Charitou, A., Aga-Spyridopoulou, R., Mylona, Z., Beck, R., McLellan, F., & Addamo, A. (2021). Investigating the knowledge and attitude of the Greek public towards marine plastic pollution and the EU Single-Use Plastics Directive. *Marine Pollution Bulletin*, *116*, 112182. doi:10.1016/j.marpolbul.2021.112182 PMID:33652246

Chen, G., Feng, Q., & Wang, J. (2020). Mini-review of microplastics in the atmosphere and their risks to humans. In Science of the Total Environment (Vol. 703). doi:10.1016/j.scitotenv.2019.135504

Chen, C.-Y., Lu, T.-H., Yang, Y.-F., & Liao, C.-M. (2021). Toxicokinetic/toxicodynamic-based risk assessment of freshwater fish health posed by microplastics at environmentally relevant concentrations. In *Science of the Total Environment* (Vol. 756). Elsevier. doi:10.1016/j.scitotenv.2020.144013

Chen, G., Li, Y., & Wang, J. (2021). Occurrence and ecological impact of microplastics in aquaculture ecosystems. *Chemosphere*, *274*, 129989. doi:10.1016/j.chemosphere.2021.129989 PMID:33979917

Chen, G.-Q. (2009). A microbial polyhydroxyalkanoates (PHA) based vio- and materials industry. *Chemical Society Reviews*, *38*(8), 2434–2446. doi:10.1039/b812677c PMID:19623359

Chen, H. L., Gibbins, C. N., Selvam, S. B., & Ting, K. N. (2021). Spatio-temporal variation of microplastic along a rural to urban transition in a tropical river. In *Environmental Pollution* (Vol. 289). Elsevier Sci Ltd. doi:10.1016/j.envpol.2021.117895

Chen, H., Jia, Q., Zhao, X., Li, L., Nie, Y., Liu, H., & Ye, J. (2020a). The occurrence of microplastics in water bodies in urban agglomerations: Impacts of drainage system overflow in wet weather, catchment land-uses, and environmental management practices. *Water Research*, *183*, 116073. doi:10.1016/j.watres.2020.116073 PMID:32599427

Chen, Q., Gundlach, M., Yang, S., Jiang, J., Velki, M., Yin, D., & Hollert, H. (2017). Quantitative investigation of the mechanisms of microplastics and nanoplastics toward zebrafish larvae locomotor activity. *The Science of the Total Environment*, *584–585*, 1022–1031. doi:10.1016/j.scitotenv.2017.01.156 PMID:28185727

Chen, Q., Yin, D., Jia, Y., Schiwy, S., Legradi, J., Yang, S., & Hollert, H. (2017). Enhanced uptake of BPA in the presence of nanoplastics can lead to neurotoxic effects in adult zebrafish. *The Science of the Total Environment*, *609*, 1312–1321. doi:10.1016/j.scitotenv.2017.07.144 PMID:28793400

Chen, X., Chen, X., Zhao, Y., Zhou, H., Xiong, X., & Wu, C. (2020). Effects of microplastic biofilms on nutrient cycling in simulated freshwater systems. *The Science of the Total Environment*, *719*, 137276. doi:10.1016/j.scitotenv.2020.137276 PMID:32114222

Chen, Y., Leng, Y., Liu, X., & Wang, J. (2020). Microplastic pollution in vegetable farmlands of suburb Wuhan, central China. *Environmental Pollution*, *257*, 113449. doi:10.1016/j.envpol.2019.113449 PMID:31706776

Chen, Y., Ling, Y., Li, X., Hu, J., Cao, C., & He, D. (2020). Size-dependent cellular internalization and effects of polystyrene microplastics in microalgae *P. helgolandica var. tsingtaoensis* and *S. quadricauda*. *Journal of Hazardous Materials*, *399*(March), 123092. doi:10.1016/j.jhazmat.2020.123092 PMID:32531675

Chen, Z., Zhao, W., Xing, R., Xie, S., Yang, X., Cui, P., Lü, J., Liao, H., Yu, Z., Wang, S., & Zhou, S. (2020). Enhanced in situ biodegradation of microplastics in sewage sludge using hyperthermophilic composting technology. *Journal of Hazardous Materials*, *384*, 121271. doi:10.1016/j.jhazmat.2019.121271 PMID:31611021

Cheung, P. K., Hung, P. L., & Fok, L. (2019). River Microplastic Contamination and Dynamics upon a Rainfall Event in Hong Kong, China. In Environmental Processes-An International Journal (Vol. 6, Issue 1, pp. 253–264). Springer International Publishing AG. doi:10.100740710-018-0345-0

Chia, W. Y., Ying Tang, D. Y., Khoo, K. S., Kay Lup, A. N., & Chew, K. W. (2020). Nature's fight against plastic pollution: Algae for plastic biodegradation and bioplastics production. *Environmental Science and Ecotechnology*, *4*, 100065. doi:10.1016/j.ese.2020.100065

Chiba, S., Saito, H., Fletcher, R., Yogi, T., Kayo, M., Miyagi, S., Ogido, M., & Fujikura, K. (2018). Human footprint in the abyss: 30 year records of deep-sea plastic debris. *Marine Policy*, *96*(March), 204–212. doi:10.1016/j.marpol.2018.03.022

Chouchene, K., Rocha-Santos, T., & Ksibi, M. (2021). Types, occurrence, and distribution of microplastics and metals contamination in sediments from south west of Kerkennah archipelago, Tunisia. *Environmental Science and Pollution Research International*, *28*(34), 46477–46487. doi:10.100711356-020-09938-z PMID:32632691

Chrisafis, A. (2016). French Law Forbids Food Waste by Supermarkets. *The Guardian*. Retrieved from https://www.theguardian .com/world/2016/feb/04/french-law-forbids-food-waste-by-supermarkets

Cinar, S. O., Chong, Z. K., Kucuker, M. A., Wieczorek, N., Cengiz, U., & Kuchta, K. (2020). Bioplastic production from microalgae: A review. *International Journal of Environmental Research and Public Health*, *17*(11), 3842. doi:10.3390/ijerph17113842 PMID:32481700

Cingotti, N., & Jensen, G. K. (2019). *Health and Environment Alliance (HEAL). Food contact materials and chemical contamination*. Health and Environment Alliance.

Clinci, D. (2021). Plastic Memories of the Anthropocene. *Metacritic Journal for Comparative Studies and Theory*, *7*(1), 83–97. doi:10.24193/mjcst.2021.11.05

Cluzard, M., Kazmiruk, T. N., Kazmiruk, V. D., & Bendell, L. I. (2015). Intertidal concentrations of microplastics and their influence on ammonium cycling as related to the shellfish industry. *Archives of Environmental Contamination and Toxicology*, *69*(3), 310–319. doi:10.100700244-015-0156-5 PMID:25916196

Colborn, T., & Clement, C. (1992). *Chemically-induced alterations in sexual and functional development: the wildlife/human connection*. Princeton Scientific Pub. Co.

Cole, M. (2016). A novel method for preparing microplastic fibers. *Scientific Reports*, *6*(1), 34519. doi:10.1038rep34519 PMID:27694820

Cole, M., & Galloway, T. S. (2015). Ingestion of nanoplastics and microplastics by Pacific oyster larvae. *Environmental Science & Technology*, *49*(24), 14625–14632. doi:10.1021/acs.est.5b04099 PMID:26580574

Cole, M., Liddle, C., Consolandi, G., Drago, C., Hird, C., Lindeque, P. K., & Galloway, T. S. (2020). Microplastics, microfibres and nanoplastics cause variable sub-lethal responses in mussels (*Mytilus* spp.). *Marine Pollution Bulletin*, *160*, 111552. doi:10.1016/j.marpolbul.2020.111552 PMID:32861936

Cole, M., Lindeque, P. K., Fileman, E., Clark, J., Lewis, C., Halsband, C., & Galloway, T. S. (2016). Microplastics alter the properties and sinking rates of zooplankton faecal pellets. *Environmental Science & Technology*, *50*(6), 3239–3246. doi:10.1021/acs.est.5b05905 PMID:26905979

Cole, M., Lindeque, P., Fileman, E., Halsband, C., & Galloway, T. S. (2015). The impact of polystyrene microplastics on feeding, function, and fecundity in the marine copepod *Calanus helgolandicus*. *Environmental Science & Technology*, *49*(2), 1130–1137. doi:10.1021/es504525u PMID:25563688

Cole, M., Lindeque, P., Fileman, E., Halsband, C., Goodhead, R., Moger, J., & Galloway, T. S. (2013). Microplastic ingestion by zooplankton. *Environmental Science & Technology*, *47*(12), 6646–6655. doi:10.1021/es400663f PMID:23692270

Cole, M., Lindeque, P., Halsband, C., & Galloway, T. S. (2011). Microplastics as contaminants in the marine environment: A review. *Marine Pollution Bulletin*, *62*(12), 2588–2597. doi:10.1016/j.marpolbul.2011.09.025 PMID:22001295

Cole, M., Webb, H., Lindeque, P. K., Fileman, E. S., Halsband, C., & Galloway, T. S. (2014). Isolation of microplastics in biota-rich seawater samples and marine organisms. *Scientific Reports*, *4*(1), 1–8. doi:10.1038rep04528 PMID:24681661

Collard, F., Gilbert, B., Eppe, G., Parmentier, E., & Das, K. (2015). Detection of Anthropogenic Particles in Fish Stomachs: An Isolation Method Adapted to Identification by Raman Spectroscopy. *Archives of Environmental Contamination and Toxicology*, *69*(3), 331–339. doi:10.100700244-015-0221-0 PMID:26289815

Coppock, R. L., Cole, M., Lindeque, P. K., Queirós, A. M., & Galloway, T. S. (2017). A small-scale, portable method for extracting microplastics from marine sediments. *Environmental Pollution*, *230*, 829–837. doi:10.1016/j.envpol.2017.07.017 PMID:28734264

Coppock, R. L., Galloway, T. S., Cole, M., Fileman, E. S., Queirós, A. M., & Lindeque, P. K. (2019). Microplastics alter feeding selectivity and faecal density in the copepod, Calanus helgolandicus. *The Science of the Total Environment*, *687*, 780–789. doi:10.1016/j.scitotenv.2019.06.009 PMID:31412481

Coppola, G., Gaudio, M. T., Lopresto, C. G., Calabro, V., Curcio, S., & Chakraborty, S. (2021). Bioplastic from Renewable Biomass: A Facile Solution for a Greener Environment. *Earth Systems and Environment*, *5*(2), 231–251. doi:10.100741748-021-00208-7

Corcoran, P. L., Biesinger, M. C., & Grifi, M. (2009). Plastics and beaches: A degrading relationship. *Marine Pollution Bulletin*, *58*(1), 80–84. doi:10.1016/j.marpolbul.2008.08.022 PMID:18834997

Corona, E., Martin, C., Marasco, R., & Duarte, C. M. (2020). Passive and Active Removal of Marine Microplastics by a Mushroom Coral (*Danafungia scruposa*). *Frontiers in Marine Science*, *7*, 128. Advance online publication. doi:10.3389/fmars.2020.00128

Corradini, F., Casado, F., Leiva, V., Huerta-Lwanga, E., & Geissen, V. (2021). Microplastics occurrence and frequency in soils under different land uses on a regional scale. *The Science of the Total Environment*, *752*, 141917. doi:10.1016/j.scitotenv.2020.141917 PMID:32892050

Corradini, F., Meza, P., Eguiluz, R., Casado, F., Huerta-Lwanga, E., & Geissen, V. (2019). Evidence of microplastic accumulation in agricultural soils from sewage sludge disposal. *The Science of the Total Environment*, *671*, 411–420. doi:10.1016/j.scitotenv.2019.03.368 PMID:30933797

Corsi, I., Bergami, E., & Caruso, G. (2021). Special issue plastics in polar regions. *Environment International*, *149*, 106203. doi:10.1016/j.envint.2020.106203 PMID:33121740

Costa, E., Gambardella, C., Piazza, V., Vassalli, M., Sbrana, F., Lavorano, S., Garaventa, F., & Faimali, M. (2020). Microplastics ingestion in the ephyra stage of Aurelia sp. triggers acute and behavioral responses. *Ecotoxicology and Environmental Safety*, *189*, 109983. doi:10.1016/j.ecoenv.2019.109983 PMID:31785944

Costa, E., Piazza, V., Lavorano, S., Faimali, M., Garaventa, F., & Gambardella, C. (2020). Trophic Transfer of Microplastics From Copepods to Jellyfish in the Marine Environment. *Frontiers in Environmental Science*, *8*, 571732. Advance online publication. doi:10.3389/fenvs.2020.571732

Courtene-Jones, W., Quinn, B., Murphy, F., Gary, S. F., & Narayanaswamy, B. E. (2017). Optimisation of enzymatic digestion and validation of specimen preservation methods for the analysis of ingested microplastics. *Analytical Methods*, *9*(9), 1437–1445. doi:10.1039/C6AY02343F

Cowger, W., Booth, A. M., Hamilton, B. M., Thaysen, C., Primpke, S., Munno, K., Lusher, A. L., Dehaut, A., Vaz, V. P., Liboiron, M., Devriese, L. I., Hermabessiere, L., Rochman, C., Athey, S. N., Lynch, J. M., Lynch, J. M., Frond, H. D., Gray, A., Jones, O. A. H., ... Nel, H. (2020). Reporting Guidelines to Increase the Reproducibility and Comparability of Research on Microplastics. *Applied Spectroscopy*, *74*(9), 1066–1077. doi:10.1177/0003702820930292 PMID:32394727

Cox, K. D., Covernton, G. A., Davies, H. L., Dower, J. F., Juanes, F., & Dudas, S. E. (2019). Human Consumption of Microplastics. *Environmental Science & Technology*, *53*(12), 7068–7074. doi:10.1021/acs.est.9b01517 PMID:31184127

Cózar, A., Echevarría, F., González-Gordillo, J. I., Irigoien, X., Úbeda, B., Hernández-León, S., Palma, A. T., Navarro, S., García-de-Lomas, J., Ruiz, A., Fernandez-de-Puelles, M. L., & Duarte, C. M. (2014). Plastic debris in the open ocean. *Proceedings of the National Academy of Sciences of the United States of America*, *111*(28), 10239–10244. doi:10.1073/pnas.1314705111 PMID:24982135

Cózar, A., Sanz-Martín, M., Martí, E., González-Gordillo, J. I., Ubeda, B., Gálvez, J. Á., Irigoien, X., & Duarte, C. M. (2015). Plastic accumulation in the Mediterranean Sea. *PLoS One*, *10*(4), e0121762. doi:10.1371/journal.pone.0121762 PMID:25831129

Crabbe, J. R., Campbell, J. R., Thompson, L., Walz, S. L., & Schultz, W. W. (1994). Biodegradation of a colloidal ester-based polyurethane by soil fungi. *International Biodeterioration & Biodegradation*, *33*(2), 103–113. doi:10.1016/0964-8305(94)90030-2

Crawford, C. B., & Quinn, B. (2016). Microplastic Pollutants. In Microplastic Pollutants. doi:10.1016/C2015-0-04315-5

Crichton, E. M., Noël, M., Gies, E. A., & Ross, P. S. (2017). A novel, density-independent and FTIR-compatible approach for the rapid extraction of microplastics from aquatic sediments. *Analytical Methods*, *9*(9), 1419–1428. doi:10.1039/C6AY02733D

Critchell, K., & Hoogenboom, M. O. (2018). Effects of microplastic exposure on the body condition and behaviour of planktivorous reef fish (*Acanthochromis polyacanthus*). *PLoS One*, *13*(3), 1–19. doi:10.1371/journal.pone.0193308 PMID:29494635

Crooks, N., Parker, H., & Pernetta, A. P. (2019). Brain food? Trophic transfer and tissue retention of microplastics by the velvet swimming crab (*Necora puber*). *Journal of Experimental Marine Biology and Ecology*, *519*(June), 151187. doi:10.1016/j.jembe.2019.151187

Crossman, J., Hurley, H. H., Futter, M., & Nizzetto, L. (2020). Transfer and transport of microplastics from biosolids to agricultural soils and the wider environment. *The Science of the Total Environment*, *724*, 138334. doi:10.1016/j.scitotenv.2020.138334 PMID:32408466

Cunha, C., Lopes, J., Paulo, J., Faria, M., Kaufmann, M., Nogueira, N., Ferreira, A., & Cordeiro, N. (2020). The effect of microplastics pollution in microalgal biomass production: A biochemical study. *Water Research*, *186*, 116370. Advance online publication. doi:10.1016/j.watres.2020.116370 PMID:32906034

Cutroneo, L., Reboa, A., Besio, G., Borgogno, F., Canesi, L., Canuto, S., Dara, M., Enrile, F., Forioso, I., Greco, G., Lenoble, V., Malatesta, A., Mounier, S., Petrillo, M., Rovetta, R., Stocchino, A., Tesan, J., Vagge, G., & Capello, M. (2020). Microplastics in seawater: Sampling strategies, laboratory methodologies, and identification techniques applied to port environment. *Environmental Science and Pollution Research International*, *27*(9), 8938–8952. doi:10.100711356-020-07783-8 PMID:32026372

Cutroneo, L., Reboa, A., Geneselli, I., & Capello, M. (2021). Considerations on salts used for density separation in the extraction of microplastics from sediments. *Marine Pollution Bulletin*, *166*(March), 112216. doi:10.1016/j.marpolbul.2021.112216 PMID:33684703

Da Costa, J. P. (2018). *Micro- and Nanoplastics in the Environment: Research and Policymaking* (Vol. 1). Elsevier.

Da Costa, J. P., Paço, A., Santos, P. S. M., Duarte, A. C., & Rocha-Santos, T. (2019). Microplastics in soils: Assessment, analytics and risks. *Environmental Chemistry*, *16*(1), 18–30. doi:10.1071/EN18150

Da Costa, J. P., Santos, P. S. M., Duarte, A. C., & Rocha-Santos, T. (2016). (Nano)plastics in the environment - Sources, fates and effects. *The Science of the Total Environment*, *566–567*, 15–26. doi:10.1016/j.scitotenv.2016.05.041 PMID:27213666

da Luz, J. M. R., Paes, S. A., Bazzolli, D. M. S., Totola, M. R., Demuner, A. J., & Kasuya, M. C. M. (2014). Abiotic and biotic degradation of oxo-biodegradable plastic bags by Pleurotus ostreatus. *PLoS One*, *9*(11), e107438. doi:10.1371/journal.pone.0107438 PMID:25419675

Dabbagh, N., & Kitsantas, A. (2012). Personal Learning Environments, social media, and self-regulated learning: A natural formula for connecting formal and informal learning. *Internet High Educ.*, *15*(1), 3–8. doi:10.1016/j.iheduc.2011.06.002

Dahms, H. T. J., van Rensburg, G. J., & Greenfield, R. (2020). The microplastic profile of an urban African stream. In *Science of the Total Environment* (Vol. 731). Elsevier. doi:10.1016/j.scitotenv.2020.138893

Dahms, H. U., Hagiwara, A., & Lee, J. S. (2011). Ecotoxicology, ecophysiology, and mechanistic studies with rotifers. *Aquatic Toxicology (Amsterdam, Netherlands)*, *101*(1), 1–12. doi:10.1016/j.aquatox.2010.09.006 PMID:20961628

Dai, H., Chang, P. R., Geng, F., Yu, J., & Ma, X. (2009). Preparation and properties of thermoplastic starch/montmorillonite nanocomposite using N-(2-Hydroxyethyl) formamide as a new additive. *Journal of Polymers and the Environment*, *17*(4), 225–232. doi:10.100710924-009-0142-y

Dantas, N. C., Duarte, O. S., Ferreira, W. C., Ayala, A. P., Rezende, C. F., & Feitosa, C. V. (2020). Plastic intake does not depend on fish eating habits: Identification of microplastics in the stomach contents of fish on an urban beach in Brazil. *Marine Pollution Bulletin*, *153*, 110959. doi:10.1016/j.marpolbul.2020.110959 PMID:32275522

Das, D. (2011). *Echinoderm*. Available in: https://www.britannica.com/animal/echinoderm

Das, K. A., Sathish, A., & Stanley, J. (2018). Production of biofuel and bioplastic from Chlorella pyrenoidosa. *Proceedings: Material Today, 5*(8), 16774-16781.

Davarpanah, E., & Guilhermino, L. (2015). Single and combined effects of microplastics and copper on the population growth of the marine microalgae *Tetraselmis chuii. Estuarine, Coastal and Shelf Science*, *167*, 269–275. doi:10.1016/j.ecss.2015.07.023

Davidson, K., & Dudas, S. E. (2016). Microplastic Ingestion by Wild and Cultured Manila Clams (Venerupis philippinarum) from Baynes Sound, British Columbia. *Archives of Environmental Contamination and Toxicology*, *71*(2), 147–156. doi:10.100700244-016-0286-4 PMID:27259879

Davis, M. D., & Rubin, B. K. (2021). Plastic Bronchitis. In *Diagnostic and Interventional Bronchoscopy in Children* (pp. 289–293). Humana. doi:10.1007/978-3-030-54924-4_23

Davison, P., & Asch, R. G. (2011). Plastic ingestion by mesopelagic fishes in the North Pacific Subtropical Gyre. *Marine Ecology Progress Series*, *432*, 173–180. doi:10.3354/meps09142

Davranche, M., Veclin, C., Pierson-Wickmann, A. C., El Hadri, H., Grassl, B., Rowenczyk, L., Dia, A., Ter Halle, A., Blancho, F., Reynaud, S., & Gigault, J. (2019). Are nanoplastics able to bind significant amount of metals? The lead example. *Environmental Pollution, 249*, 940–948. doi:10.1016/j.envpol.2019.03.087 PMID:30965546

De Falco, F., Gullo, M. P., Gentile, G., Di Pace, E., Cocca, M., Gelabert, L., Brouta-Agnésa, M., Rovira, A., Escudero, R., Villalba, R., Mossotti, R., Montarsolo, A., Gavignano, S., Tonin, C., & Avella, M. (2018). Evaluation of microplastic release caused by textile washing processes of synthetic fabrics. *Environmental Pollution, 236*, 916–925. doi:10.1016/j.envpol.2017.10.057 PMID:29107418

de Jesus Pinon-Colin, T., Rodriguez-Jimenez, R., Rogel-Hernandez, E., Alvarez-Andrade, A., & Wakida, F. T. (2020). Microplastics in stormwater runoff in a semiarid region, Tijuana, Mexico. In *Science of the Total Environment* (Vol. 704). Elsevier. doi:10.1016/j.scitotenv.2019.135411

de Jong, E., Dam, M. A., Sipos, L., & Gruter, G.-J. M. (2012). *Biobased Monomers, Polymers, and Materials*. American Chemical Society.

de Lorenzo, V. (2018). Environmental Microbiology to the Rescue of Planet Earth. *Environmental Microbiology, 20*(6), 1910–1916. doi:10.1111/1462-2920.14105 PMID:29575463

de Sá, L. C., Luís, L. G., & Guilhermino, L. (2015). Effects of microplastics on juveniles of the common goby (Pomatoschistus microps): Confusion with prey, reduction of the predatory performance and efficiency, and possible influence of developmental conditions. *Environmental Pollution, 196*, 359–362. doi:10.1016/j.envpol.2014.10.026 PMID:25463733

de Souza Machado, A. A., Lau, C. W., Kloas, W., Bergmann, J., Bacheher, J. B., Faltin, E., Becker, R., Goerlich, A. S., & Rillig, M. C. (2019). Microplastics can change soil properties and affect plant performance. *Environmental Science & Technology, 53*(10), 6044–6052. doi:10.1021/acs.est.9b01339 PMID:31021077

de Souza Machado, A. A., Lau, C. W., Till, J., Kloas, W., Lehmann, A., Becker, R., & Rillig, M. C. (2018). Impacts of microplastics on the soil biophysical environment. *Environmental Science & Technology, 52*(17), 9656–9665. doi:10.1021/acs.est.8b02212 PMID:30053368

de Wit, W., & Bigaud, N. (2019). No Plastic In Nature: Assessing plastic ingestion from nature to people (AN ANALYSIS for WWF). *World Wide Fund For Nature*, 7.

Debrah, J., Vidal, D., & Dinis, M. (2021). Raising Awareness on Solid Waste Management through Formal Education for Sustainability: Developing Countries Evidence Review. *Recycling, 6*(6).

Defontaine, S., Sous, D., Tesan, J., Monperrus, M., Lenoble, V., & Lanceleur, L. (2020). Microplastics in a salt-wedge estuary: Vertical structure and tidal dynamics. In *Marine Pollution Bulletin* (Vol. 160). Pergamon-Elsevier Science Ltd. doi:10.1016/j.marpolbul.2020.111688

Dehaut, A., Cassone, A. L., Frère, L., Hermabessiere, L., Himber, C., Rinnert, E., Rivière, G., Lambert, C., Soudant, P., Huvet, A., Duflos, G., & Paul-Pont, I. (2016). Microplastics in seafood: Benchmark protocol for their extraction and characterization. *Environmental Pollution, 215*(August), 223–233. doi:10.1016/j.envpol.2016.05.018 PMID:27209243

Dehghani, S., Moore, F., & Akhbarizadeh, R. (2017). Microplastic pollution in deposited urban dust, Tehran metropolis, Iran. *Environmental Science and Pollution Research International, 24*(25), 20360–20371. doi:10.100711356-017-9674-1 PMID:28707239

Deidda, I., Russo, R., Bonaventura, R., Costa, C., Zito, F., & Lampiasi, N. (2021). Neurotoxicity in marine invertebrates: An update. *Biology (Basel), 10*(2), 161. doi:10.3390/biology10020161 PMID:33670451

De-la-Torre, G. E., Dioses-Salinas, D. C., Pizarro-Ortega, C. I., & Santillán, L. (2021). New plastic formations in the Anthropocene. *The Science of the Total Environment*, *754*, 142216. doi:10.1016/j.scitotenv.2020.142216 PMID:33254855

Della Torre, C., Bergami, E., Salvati, A., Faleri, C., Cirino, P., Dawson, K. A., & Corsi, I. (2014). Accumulation and embryotoxicity of polystyrene nanoparticles at early stage of development of sea urchin embryos Paracentrotus lividus. *Environmental Science & Technology*, *48*(20), 12302–12311. doi:10.1021/es502569w PMID:25260196

Deng, Y., Zhang, Y., Lemos, B., & Ren, H. (2017). Tissue accumulation of microplastics in mice and biomarker responses suggest widespread health risks of exposure. *Scientific Reports*, *7*(1), 1–10. doi:10.1038rep46687 PMID:28436478

Derraik, J. G. (2002). The pollution of the marine environment by plastic debris: A review. *Marine Pollution Bulletin*, *44*(9), 842–852. doi:10.1016/S0025-326X(02)00220-5 PMID:12405208

Desforges, J. P. W., Galbraith, M., & Ross, P. S. (2015). Ingestion of microplastics by zooplankton in the Northeast Pacific Ocean. *Archives of Environmental Contamination and Toxicology*, *69*(3), 320–330. doi:10.100700244-015-0172-5 PMID:26066061

Desforges, J. W., Galbraith, M., Dangerfield, N., & Ross, P. S. (2014). Widespread distribution of microplastics in subsurface seawater in the NE Pacific Ocean. *Marine Pollution Bulletin*, *79*(1-2), 94–99. Advance online publication. doi:10.1016/j.marpolbul.2013.12.035 PMID:24398418

Détrée, C., & Gallardo-Escárate, C. (2017). Polyethylene microbeads induce transcriptional responses with tissue-dependent patterns in the mussel *Mytilus galloprovincialis. The Journal of Molluscan Studies*, *83*(2), 220–225. doi:10.1093/mollus/eyx005

Di Dong, C., Chen, C. W., Chen, Y. C., Chen, H. H., Lee, J. S., & Lin, C. H. (2020). Polystyrene microplastic particles: In vitro pulmonary toxicity assessment. *Journal of Hazardous Materials*, *385*, 121575. doi:10.1016/j.jhazmat.2019.121575 PMID:31727530

Di Renzo, L., Mascilongo, G., Berti, M., Bogdanović, T., Listeš, E., Brkljača, M., Notarstefano, V., Gioacchini, G., Giorgini, E., Olivieri, V., Silvestri, C., Matiddi, M., D'Alterio, N., Ferri, N., & Di Giacinto, F. (2021). Potential Impact of Microplastics and Additives on the Health Status of Loggerhead Turtles (Caretta caretta) Stranded Along the Central Adriatic Coast. *Water, Air, and Soil Pollution*, *232*(3), 98. Advance online publication. doi:10.100711270-021-04994-8

Diana, Z., Sawickij, N., Rivera, N. A. Jr, Hsu-Kim, H., & Rittschof, D. (2020). Plastic pellets trigger feeding responses in sea anemones. *Aquatic Toxicology (Amsterdam, Netherlands)*, *222*, 105447. doi:10.1016/j.aquatox.2020.105447 PMID:32145485

Diaz-Basantes, M. F., Conesa, J. A., & Fullana, A. (2020). Microplastics in honey, beer, milk and refreshments in Ecuador as emerging contaminants. *Sustainability (Switzerland)*, *12*(12), 5514. Advance online publication. doi:10.3390u12145514

Didier, B. (2015). *Briefing of the European Parliament*. https://www.europarl.europa.eu/RegData/etudes/BRIE/2015/559493/EPRS_BRI(2015)559493_EN.pdf

DiGregorio, B. E. (2009). Biobased performance bioplastic: Mirel. *Chemistry & Biology*, *16*(1), 1–2. doi:10.1016/j.chembiol.2009.01.001 PMID:19171300

Di, M., & Wang, J. (2018). Microplastics in surface waters and sediments of the Three Gorges Reservoir, China. *The Science of the Total Environment*, *616–617*, 1620–1627. doi:10.1016/j.scitotenv.2017.10.150 PMID:29050832

Ding, N., Jiang, L., Wang, X., Wang, C., Geng, Y., Zhang, J., Sun, Y., Zhang, Y., Yuan, Q. & Liu, H. (2021). *The Toxicity of Polyethylene Microplastic Exposure and Its Concurrent Effect With Aeromonas Hydrophila Infection To Zebrafish.* Academic Press.

Ding, Y., Zhang, R., Li, B., Du, Y., Li, J., Tong, X., Wu, Y., Ji, X., & Zhang, Y. (2021). Tissue distribution of polystyrene nanoplastics in mice and their entry, transport, and cytotoxicity to GES-1 cells. *Environmental Pollution*, *280*, 116974. doi:10.1016/j.envpol.2021.116974 PMID:33784569

Dong, Y., Gao, M., Qiu, W., & Song, Z. (2021). Effect of microplastics and arsenic on nutrients and microorganisms in rice rhizosphere soil. *Ecotoxicology and Environmental Safety*, *211*, 111899. doi:10.1016/j.ecoenv.2021.111899 PMID:33453641

Donohue, M. J., Masura, J., Gelatt, T., Ream, R., Baker, J. D., Faulhaber, K., & Lerner, D. T. (2019). Evaluating exposure of northern fur seals, Callorhinus ursinus, to microplastic pollution through fecal analysis. *Marine Pollution Bulletin*, *138*, 213–221. doi:10.1016/j.marpolbul.2018.11.036 PMID:30660265

Dowarah, K., Patchaiyappan, A., Thirunavukkarasu, C., Jayakumar, S., & Devipriya, S. P. (2020). Quantification of microplastics using Nile Red in two bivalve species Perna viridis and Meretrix meretrix from three estuaries in Pondicherry, India and microplastic uptake by local communities through bivalve diet. *Marine Pollution Bulletin*, *153*(February), 110982. doi:10.1016/j.marpolbul.2020.110982 PMID:32275539

Dris, R., Gasperi, J., Mirande, C., Mandin, C., Guerrouache, M., Langlois, V., & Tassin, B. (2017). A first overview of textile fibers, including microplastics, in indoor and outdoor environments. *Environmental Pollution*, *221*, 453–458. doi:10.1016/j.envpol.2016.12.013 PMID:27989388

Dris, R., Gasperi, J., Rocher, V., Saad, M., Renault, N., & Tassin, B. (2015). Microplastic contamination in an urban area: A case study in Greater Paris. *Environmental Chemistry*, *12*(5), 592–599. doi:10.1071/EN14167

Dris, R., Gasperi, J., Saad, M., Mirande, C., & Tassin, B. (2016). Synthetic fibers in atmospheric fallout: A source of microplastics in the environment? *Marine Pollution Bulletin*, *104*(1–2), 290–293. doi:10.1016/j.marpolbul.2016.01.006 PMID:26787549

Duan, J., Bolan, N., Li, Y., Ding, S., Atugoda, T., Vithanage, M., Sarkar, B., Tsang, D. C. W., & Kirkham, M. B. (2021). Weathering of microplastics and interaction with other coexisting constituents in terrestrial and aquatic environments. *Water Research*, *196*, 117011. doi:10.1016/j.watres.2021.117011 PMID:33743325

Du, J., Xu, S., Zhou, Q., Li, H., Fu, L., Tang, J., Wang, Y., Peng, X., Xu, Y., & Du, X. (2020). A review of microplastics in the aquatic environmental: Distribution, transport, ecotoxicology, and toxicological mechanisms. *Environmental Science and Pollution Research International*, *27*(11), 11494–11505. doi:10.100711356-020-08104-9 PMID:32088821

Dümichen, E., Barthel, A. K., Braun, U., Bannick, C. G., Brand, K., Jekel, M., & Senz, R. (2015). Analysis of polyethylene microplastics in environmental samples, using a thermal decomposition method. *Water Research*, *85*, 451–457. doi:10.1016/j.watres.2015.09.002 PMID:26376022

Dunlap, R. E., & Scarce, R. (1991). Poll trends: Environmental problems and protection. *Public Opinion Quarterly*, *55*(4), 651–672. doi:10.1086/269288

Ebbesen, M. F., Gerke, C., Hartwig, P., & Hartmann, L. (2016). Biodegradable poly(amidoamine)s with uniform degradation fragments via sequence-controlled macromonomers. *Polymer Chemistry*, *7*(46), 7086–7093. doi:10.1039/C6PY01700B

Ebere, E. C., Wirnkor, V. A., & Ngozi, V. E. (2019). Uptake of microplastics by plant: A reason to worry or to be happy? *World Scientific News*, *131*, 256–267.

EC (European Commission). (2018). *A European Strategy for Plastics in a Circular Economy*. https://ec.europa.eu/environment/strategy/plastics-strategy_en

EC (European Commission). (2019). *Directive on single-use plastics.* https://eur-lex.europa.eu/legal-content/EN/TXT/PDF/?uri=CELEX:32019L0904&from=EN

Eckelman, M. J., Ashton, W., Arakaki, Y., Hanaki, K., Nagashima, S., & Malone-Lee, L. C. (2014). Island waste management systems: Statistics, challenges, and opportunities for applied industrial ecology. *Journal of Industrial Ecology, 18*(2), 306–317. doi:10.1111/jiec.12113

ECORYS (2016). *Study on Specific Challenges for a Sustainable Development of Coastal and Maritime Tourism in Europe.* doi:10.2826/94993

ECORYS. (2013). *Study in Support of Policy Measures for Maritime and Coastal Tourism at EU Level.* ECORYS.

EEA (European Environmental Agency). (2016). *Restoring European rivers and lakes in cities improves quality of life.* https://www.eea.europa.eu/highlights/restoring-european-rivers-and-lakes

Eerkes-Medrano, D., Thompson, R. C., & Aldridge, D. C. (2015). Microplastics in freshwater systems: A review of the emerging threats, identification of knowledge gaps and prioritisation of research needs. *Water Research, 75*, 63–82. doi:10.1016/j.watres.2015.02.012 PMID:25746963

Egessa, R., Nankabirwa, A., Ocaya, H., & Pabire, W. G. (2020). Microplastic pollution in surface water of Lake Victoria. In *Science of the Total Environment* (Vol. 741). Elsevier. doi:10.1016/j.scitotenv.2020.140201

Eggink, G., deWaard, P., & Huijberts, G. N. (1995). Formation of novel poly(hydroxyalkanoates) from long-chain fatty acids. *Canadian Journal of Microbiology, 41*(13), 14–21. doi:10.1139/m95-163 PMID:7606658

Eldsäter, C., Albertsson, A. C., & Karlsson, S. (1997). Impact of degradation mechanisms on poly(3-hydroxybutyrate-co-3-hydroxyvalerate) during composting. *Acta Polymerica, 48*(11), 478–483. doi:10.1002/actp.1997.010481103

Elizalde-Velázquez, G. A., & Gómez-Oliván, L. M. (2021). Microplastics in aquatic environments: A review on occurrence, distribution, toxic effects, and implications for human health. *The Science of the Total Environment, 780*, 146551. doi:10.1016/j.scitotenv.2021.146551 PMID:33773347

Elkhatib, D., & Oyanedel-Craver, V. (2020). A Critical Review of Extraction and Identification Methods of Microplastics in Wastewater and Drinking Water. *Environmental Science & Technology, 54*(12), 7037–7049. doi:10.1021/acs.est.9b06672 PMID:32432459

Enders, A. C., & Blankenship, T. N. (1999). Comparative placental structure. *Advanced Drug Delivery Reviews, 38*(1), 3–15. doi:10.1016/S0169-409X(99)00003-4 PMID:10837743

Enders, K., Lenz, R., Beer, S., & Stedmon, C. A. (2017). Extraction of microplastic from biota: Recommended acidic digestion destroys common plastic polymers. *ICES Journal of Marine Science, 74*(1), 326–331. doi:10.1093/icesjms/fsw173

Engler, R. E. (2012). Chemicals in the Ocean. *Environmental Science & Technology, 46*, 302–315. PMID:23088563

Eo, S., Hong, S. H., Song, Y. K., Han, G. M., & Shim, W. J. (2019). Spatiotemporal distribution and annual load of microplastics in the Nakdong River, South Korea. In *Water Research* (Vol. 160, pp. 228–237). Pergamon-Elsevier Science Ltd. doi:10.1016/j.watres.2019.05.053

EPA. (2021). *EPA Research about Coral Reefs.* https://www.epa.gov/coral-reefs/epa-research-about-coral-reefs#Biological-Criteria

Eppehimer, D. E., Hamdhani, H., Hollien, K. D., Nemec, Z. C., Lee, L. N., Quanrud, D. M., & Bogan, M. T. (2021). Impacts of baseflow and flooding on microplastic pollution in an effluent-dependent arid land river in the USA. In Environmental Science and Pollution Research (Vol. 28, Issue 33, pp. 45375–45389). Springer Heidelberg. doi:10.100711356-021-13724-w

Eriksen, M., Lebreton, L. C., Carson, H. S., Thiel, M., Moore, C. J., Borerro, J. C., Galgani, F., Ryan, P. G., & Reisser, J. (2014). Plastic pollution in the world's oceans: More than 5 trillion plastic pieces weighing over 250,000 tons afloat at sea. *PLoS One*, *9*(12), e111913. doi:10.1371/journal.pone.0111913 PMID:25494041

Eriksson, C., & Burton, H. (2003). Origins and biological accumulation of small plastic particles in fur seals from Macquarie Island. *Ambio*, *32*(6), 380–384. doi:10.1579/0044-7447-32.6.380 PMID:14627365

Eriksson, C., Burton, H., Fitch, S., Schulz, M., & van den Hoff, J. (2013). Daily accumulation rates of marine debris on sub-Antarctic island beaches. *Marine Pollution Bulletin*, *66*(1-2), 199–208. doi:10.1016/j.marpolbul.2012.08.026 PMID:23219394

Erni-Cassola, G., Zadjelovic, V., Gibson, M. I., & Christie-Oleza, J. A. (2019). Distribution of plastic polymer types in the marine environment; A meta-analysis. *Journal of Hazardous Materials*, *369*, 691–698. Advance online publication. doi:10.1016/j.jhazmat.2019.02.067 PMID:30826562

Espinosa, C., Cuesta, A., & Esteban, M. Á. (2017). Effects of dietary polyvinylchloride microparticles on general health, immune status and expression of several genes related to stress in gilthead seabream (*Sparus aurata L.*). *Fish & Shellfish Immunology*, *68*, 251–259. doi:10.1016/j.fsi.2017.07.006 PMID:28684324

Espinosa, C., García Beltrán, J. M., Esteban, M. A., & Cuesta, A. (2018). In vitro effects of virgin microplastics on fish head-kidney leucocyte activities. *Environmental Pollution*, *235*, 30–38. doi:10.1016/j.envpol.2017.12.054 PMID:29274535

Essefi, E. (2021a). Parallel evolution of energy consumption and environmental pollution during the Anthropocene. *Journal of Global Ecology and Environment*, 36-42.

Essefi, E. (2021b). Record of the Anthropocene-Great Acceleration along a core from the coast of Sfax, southeastern Tunisia. *Turkish Journal of Earth Science*, 1-16.

Essefi, E. (2022b). Millennial to Centennial Cyclicity Within the Exoreic Saline System of Boujmel, Southern Tunisia. In Handbook of Research on Monitoring and Evaluating the Ecological Health of Wetlands (pp. 230-251). IGI Global.

Essefi, E., & Hajji, S. (2022a). Response of Erosion to Environmental and Climate Changes During the Anthropocene Within the Endorheic System of Mhabeul, Southeastern Tunisia. In Prevention and Management of Soil Erosion and Torrential Floods (pp. 217-234). IGI Global.

Essefi, E. (2020). On the Geochemistry and Mineralogy of the Anthropocene. *Int J Water Wastewater Treat*, *6*(2).

Essefi, E. (2021c). Homo Sapiens Sapiens Progressive Defaunation During The Great Acceleration: The Cli-Fi Apocalypse Hypothesis. *International Journal of Toxicology and Toxicity Assessment*, *1*(1), 1–6.

Eubeler, J. P., Bernhard, M., & Knepper, T. P. (2010). Environmental biodegradation of synthetic polymers II. Biodegradation of different polymer groups. Trends in Analytical Chemistry (Reference Ed.), 29, 84–100.

EUNOMIA. (2016). *Plastics in the Marine Environment*. https://www.eunomia.co.uk/reports-tools/plastics-in-the-marine-environment/

Europe, P. (2020). *Plastics – the Facts 2019, an Analysis of European Plastics Production, Demand and Waste Data.* https://www.plasticseurope.org/en/resources/market-data

European Chemicals Agency (ECHA). (2019). *Annex XV Restriction Report. Proposal for a Restriction.* Intentionally Added Microplastics. ECHA.

European Commission. (2013). *MSDF Guidance on Monitoring Marine Litter.* doi:10.2788/99475

Europen. (2009). *The European Shopping Baskets – Packaging trends for Fast Moving Consumer Goods in Selected European Countries*. Europen, The European Organization for packaging and the environment. https://www.leanbusinessireland.ie/includes/documents/Public%2520Phase%2520I%2520ESB%2520Report%5B1%5D.pdf

Europe, P. (2020). Plastics–the facts 2020. *PlasticEurope*, *1*, 1–64.

Everaert, G., Van Cauwenberghe, L., De Rijcke, M., Koelmans, A. A., Mees, J., Vandegehuchte, M., & Janssen, C. R. (2018). Risk assessment of microplastics in the ocean: Modelling approach and first conclusions. *Environmental Pollution*, *242*, 1930–1938. doi:10.1016/j.envpol.2018.07.069 PMID:30061084

Facciolà, A., Visalli, G., Pruiti Ciarello, M., & Di Pietro, A. (2021). Newly Emerging Airborne Pollutants: Current Knowledge of Health Impact of Micro and Nanoplastics. *International Journal of Environmental Research and Public Health*, *18*(6), 2997. doi:10.3390/ijerph18062997 PMID:33803962

Fan, J., Zou, L., & Zhao, G. (2021). Microplastic abundance, distribution, and composition in the surface water and sediments of the Yangtze River along Chongqing City, China. In Journal of Soils and Sediments (Vol. 21, Issue 4, pp. 1840–1851). Springer heidelberg. doi:10.100711368-021-02902-5

Fan, Y., Zheng, K., Zhu, Z., Chen, G., & Peng, X. (2019). Distribution, sedimentary record, and persistence of microplastics in the Pearl River catchment, China. In *Environmental Pollution* (Vol. 251, pp. 862–870). Elsevier Sci Ltd. doi:10.1016/j.envpol.2019.05.056

FAO (Food and Agriculture Organization of the United Nations). (2017). *Microplastics in fisheries and aquaculture. Status of knowledge on their occurrence and implications for aquatic organisms and food safety.* FAO. https://www.fao.org/3/I7677E/I7677E.pdf

Farrell, P., & Nelson, K. (2013). Trophic level transfer of microplastic: *Mytilus edulis* (L.) to *Carcinus maenas* (L.). *Environmental Pollution*, *177*, 1–3. doi:10.1016/j.envpol.2013.01.046 PMID:23434827

Felsing, S., Kochleus, C., Buchinger, S., Brennholt, N., Stock, F., & Reifferscheid, G. (2018). A new approach in separating microplastics from environmental samples based on their electrostatic behavior. *Environmental Pollution*, *234*, 20–28. doi:10.1016/j.envpol.2017.11.013 PMID:29154206

Fendall, L. S., & Sewell, M. A. (2009). Contributing to marine pollution by washing your face: Microplastics in facial cleansers. *Marine Pollution Bulletin*, *58*(8), 1225–1228. doi:10.1016/j.marpolbul.2009.04.025 PMID:19481226

Feng, X., Wang, Q., Sun, Y., Zhang, S., & Wang, F. (2022). Microplastics change soil properties, heavy metal availability and bacterial community in a Pb-Zn contaminated soil. *Journal of Hazardous Materials*, *424*, 127364. doi:10.1016/j.jhazmat.2021.127364 PMID:34879561

Feng, Z., Zhang, T., Wang, J., Huang, W., Wang, R., Xu, J., Fu, G., & Gao, G. (2020). Spatio-temporal features of microplastics pollution in macroalgae growing in an important mariculture area, China. *The Science of the Total Environment*, *719*, 137490. doi:10.1016/j.scitotenv.2020.137490 PMID:32143099

Ferraro, G., & Failler, P. (2020). Governing plastic pollution in the oceans: Institutional challenges and areas. *Environmental Science & Policy*, *112*, 453–460. doi:10.1016/j.envsci.2020.06.015

Ferraz, M., Bauer, A. L., Valiati, V. H., & Schulz, U. H. (2020). Microplastic Concentrations in Raw and Drinking Water in the Sinos River, Southern Brazil. In Water (Vol. 12, Issue 11). MDPI. doi:10.3390/w12113115

Ferreira, I., Venâncio, C., Lopes, I., & Oliveira, M. (2019). Nanoplastics and marine organisms: What has been studied? *Environmental Toxicology and Pharmacology*, *67*, 1–7. doi:10.1016/j.etap.2019.01.006 PMID:30685594

Filiciotto, L., & Rothenberg, G. (2021). Biodegradable plastics: Standards, policies, and impacts. *ChemSusChem*, *14*(1), 56–72. doi:10.1002/cssc.202002044 PMID:33112051

Fischer, E. K., Paglialonga, L., Czech, E., & Tamminga, M. (2016). Microplastic pollution in lakes and lake shoreline sediments - A case study on Lake Bolsena and Lake Chiusi (central Italy). *Environmental Pollution*, *213*, 648–657. doi:10.1016/j.envpol.2016.03.012 PMID:27104923

Fischer, M., & Scholz-Böttcher, B. M. (2017). Simultaneous Trace Identification and Quantification of Common Types of Microplastics in Environmental Samples by Pyrolysis-Gas Chromatography-Mass Spectrometry. *Environmental Science & Technology*, *51*(9), 5052–5060. doi:10.1021/acs.est.6b06362 PMID:28391690

Fleming, S. (2020). *Scientists find plastic pollution in the rain and in the air we breathe.* https://www.weforum.org/agenda/2020/07/scientists-find-plastic-pollution-in-the-rain-and-in-the-air-we-breathe/

Flury, M., & Narayan, R. (2021). Biodegradable plastic as an integral part of the solution to plastic waste pollution of the environment. *Current Opinion in Green and Sustainable Chemistry, 30.*

Foekema, E. M., De Gruijter, C., Mergia, M. T., Van Franeker, J. A., Murk, A. J., & Koelmans, A. A. (2013). Plastic in north sea fish. *Environmental Science & Technology*, *47*(15), 8818–8824. doi:10.1021/es400931b PMID:23777286

Folke, C., Polasky, S., Rockström, J., Galaz, V., Westley, F., Lamont, M., ... Walker, B. H. (2021). Our future in the Anthropocene biosphere. *Ambio*, 1–36. PMID:33715097

Fonte, E., Ferreira, P., & Guilhermino, L. (2016). Temperature rise and microplastics interact with the toxicity of the antibiotic cefalexin to juveniles of the common goby (*Pomatoschistus microps*): Post-exposure predatory behaviour, acetylcholinesterase activity and lipid peroxidation. *Aquatic Toxicology (Amsterdam, Netherlands)*, *180*, 173–185. doi:10.1016/j.aquatox.2016.09.015 PMID:27721112

Forrest, A. K., & Hindell, M. (2018). Ingestion of plastic by fish destined for human consumption in remote South Pacific Islands. *Australian Journal of Maritime and Ocean Affairs*, *10*(2), 81–97. doi:10.1080/18366503.2018.1460945

Forte, M., Iachetta, G., Tussellino, M., Carotenuto, R., Prisco, M., De Falco, M., Laforgia, V., & Valiante, S. (2016). Polystyrene nanoparticles internalization in human gastric adenocarcinoma cells. *Toxicology in Vitro: An International Journal, 31*, 126–136.

Fotopoulou, K. N., & Karapanagioti, H. K. (2012). Surface properties of beached plastic pellets. *Marine Environmental Research*, *81*, 70–77. doi:10.1016/j.marenvres.2012.08.010 PMID:23013745

Fraissinet, S., Pennetta, A., Rossi, S., De Benedetto, G. E., & Malitesta, C. (2021). Optimization of a new multi-reagent procedure for quantitative mussel digestion in microplastic analysis. *Marine Pollution Bulletin, 173*(PA), 112931. doi:10.1016/j.marpolbul.2021.112931

Franco, A. A., Arellano, J. M., Albendin, G., Rodriguez-Barroso, R., Quiroga, J. M., & Coello, M. D. (2021). Microplastic pollution in wastewater treatment plants in the city of C?diz: Abundance, removal efficiency and presence in receiving water body. In *Science of the Total Environment* (Vol. 776). Elsevier. doi:10.1016/j.scitotenv.2021.145795

Franzellitti, S., Canesi, L., Auguste, M., Wathsala, R., & Fabbri, E. (2019). Microplastic exposure and effects in aquatic organisms: A physiological perspective. *Environmental Toxicology and Pharmacology*, *68*, 37–51. doi:10.1016/j.etap.2019.03.009 PMID:30870694

Free, C. M., Jensen, O. P., Mason, S. A., Eriksen, M., Williamson, N. J., & Boldgiv, B. (2014). High-levels of microplastic pollution in a large, remote, mountain lake. *Marine Pollution Bulletin, 85*(1), 156–163. doi:10.1016/j.marpolbul.2014.06.001 PMID:24973278

Frias, J. P. G. L., & Nash, R. (2019). Microplastics: Finding a consensus on the definition. *Marine Pollution Bulletin, 138*(November), 145–147. doi:10.1016/j.marpolbul.2018.11.022

Frias, J., Pagter, E., Nash, R., O'Connor, I., Carretero, O., Filgueiras, A., Viñas, L., Gago, J., Antunes, J., Bessa, F., Sobral, P., Goruppi, A., Tirelli, V., Pedrotti, M. L., Suaria, G., Aliani, S., Lopes, C., Raimundo, J., Caetano, M., … Gerdts, G. (2018). Standardised protocol for monitoring microplastics in sediments. *JPI-Oceans BASEMAN Project,* 33. doi:10.13140/RG.2.2.36256.89601/1

Fries, E., Deki, H., Willmeyer, J., Nuelle, M., & Remy, D. (2013). *Environmental Science Processes & Impacts scanning electron microscopy*. doi:10.1039/c3em00214d

Fukuzaki, H., Yoshida, M., Asano, M., & Kumakura, M. (1989). Synthesis of copoly(d, l-lactic acid) with relative low molecular weight and in vitro degradation. *European Polymer Journal, 25*(10), 1019–1026. doi:10.1016/0014-3057(89)90131-6

Fuller, S., & Gautam, A. (2016). A Procedure for Measuring Microplastics using Pressurized Fluid Extraction. *Environmental Science & Technology, 50*(11), 5774–5780. doi:10.1021/acs.est.6b00816 PMID:27172172

Furukuma, S. (2021). A study of 'new plastic formations' found in the Seto Inland Sea, Japan. *Int. J. Sci. Res. Publ., 11*(6), 185–188. doi:10.29322/IJSRP.11.06.2021.p11427

G20 Germany. (2017). *G20 Action Plan on Marine litter.* G20 Germany.

G20. (2017). *G20 Action Plan on Marine Litter.* Retrieved from https://www.mofa.go.jp/mofaj/files/000272290.pdf

G7, Annex to the Leaders' Declaration. (2015.). *G7 Summit 7–8 June 2015. Think ahead Act together.* An morgen denken. Gemeinsam handeln.

Galgani, F., Brien, A. S., Weis, J., Ioakeimidis, C., Schuyler, Q., Makarenko, I., Griffiths, H., Bondareff, J., Vethaak, D., Deidun, A., Sobral, P., Topouzelis, K., Vlahos, P., Lana, F., Hassellov, M., Gerigny, O., Arsonina, B., Ambulkar, A., Azzaro, M., & Bebianno, M. J. (2021). Are litter, plastic and microplastic quantities increasing in the ocean? *Microplastics and Nanoplastics, 1*(1), 8–11. doi:10.118643591-020-00002-8

Galgani, L., Engel, A., Rossi, C., Donati, A., & Loiselle, S. A. (2018). Polystyrene microplastics increase microbial release of marine Chromophoric Dissolved Organic Matter in microcosm experiments. *Scientific Reports, 8*(1), 1–11. doi:10.103841598-018-32805-4 PMID:30279474

Galgani, L., & Loiselle, S. A. (2021). Plastic pollution impacts on marine carbon biogeochemistry. *Environmental Pollution, 268,* 115598. doi:10.1016/j.envpol.2020.115598 PMID:33158618

Galloway, T. S., Cole, M., & Lewis, C. (2017). Interactions of microplastic debris throughout the marine ecosystem. *Nature Ecology & Evolution, 1*(5), 1–8. doi:10.103841559-017-0116 PMID:28812686

Gamaralalage, P., & Onogawa, K. (2019). *Strategies to Reduce Marine Plastic Pollution from Land-based Sources in Low and Middle - Income Countries*. UNEP.

Gambardella, C., Morgana, S., Bramini, M., Rotini, A., Manfra, L., Migliore, L., Piazza, V., Garaventa, F., & Faimali, M. (2018). Ecotoxicological effects of polystyrene microbeads in a battery of marine organisms belonging to different trophic levels. *Marine Environmental Research, 141,* 313–321. Advance online publication. doi:10.1016/j.marenvres.2018.09.023 PMID:30274720

Gambardella, C., Morgana, S., Ferrando, S., Bramini, M., Piazza, V., Costa, E., Garaventa, F., & Faimali, M. (2017). Effects of polystyrene microbeads in marine planktonic crustaceans. *Ecotoxicology and Environmental Safety, 145*, 250–257. doi:10.1016/j.ecoenv.2017.07.036 PMID:28750293

Ganapathy, V., Prasad, P. D., Ganapathy, M. E., & Leibach, F. H. (2000). Placental transporters relevant to drug distribution across the maternal-fetal interface. *The Journal of Pharmacology and Experimental Therapeutics, 294*, 413–420. PMID:10900213

Gao, B., Yao, H., Li, Y., & Zhu, Y. (2021). Microplastic addition alters the microbial community structure and stimulates soil carbon dioxide emissions in vegetable-growing soil. *Environmental Toxicology and Chemistry, 40*(2), 352–365. doi:10.1002/etc.4916 PMID:33105038

Gao, M., Liu, Y., & Song, Z. (2019). Effects of polyethylene microplastic on the phytotoxicity of di-n-butyl phthalate in lettuce (*Lactuca sativa* L. *var. ramosa Hort*). *Chemosphere, 237*, 124482. doi:10.1016/j.chemosphere.2019.124482 PMID:31398608

Garcia, A. G., Suarez, D. C., Li, J., & Rotchell, J. M. (2021). A comparison of microplastic contamination in freshwater fish from natural and farmed sources. In Environmental Science and Pollution Research (Vol. 28, Issue 12, pp. 14488–14497). Springer Heidelberg. doi:10.100711356-020-11605-2

Gardon, T., Morvan, L., Huvet, A., Quillien, V., Soyez, C., Le Moullac, G., & Le Luyer, J. (2020). Microplastics induce dose-specific transcriptomic disruptions in energy metabolism and immunity of the pearl oyster *Pinctada margaritifera. Environmental Pollution, 115180.* Advance online publication. doi:10.1016/j.envpol.2020.115180 PMID:32673975

Gardon, T., Reisser, C., Soyez, C., Quillien, V., & Le Moullac, G. (2018). Microplastics Affect Energy Balance and Gametogenesis in the Pearl Oyster *Pinctada margaritifera. Environmental Science & Technology, 52*(9), 5277–5286. doi:10.1021/acs.est.8b00168 PMID:29620881

Garg, A., Basu, S., Shetti, N. P., & Reddy, K. R. (2021). 2D materials and its heterostructured photocatalysts: Synthesis, properties, functionalization and applications in environmental remediation. *Journal of Environmental Chemical Engineering, 9*(6), 106408. doi:10.1016/j.jece.2021.106408

Gasperi, J., Wright, S. L., Dris, R., Collard, F., Mandin, C., Guerrouache, M., Langlois, V., Kelly, F. J., & Tassin, B. (2018). Microplastics in air: Are we breathing it in? *Current Opinion in Environmental Science & Health, 1*, 1–5. doi:10.1016/j.coesh.2017.10.002

Geiser, M., Rothen-Rutishauser, B., Kapp, N., Schurch, S., Kreyling, W., Schulz, H., Semmler, M., Im Hof, V., Heyder, J., & Gehr, P. (2005). Ultrafine particles cross cellular membranes by nonphagocytic mechanisms in lungs and in cultured cells. *Environmental Health Perspectives, 113*(11), 1555–1560. doi:10.1289/ehp.8006 PMID:16263511

Ge, J., Li, H., Liu, P., Zhang, Z., Ouyang, Z., & Guo, X. (2021). Review of the toxic effect of microplastics on terrestrial and aquatic plants. *The Science of the Total Environment, 791*, 148333. doi:10.1016/j.scitotenv.2021.148333 PMID:34412379

Geng, X., Wang, J., Zhang, Y., & Jiang, Y. (2021). How do microplastics affect the marine microbial loop? Predation of microplastics by microzooplankton. *The Science of the Total Environment, 758*, 144030. doi:10.1016/j.scitotenv.2020.144030 PMID:33340809

George, M., & Fabre, P. (2021). Floating plastics in oceans: A matter of size. *Current Opinion in Green and Sustainable Chemistry, 32*, 100543. doi:10.1016/j.cogsc.2021.100543

GESAMP Joint Group of Experts on the Scientific Aspects of Marine Environmental Protection. (2016). Sources, fate and effects of microplastics in the marine environment: part 2 of a global assessment. IMO, FAO/UNESCO-IOC/UNIDO/WMO/IAEA/UN/UNEP/UNDP.

GESAMP. (2015). *Sources, fate and effects of microplastics in the marine environment: A global assessment.* GESAMP. https://ec.europa.eu/environment/marine/good-environmental-status/descriptor-10/pdf/GESAMP_microplastics%20 full%20study.pdf

GESAMP. (2016). *Sources, fate and effects of microplastics in the marine environment: Part 2 of a global assessment.* GESAMP. http://www.gesamp.org/publications/microplastics-in-the-marine-environment-part-2

GESAMP. (2016). Sources, fate and effects of microplastics in the marine environment: part two of a global assessment. IMO/FAO/UNESCO-IOC/UNIDO/WMO/IAEA/UN/ UNEP/UNDP Joint Group of Experts on the Scientific Aspects of Marine Environmental Protection.

Gewert, B., MacLeod, M., & Breitholtz, M. (2021). Variability in Toxicity of Plastic Leachates as a Function of Weathering and Polymer Type: A Screening Study with the Copepod *Nitocra spinipes. The Biological Bulletin, 240*(3), 191–199. doi:10.1086/714506 PMID:34129442

Gewert, B., Plassmann, M. M., & MacLeod, M. (2015). Pathways for degradation of plastic polymers floating in the marine environment. *Environmental Science. Processes & Impacts, 17*(9), 1513–1521. doi:10.1039/C5EM00207A PMID:26216708

Geyer, R., Jambeck, J. R., & Law, K. L. (2017). Production, use, and fate of all plastics ever made. *Science Advances, 3*(7), e1700782. doi:10.1126ciadv.1700782 PMID:28776036

Ghaffari, S., Bakhtiari, A. R., Ghasempouri, S. M., & Nasrolahi, A. (2019). The influence of human activity and morphological characteristics of beaches on plastic debris distribution along the Caspian Sea as a closed water body. In Environmental Science and Pollution Research (Vol. 26, Issue 25, pp. 25712–25724). Springer Heidelberg. doi:10.100711356-019-05790-y

Ghatge, S., Yang, Y., Ahn, J. H., & Hur, H.-G. (2020). Biodegradation of polyethylene: A brief review. *Applied Biological Chemistry, 63*(1), 27. doi:10.118613765-020-00511-3

Ghosh, S. K., Pal, S., & Ray, S. (2013). Study of microbes having potentiality for biodegradation of plastics. *Environmental Science and Pollution Research International, 20*(7), 4339–4355. doi:10.100711356-013-1706-x PMID:23613206

Gigault, J., Halle, A. T., Baudrimont, M., Pascal, P. Y., Gauffre, F., Phi, T. L., El Hadri, H., Grassl, B., & Reynaud, S. (2018). Current opinion: What is a nanoplastic? *Environmental Pollution, 235*, 1030–1034.

Gigault, J., ter Halle, A., Baudrimont, M., Pascal, P. Y., Gauffre, F., Phi, T. L., El Hadri, H., Grassl, B., & Reynaud, S. (2018). Current opinion: What is a nanoplastic? *Environmental Pollution, 235*, 1030–1034. doi:10.1016/j.envpol.2018.01.024 PMID:29370948

Gillibert, R., Balakrishnan, G., Deshoules, Q., Tardivel, M., Magazzu, A., Donato, M. G., Marago, O. M., Lamy, M., Chapelle, D. La, Colas, F., Lagarde, F., & Gucciardi, P. G. (2019). *Raman Tweezers for Small Microplastics and Nanoplastics Identi fi cation in Seawater.* doi:10.1021/acs.est.9b03105

Gilman, E. (2015). Status of international monitoring and management of abandoned, lost and discarded fishing gear and ghost fishing. *Marine Policy, 60*, 225–239. doi:10.1016/j.marpol.2015.06.016

Gkoutselis, G., Rohrbach, S., Harjes, J., Obst, M., Brachmann, A., Horn, M. A., & Rambold, G. (2021). Microplastics accumulate fungal pathogens in terrestrial ecosystems. *Scientific Reports, 11*(1), 1–13. doi:10.103841598-021-92405-7 PMID:34267241

Gokce, E. (2018). Rethinking sustainability: A research on starch based bioplastic. *Journal of Sustainable Construction Materials and Technologies, 3*(3), 249–260. doi:10.29187/jscmt.2018.28

Goldsworthy, S. D., Hindell, M. A., & Crowley, H. M. (1997). *Diet and diving behaviour of sympatric fur seals Arctocephalus gazella and A. tropicalis at Macquarie Island, Marine Mammal Research in the Southern Hemisphere* (Vol. 1). Status, Ecology and Medicine.

Golwala, H., Zhang, X., Iskander, S. M., & Smith, A. L. (2021). Solid waste: An overlooked source of microplastics to the environment. *The Science of the Total Environment*, *769*, 144581. doi:10.1016/j.scitotenv.2020.144581 PMID:33482549

Gomes, T., Almeida, A. C., & Georgantzopoulou, A. (2020). Characterization of cell responses in *Rhodomonas baltica* exposed to PMMA nanoplastics. *The Science of the Total Environment*, *726*, 138547. doi:10.1016/j.scitotenv.2020.138547 PMID:32320882

Gonçalves, H. C., Mercante, M. A., & Santos, E. T. (2011). Hydrological cycle. *Brazilian Journal of Biology*, *71*(1), 241–253. doi:10.1590/S1519-69842011000200003 PMID:21537597

Gonçalves, J. M., Sousa, V. S., Teixeira, M. R., & Bebianno, M. J. (2022, January). Chronic toxicity of polystyrene nanoparticles in the marine mussel *Mytilus galloprovincialis. Chemosphere*, *287*, 132356. doi:10.1016/j.chemosphere.2021.132356 PMID:34600009

Gong, Y., Putnam, E., You, W., & Zhao, C. (2020). Investigation into circular economy of plastics: The case of the UK fast moving consumer goods industry. *Journal of Cleaner Production*, *244*, 118941. doi:10.1016/j.jclepro.2019.118941

González, D., Hanke, G., Tweehuysen, G., Bellert, B., Holzhauer, M., Palatinus, A., Hohenblum, P., & Oosterbaan, L. (2016). Riverine Litter Monitoring - Options and Recommendations - Thematic Report. In *JRC Scientific and Technical Reports*. doi:10.2788/461233

González-Fernández, C., Le Grand, F., Bideau, A., Huvet, A., Paul-Pont, I., & Soudant, P. (2020). Nanoplastics exposure modulate lipid and pigment compositions in diatoms. *Environmental Pollution*, *262*, 114274. Advance online publication. doi:10.1016/j.envpol.2020.114274 PMID:32135430

González-Fernández, C., Tallec, K., Le Goïc, N., Lambert, C., Soudant, P., Huvet, A., Suquet, M., Berchel, M., & Paul-Pont, I. (2018). Cellular responses of Pacific oyster (Crassostrea gigas) gametes exposed in vitro to polystyrene nanoparticles. *Chemosphere*, *208*, 764–772. doi:10.1016/j.chemosphere.2018.06.039 PMID:29902761

Gopinath, K., Seshachalam, S., Neelavannan, K., Anburaj, V., Rachel, M., Ravi, S., Bharath, M., & Achyuthan, H. (2020). Quantification of microplastic in Red Hills Lake of Chennai city, Tamil Nadu, India. In Environmental Science and Pollution Research (Vol. 27, Issues 26, SI, pp. 33297–33306). Springer Heidelberg. doi:10.100711356-020-09622-2

Gorrasi, G., Sorrentino, A., & Lichtfouse, E. (2021). Back to plastic pollution in COVID times. *Environmental Chemistry Letters*, *19*(1), 1–4. doi:10.100710311-020-01129-z PMID:33192208

Goss, H., Jaskiel, J., & Rotjan, R. (2018). Thalassia testudinum as a potential vector for incorporating microplastics into benthic marine food webs. *Marine Pollution Bulletin*, *135*, 1085–1089. doi:10.1016/j.marpolbul.2018.08.024 PMID:30301005

Government Communication Unit. (2019). *Notice to travellers planning to visit Tanzania*. The United Republic of Tanzania Vice President's Office.

Govil, T., Wang, J., Samanta, D., David, A., Tripathi, A., Rauniyar, S., Salem, D. R., & Sani, R. K. (2020). Lignocellulosic feedstock: A review of a sustainable platform for cleaner production of nature's plastics. *Journal of Cleaner Production*, *270*, 122521. doi:10.1016/j.jclepro.2020.122521

Grafmuller, S., Manser, P., Krug, H. F., Wick, P., & von Mandach, U. (2013). Determination of the transport rate of xenobiotics and nanomaterials across the placenta using the *ex vivo* human placental perfusion model. *Journal of Visualized Experiments, 18*(76), 76. doi:10.3791/50401 PMID:23851364

Graham, E. R., & Thompson, J. T. (2009). Deposit-and suspension-feeding sea cucumbers (Echinodermata) ingest plastic fragments. *Journal of Experimental Marine Biology and Ecology, 368*(1), 22–29. doi:10.1016/j.jembe.2008.09.007

Green, D. S. (2016). Effects of microplastics on European flat oysters, Ostrea edulis and their associated benthic communities. *Environmental Pollution, 216*, 95–103. doi:10.1016/j.envpol.2016.05.043 PMID:27239693

Green, D. S., Boots, B., O'Connor, N. E., & Thompson, R. (2016). Microplastics Affect the Ecological Functioning of an Important Biogenic Habitat. *Environmental Science & Technology, 51*(1), 68–77. doi:10.1021/acs.est.6b04496 PMID:27936642

Green, D. S., Boots, B., Sigwart, J., Jiang, S., & Rocha, C. (2016). Effects of conventional and biodegradable microplastics on a marine ecosystem engineer (Arenicola marina) and sediment nutrient cycling. *Environmental Pollution, 208*, 426–434. doi:10.1016/j.envpol.2015.10.010 PMID:26552519

Greene, J. P. (2014). *Sustainable Plastics.* John Wiley & Sons, Ltd. doi:10.1002/9781118899595

Greenpeace. (2020). *34 Plastic Bans in Africa. A Reality Check.* https://www.greenpeace.org/africa/

Gregory, M. R. (2009). Environmental implications of plastic debris in marine settings—Entanglement, ingestion, smothering, hangers-on, hitch-hiking and alien invasions. Philos. Trans. R. Soc. Lond. Ser. B Biol. *Sci., 364*(1526), 2013–2025. PMID:19528053

Greven, A. C., Merk, T., Karagöz, F., Mohr, K., Klapper, M., Jovanović, B., & Palić, D. (2016). Polycarbonate and polystyrene nanoplastic particles act as stressors to the innate immune system of fathead minnow (*Pimephales promelas*). *Environmental Toxicology and Chemistry, 35*(12), 3093–3100. doi:10.1002/etc.3501 PMID:27207313

Grillo, J. F., Sabino, M. A., & Ramos, R. (2021). Short-term ingestion and tissue incorporation of Polystyrene microplastic in the scleractinian coral *Porites porites. Regional Studies in Marine Science, 43*, 101697. doi:10.1016/j.rsma.2021.101697

Gruber, M. M., Hirschmugl, B., Berger, N., Holter, M., Radulović, S., Leitinger, G., & Wadsack, C. (2020). Plasma proteins facilitates placental transfer of polystyrene particles. *Journal of Nanobiotechnology, 18*(1), 1–14. doi:10.118612951-020-00676-5 PMID:32907583

Guerranti, C., Perra, G., Martellini, T., Giari, L., & Cincinelli, A. (2020). Knowledge about microplastic in mediterranean tributary river ecosystems: Lack of data and research needs on such a crucial marine pollution source. *Journal of Marine Science and Engineering, 8*(3), 216. Advance online publication. doi:10.3390/jmse8030216

Guglielmi, G. (2017). *In the next 30 years, we'll make four times more plastic waste than we ever have.* https://www.sciencemag.org/news/2017/07/next-30-years-we-ll-make-four-times-more-plastic-waste-we-ever-have

Gu, H., Wei, S., Hu, M., Wei, H., Wang, X., Shang, Y., Li, L., Shi, H., & Wang, Y. (2020). Microplastics aggravate the adverse effects of BDE-47 on physiological and defence performance in mussels. *Journal of Hazardous Materials, 122909*, 122909. Advance online publication. doi:10.1016/j.jhazmat.2020.122909 PMID:32460126

Guilhermino, L., Vieira, L. R., Ribeiro, D., Tavares, A. S., Cardoso, V., Alves, A., & Almeida, J. M. (2018). Uptake and effects of the antimicrobial florfenicol, microplastics and their mixtures on freshwater exotic invasive bivalve *Corbicula fluminea. The Science of the Total Environment, 622-623*, 1131–1142. doi:10.1016/j.scitotenv.2017.12.020 PMID:29890582

Guillard, V., Gaucel, S., Fornaciari, C., Angellier-Coussy, H., Buche, P., & Gontard, N. (2018). The next generation of sustainable food packaging to preserve our environment in a circular economy context. *Frontiers in Nutrition*, *5*(121), 121. doi:10.3389/fnut.2018.00121 PMID:30564581

Gunaalan, K., Fabbri, E., & Capolupo, M. (2020). The hidden threat of plastic leachates: A critical review on their impacts on aquatic organisms. *Water Research*, *116170*. Advance online publication. doi:10.1016/j.watres.2020.116170 PMID:32698093

Gunasekaran, D., Chandrasekaran, N., Jenkins, D., & Mukherjee, A. (2020). Plain polystyrene microplastics reduce the toxic effects of ZnO particles on marine microalgae *Dunaliella salina*. *Journal of Environmental Chemical Engineering*, *8*(5), 104250. doi:10.1016/j.jece.2020.104250

Gupta, A. K., & Gupta, M. (2005). Synthesis and surface engineering of iron oxide nanoparticles for biomedical applications. *Biomaterials*, *26*(18), 3995–4021. doi:10.1016/j.biomaterials.2004.10.012 PMID:15626447

Guterres, S. S., Alves, M. P., & Pohlmann, A. R. (2007). Polymeric Nanoparticles, Nanospheres and Nanocapsules, for Cutaneous Applications. *Drug Target Insights*, *2*. doi:10.1177/117739280700200002 PMID:21901071

Gutow, L., Eckerlebe, A., Giménez, L., & Saborowski, R. (2016). Experimental Evaluation of Seaweeds as a Vector for Microplastics into Marine Food Webs. *Environmental Science & Technology*, *50*(2), 915–923. doi:10.1021/acs.est.5b02431 PMID:26654910

Gu, Y. Y., Wei, Q., Wang, L. Y., Zhang, Z. M., Zhang, X. Q., Sun, A. L., Chen, J., & Shi, X. Z. (2021). A comprehensive study of the effects of phthalates on marine mussels: Bioconcentration, enzymatic activities and metabolomics. *Marine Pollution Bulletin*, *168*(January), 112393. doi:10.1016/j.marpolbul.2021.112393 PMID:33932843

Guzzetti, E., Sureda, A., Tejada, S., & Faggio, C. (2018). Microplastic in marine organism: Environmental and toxicological effects. *Environmental Toxicology and Pharmacology*, *64*, 164–171. doi:10.1016/j.etap.2018.10.009 PMID:30412862

Haberstroh, C. J., Arias, M. E., Yin, Z., & Wang, M. C. (2021). Effects of Urban Hydrology on Plastic Transport in a Subtropical River. In ACS ES&T WATER (Vol. 1, Issue 8, pp. 1714–1727). Amer Chemical Soc. doi:10.1021/acsestwater.1c00072

Haberstroh, C. J., Arias, M. E., Yin, Z., Sok, T., & Wang, M. C. (2021). Plastic transport in a complex confluence of the Mekong River in Cambodia. In Environmental Research Letters (Vol. 16, Issue 9). IOP Publishing Ltd. doi:10.1088/1748-9326/ac2198

Hahladakis, J. N., Velis, C. A., Weber, R., Iacovidou, E., & Purnell, P. (2018). An overview of chemical additives present in plastics: Migration, release, fate and environmental impact during their use, disposal and recycling. *Journal of Hazardous Materials*, *344*, 179–199. doi:10.1016/j.jhazmat.2017.10.014 PMID:29035713

Haider, T. P., Völker, C., Kramm, J., Landfester, K., & Wurm, F. R. (2019). Plastics of the future? The impact of biodegradable polymers on the environment and on society. *Angewandte Chemie International Edition*, *58*(1), 50–62. doi:10.1002/anie.201805766 PMID:29972726

Hakkarainen, M. (2002). Aliphatic polyesters: Abiotic and biotic degradation products. *Advances in Polymer Science*, *157*, 113–138. doi:10.1007/3-540-45734-8_4

Halden, R. U., Rolsky, C., & Khan, F. R. (2021). Time: A Key Driver of Uncertainty When Assessing the Risk of Environmental Plastics to Human Health. *Environmental Science & Technology*, *55*(19), 12766–12769. doi:10.1021/acs.est.1c02580 PMID:34520666

Hale, R. C., Seeley, M. E., La Guardia, M. J., Mai, L., & Zeng, E. Y. (2020). A global perspective on microplastics. *Journal of Geophysical Research: Oceans, 125*(1), e2018JC014719.

Halfar, J., Cabanov, K., Hevi, S., & Kašp, A. (2021). *Disparities in Methods Used to Determine Microplastics in the Aquatic Environment : A Review of Legislation*. Sampling Process and Instrumental Analysis.

Hall, N. M., Berry, K. L. E., Rintoul, L., & Hoogenboom, M. O. (2015). Microplastic ingestion by scleractinian corals. *Marine Biology, 162*(3), 725–732. doi:10.100700227-015-2619-7

Hamed, M., Soliman, H. A., Osman, A. G., & Sayed, A. E. D. H. (2020). Antioxidants and molecular damage in Nile Tilapia (Oreochromis niloticus) after exposure to microplastics. *Environmental Science and Pollution Research International, 27*(13), 14581–14588. doi:10.100711356-020-07898-y PMID:32048193

Hämer, J., Gutow, L., Köhler, A., & Saborowski, R. (2014). Fate of microplastics in the marine isopod *idotea emarginata. Environmental Science & Technology, 48*(22), 13451–13458. doi:10.1021/es501385y PMID:25289587

Hamidian, A. H., Ozumchelouei, E. J., Feizi, F., Wu, C., Zhang, Y., & Yang, M. (2021). A review on the characteristics of microplastics in wastewater treatment plants: A source for toxic chemicals. *Journal of Cleaner Production, 295*, 126480. doi:10.1016/j.jclepro.2021.126480

Hamidon, N. (2018). Potential of production bioplastic from potato starch. *Sustainable Environmental Technology, 1*, 115–123.

Hamlin, H. J., Marciano, K., & Downs, C. A. (2015). Migration of nonylphenol from food-grade plastic is toxic to the coral reef fish species *Pseudochromis fridmani. Chemosphere, 139*, 223–228. doi:10.1016/j.chemosphere.2015.06.032 PMID:26134675

Hancock, L. (2019). *Our oceans are haunted by ghost nets: Why that's scary and what we can do.* WWF. https://www.worldwildlife.org/stories/our-oceans-are-haunted-by-ghost-nets-why-that-s-scary-and-what-we-can-do--23

Hankins, C., Duffy, A., & Drisco, K. (2018). Scleractinian coral microplastic ingestion: Potential calcification effects, size limits, and retention. *Marine Pollution Bulletin, 135*, 587–593. doi:10.1016/j.marpolbul.2018.07.067 PMID:30301077

Hankins, C., Moso, E., & Lasseigne, D. (2021). Microplastics impair growth in two atlantic scleractinian coral species, Pseudodiploria clivosa and Acropora cervicornis. *Environmental Pollution, 275*, 116649. doi:10.1016/j.envpol.2021.116649 PMID:33571858

Hann, S., Scholes, R., Briedis, R., & Kirkevaag, K. (2018). *Bio-Based and Biodegradable Plastics: An Assessment of the Value Chain for Bio-Based and Biodegradable Plastics in Norway*. Eunomia For The Norwegian Environment Agency.

Harding, K., Gounden, T., & Pretorius, S. (2017). Biodegradable" plastics: A myth of marketing? *Procedia Manufacturing, 7*, 106–110. doi:10.1016/j.promfg.2016.12.027

Hariharan, G., Purvaja, R., Anandavelu, I., Robin, R. S., & Ramesh, R. (2021). Accumulation and ecotoxicological risk of weathered polyethylene (wPE) microplastics on green mussel (*Perna viridis*). *Ecotoxicology and Environmental Safety, 208*, 111765. doi:10.1016/j.ecoenv.2020.111765 PMID:33396084

Haritash, A. K., & Kaushik, C. P. (2009). Biodegradation aspects of Polycyclic Aromatic Hydrocarbons (PAHs): A review. *Journal of Hazardous Materials, 169*(1–3), 1–15. doi:10.1016/j.jhazmat.2009.03.137 PMID:19442441

Haro, P., Ollero, P., & Trippe, F. (2013). Technoeconomic assessment of potential processes for bio-ethylene production. *Fuel Processing Technology, 114*, 35–48. doi:10.1016/j.fuproc.2013.03.024

Harris, L., Liboiron, M., Charron, L., & Mather, C. (2021). Using citizen science to evaluate extended producer responsibility policy to reduce marine plastic debris shows no reduction in pollution levels. *Marine Policy*, *123*, 104319. doi:10.1016/j.marpol.2020.104319

Hart, M. W. (1991). Particle Captures and the Method of Suspension Feeding by Echinoderm Larvae. *The Biological Bulletin*, *180*(1), 12–27. doi:10.2307/1542425 PMID:29303636

Hartmann, N. B., Hüffer, T., Thompson, R. C., Hassellöv, M., Verschoor, A., Daugaard, A. E., Rist, S., Karlsson, T., Brennholt, N., Cole, M., Herrling, M. P., Hess, M. C., Ivleva, N. P., Lusher, A. L., & Wagner, M. (2019). Are We Speaking the Same Language? Recommendations for a Definition and Categorization Framework for Plastic Debris. *Environmental Science & Technology*, *53*(3), 1039–1047. doi:10.1021/acs.est.8b05297 PMID:30608663

Harunsyah, Y. M., & Fauzan, R. (2017). Mechanical properties of bioplastics cassava starch film with Zinc Oxide nanofiller as reinforcement. *IOP Conference Series. Materials Science and Engineering*, *210*, 012015. doi:10.1088/1757-899X/210/1/012015

Hasan, S. (2004). Public awareness is key to successful waste management. *Journal of Environmental Science and Health. Part A, Toxic/Hazardous Substances & Environmental Engineering*, *39*(2), 483–492. doi:10.1081/ESE-120027539 PMID:15027831

Haward, M. (2018). Plastic pollution of the world's seas and oceans as a contemporary challenge in ocean governance. *National Commun.*, 667.

Haward, M. (2018). Plastic pollution of the world's seas and oceans as a contemporary challenge in ocean governance. *Nature Communications*, *9*(1), 1–3. doi:10.103841467-018-03104-3 PMID:29445166

Hayes, A., Kirkbride, K. P., & Leterme, S. C. (2021). Variation in polymer types and abundance of microplastics from two rivers and beaches in Adelaide, South Australia. In *Marine Pollution Bulletin* (Vol. 172). Pergamon-Elsevier Science Ltd. doi:10.1016/j.marpolbul.2021.112842

He, B., Duodu, G. O., Rintoul, L., Ayoko, G. A., & Goonetilleke, A. (2020). Influence of microplastics on nutrients and metal concentrations in river sediments. In Environmental Pollution (Vol. 263, Issue A). Elsevier Sci Ltd. doi:10.1016/j.envpol.2020.114490

He, D., Zhang, X., & Hu, J. (2020). Jo u rn a l P of. *Journal of Hazardous Materials*, *124640*. Advance online publication. doi:10.1016/j.jhazmat.2020.124640 PMID:33246814

He, L., Wu, D., Rong, H., Li, M., Tong, M., & Kim, H. (2018). Influence of nano- and microplastic particles on the transport and deposition behaviors of bacteria in quartz sand. *Environmental Science & Technology*, *52*, 11545–1155. doi:10.1021/acs.est.8b01673 PMID:30204419

Helcoski, R., Yonkos, L. T., Sanchez, A., & Baldwin, A. H. (2020). Wetland soil microplastics are negatively related to vegetation cover and stem density. *Environmental Pollution*, *256*, 113391. doi:10.1016/j.envpol.2019.113391 PMID:31662247

Helinski, K., Poor, J., & Wolfand, M. (2021). Ridding our rivers of plastic: A framework for plastic pollution capture device selection. *Marine Pollution Bulletin*, *165*, 112095. doi:10.1016/j.marpolbul.2021.112095 PMID:33561713

Hendrickson, E., Minor, E. C., & Schreiner, K. (2018). *Microplastic Abundance and Composition in Western Lake Superior As Determined via Microscopy*. Pyr-GC/MS, and FTIR. doi:10.1021/acs.est.7b05829

Henry, B., Laitala, K., & Klepp, I. G. (2019). Microfibres from apparel and home textiles: Prospects for including microplastics in environmental sustainability assessment. *The Science of the Total Environment*, *652*, 483–494. doi:10.1016/j.scitotenv.2018.10.166 PMID:30368178

Herbort, A. F., & Schuhen, K. (2017). A concept for the removal of microplastics from the marine environment with innovative host-guest relationships. *Environmental Science and Pollution Research International*, *24*(12), 11061–11065. doi:10.100711356-016-7216-x PMID:27421855

Herbort, A. F., Sturm, M. T., Fiedler, S., Abkai, G., & Schuhen, K. (2018). Alkoxy-silyl Induced Agglomeration: A New Approach for the Sustainable Removal of Microplastic from Aquatic Systems. *Journal of Polymers and the Environment*, *26*(11), 4258–4270. doi:10.100710924-018-1287-3

Hermsen, E., Mintenig, S. M., Besseling, E., & Koelmans, A. A. (2018). Quality Criteria for the Analysis of Microplastic in Biota Samples. *Critical Reviews in Environmental Science and Technology*, *52*(18), 10230–10240. doi:10.1021/acs.est.8b01611 PMID:30137965

Hernandez, L. M., Xu, E. G., Larsson, H., Tahara, R., Maisuria, V. B., & Tufenkji, N. (2019). Plastic Teabags Release Billions of Microparticles and Nanoparticles into Tea. *Environmental Science & Technology*, *53*(21), 12300–12310. doi:10.1021/acs.est.9b02540 PMID:31552738

Hernandez, L. M., Yousefi, N., & Tufenkji, N. (2017). Are There Nanoplastics in Your Personal Care Products? *Environmental Science & Technology Letters*, *4*(7), 280–285. doi:10.1021/acs.estlett.7b00187

Heshmati, S., Makhdoumi, P., Pirsaheb, M., Hossini, H., Ahmadi, S., & Fattahi, H. (2021). Occurrence and characterization of microplastic content in the digestive system of riverine fishes. In *Journal of Environmental Management* (Vol. 299). Academic Press Ltd- Elsevier Science Ltd. doi:10.1016/j.jenvman.2021.113620

Hidalgo-Ruz, V., Gutow, L., Thompson, R. C., & Thiel, M. (2012). Thompson, R.C.; Thiel, M. Microplastics in the marine environment: A review of the methods used for identification and quantification. *Environmental Science & Technology*, *2012*(46), 3060–3075. doi:10.1021/es2031505 PMID:22321064

Hintersteiner, I., Himmelsbach, M., & Buchberger, W. W. (2015). Characterization and quantitation of polyolefin microplastics in personal-care products using high-temperature gel-permeation chromatography. *Analytical and Bioanalytical Chemistry*, *407*(4), 1253–1259. doi:10.100700216-014-8318-2 PMID:25410643

Hitchcock, J. N. (2020). Storm events as key moments of microplastic contamination in aquatic ecosystems. In *Science of the Total Environment* (Vol. 734). Elsevier. doi:10.1016/j.scitotenv.2020.139436

Hoffmann, L., Eggers, S. L., Allhusen, E., Katlein, C., & Peeken, I. (2020). Interactions between the ice algae *Fragillariopsis cylindrus* and microplastics in sea ice. *Environment International*, *139*(April), 105697. Advance online publication. doi:10.1016/j.envint.2020.105697 PMID:32334123

Hojabri, L., Kong, X., & Narine, S. S. (2009). Fatty Acid-Derived Diisocyanate and Biobased Polyurethane Produced from Vegetable Oil: Synthesis, Polymerization, and Characterization. *Biomacromolecules*, *10*(4), 884–891. doi:10.1021/bm801411w PMID:19281152

Hopewell, J., Dvorak, R., & Kosior, E. (2009). Plastics recycling: Challenges and opportunities. *Philosophical Transactions of the Royal Society of London. Series B, Biological Sciences*, *364*(1526), 2115–2126. doi:10.1098/rstb.2008.0311 PMID:19528059

Horn, D. A., Granek, E. F., & Steele, C. L. (2020). Effects of environmentally relevant concentrations of microplastic fibers on Pacific mole crab (*Emerita analoga*) mortality and reproduction. *Limnology and Oceanography Letters*, *5*(1), 74–83. doi:10.1002/lol2.10137

Horodytska, O., Cabanes, A., & Fullana, A. (2019). *The Handbook of Environmental Chemistry*. Springer.

Horton, A. A., Svendsen, C., Williams, R. J., Spurgeon, D. J., & Lahive, E. (2017). Large microplastic particles in sediments of tributaries of the River Thames, UK - Abundance, sources and methods for effective quantification. In Marine Pollution Bulletin (Vol. 114, Issue 1, pp. 218–226). Pergamon-Elsevier Science Ltd. doi:10.1016/j.marpolbul.2016.09.004

Horton, A. A., Walton, A., Spurgeon, D. J., Lahive, E., & Svendsen, C. (2017). Microplastics in freshwater and terrestrial environments: Evaluating the current understanding to identify the knowledge gaps and future research priorities. *The Science of the Total Environment*, *586*, 127–141. doi:10.1016/j.scitotenv.2017.01.190 PMID:28169032

Hossain, M. S., Rahman, M. S., Uddin, M. N., Sharifuzzaman, S. M., Chowdhury, S. R., Sarker, S., & Chowdhury, M. S. N. (2020). Microplastic contamination in Penaeid shrimp from the Northern Bay of Bengal. *Chemosphere*, *238*, 124688. doi:10.1016/j.chemosphere.2019.124688 PMID:31524623

Hou, L., McMahan, C. D., McNeish, R. E., Munno, K., Rochman, C. M., & Hoellein, T. J. (2021). A fish tale: A century of museum specimens reveal increasing microplastic concentrations in freshwater fish. In Ecological Applications (Vol. 31, Issue 5). Wiley. doi:10.1002/eap.2320

Hou, J., Xu, X., Yu, H., Xi, B., & Tan, W. (2021). Comparing the long-term responses of soil microbial structures and diversities to polyethylene microplastics in different aggregate fractions. *Environment International*, *149*, 106398. doi:10.1016/j.envint.2021.106398 PMID:33503554

Howard, G. T. (2002). Biodegradation of polyurethane: A review. *International Biodeterioration & Biodegradation*, *49*(4), 245–252. doi:10.1016/S0964-8305(02)00051-3

Huang, S., Peng, C., Wang, Z., Xiong, X., Bi, Y., Liu, Y., & Li, D. (2021). Spatiotemporal distribution of microplastics in surface water, biofilms, and sediments in the world's largest drinking water diversion project. In *Science of the Total Environment* (Vol. 789). Elsevier. doi:10.1016/j.scitotenv.2021.148001

Huang, W., Chen, M., Song, B., Deng, J., Shen, M., Chen, Q., Zeng, G., & Liang, J. (2021). Microplastics in the coral reefs and their potential impacts on corals: A mini-review. *The Science of the Total Environment*, *762*, 143112. doi:10.1016/j.scitotenv.2020.143112 PMID:33172634

Huang, W., Wang, X., Chen, D., Xu, E. G., Luo, X., Zeng, J., Huan, T., Li, L., & Wang, Y. (2021). Toxicity mechanisms of polystyrene microplastics in marine mussels revealed by high-coverage quantitative metabolomics using chemical isotope labeling liquid chromatography mass spectrometry. *Journal of Hazardous Materials*, *417*, 126003. doi:10.1016/j.jhazmat.2021.126003 PMID:33992921

Huang, Y., Zhao, Y., Wang, J., Zhang, M., Jia, W., & Qin, X. (2020). LDPE microplastic films alter microbial community composition and enzymatic activities in soil. *Environmental Pollution*, *254*, 112983. doi:10.1016/j.envpol.2019.112983 PMID:31394342

Hu, E., Shang, S., Fu, Z., Zhao, X., Nan, X., Du, Y., & Chen, X. (2020). Cotransport of naphthalene with polystyrene nanoplastics (PSNP) in saturated porous media: Effects of PSNP/naphthalene ratio and ionic strength. *Chemosphere*, *245*, 125602. doi:10.1016/j.chemosphere.2019.125602 PMID:31864042

Huerta Lwanga, E., Gertsen, H., Gooren, H., Peters, P., Salanki, T., van der Ploeg, M., Besseling, E., Koelmans, A. A., & Geissen, V. (2017). Incorporation of microplastics from litter into burrows of Lumbricus terrestris. *Environmental Pollution*, *220*, 523–531. doi:10.1016/j.envpol.2016.09.096 PMID:27726978

Huerta Lwanga, E., Gertsen, H., Gooren, H., Peters, P., Salánki, T., Van, P. M., Besseling, E., Koelmans, A. A., & Geissen, V. (2016). Microplastics in the terrestrial ecosystem: Implications for Lumbricus terrestris (*Oligochaeta, Lumbricidae*). *Environmental Science & Technology*, *50*(5), 2685–2691. doi:10.1021/acs.est.5b05478 PMID:26852875

Huerta Lwanga, E., Mendoza Vega, J., Ku Quej, V., Chi, J., Sanchez Del Cid, L., Chi, C., Escalona Segura, G., Gertsen, H., Salánki, T., van der Ploeg, M., Koelmans, A. A., & Geissen, V. (2017). Field evidence for transfer of plastic debris along a terrestrial food chain. *Scientific Reports*, *7*(1), 14071. doi:10.103841598-017-14588-2 PMID:29074893

Hu, L., Chernick, M., Lewis, A. M., Ferguson, P. L., & Hinton, D. E. (2020). Chronic microfiber exposure in adult Japanese medaka (Oryzias latipes). *PLoS One*, *15*(3), e0229962. doi:10.1371/journal.pone.0229962 PMID:32150587

Hu, L., Su, L., Xue, Y., Mu, J., Zhu, J., Xu, J., & Shi, H. (2016). Uptake, accumulation and elimination of polystyrene microspheres in tadpoles of Xenopus tropicalis. *Chemosphere*, *164*, 611–617. doi:10.1016/j.chemosphere.2016.09.002 PMID:27635643

Huppertsberg, S., & Knepper, T. P. (2018). *Instrumental analysis of microplastics — benefits and challenges*. Academic Press.

Hurley, R. R., Woodward, J. C., & Rothwell, J. J. (2017). Ingestion of Microplastics by Freshwater Tubifex Worms. In Environmental Science & Technology (Vol. 51, Issue 21, pp. 12844–12851). Amer Chemical Soc. doi:10.1021/acs.est.7b03567

Hurley, R., Woodward, J., & Rothwell, J. J. (2018). Microplastic contamination of river beds significantly reduced by catchment-wide flooding. In Nature Geoscience (Vol. 11, Issue 4, p. 251+). Nature Publishing Group. doi:10.103841561-018-0080-1

Hurley, R. R., Lusher, A. L., Olsen, M., & Nizzetto, L. (2018). Validation of a Method for Extracting Microplastics from Complex, Organic-Rich, Environmental Matrices. *Environmental Science & Technology*, *52*(13), 7409–7417. doi:10.1021/acs.est.8b01517 PMID:29886731

Hussein, B. A., Tsegaye, A. A., & Abdulahi, A. (2021). Assessment of the environmental and health impacts of disposal plastics in Gode town, Somali regional state, Eastern Ethiopia. *J Mater Environ Sci*, *12*(3), 455–471.

Hwang, J., Choi, D., Han, S., Choi, J., & Hong, J. (2019). An assessment of the toxicity of polypropylene microplastics in human derived cells. *The Science of the Total Environment*, *684*, 657–669. doi:10.1016/j.scitotenv.2019.05.071 PMID:31158627

ICES. (2015). OSPAR request on development of a common monitoring protocol for plastic particles in fish stomachs and selected shellfish on the basis of existing fish disease surveys. *IICES Advice,* 1–6.

Id, A. K. B., Spanjer, A. R., Id, M. R. R., & Thom, T. (2020). *Microplastics in Lake Mead National Recreation Area, USA : Occurrence and biological uptake*. doi:10.1371/journal.pone.0228896

Igarashi, M., de Boer, L., & Fet, A. (2013). What is required for greener supplier selection? A literature review and conceptual model development. *Journal of Purchasing and Supply Management*, *19*(4), 247–263. doi:10.1016/j.pursup.2013.06.001

Imasha, H. U. E., & Babel, S. (2021). Microplastics Contamination in Commercial Green Mussels from Selected Wet Markets in Thailand. *Archives of Environmental Contamination and Toxicology*, (3), 449–459. Advance online publication. doi:10.100700244-021-00886-4 PMID:34508277

Imhof, H. K., Schmid, J., Niessner, R., Ivleva, N. P., & Laforsch, C. (2012). A novel, highly efficient method for the separation and quantification of plastic particles in sediments of aquatic environments. *Limnology and Oceanography, Methods*, *10*(July), 524–537. doi:10.4319/lom.2012.10.524

Inkielewicz-Stepniak, I., Tajber, L., Behan, G., Zhang, H., Radomski, M. W., Medina, C., & Santos-Martinez, M. J. (2018). The Role of Mucin in the Toxicological Impact of Polystyrene Nanoparticles. *Materials (Basel, Switzerland), 11*(5), 724. doi:10.3390/ma11050724 PMID:29751544

Irfan, M., Qadir, A., Mumtaz, M., & Ahmad, S. R. (2020). An unintended challenge of microplastic pollution in the urban surface water system of Lahore, Pakistan. In Environmental Science And Pollution Research (Vol. 27, Issue 14, pp. 16718–16730). Springer heidelberg. doi:10.100711356-020-08114-7

Ishangulyyev, R., Kim, S., & Lee, S. H. (2019). Understanding food loss and waste – why are we losing and wasting food? *Foods, 8*(8), 297. doi:10.3390/foods8080297 PMID:31362396

Islam, N., Garcia da Fonseca, T., Vilke, J., Gonçalves, J. M., Pedro, P., Keiter, S., Cunha, S. C., Fernandes, J. O., & Bebianno, M. J. (2021). Perfluorooctane sulfonic acid (PFOS) adsorbed to polyethylene microplastics: Accumulation and ecotoxicological effects in the clam *Scrobicularia plana. Marine Environmental Research, 164*, 105249. doi:10.1016/j.marenvres.2020.105249 PMID:33477023

Issac, M. N., & Kandasubramanian, B. (2021). Effect of microplastics in water and aquatic systems. *Environmental Science and Pollution Research, 28*(16), 19544–19562. doi:10.1007/s11356-021-13184-2

ISWA (International Solid Waste Association). (2017). *Prevent marine plastic litter - now!* ISWA Marine Task Force. https://marinelitter.iswa.org/fileadmin/user_upload/Marine_Task_Force_Report_2017/ISWA_report170927_interactive_lowres.pdf

Iwalaye, O. A., Moodley, G. K., & Robertson-Andersson, D. V. (2020). The possible routes of microplastics uptake in sea cucumber *Holothuria cinerascens* (Brandt, 1835). *Environmental Pollution, 114644*. Advance online publication. doi:10.1016/j.envpol.2020.114644 PMID:32559857

Iwalaye, O. A., Moodley, G. K., & Robertson-Andersson, D. V. (2021). Water Temperature and Microplastic Concentration Influenced Microplastic Ingestion and Retention Rates in Sea Cucumber (*Holothuria cinerascens* Brandt, 1835). *Ocean Science Journal, 56*(2), 141–155. doi:10.100712601-021-00013-3

Jambeck, J. R., Geyer, R., Wilcox, C., Siegler, T. R., Perryman, M., Andrady, A., Narayan, R., & Law, K. L. (2015). Plastic waste inputs from land into the ocean. *Science, 347*(6223), 768–771. doi:10.1126cience.1260352 PMID:25678662

James, G. (2019). *The Plastics Landscape: Risk and opportunities along the value chain.* Principles for Responsible Investment. https://www.unpri.org/plastics/risks-and-opportunities-along-the-plastics-value-chain/4774.article

James, W. D., Berger, T. G., & Elston, D. M. (2006). *Andrews' diseases of the skin: Clinical dermatology* (10th ed.). Elsevier Saunders.

Jamieson, A. J., Brooks, L. S. R., Reid, W. D. K., Piertney, S. B., Narayanaswamy, B. E., & Linley, T. D. (2019). Microplastics and Synthetic Particles Ingested by Deep-Sea Amphipods in Six of the Deepest Marine Ecosystems on Earth. *Royal Society Open Science, 6*(2), 180667. doi:10.1098/rsos.180667 PMID:30891254

Jang, Y. C., Lee, J., Hong, S., Lee, J. S., Shim, W. J., & Song, Y. K. (2014). Sources of plastic marine debris on beaches of Korea: More from the ocean than the land. *Ocean Science Journal, 49*(2), 151–162. doi:10.1007/s12601-014-0015-8

Jang, Y. C., Hong, S., Lee, J., Lee, M. J., & Shim, W. J. (2014). Estimation of lost tourism revenue in Geoje Island from the 2011 marine debris pollution event in South Korea. *Marine Pollution Bulletin, 81*(1), 49–54. doi:10.1016/j.marpolbul.2014.02.021 PMID:24635983

Jeong, C.-B., Won, E.-J., Kang, H.-M., Lee, M.-C., Hwang, D.-S., Hwang, U.-K., Zhou, B., Souissi, S., Lee, S.-J., & Lee, J.-S. (2016). Microplastic size-dependent toxicity, oxidative stress induction, and p-JNK and p-p38 activation in the monogonont rotifer (Brachionus koreanus). *Environmental Science & Technology*, *50*(16), 8849–8857. doi:10.1021/acs.est.6b01441 PMID:27438693

Jeong, J., & Choi, J. (2019). Adverse outcome pathways potentially related to hazard identification of microplastics based on toxicity mechanisms. *Chemosphere*, *231*, 249–255. doi:10.1016/j.chemosphere.2019.05.003 PMID:31129406

Jerez, A., Partal, P., Martínez, I., Gallegos, C., & Guerrero, A. (2005). Rheology and processing of gluten based bioplastics. *Biochemical Engineering Journal*, *26*(2-3), 131–138. doi:10.1016/j.bej.2005.04.010

Ji, X., Ma, Y., Zeng, G., Xu, X., Mei, K., Wang, Z., Chen, Z., Dahlgren, R., Zhang, M., & Shang, X. (2021). Transport and fate of microplastics from riverine sediment dredge piles: Implications for disposal. In Journal of Hazardous Materials (Vol. 404, Issue A). Elsevier. doi:10.1016/j.jhazmat.2020.124132

Jiang, B., Kauffman, A. E., Li, L., McFee, W., Cai, B., Weinstein, J., Lead, J. R., Chatterjee, S., Scott, G. I., & Xiao, S. (2020). Health impacts of environmental contamination of micro- and nanoplastics: A review. *Environmental Health and Preventive Medicine*, *25*(1), 29. doi:10.118612199-020-00870-9 PMID:32664857

Jiang, T., Ma, X., Tang, Q., Yang, J., Li, G., & Schuchardt, F. (2016). Combined use of nitrification inhibitor and struvite crystallization to reduce the NH_3 and N_2O emissions during composting. *Bioresource Technology*, *217*, 210–218. doi:10.1016/j.biortech.2016.01.089 PMID:26865057

Jiang, X., Chen, H., Liao, Y., Ye, Z., Li, M., & Klobučar, G. (2019). Ecotoxicity and genotoxicity of polystyrene microplastics on higher plant Vicia faba. *Environmental Pollution*, *250*, 831–838. doi:10.1016/j.envpol.2019.04.055 PMID:31051394

Jimenez-Rosado, M., Bouroudian, E., Perez-Puyana, V., Guerrero, A., & Romero, A. (2020). Evaluation of different strengthening methods in the mechanical and functional properties of soy proteinbased bioplastics. *Journal of Cleaner Production*, *262*, 121517. doi:10.1016/j.jclepro.2020.121517

Jin, H., Ma, T., Sha, X., Liu, Z., Zhou, Y., Meng, X., Chen, Y., Han, X., & Ding, J. (2021). Polystyrene microplastics induced male reproductive toxicity in mice. *Journal of Hazardous Materials*, *401*, 123430. doi:10.1016/j.jhazmat.2020.123430 PMID:32659591

Jin, Y., Lu, L., Tu, W., Luo, T., & Fu, Z. (2019). Impacts of polystyrene microplastic on the gut barrier, microbiota and metabolism of mice. *The Science of the Total Environment*, *649*, 308–317. doi:10.1016/j.scitotenv.2018.08.353 PMID:30176444

Jõgi, K., & Bhat, R. (2020). Valorization of food processing wastes and by-products for bioplastic production. *Sustainable Chemistry and Pharmacy*, *18*, 100326. doi:10.1016/j.scp.2020.100326

Johnson, S. (2019). *'It is raining plastic': Microplastics found in U.S. rainwater.* https://bigthink.com/the-present/microplastics-rainwater/

Johnson, N. G., Burnett, L. E., & Burnett, K. G. (2011). Properties of bacteria that trigger hemocytopenia in the Atlantic blue crab, Callinectes sapidus. *The Biological Bulletin*, *221*(2), 164–175. doi:10.1086/BBLv221n2p164 PMID:22042435

Joon, M. (2019). Trophic transfer of microplastics in zooplanktons towards its speculations on human health: A review. *Journal of Biomedical and Therapeutic Sciences*, *6*(1), 8-14.

Joseph, B., James, J., Kalarikkal, N., & Thomas, S. (2021). Recycling of medical plastics. *Advanced Industrial and Engineering Polymer Research*, *4*(3), 199–208. doi:10.1016/j.aiepr.2021.06.003

Jovanović, B. (2017). Ingestion of microplastics by fish and its potential consequences from a physical perspective. *Integrated Environmental Assessment and Management, 13*(3), 510–515. doi:10.1002/ieam.1913 PMID:28440941

Jovanović, B., Gökdağ, K., Güven, O., Emre, Y., Whitley, E. M., & Kideys, A. E. (2018). Virgin microplastics are not causing imminent harm to fish after dietary exposure. *Marine Pollution Bulletin, 130*, 123–131. doi:10.1016/j.marpolbul.2018.03.016 PMID:29866538

JRC. (2013). *Guidance on Monitoring of Marine Litter in European Seas*. Joint Research Centre of the European Commission, Ispra, EUR 26113 EN. https://mcc.jrc.ec.europa.eu/documents/201702074014.pdf

Judy, J. D., Williams, M., Gregg, A., Oliver, D., Kumar, A., Kookana, R., & Kirby, J. K. (2019). Microplastics in municipal mixed-waste organic outputs induce minimal short to long-term toxicity in key terrestrial biota. *Environmental Pollution, 252*, 522–531. doi:10.1016/j.envpol.2019.05.027 PMID:31167160

Jung, S., Cho, S. H., Kim, K. H., & Kwon, E. E. (2021). Progress in quantitative analysis of microplastics in the environment: A review. *Chemical Engineering Journal, 422*(April), 130154. doi:10.1016/j.cej.2021.130154

Kaiser, D., Kowalski, N., & Waniek, J. J. (2017). Effects of biofouling on the sinking behavior of microplastics. *Environmental Research Letters, 12*(12), 124003. doi:10.1088/1748-9326/aa8e8b

Kalambur, S., & Rizvi, S. S. H. (2006). An overview of starch-based plastic blends from reactive extrusion. *Journal of Plastic Film & Sheeting, 22*(1), 39–58. doi:10.1177/8756087906062729

Kalogerakis, N., Karkanorachaki, K., Kalogerakis, G. C., Triantafyllidi, E. I., Gotsis, A. D., Partsinevelos, P., & Fava, F. (2017). Microplastics generation: Onset of fragmentation of polyethylene films in marine environment mesocosms. *Frontiers in Marine Science, 4*, 84. doi:10.3389/fmars.2017.00084

Kang, H.-M., Byeon, E., Jeong, H., Lee, Y., Hwang, U.-K., Jeong, C.-B., Yoon, C., & Lee, J.-S. (2021). Arsenic exposure combined with nano- or microplastic induces different effects in the marine rotifer *Brachionus plicatilis. Aquatic Toxicology (Amsterdam, Netherlands), 233*, 105772. doi:10.1016/j.aquatox.2021.105772 PMID:33618324

Kang, J. H., Kwon, O. Y., Lee, K. W., Song, Y. K., & Shim, W. J. (2015). Marine neustonic microplastics around the southeastern coast of Korea. *Marine Pollution Bulletin, 96*(1–2), 304–312. doi:10.1016/j.marpolbul.2015.04.054 PMID:25979811

Kang, J., Zhou, L., Duan, X., Sun, H., Ao, Z., & Wang, S. (2019). Degradation of cosmetic microplastics via functionalized carbon nanosprings. *Matter, 1*(3), 745–758. doi:10.1016/j.matt.2019.06.004

Kanhai, L. D. K., Gardfeldt, K., Krumpen, T., Thompson, R. C., & O'Connor, I. (2020). Microplastics in sea ice and seawater beneath ice floes from the Arctic Ocean. *Scientific Reports, 10*(1), 1–11. doi:10.103841598-020-61948-6 PMID:32193433

Kanhai, L. D. K., Johansson, C., Frias, J. P. G. L., Gardfeldt, K., Thompson, R. C., & O'Connor, I. (2019). Deep sea sediments of the Arctic Central Basin: A potential sink for microplastics. *Deep-sea Research. Part I, Oceanographic Research Papers, 145*, 137–142. doi:10.1016/j.dsr.2019.03.003

Kanhai, L. D. K., Officer, R., Lyashevska, O., Thompson, R. C., & O'Connor, I. (2017). Microplastic abundance, distribution and composition along a latitudinal gradient in the Atlantic Ocean. *Marine Pollution Bulletin, 115*(1–2), 307–314. doi:10.1016/j.marpolbul.2016.12.025 PMID:28007381

Kankanige, D., & Babel, S. (2020). Smaller-sized micro-plastics (MPs) contamination in single-use PET-bottled water in Thailand. *The Science of the Total Environment, 717*, 137232. doi:10.1016/j.scitotenv.2020.137232 PMID:32062244

Kaposi, K. L., Mos, B., Kelaher, B. P., & Dworjanyn, S. A. (2014). Ingestion of microplastic has limited impact on a marine larva. *Environmental Science & Technology*, *48*(3), 1638–1645. doi:10.1021/es404295e PMID:24341789

Käppler, A., Fischer, D., Oberbeckmann, S., Schernewski, G., Labrenz, M., Eichhorn, K., & Voit, B. (2016). Analysis of environmental microplastics by vibrational microspectroscopy : FTIR, Raman or both? *Analytical and Bioanalytical Chemistry*, *408*(29), 8377–8391. doi:10.100700216-016-9956-3 PMID:27722940

Karami, A., Golieskardi, A., Choo, C. K., Romano, N., Ho, Y., & Salamatinia, B. (2017). A high-performance protocol for extraction of microplastics in fish. *The Science of the Total Environment*, *578*, 485–494. doi:10.1016/j.scitotenv.2016.10.213 PMID:27836345

Karami, A., Golieskardi, A., Ho, Y. B., Larat, V., & Salamatinia, B. (2017). Microplastics in eviscerated flesh and excised organs of dried fish. *Scientific Reports*, *7*(1), 5473. doi:10.103841598-017-05828-6 PMID:28710445

Karbalaei, S., Hanachi, P., Walker, T. R., & Cole, M. (2018). Occurrence, sources, human health impacts and mitigation of microplastic pollution. *Environmental Science and Pollution Research International*, *25*(36), 36046–36063. doi:10.100711356-018-3508-7 PMID:30382517

Karlsson, T. M., Vethaak, A. D., Almroth, B. C., Ariese, F., van Velzen, M., Hassellöv, M., & Leslie, H. A. (2017). Screening for microplastics in sediment, water, marine invertebrates and fish: Method development and microplastic accumulation. *Marine Pollution Bulletin*, *122*(1–2), 403–408. doi:10.1016/j.marpolbul.2017.06.081 PMID:28689849

Katija, K., Sherlock, R. E., Sherman, A. D., & Robison, B. H. (2017). New technology reveals the role of giant larvaceans in oceanic carbon cycling. *Science Advances*, *3*(5), e1602374. doi:10.1126ciadv.1602374 PMID:28508058

Kawaguchi, H., Hasunuma, T., Ogino, C., & Kondo, A. (2016). Bioprocessing of biobased chemicals produced from lignocellulosic feedstocks. *Current Opinion in Biotechnology*, *42*, 30–39. doi:10.1016/j.copbio.2016.02.031 PMID:26970511

Kaza, S., Yao, L., Bhada-Tata, P., & Woerden, F. V. (2018). 2018. What a Waste 2.0: A Global Snapshot of Solid Waste Management to 2050. Urban Development Series. Washington, DC: World Bank. doi:10.1596/978-1-4648-1329-0

Keenan, T. M., Nakas, J. P., & Tanenbaum, S. W. (2006). Polyhydroxyalkanoate copolymers from forest biomass. *Journal of Industrial Microbiology & Biotechnology*, *33*(7), 616–626. doi:10.100710295-006-0131-2 PMID:16761168

Kentin, E., & Kaarto, H. (2018). An EU ban on microplastics in cosmetic products and the right to regulate. *Review of European, Comparative & International Environmental Law*, *27*(3), 254–266. doi:10.1111/reel.12269

Kershaw, P. (2015). Sources, fate and effects of microplastics in the marine environment: A global assessment. *Reports and Studies GESAMP.*, *90*, 96.

Khalid, N., Aqeel, M., Noman, A., Hashem, M., Mostafa, Y. S., Alhaithloul, H. A. S., & Alghanem, S. M. (2021). Linking effects of microplastics to ecological impacts in marine environments. *Chemosphere*, *264*, 128541. doi:10.1016/j.chemosphere.2020.128541 PMID:33059282

Kim, J. S., Lee, H. J., Kim, S. K., & Kim, H. J. (2018). Global Pattern of Microplastics (MPs) in Commercial Food-Grade Salts: Sea Salt as an Indicator of Seawater MP Pollution. *Environmental Science & Technology*, *52*(21), 12819–12828. doi:10.1021/acs.est.8b04180 PMID:30285421

Kim, J.-Y., Lee, H. W., Lee, S. M., Jae, J., & Park, Y.-K. (2019). Overview of the recent advances in lignocellulose liquefaction for producing biofuels, bio-based materials and Chemicals. *Bioresource Technology*, *279*, 373–384. doi:10.1016/j.biortech.2019.01.055 PMID:30685133

Kim, S. K., Kim, J. S., Lee, H., & Lee, H. J. (2021). Abundance and characteristics of microplastics in soils with different agricultural practices: Importance of sources with internal origin and environmental fate. *Journal of Hazardous Materials*, *403*, 123997.

Kitahara, K. I., & Nakata, H. (2020). Plastic additives as tracers of microplastic sources in Japanese road dusts. *The Science of the Total Environment*, *736*, 139694. doi:10.1016/j.scitotenv.2020.139694 PMID:32502788

Klaine, S. J., Koelmans, A. A., Horne, N., Carley, S., Handy, R. D., Kapustka, L., Nowack, B., & von der Kammer, F. (2012). Paradigms to assess the environmental impact of manufactured nanomaterials. *Environmental Toxicology and Chemistry*, *31*(1), 3–14. doi:10.1002/etc.733 PMID:22162122

Klein, S., D. I. K., J., E., & T.P., K. (2018). Analysis, Occurrence, and Degradation of Microplastics in the Aqueous Environment. In Freshwater Microplastics. The Handbook of Environmental Chemistry (p. 302). Springer. doi:10.1007/978-3-319-61615-5

Klein, M., & Fischer, E. K. (2019). Microplastic abundance in atmospheric deposition within the Metropolitan area of Hamburg, Germany. *The Science of the Total Environment*, *685*, 96–103. doi:10.1016/j.scitotenv.2019.05.405 PMID:31174127

Klein, S., Dimzon, I. K., Eubeler, J., & Knepper, T. P. (2018). Analysis, occurrence, and degradation of microplastics in the aqueous environment. In *Freshwater microplastics* (pp. 51–67). Springer. doi:10.1007/978-3-319-61615-5_3

Klein, S., Worch, E., & Knepper, T. P. (2015). Occurrence and spatial distribution of microplastics in river shore sediments of the Rhine-main area in Germany. *Environmental Science & Technology*, *49*(10), 6070–6076. doi:10.1021/acs.est.5b00492 PMID:25901760

Kobayashi, T., Uchino, K., Abe, T., Yamazaki, Y., & Saito, T. (2005). Novel intracellular 3-hydroxybutyrate-oligomer hydrolase in Wautersia eutropha H16. *Journal of Bacteriology*, *187*(15), 5129–5135. doi:10.1128/JB.187.15.5129-5135.2005 PMID:16030206

Koelmans, A. A., Bakir, A., Burton, G. A., & Janssen, C. R. (2016). Microplastic as a vector for chemicals in the aquatic environment: Critical review and model-supported reinterpretation of empirical studies. *Environmental Science & Technology*, *50*(7), 3315–3326. doi:10.1021/acs.est.5b06069 PMID:26946978

Koelmans, A. A., Nor, N. H. M., Hermsen, E., Kooi, M., Mintenig, S. M., & De France, J. (2019). Microplastics in freshwaters and drinking water: Critical review and assessment of data quality. *Water Research*, *155*, 410–422. doi:10.1016/j.watres.2019.02.054 PMID:30861380

Kögel, T., Bjorøy, Ø., Toto, B., Bienfait, A. M., & Sanden, M. (2020). Micro- and nanoplastic toxicity on aquatic life: Determining factors. *The Science of the Total Environment*, *709*(5817), 136050. doi:10.1016/j.scitotenv.2019.136050 PMID:31887526

Köhler, A. (2010). *Cellular fate of organic compounds in marine invertebrates*. Comparative Biochemistry and Physiology Part A: Molecular & Integrative Physiology; 27th Congress of the new European Society of Comparative Biochemistry and Physiology, Alessandria, Italy. 10.1016/j.cbpa.2010.06.020

Kokalj, A. J., Kunej, U., & Skalar, T. (2018). Screening study of four environmentally relevant microplastic pollutants: Uptake and effects on Daphnia magna and Artemia franciscana. *Chemosphere*, *208*, 522–529. doi:10.1016/j.chemosphere.2018.05.172 PMID:29890490

Koller, M., & Braunegg, G. (2018). Advanced approaches to produce polyhydroxyalkanoate (PHA) biopolyesters in a sustainable and economic fashion. *The EuroBiotech Journal*, *2*(2), 89–103. doi:10.2478/ebtj-2018-0013

Kowalski, N., Reichardt, A. M., & Waniek, J. J. (2016). Sinking rates of microplastics and potential implications of their alteration by physical, biological, and chemical factors. *Marine Pollution Bulletin*, *109*(1), 310–319. doi:10.1016/j.marpolbul.2016.05.064 PMID:27297594

Krelling, A., Williams, A., & Turra, A. (2017). Differences in perception and reaction of tourist groups to beach marine debris that can influence a loss of tourism revenue in coastal areas. *Marine Policy*, *85*, 87–99. doi:10.1016/j.marpol.2017.08.021

Kreyling, W. G., Semmler-Behnke, M., Seitz, J., Scymczak, W., Wenk, A., Mayer, P., Takenaka, S., & Oberdörster, G. (2009). Size dependence of the translocation of inhaled iridium and carbon nanoparticle aggregates from the lung of rats to the blood and secondary target organs. *Inhalation Toxicology*, *21*(sup1, Suppl 1), 55–60. doi:10.1080/08958370902942517 PMID:19558234

Krishnamurthy, A., & Amritkumar, P. (2019). Synthesis and characterization of eco-friendly bioplastic from low-cost plant resources. *SN Applied Sciences*, *1*(11), 1432. doi:10.100742452-019-1460-x

Krüger, L., Casado-Coy, N., Valle, C., Ramos, M., Sánchez-Jerez, P., Gago, J., Carretero, O., Beltran-Sanahuja, A., & Sanz-Lazaro, C. (2020). Plastic debris accumulation in the seabed derived from coastal fish farming. *Environmental Pollution*, *257*, 113336. doi:10.1016/j.envpol.2019.113336 PMID:31753624

Kubowicz, S., & Booth, A. M. (2017). Biodegradability of Plastics: Challenges and Misconceptions. *Environmental Science & Technology*, *51*(21), 12058–12060. doi:10.1021/acs.est.7b04051 PMID:29022342

Kukulka, T., Proskurowski, G., Morét-Ferguson, S., Meyer, D. W., & Law, K. L. (2012). The effect of wind mixing on the vertical distribution of buoyant plastic debris. *Geophysical Research Letters*, *39*(7), n/a. Advance online publication. doi:10.1029/2012GL051116

Kumar, M., Xiong, X., He, M., Tsang, D. C. W., Gupta, J., Khan, E., Harrad, S., Hou, D., Ok, Y. S., & Bolan, N. S. (2020). Microplastics as pollutants in agricultural soils. *Environmental Pollution*, *265*, 114980. doi:10.1016/j.envpol.2020.114980 PMID:32544663

Kummu, M., De Moel, H., Ward, P. J., & Varis, O. (2011). How close do we live to water? A global analysis of population distance to freshwater bodies. *PLoS One*, *6*(6), e20578. doi:10.1371/journal.pone.0020578 PMID:21687675

Kundu, A., Sharma, S., & Basu, S. (2021). Modulated BiOCl Nanoplates with Porous g-C3N4 Nanosheets for photocatalytic degradation of Color/Colorless Pollutants in Natural Sunlight. *Journal of Physics and Chemistry of Solids*, *154*, 110064. doi:10.1016/j.jpcs.2021.110064

Kundu, A., Shetti, N. P., Basu, S., Reddy, K. R., Nadagouda, M. N., & Aminabhavi, T. M. (2021). Identification and removal of micro- and nano-plastics: Efficient and cost-effective methods. *Chemical Engineering Journal*, *421*, 129816.

Kundu, A., Shetti, N. P., Basu, S., Reddy, K. R., Nadagouda, M. N., & Aminabhavi, T. M. (2021). Identification and removal of micro-and nano-plastics: Efficient and cost-effective methods. *Chemical Engineering Journal*, *421*, 129816. doi:10.1016/j.cej.2021.129816 PMID:34504393

Kwak, J. I., & An, Y. J. (2021). Microplastic digestion generates fragmented nanoplastics in soils and damages earthworm spermatogenesis and coelomocyte viability. *Journal of Hazardous Materials*, *402*, 124034. doi:10.1016/j.jhazmat.2020.124034 PMID:33254833

Lagarde, F., Olivier, O., Zanella, M., Daniel, P., Hiard, S., & Caruso, A. (2016). Microplastic interactions with freshwater microalgae: Hetero-aggregation and changes in plastic density appear strongly dependent on polymer type. *Environmental Pollution*, *215*, 331–339. doi:10.1016/j.envpol.2016.05.006 PMID:27236494

Lahens, L., Strady, E., Kieu-Le, T. C., Dris, R., Boukerma, K., Rinnert, E., Gasperi, J., & Tassin, B. (2018). Macroplastic and microplastic contamination assessment of a tropical river (Saigon River, Vietnam) transversed by a developing megacity. *Environmental Pollution, 236*, 661–671. doi:10.1016/j.envpol.2018.02.005 PMID:29438952

Laist, D. W. (1997). Impacts of marine debris: entanglement of marine life in marine debris including a comprehensive list of species with entanglement and ingestion records. In Marine Debris —Sources, Impacts and Solutions. SpringerVerlag. doi:10.1007/978-1-4613-8486-1_10

Lambert, S., & Wagner, M. (2016). Formation of microscopic particles during the degradation of different polymers. *Chemosphere, 161*, 510–517. doi:10.1016/j.chemosphere.2016.07.042 PMID:27470943

Lambert, S., & Wagner, M. (2017). Environmental performance of bio-based and biodegradable plastics: The road ahead. *Chemical Society Reviews, 46*(22), 6855–6871. doi:10.1039/C7CS00149E PMID:28932844

Lamb, J. B., Willis, B. L., Fiorenza, E. A., Couch, C. S., Howard, R., Rader, D. N., True, J. D., Kelly, L. A., Ahamd, A., Jompa, J., & Harvell, C. D. (2018). Plastic waste associated with disease on coral reefs. *Science, 359*(6374), 460–462. doi:10.1126cience.aar3320 PMID:29371469

Lamprecht, A. (2013). *The abundance, distribution and accumulation of plastic debris in Table Bay, Cape Town, South Africa* [Master's dissertation]. University of Cape Town. http://hdl.handle.net/11427/6633

Lanctôt, C. M., Bednarz, V. N., Melvin, S., Jacob, H., Oberhaensli, F., Swarzenski, P. W., Ferrier-Pagès, C., Carroll, A. R., & Metian, M. (2020). Physiological stress response of the scleractinian coral *Stylophora pistillata* exposed to polyethylene microplastics. *Environmental Pollution, 114559*. Advance online publication. doi:10.1016/j.envpol.2020.114559 PMID:32325355

Lange, G. M. (2015). Tourism in Zanzibar: Incentives for sustainable management of the coastal environment. *Ecosystem Services, 11*, 5–11. doi:10.1016/j.ecoser.2014.11.009

Langner, S., Rakers, S., Ciba, P., Petschnik, A. E., Rapoport, D. H., & Kruse, C. (2011). New cell line from adipopancreatic tissue of Atlantic herring *Clupea harengus*. *Aquatic Biology, 11*(3), 271–278. doi:10.3354/ab00317

Lan, R., Wei, Y., & Xue, R. (2021). Uptake of polystyrene microplastics by marine rotifers under different experimental conditions. *IOP Conference Series. Earth and Environmental Science, 687*(1), 012071. doi:10.1088/1755-1315/687/1/012071

Lasprilla, A. J. R., Martinez, G. A. R., Lunelli, B. H., Jardini, A. L., & Filho, R. M. (2012). Poly-lactic acid synthesis for application in biomedical devices – A review. *Biotechnology Advances, 30*(1), 321–328. doi:10.1016/j.biotechadv.2011.06.019 PMID:21756992

Lau, W. W. Y., Shiran, Y., Bailey, R. M., Cook, E., Stuchtey, M. R., Koskella, J., Velis, C. A., Godfrey, L., Boucher, J., Murphy, M. B., Thompson, R. C., Jankowska, E., Castillo Castillo, A., Pilditch, T. D., Dixon, B., Koerselman, L., Kosior, E., Favoino, E., Gutberlet, J., ... Palardy, J. E. (2020). Evaluating scenarios toward zero plastic pollution. *Science, 369*(6510), 1455–1461. doi:10.1126cience.aba9475 PMID:32703909

Laville, S. (2019). Dumped fishing gear is biggest plastic polluter in ocean, finds report. *The Gardian*. https://www.theguardian.com/environment/2019/nov/06/dumped-fishing-gear-is-biggest-plastic-polluter-in-ocean-finds-report

Law, K. L. (2017). Plastics in the Marine Environment. *Annual Review of Marine Science, 9*(1), 205–229. doi:10.1146/annurev-marine-010816-060409 PMID:27620829

Law, K. L., Morét-Ferguson, S. E., Goodwin, D. S., Zettler, E. R., DeForce, E., Kukulka, T., & Proskurowski, G. (2014). Distribution of surface plastic debris in the eastern Pacific Ocean from an 11-year data set. *Environmental Science & Technology, 48*(9), 4732–4738. doi:10.1021/es4053076 PMID:24708264

Law, K. L., Morét-Ferguson, S., Maximenko, N. A., Proskurowski, G., Peacock, E. E., Hafner, J., & Reddy, C. M. (2010). Plastic accumulation in the North Atlantic subtropical gyre. *Science*, *329*(5996), 1185–1188. doi:10.1126cience.1192321 PMID:20724586

Law, K. L., & Thompson, R. C. (2014). Oceans: Microplastics in the seas. *Science*, *345*(6193), 144–145. doi:10.1126cience.1254065 PMID:25013051

Lazarevic, D., Aoustin, E., Buclet, N., & Brandt, N. (2010). Plastic waste management in the context of a European recycling society: Comparing results and uncertainties in a life cycle perspective. *Resources, Conservation and Recycling*, *55*(2), 246–259. doi:10.1016/j.resconrec.2010.09.014

Le Guern, C. (2018). *When the mermaids cry: The great plastic tide. Coastal Care.* Retrieved from https://coastalcare.org

Lebreton, L. C., Van Der Zwet, J., Damsteeg, J. W., Slat, B., Andrady, A., & Reisser, J. (2017). River plastic emissions to the world's oceans. *Nature Communications*, *8*(1), 1–10. doi:10.1038/ncomms15611 PMID:28589961

Lebreton, L., & Andrady, A. (2019). Future scenarios of global plastic waste generation and disposal. *Palgrave Communications*, *5*(1), 6. Advance online publication. doi:10.105741599-018-0212-7

Lechner, A., & Ramler, D. (2015). The discharge of certain amounts of industrial microplastic from a production plant into the River Danube is permitted by the Austrian legislation. *Environmental Pollution*, *200*, 159–160. doi:10.1016/j.envpol.2015.02.019 PMID:25734504

Lee, G. E., & Lee, J. H. (2021). Spatial correlation analysis using the indicators of the anthropocene focusing on atmospheric pollution: A case study of Seoul. *Ecological Indicators*, *125*, 107535. doi:10.1016/j.ecolind.2021.107535

Lee, H., Byun, D.-E., Kim, J. M., & Kwon, J.-H. (2018). Desorption of Hydrophobic Organic Chemicals from Fragment-Type Microplastics. *Ocean Science Journal*, *53*(4), 631–639. doi:10.100712601-018-0051-x

Lee, H., Kunz, A., Shim, W. J., & Walther, B. A. (2019). Microplastic contamination of table salts from Taiwan, including a global review. *Scientific Reports*, *9*(1), 1–9. doi:10.103841598-019-46417-z PMID:31300670

Lee, H., Shim, W. J., & Kwon, J. H. (2014). Sorption capacity of plastic debris for hydrophobic organic chemicals. *The Science of the Total Environment*, *470–471*, 1545–1552. doi:10.1016/j.scitotenv.2013.08.023 PMID:24012321

Lee, K. W., Shim, W. J., Kwon, O. Y., & Kang, J. H. (2013). Size-dependent effects of micro polystyrene particles in the marine copepod tigriopus japonicus. *Environmental Science & Technology*, *47*(19), 11278–11283. doi:10.1021/es401932b PMID:23988225

Lee, S., Gounley, J., Randles, A., & Vetter, J. S. (2019). Performance portability study for massively parallel computational fluid dynamics application on scalable heterogeneous architectures. *Journal of Parallel and Distributed Computing*, *129*, 1–13. doi:10.1016/j.jpdc.2019.02.005

Lehel, J., & Murphy, S. (2021). Microplastics in the Food Chain: Food Safety and Environmental Aspects. *Reviews of Environmental Contamination and Toxicology*, *259*, 1–49. PMID:34611754

Lehmann, A., Leifheit, E. F., Feng, L., Bergmann, J., Wulf, A., & Rillig, M. C. (2020). *Microplastic fiber and drought effects on plants and soil are only slightly modified by arbuscular mycorrhizal fungi.* Soil Ecology Letters., doi:10.100742832-020-0060-4

Lehner, R., Weder, C., Petri-Fink, A., & Rothen-Rutishauser, B. (2019). Emergence of Nanoplastic in the Environment and Possible Impact on Human Health. *Environmental Science & Technology*, *53*(4), 1748–1765. doi:10.1021/acs.est.8b05512 PMID:30629421

Lehtiniemi, M., Hartikainen, S., Turja, R., Lehtonen, K. K., Vepsäläinen, J., Peräniemi, S., Leskinen, J., & Setälä, O. (2021). Exposure to leachates from post-consumer plastic and recycled rubber causes stress responses and mortality in a copepod Limnocalanus macrurus. *Marine Pollution Bulletin, 173*, 113103. doi:10.1016/j.marpolbul.2021.113103 PMID:34741928

Lei, L., Wu, S., Lu, S., Liu, M., Song, Y., Fu, Z., Shi, H., Raley-Susman, K. M., & He, D. (2018). Microplastic particles cause intestinal damage and other adverse effects in zebrafish Danio rerio and nematode Caenorhabditis elegans. *The Science of the Total Environment, 619-620*, 1–8. doi:10.1016/j.scitotenv.2017.11.103 PMID:29136530

Lenz, R., Enders, K., Stedmon, C. A., MacKenzie, D. M. A., & Nielsen, T. G. (2015). A critical assessment of visual identification of marine microplastic using Raman spectroscopy for analysis improvement. *Marine Pollution Bulletin, 100*(1), 82–91. doi:10.1016/j.marpolbul.2015.09.026 PMID:26455785

Leslie, H. A. (2014). Review of microplastics in cosmetics. *IVM Institute for Environmental Studies, 476*, 1–33.

Leslie, H. A., Brandsma, S. H., van Velzen, M. J. M., & Vethaak, A. D. (2017). Microplastics en route: Field measurements in the Dutch river delta and Amsterdam canals, wastewater treatment plants, North Sea sediments and biota. *Environment International, 101*, 133–142. doi:10.1016/j.envint.2017.01.018 PMID:28143645

Li, Q., Feng, Z., Zhang, T., Ma, C., & Shi, H. (2020). Microplastics in the commercial seaweed nori. *Journal of Hazardous Materials, 388*(December), 122060. doi:10.1016/j.jhazmat.2020.122060

Lian, J., Liu, W., Meng, L., Wu, J., Zeb, A., Cheng, L., Lian, Y., & Sun, H. (2021). Effects of microplastics derived from polymer-coated fertilizer on maize growth, rhizosphere, and soil properties. *Journal of Cleaner Production, 318*, 128571. doi:10.1016/j.jclepro.2021.128571

Liao, B., Wang, J., Xiao, B., Yang, X., Xie, Z., Li, D., & Li, C. (2021). Effects of acute microplastic exposure on physiological parameters in *Tubastrea aurea* corals. *Marine Pollution Bulletin, 165*, 112173. doi:10.1016/j.marpolbul.2021.112173 PMID:33621903

Liebezeit, G., & Dubaish, F. (2012). Microplastics in beaches of the East Frisian Islands Spiekeroog and Kachelotplate. *Bulletin of Environmental Contamination and Toxicology, 89*(1), 213–217. doi:10.100700128-012-0642-7 PMID:22526995

Liebezeit, G., & Liebezeit, E. (2014). Synthetic particles as contaminants in German beers. *Food Additives & Contaminants. Part A, Chemistry, Analysis, Control, Exposure & Risk Assessment, 31*(9), 1574–1578. doi:10.1080/19440049.2014.945099 PMID:25056358

Li, H.-X., Getzinger, G. J., Ferguson, P. L., Orihuela, B., Zhu, M., & Rittschof, D. (2015). Effects of Toxic Leachate from Commercial Plastics on Larval Survival and Settlement of the Barnacle *Amphibalanus amphitrite. Environmental Science & Technology, 50*(2), 924–931. doi:10.1021/acs.est.5b02781 PMID:26667586

Li, J., Green, C., Reynolds, A., Shi, H., & Rotchell, J. M. (2018). Microplastics in mussels sampled from coastal waters and supermarkets in the United Kingdom. *Environmental Pollution, 241*, 35–44. doi:10.1016/j.envpol.2018.05.038 PMID:29793106

Li, J., Liu, H., & Chen, J. P. (2018). Microplastics in freshwater systems: A review on occurrence, environmental effects, and methods for microplastics detection. *Water Research, 137*, 362–374. doi:10.1016/j.watres.2017.12.056 PMID:29580559

Li, J., Song, Y., & Cai, Y. (2020). Focus topics on microplastics in soil: Analytical methods, occurrence, transport, and ecological risks. *Environmental Pollution, 257*, 113570. doi:10.1016/j.envpol.2019.113570 PMID:31767234

Li, J., Wang, Z., Rotchell, J. M., Shen, X., Li, Q., & Zhu, J. (2021). Where are we? Towards an understanding of the selective accumulation of microplastics in mussels. *Environmental Pollution*, *286*(June), 117543. doi:10.1016/j.envpol.2021.117543 PMID:34119866

Li, J., Yang, D., Li, L., Jabeen, K., & Shi, H. (2015). Microplastics in commercial bivalves from China. *Environmental Pollution*, *207*, 190–195. doi:10.1016/j.envpol.2015.09.018 PMID:26386204

Li, L., Geng, S., Wu, C., Song, K., Sun, F., Visvanathan, C., Xie, F., & Wang, Q. (2019). Microplastics contamination in different trophic state lakes along the middle and lower reaches of Yangtze River Basin. *Environmental Pollution*, *254*, 112951. doi:10.1016/j.envpol.2019.07.119 PMID:31374488

Lim, X. (2021). *Microplastics are everywhere—but are they harmful?* Academic Press.

Lim, L.-T., Auras, R., & Rubino, M. (2008). Processing technologies for poly(lactic acid). *Progress in Polymer Science*, *33*(8), 820–852. doi:10.1016/j.progpolymsci.2008.05.004

Lindhqvist, T. (2000). *Extended Producer Responsibility in Cleaner Production' The International Institute for Industrial Environmental Economics*. Lund University.

Lin, L., Zuo, L. Z., Peng, J. P., Cai, L. Q., Fok, L., Yan, Y., Li, H. X., & Xu, X. R. (2018). Occurrence and distribution of microplastics in an urban river: A case study in the Pearl River along Guangzhou City, China. *The Science of the Total Environment*, *644*, 375–381. doi:10.1016/j.scitotenv.2018.06.327 PMID:29981986

Lippiatt, S., Opfer, S., & Arthur, C. (2013). *Marine debris monitoring and assessment: recommendations for monitoring debris trends in the marine environment*. NOAA. https://repository.library.noaa.gov/view/noaa/2681

Li, Q., Wu, J., Zhao, X., Gu, X., & Ji, R. (2019). Separation and identification of microplastics from soil and sewage sludge. *Environmental Pollution*, *254*, 113076. doi:10.1016/j.envpol.2019.113076 PMID:31472456

Lithner, D., Damberg, J., Dave, G., & Larsson, Å. (2009). Leachates from plastic consumer products - Screening for toxicity with *Daphnia magna*. *Chemosphere*, *74*(9), 1195–1200. doi:10.1016/j.chemosphere.2008.11.022 PMID:19108869

Liu, B., Jiang, L., & Zhang, J. (2010). *Development of soy protein/poly (lacctic acid) bioplastics*. Society of Plastic Engineers.

Liu, M., Lu, S., Chen, Y., Cao, C., Bigalke, M., & He, D. (2020). Analytical Methods for Microplastics in Environments: Current Advances and Challenges. In Handbook of Environmental Chemistry (Vol. 95, pp. 3–24). doi:10.1007/698_2019_436

Liu, E., He, W. Q., & Yan, C. (2014). 'White revolution' to 'white pollution' - agricultural plastic film mulch in China. *Environmental Research Letters*, *9*(9), 091001. doi:10.1088/1748-9326/9/9/091001

Liu, F., Olesen, K. B., Borregaard, A. R., & Vollertsen, J. (2019). Microplastics in urban and highway stormwater retention ponds. *The Science of the Total Environment*, *671*, 992–1000. doi:10.1016/j.scitotenv.2019.03.416 PMID:31604201

Liu, H. F., Yang, X. M., Liu, G. B., Liang, C. T., Xue, S., Chen, H., Ritsema, C. J., & Geissen, V. (2017). Response of soil dissolved organic matter to microplastic addition in Chinese loess soil. *Chemosphere*, *185*, 907–917. doi:10.1016/j.chemosphere.2017.07.064 PMID:28747000

Liu, J., Lezama, N., Gasper, J., Kawata, J., Morley, S., Helmer, D., & Ciminera, P. (2016). Burn Pit Emissions Exposure and Respiratory and Cardiovascular Conditions Among Airborne Hazards and Open Burn Pit Registry Participants. *Journal of Occupational and Environmental Medicine*, *58*(7), e249–e255. doi:10.1097/JOM.0000000000000776 PMID:27218278

Liu, J., Yang, Y., Ding, J., Zhu, B., & Gao, W. (2019). Microfibers: A preliminary discussion on their definition and sources. *Environmental Science and Pollution Research International, 26*(28), 29497–29501. doi:10.100711356-019-06265-w PMID:31444725

Liu, K., Wang, X., Fang, T., Xu, P., Zhu, L., & Li, D. (2019). Source and potential risk assessment of suspended atmospheric microplastics in Shanghai. *The Science of the Total Environment, 675*, 462–471. doi:10.1016/j.scitotenv.2019.04.110 PMID:31030152

Liu, K., Wang, X., Song, Z., Wei, N., & Li, D. (2020). Terrestrial plants as a potential temporary sink of atmospheric microplastics during transport. *The Science of the Total Environment, 742*, 140523.

Liu, K., Wang, X., Wei, N., Song, Z., & Li, D. (2019). Accurate quantification and transport estimation of suspended atmospheric microplastics in megacities: Implications for human health. *Environment International, 132*, 105127. doi:10.1016/j.envint.2019.105127 PMID:31487610

Liu, K., Wu, T., Wang, X., Song, Z., Zong, C., Wei, N., & Li, D. (2019). Consistent Transport of Terrestrial Microplastics to the Ocean through Atmosphere. *Environmental Science & Technology, 53*(18), 10612–10619. doi:10.1021/acs.est.9b03427 PMID:31408609

Liu, L., Fokkink, R., & Koelmans, A. A. (2016). Sorption of polycyclic aromatic hydrocarbons to polystyrene nanoplastic. *Environmental Toxicology and Chemistry, 35*(7), 1650–1655. doi:10.1002/etc.3311 PMID:26588181

Liu, M., Lu, S., Song, Y., Lei, L., Hu, J., Lv, W., Zhou, W., Cao, C., Shi, H., Yang, X., & He, D. (2018). Microplastic and mesoplastic pollution in farmland soils in suburbs of Shanghai, China. *Environmental Pollution, 242*, 855–862. doi:10.1016/j.envpol.2018.07.051 PMID:30036839

Liu, X., Shi, H., Xie, B., Dionysiou, D. D., & Zhao, Y. (2019). Microplastics as both a sink and a source of bisphenol A in the marine environment. *Environmental Science & Technology, 53*(17), 10188–10196. doi:10.1021/acs.est.9b02834 PMID:31393116

Liu, Z., Adams, M., & Walker, T. (2018). Are exports of recyclables from developed to developing countries waste pollution transfer or part of the global circular economy? *Resources, Conservation and Recycling, 136*, 22–23. doi:10.1016/j.resconrec.2018.04.005

Liu, Z., Yu, P., Cai, M., Wu, D., Zhang, M., Chen, M., & Zhao, Y. (2019). Effects of microplastics on the innate immunity and intestinal microflora of juvenile *Eriocheir sinensis. The Science of the Total Environment, 685*, 836–846. doi:10.1016/j.scitotenv.2019.06.265 PMID:31247433

Li, W. C., Tse, H. F., & Fok, L. (2016). Plastic waste in the marine environment: A review of sources, occurrence and effects. *The Science of the Total Environment, 566*, 333–349. doi:10.1016/j.scitotenv.2016.05.084 PMID:27232963

Li, W., Wufuer, R., Duo, J., Wang, S., Luo, Y., Zhang, D., & Pan, X. (2020). Microplastics in agricultural soils: Extraction and characterization after different periods of polythene film mulching in an arid region. *The Science of the Total Environment, 749*, 141420. doi:10.1016/j.scitotenv.2020.141420 PMID:32836118

Li, Y., Zhang, H., & Tang, C. (2020). *A review of possible pathways of marine microplastics transport in the ocean.* Anthropocene Coasts. doi:10.1139/anc-2018-0030

Lizárraga, D., Danihel, A., & Pernet, B. (2017). Low concentrations of large inedible particles reduce feeding rates of echinoderm larvae. *Marine Biology, 164*(5), 102. Advance online publication. doi:10.100700227-017-3134-9

Long, M., Paul-Pont, I., Hégaret, H., Moriceau, B., Lambert, C., Huvet, A., & Soudant, P. (2017). Interactions between polystyrene microplastics and marine phytoplankton lead to species-specific hetero-aggregation. *Environmental Pollution, 228*, 454–463. doi:10.1016/j.envpol.2017.05.047 PMID:28558286

Long, Z., Pan, Z., Wang, W., Ren, J., Yu, X., Lin, L., Lin, H., Chen, H., & Jin, X. (2019). Microplastic abundance, characteristics, and removal in wastewater treatment plants in a coastal city of China. *Water Research, 155*, 255–265. doi:10.1016/j.watres.2019.02.028 PMID:30852313

Lönnstedt, O. M., & Eklöv, P. (2016). Environmentally relevant concentrations of microplastic particles influence larval fish ecology. *Science, 352*(6290), 1213–1216. doi:10.1126cience.aad8828 PMID:27257256

López Rocha, C. J., Álvarez-Castillo, E., Estrada Yáñez, M. R., Bengoechea, C., Guerrero, A., & Orta Ledesma, M. T. (2020). Development of bioplastics from a microalgae consortium from wastewater. *Journal of Environmental Management, 263*, 110353. doi:10.1016/j.jenvman.2020.110353 PMID:32883472

Lots, F. A. E., Behrens, P., Vijver, M. G., Horton, A. A., & Bosker, T. (2017). A large-scale investigation of microplastic contamination: Abundance and characteristics of microplastics in European beach sediment. *Marine Pollution Bulletin, 123*(1–2), 219–226. doi:10.1016/j.marpolbul.2017.08.057 PMID:28893402

Lozano, Y. M., Aguilar-Trigueros, C. A., Onandia, G., Maaß, S., Zhao, T., & Rillig, M. C. (2021). Effects of microplastics and drought on soil ecosystem functions and multifunctionality. *Journal of Applied Ecology, 00*(5), 1–9. doi:10.1111/1365-2664.13839

Lozano, Y. M., & Rillig, M. C. (2020). Effects of microplastic fibers and drought on plant communities. *Environmental Science & Technology, 54*(10), 6166–6173. doi:10.1021/acs.est.0c01051 PMID:32289223

Luigi, P., Chiara, A., Elisabetta, G., Alessandra, S., & Luigi, M. G. (2012). Utilization of marine crustaceans as study models: A new approach in marine ecotoxicology for European (REACH) regulation. Academic Press.

Lu, L., Luo, T., Zhao, Y., Cai, C., Fu, Z., & Jin, Y. (2019). Interaction between microplastics and microorganism as well as gut microbiota: A consideration on environmental animal and human health. *The Science of the Total Environment, 667*, 94–100. doi:10.1016/j.scitotenv.2019.02.380 PMID:30826685

Lu, L., Wan, Z., Luo, T., Fu, Z., & Jin, Y. (2018). Polystyrene microplastics induce gut microbiota dysbiosis and hepatic lipid metabolism disorder in mice. *The Science of the Total Environment, 631-632*, 449–458. doi:10.1016/j.scitotenv.2018.03.051 PMID:29529433

Luo, H., Liu, C., He, D., Xu, J., Sun, J., Li, J., & Pan, X. (2022). Environmental behaviors of microplastics in aquatic systems: A systematic review on degradation, adsorption, toxicity and biofilm under aging conditions. *Journal of Hazardous Materials, 423*, 126915. doi:10.1016/j.jhazmat.2021.126915 PMID:34461541

Luo, K., Yang, J., Kopečkova, P., & Kopeček, J. (2011). Biodegradable multiblock poly[N-(2-hydroxypropyl)methacrylamide] via reversible addition-fragmentation chain transfer polymerization and click chemistry. *Macromolecules, 44*(8), 2481–2488. doi:10.1021/ma102574e PMID:21552355

Luo, T., Zhang, Y., Wang, C., Wang, X., Zhou, J., Shen, M., Zhao, Y., Fu, Z., & Jin, Y. (2019). Maternal exposure to different sizes of polystyrene microplastics during gestation causes metabolic disorders in their offspring. *Environmental Pollution, 255*, 113122. doi:10.1016/j.envpol.2019.113122 PMID:31520900

Luo, W., Su, L., Craig, N. J., Du, F., Wu, C., & Shi, H. (2019). Comparison of microplastic pollution in different water bodies from urban creeks to coastal waters. In *Environmental Pollution* (Vol. 246, pp. 174–182). Elsevier Sci Ltd. doi:10.1016/j.envpol.2018.11.081

Lusher, A. L., Munno, K., Hermabessiere, L., & Carr, S. (2020). Isolation and Extraction of Microplastics from Environmental Samples: An Evaluation of Practical Approaches and Recommendations for Further Harmonization. In Applied Spectroscopy (Vol. 74, Issue 9). doi:10.1177/0003702820938993

Lusher, A. L., McHugh, M., & Thompson, R. C. (2013). Occurrence of microplastics in the gastrointestinal tract of pelagic and demersal fish from the English Channel. *Marine Pollution Bulletin*, *67*(1–2), 94–99. doi:10.1016/j.marpolbul.2012.11.028 PMID:23273934

Lusher, A. L., Tirelli, V., O'Connor, I., & Officer, R. (2015). Microplastics in Arctic polar waters: The first reported values of particles in surface and sub-surface samples. *Scientific Reports*, *5*(September), 1–9. doi:10.1038rep14947 PMID:26446348

Lusher, A. L., Welden, N. A., Sobral, P., & Cole, M. (2017). Sampling, isolating and identifying microplastics ingested by fish and invertebrates. *Analytical Methods*, *9*(9), 1346–1360. doi:10.1039/C6AY02415G

Lusher, A., Hollman, P., & Mendozal, J. (2017). Microplastics in fisheries and aquaculture: Status of knowledge on their occurrence and implications for aquatic organisms and food safety. *FAO Fisheries and Aquaculture Technical Paper*, *615*, 147.

Lu, Y., Zhang, Y., Deng, Y., Jiang, W., Zhao, Y., Geng, J., Ding, L., & Ren, H. (2016). Uptake and accumulation of polystyrene microplastics in zebrafish (Danio rerio) and toxic effects in liver. *Environmental Science & Technology*, *50*(7), 4054–4060. doi:10.1021/acs.est.6b00183 PMID:26950772

lvarez-Román, R., Naik, A., Kalia, Y. N., Guy, R. H., & Fessi, H. (2004). Skin penetration and distribution of polymeric nanoparticles. *Journal of Controlled Release, 99*(1), 53-62.

Lv, L., Qu, J., Yu, Z., Chen, D., Zhou, C., Hong, P., Sun, S., & Li, C. (2019). A simple method for detecting and quantifying microplastics utilizing fluorescent dyes - Safranine T, fluorescein isophosphate, Nile red based on thermal expansion and contraction property. *Environmental Pollution*, *255*, 113283. doi:10.1016/j.envpol.2019.113283 PMID:31580990

Lv, L., Yan, X., Feng, L., Jiang, S., Lu, Z., Xie, H., Sun, S., Chen, J., & Li, C. (2021). Challenge for the detection of microplastics in the environment. *Water Environment Research*, *93*(1), 5–15. doi:10.1002/wer.1281 PMID:31799785

Lyakurwa, D. J. (2017). *Uptake and effects of microplastic particles in selected marine microalgae species: Oxyrrhis marina* and *Rhodomonas baltica*. Academic Press.

Lydon, T. (2021). *3,000 Shipping Containers Fell Into the Pacific Ocean Last Winter.* https://therevelator.org/container-ship-accidents/

Maaghloud, H., Houssa, R., Bellali, F., El Bouqdaoui, K., Ouansafi, S., Loulad, S., & Fahde, A. (2021). Microplastic ingestion by Atlantic horse mackerel (Trachurus trachurus) in the North and central Moroccan Atlantic coast between Larache (35 degrees 30 ` N) and Boujdour (26 degrees 30 ` N). In *Environmental Pollution* (Vol. 288). Elsevier Sci Ltd. doi:10.1016/j.envpol.2021.117781

Ma, B., Xue, W., Ding, Y., Hu, C., Liu, H., & Qu, J. (2019). Removal characteristics of microplastics by Fe-based coagulants during drinking water treatment. *Journal of Environmental Sciences (China)*, *78*, 267–275. doi:10.1016/j.jes.2018.10.006 PMID:30665645

Macali, A., Semenov, A., Venuti, V., Crupi, V., D'Amico, F., Rossi, B., Corsi, I., & Bergami, E. (2018). Episodic records of jellyfish ingestion of plastic items reveal a novel pathway for trophic transference of marine litter. *Scientific Reports*, *8*(1), 1–5. doi:10.103841598-018-24427-7 PMID:29666447

Mack, C. (2018). *How to Write a Good Scientific Paper*. SPIE. doi:10.1117/3.2317707

Magara, G., Elia, A. C., Syberg, K., & Khan, F. R. (2018). Single contaminant and combined exposures of polyethylene microplastics and fluoranthene: Accumulation and oxidative stress response in the blue mussel, Mytilus edulis. *Journal of Toxicology and Environmental Health. Part A.*, *81*(16), 761–773. doi:10.1080/15287394.2018.1488639 PMID:29969377

Magar, S. P., Ingle, A. B., & Ganorkar, R. N. (2015). Production of bioplastic (PHA) from emulsified cotton seed oil medium by Ralstonia Spp. *International Journal of Engineering Research and General Science*, *3*(1), 436–441.

Magnusson, K., & Norén, F. (2014). Screening of microplastic particles in and down-stream a wastewater treatment plant. *IVL Swedish Environmental Research Institute, 55*(C), 22.

Magnusson, K., Eliaeson, K., Fråne, A., Haikonen, K., Olshammar, M., Stadmark, J., & Hultén, J. (2016). *Swedish sources and pathways for microplastics to the marine environment.* https://www.diva-portal.org/smash/record.jsf?pid=diva2%3A1549783&dswid=4554

Mai, L., You, S.-N., He, H., Bao, L.-J., Liu, L.-Y., & Zeng, E. Y. (2019). Riverine Microplastic Pollution in the Pearl River Delta, China: Are Modeled Estimates Accurate? In Environmental Science & Technology (Vol. 53, Issue 20, pp. 11810–11817). Amer Chemical Soc. doi:10.1021/acs.est.9b04838

Mai, L., Bao, L. J., Shi, L., Wong, C. S., & Zeng, E. Y. (2018). A review of methods for measuring microplastics in aquatic environments. *Environmental Science and Pollution Research International*, *25*(12), 11319–11332. doi:10.100711356-018-1692-0 PMID:29536421

Maione, C. (2019). *Emergence of plastic pollution on tourism beaches in Zanzibar, Tanzania* [Master's Thesis]. University of Michigan. http://hdl.handle.net/2027.42/148801

Maione, C. (2021). Quantifying plastics waste accumulations on coastal tourism sites in Zanzibar, Tanzania. *Marine Pollution Bulletin, 168*, 112418. doi:10.1016/j.marpolbul.2021.112418 PMID:33930645

Maione, C., & Fernandez, G. (2021). Plastic Detection Using a Multi-method Approach: Comparative Case Studies from Coastal Tourism Sites. In *Abstracts of 1st International Symposium on Plastic Pollution: Removal, Analysis, and Risk Assessment of Microplastics* (pp. 23-27). AIJR. 10.21467/abstracts.119

Malek, A., Willi, A., Muller, J., Sager, R., Hanggi, W., & Bersinger, N. (2001). Capacity for hormone production of cultured trophoblast cells obtained from placentae at term and in early pregnancy. *Journal of Assisted Reproduction and Genetics*, *18*(5), 299–304. doi:10.1023/A:1016674503298 PMID:11464582

Malik, S., Suchal, K., Gamad, N., Dinda, A. K., Arya, D. S., & Bhatia, J. (2015). Telmisartan ameliorates cisplatin-induced nephrotoxicity by inhibiting MAPK mediated inflammation and apoptosis. *European Journal of Pharmacology*, *748*, 54–60. doi:10.1016/j.ejphar.2014.12.008 PMID:25510231

Manfra, L., Rotini, A., Bergami, E., Grassi, G., Faleri, C., & Corsi, I. (2017). Comparative ecotoxicity of polystyrene nanoparticles in natural seawater and reconstituted seawater using the rotifer *Brachionus plicatilis. Ecotoxicology and Environmental Safety*, *145*, 557–563. doi:10.1016/j.ecoenv.2017.07.068 PMID:28800530

Mani, T., Hauk, A., Walter, U., & Burkhardt-Holm, P. (2015). Microplastics profile along the Rhine River. *Scientific Reports*, *5*(1), 1–7. doi:10.1038rep17988 PMID:26644346

Mao, Y., Ai, H., Chen, Y., Zhang, Z., Zeng, P., Kang, L., Li, W., Gu, W., He, Q., & Li, H. (2018). Phytoplankton response to polystyrene microplastics: Perspective from an entire growth period. *Chemosphere*, *208*, 59–68. doi:10.1016/j.chemosphere.2018.05.170 PMID:29860145

Mao, Y., Li, H., Huangfu, X., Liu, Y., & He, Q. (2020). Nanoplastics display strong stability in aqueous environments: Insights from aggregation behaviour and theoretical calculations. *Environmental Pollution*, *258*, 113760. doi:10.1016/j.envpol.2019.113760 PMID:31855670

Martin, C., Corona, E., Mahadik, G. A., & Duarte, C. M. (2019). Adhesion to coral surface as a potential sink for marine microplastics. *Environmental Pollution*, *255*, 113281. doi:10.1016/j.envpol.2019.113281 PMID:31600700

Martínez-Gómez, C., León, V. M., Calles, S., Gomáriz-Olcina, M., & Vethaak, A. D. (2017). The adverse effects of virgin microplastics on the fertilization and larval development of sea urchins. *Marine Environmental Research*, *130*, 69–76. doi:10.1016/j.marenvres.2017.06.016 PMID:28716299

Martin, J., Lusher, A. L., & Nixon, F. C. (2022). A review of the use of microplastics in reconstructing dated sedimentary archives. *The Science of the Total Environment*, *806*, 150818. doi:10.1016/j.scitotenv.2021.150818 PMID:34637878

Mason, S. A., Kammin, L., Eriksen, M., Aleid, G., Wilson, S., Box, C., Williamson, N., & Riley, A. (2016). Pelagic plastic pollution within the surface waters of Lake Michigan, USA. In Journal of Great Lakes Research (Vol. 42, Issue 4, pp. 753–759). Elsevier Sci Ltd. doi:10.1016/j.jglr.2016.05.009

Masura, J., Baker, J., Foster, G., & Arthur, C. (2015). Laboratory Methods for the Analysis of Microplastics in the Marine Environment. *NOAA Marine Debris Program National*, (July), 1–39. doi:10.1016/j.jjcc.2016.11.011

Mathalon, A., & Hill, P. (2014). Microplastic fibers in the intertidal ecosystem surrounding Halifax Harbor, Nova Scotia. *Marine Pollution Bulletin*, *81*(1), 69–79. doi:10.1016/j.marpolbul.2014.02.018 PMID:24650540

Mathiot, C., Ponge, P., Gallard, B., Sassi, J. F., Delrue, F., & Le Moigne, N. (2019). Microalgae starch-based bioplastics: Screening of ten strains and plasticization of unfractionated microalgae by extrusion. *Carbohydrate Polymers*, *208*, 142–151. doi:10.1016/j.carbpol.2018.12.057 PMID:30658785

Mato, Y., Isobe, T., Takada, H., Kanehiro, H., Ohtake, C., & Kaminuma, T. (2001). Plastic resin pellets as a transport medium for toxic chemicals in the marine environment. *Environmental Science & Technology*, *35*(2), 318–324. doi:10.1021/es0010498 PMID:11347604

Matsuguma, Y., Takada, H., Kumata, H., Kanke, H., Sakurai, S., Suzuki, T., Itoh, M., Okazaki, Y., Boonyatumanond, R., Zakaria, M. P., Weerts, S., & Newman, B. (2017). Microplastics in Sediment Cores from Asia and Africa as Indicators of Temporal Trends in Plastic Pollution. In Archives of Environmental Contamination and Toxicology (Vol. 73, Issues 2, SI, pp. 230–239). Springer. doi:10.100700244-017-0414-9

Matsui, K., Ishimura, T., Mattonai, M., Iwai, I., Watanabe, A., Teramae, N., Ohtani, H., & Watanabe, C. (2020). Journal of Analytical and Applied Pyrolysis Identification algorithm for polymer mixtures based on Py-GC / MS and its application for microplastic analysis in environmental samples. *Journal of Analytical and Applied Pyrolysis*, *149*(April), 104834. doi:10.1016/j.jaap.2020.104834

Mattsson, K., Ekvall, M. T., Hansson, L. A., Linse, S., Malmendal, A., & Cedervall, T. (2015). Altered behavior, physiology, and metabolism in fish exposed to polystyrene nanoparticles. *Environmental Science & Technology*, *49*(1), 553–561. doi:10.1021/es5053655 PMID:25380515

Mattsson, K., Hansson, L. A., & Cedervall, T. (2015). Nano-plastics in the aquatic environment. *Environmental Science. Processes & Impacts*, *17*(10), 1712–1721. doi:10.1039/C5EM00227C PMID:26337600

Mattsson, K., Jocic, S., Doverbratt, I., & Hansson, L. A. (2018). Nanoplastics in the aquatic environment. In *Microplastic Contamination in Aquatic Environments: An Emerging Matter of Environmental Urgency*. Elsevier Inc. doi:10.1016/B978-0-12-813747-5.00013-8

Mazurais, D., Ernande, B., Quazuguel, P., Severe, A., Huelvan, C., Madec, L., Mouchel, O., Soudant, P., Robbens, J., Huvet, A., & Zambonino-Infante, J. (2015). Evaluation of the impact of polyethylene microbeads ingestion in European sea bass (*Dicentrarchus labrax*) larvae. *Marine Environmental Research*, *112*, 78–85. doi:10.1016/j.marenvres.2015.09.009 PMID:26412109

McDevitt, J. P., Criddle, C. S., Morse, M., Hale, R. C., Bott, C. B., & Rochman, C. M. (2017). Addressing the Issue of Microplastics in the Wake of the Microbead-Free Waters Act - A New Standard Can Facilitate Improved Policy. In Environmental Science and Technology (Vol. 51, Issue 12, pp. 6611–6617). ACS Publications. doi:10.1021/acs.est.6b05812

McIlgorm, A., Campbell, H. F., & Rule, M. J. (2011). The economic cost and control of marine debris damage in the Asia-Pacific region. *Ocean and Coastal Management*, *54*(9), 643–651. doi:10.1016/j.ocecoaman.2011.05.007

McMahon, C. R., Holley, D., & Robinson, S. (1999). The diet of itinerant male Hooker's sea lions, *Phocarctos hookeri*, at sub-Antarctic Macquarie Island. *Wildlife Research*, *26*(6), 839. doi:10.1071/WR98079

Meereboer, K. W., Misra, M., & Mohanty, A. K. (2020). Review of recent advances in the biodegradability of polyhydroxyalkanoate (PHA) bioplastics and their composites. *Green Chemistry*, *22*(17), 5519–5558. doi:10.1039/D0GC01647K

Mendrik, F. M., Henry, T. B., Burdett, H., Hackney, C. R., Waller, C., Parsons, D. R., & Hennige, S. J. (2021). Species-specific impact of microplastics on coral physiology. *Environmental Pollution*, *269*, 116238. doi:10.1016/j.envpol.2020.116238 PMID:33321308

Menéndez-Pedriza, A., Jaumot, J., & Bedia, C. (2022). Lipidomic analysis of single and combined effects of polyethylene microplastics and polychlorinated biphenyls on human hepatoma cells. *Journal of Hazardous Materials*, *421*, 126777. doi:10.1016/j.jhazmat.2021.126777 PMID:34364209

Menicagli, V., Balestri, E., & Lardicci, C. (2019). Exposure of coastal dune vegetation to plastic bag leachates: A neglected impact of plastic litter. *The Science of the Total Environment*, *683*, 737–748. doi:10.1016/j.scitotenv.2019.05.245 PMID:31150894

Messinetti, S., Mercurio, S., Parolini, M., Sugni, M., & Pennati, R. (2018). Effects of polystyrene microplastics on early stages of two marine invertebrates with different feeding strategies. *Environmental Pollution*, *237*, 1080–1087. doi:10.1016/j.envpol.2017.11.030 PMID:29146202

Miller, E., Sedlak, M., Lin, D., Box, C., Holleman, C., Rochman, C. M., & Sutton, R. (2021). Recommended best practices for collecting, analyzing, and reporting microplastics in environmental media: Lessons learned from comprehensive monitoring of San Francisco Bay. *Journal of Hazardous Materials, 409*(November), 124770. doi:10.1016/j.jhazmat.2020.124770

Mincer, J. (2021). *Aftershocks of SARS-CoV-2: A plastic pandemic*. Canadian Family Physician.

Mintenig, S. M., Int-Veen, I., Löder, M. G. J., Primpke, S., & Gerdts, G. (2017). Identification of microplastic in effluents of waste water treatment plants using focal plane array-based micro-Fourier-transform infrared imaging. *Water Research*, *108*, 365–372. doi:10.1016/j.watres.2016.11.015 PMID:27838027

Mintenig, S. M., Kooi, M., Erich, M. W., Primpke, S., Redondo- Hasselerharm, P. E., Dekker, S. C., Koelmans, A. A., & van Wezel, A. P. (2020). A systems approach to understand microplastic occurrence and variability in Dutch riverine surface waters. *Water Research*, *176*, 115723. doi:10.1016/j.watres.2020.115723 PMID:32220661

Miranda, D. de A., & de Carvalho-Souza, G. F. (2016). Are we eating plastic-ingesting fish? *Marine Pollution Bulletin*, *103*(1–2), 109–114. doi:10.1016/j.marpolbul.2015.12.035 PMID:26763323

Mirtha, E.F., & Lopez, N.I., Mendez, B.S., Furst, U.P., & Steinbuchel, A. (1995). Isolation and partial characterization of Bacillus megaterium mutants deficient in poly(3-hydroxybutyrate) synthesis. *Canadian Journal of Microbiology, 41*(1), 77–79.

Miyagawa, S., Sato, T., & Iguchi, T. (2016). Handbook of Hormones. Academic Press.

Mohammed, S. M. (2002). Pollution management in Zanzibar: The need for a new approach. *Ocean and Coastal Management, 45*(4-5), 301–311. doi:10.1016/S0964-5691(02)00060-1

Mohanan, N., Montazer, Z., Sharma, P. K., & Levin, D. B. (2020). Microbial and Enzymatic Degradation of Synthetic Plastics. *Frontiers in Microbiology, 11*, 580709. doi:10.3389/fmicb.2020.580709 PMID:33324366

Mohee, R., Mauthoor, S., Bundhoo, Z. M., Somaroo, G., Soobhany, N., & Gunasee, S. (2015). Current status of solid waste management in small island developing states: A review. *Waste Management (New York, N.Y.), 43*, 539–549. doi:10.1016/j.wasman.2015.06.012 PMID:26116009

Mohsen, M., Sun, L., Lin, C., Huo, D., & Yang, H. (2021). Mechanism underlying the toxicity of the microplastic fibre transfer in the sea cucumber *Apostichopus japonicus. Journal of Hazardous Materials, 416*, 125858. doi:10.1016/j.jhazmat.2021.125858 PMID:34492807

Mohsen, M., Zhang, L., Sun, L., Lin, C., Wang, Q., & Yang, H. (2019). Microplastic fibers transfer from the water to the internal fluid of the sea cucumber *Apostichopus japonicus. Environmental Pollution, 113606*. Advance online publication. doi:10.1016/j.envpol.2019.113606 PMID:31761598

Möller, J. N., Löder, M. G. J., & Laforsch, C. (2020). Finding Microplastics in Soils: A Review of Analytical Methods. *Environmental Science & Technology, 54*(4), 2078–2090. doi:10.1021/acs.est.9b04618 PMID:31999440

Moore, C. J. (2008). Synthetic polymers in the marine environment: A rapidly increasing, long-term threat. *Environmental Research, 108*(2), 131–139. doi:10.1016/j.envres.2008.07.025 PMID:18949831

Morales-Cerrada, R., Tavernier, R., & Caillol, S. (2021). Fully bio-based thermosetting polyurethanes from bio-based polyols and isocyanates. *Polymers, 13*(8), 1255. doi:10.3390/polym13081255 PMID:33924399

Morcillo, P., Chaves-Pozo, E., Meseguer, J., Esteban, M. Á., & Cuesta, A. (2017). Establishment of a new teleost brain cell line (DLB-1) from the European sea bass and its use to study metal toxicology. *Toxicology In Vitro, 38*, 91–100. doi:10.1016/j.tiv.2016.10.005 PMID:27746373

Morét-Ferguson, S., Law, K. L., Proskurowski, G., Murphy, E. K., Peacock, E. E., & Reddy, C. M. (2010). The size, mass, and composition of plastic debris in the western North Atlantic Ocean. *Marine Pollution Bulletin, 60*(10), 1873–1878. doi:10.1016/j.marpolbul.2010.07.020 PMID:20709339

Morgana, S., Ghigliotti, L., Estévez-Calvar, N., Stifanese, R., Wieckzorek, A., Doyle, T., Christiansen, J. S., Faimali, M., & Garaventa, F. (2018). Microplastics in the Arctic: A case study with sub-surface water and fish samples off Northeast Greenland. *Environmental Pollution, 242*, 1078–1086. doi:10.1016/j.envpol.2018.08.001 PMID:30096546

Mortillaro, N. (2017). *Humans have produced 8.3 billion tonnes of plastic, researchers say*. Retrieved from https://www.cbc.ca/amp/1.4210279

Mostafa, N. A., Farag, A. A., Abo-dief, H. M., & Tayeb, A. M. (2014). Production of biodegradable plastic from agricultural wastes. *Arabian Journal of Chemistry*, 4–11.

Mouchi, V., Chapron, L., Peru, E., Pruski, A. M., Meistertzheim, A.-L., Vétion, G., Galand, P. E., & Lartaud, F. (2019). Long-term aquaria study suggests species-specific responses of two cold-water corals to macro-and microplastics exposure. *Environmental Pollution, 253*, 322–329. Advance online publication. doi:10.1016/j.envpol.2019.07.024 PMID:31323615

Moyce, S. C., & Schenker, M. (2018). Migrant workers and their occupational health and safety. *Annual Review of Public Health*, *39*(1), 351–365. doi:10.1146/annurev-publhealth-040617-013714 PMID:29400993

Murano, C., Agnisola, C., Caramiello, D., Castellano, I., Casotti, R., Corsi, I., & Palumbo, A. (2020). How sea urchins face microplastics: Uptake, tissue distribution and immune system response. *Environmental Pollution*, *114685*. Advance online publication. doi:10.1016/j.envpol.2020.114685 PMID:32402714

Murphy, F., Ewins, C., Carbonnier, F., & Quinn, B. (2016). Wastewater treatment works (WwTW) as a source of microplastics in the aquatic environment. *Environmental Science & Technology*, *50*(11), 5800–5808. doi:10.1021/acs.est.5b05416 PMID:27191224

Murray, F., & Cowie, P. R. (2011). Plastic contamination in the decapod crustacean Nephrops norvegicus (Linnaeus, 1758). *Marine Pollution Bulletin*, *62*(6), 1207–1217. doi:10.1016/j.marpolbul.2011.03.032 PMID:21497854

Muthukumar, A., & Veerappapillai, S. (2015). Biodegradation of Plastics - A Brief Review. *International Journal of Pharmaceutical Sciences Review and Research*, *31*(2), 204–209.

Mwanza, B. (2018). *An African Reverse Logistics Model for Plastic Solid Wastes* [PhD Thesis]. University of Johannesburg.

Mwanza, B. G. (2020). Introduction to Recycling. In Recent Developments in Pastics Recycling (pp. 1-13). Springer.

Mwanza, B. G., & Mbohwa, C. (2019). Knowledge and awareness on Plastic Solid Waste (PSW) management in Zambia: where are we? Procs West Africa Built Environment Research (WABER) Conference, 749-756.

Mwanza, B. G. (2018). *An Afriacn Reverse Logistics Model for Plastic Solid Wastes*. University of Johannesburg.

Myllynen, P. K., Loughran, M. J., Howard, C. V., Sormunen, R., Walsh, A. A., & Vahakangas, K. H. (2008). Kinetics of gold nanoparticles in the human placenta. *Reproductive Toxicology (Elmsford, N.Y.)*, *26*(2), 130–137. doi:10.1016/j.reprotox.2008.06.008 PMID:18638543

Nakajima-Kambe, T., Shigeno-Akutsu, Y., Nomura, N., Onuma, F., & Nakahara, T. (1999). Microbial degradation of polyurethane, polyester polyurethanes and polyether polyurethanes. *Applied Microbiology and Biotechnology*, *51*(2), 134–140. doi:10.1007002530051373 PMID:10091317

Nakamiya, K., Ooi, T., & Kinoshita, S. (1997). Non-heme hydroquinone peroxidase from Azotobacter beijerinckii HM121. *Journal of Fermentation and Bioengineering*, *84*(1), 14–21. doi:10.1016/S0922-338X(97)82780-8

Nanninga, G. B., Horswill, C., Lane, S. M., Manica, A., & Briffa, M. (2020). Microplastic exposure increases predictability of predator avoidance strategies in hermit crabs. *Journal of Hazardous Materials Letters*, *1*(October), 100005. doi:10.1016/j.hazl.2020.100005

Nanninga, G. B., Pertzelan, A., Kiflawi, M., Holzman, R., Plakolm, I., & Manica, A. (2021). Treatment-level impacts of microplastic exposure may be confounded by variation in individual-level responses in juvenile fish. *Journal of Hazardous Materials*, *416*, 126059. doi:10.1016/j.jhazmat.2021.126059 PMID:34492894

Napper, I. E., Davies, B. F., Clifford, H., Elvin, S., Koldewey, H. J., Mayewski, P. A., Miner, K. R., Potocki, M., Elmore, A. C., Gajurel, A. P., & Thompson, R. C. (2020). Reaching new heights in plastic pollution—Preliminary findings of microplastics on Mount Everest. *One Earth*, *3*(5), 621–630. doi:10.1016/j.oneear.2020.10.020

Neis, E. P., Dejong, C. H., & Rensen, S. S. (2015). The role of microbial amino acid metabolism in host metabolism. *Nutrients*, *7*(4), 2930–2946. doi:10.3390/nu7042930 PMID:25894657

Nel, H. A., & Froneman, P. W. (2015). A quantitative analysis of microplastic pollution along the south-eastern coastline of South Africa. *Marine Pollution Bulletin*, *101*(1), 274–279. doi:10.1016/j.marpolbul.2015.09.043 PMID:26433774

Nelms, S. E., Barnett, J., Brownlow, A., Davison, N. J., Deaville, R., Galloway, T. S., Lindeque, P. K., Santillo, D., & Godley, B. J. (2019). Microplastics in marine mammals stranded around the British coast: Ubiquitous but transitory? *Scientific Reports*, *9*(1), 1–8. doi:10.103841598-018-37428-3 PMID:30705316

Nelms, S. E., Duncan, E. M., Broderick, A. C., Galloway, T. S., Godfrey, M. H., Hamann, M., Lindeque, P. K., & Godley, B. J. (2016). Plastic and marine turtles: A review and call for research. *ICES Journal of Marine Science*, *73*(2), 165–181. doi:10.1093/icesjms/fsv165

Nelms, S. E., Galloway, T. S., Godley, B. J., Jarvis, D. S., & Lindeque, P. K. (2018). Investigating microplastic trophic transfer in marine top predators. *Environmental Pollution*, *238*, 999–1007. doi:10.1016/j.envpol.2018.02.016 PMID:29477242

Ng, E. L., Huerta Lwanga, E., Eldridge, S. M., Johnston, P., Hu, H. W., Geissen, V., & Chen, D. (2018). An overview of microplastic and nanoplastic pollution in agroecosystems. *The Science of the Total Environment*, *627*, 1377–1388.

Ng, E. L., Lin, S. Y., Dungan, A. M., Colwell, J. M., Ede, S., Lwanga, E. H., Meng, K., Geissen, V., Blackall, L. L., & Chen, D. (2021). Microplastic pollution alters forest soil microbiome. *Journal of Hazardous Materials*, *409*, 124606. doi:10.1016/j.jhazmat.2020.124606 PMID:33246819

Ng, Y. T., Lu, W. F., & Song, B. (2014). Quantification of end-of-life product condition to support product recovery decision. *Procedia CIRP*, *15*, 257–262. doi:10.1016/j.procir.2014.06.086

Nielsen, T. D., Hasselbalch, J., Holmberg, K., & Stripple, J. (2020). Politics and the plastic crisis: A review throughout the plastic life cycle. *Wiley Interdisciplinary Reviews. Energy and Environment*, *9*(1), e360. doi:10.1002/wene.360

Nihei, Y., Yoshida, T., Kataoka, T., & Ogata, R. (2020). High-Resolution Mapping of Japanese Microplastic and Macroplastic Emissions from the Land into the Sea. In Water (Vol. 12, Issue 4). MDPI. doi:10.3390/w12040951

Ning, Q., Wang, D., An, J., Ding, Q., Huang, Z., Zou, Y., Wu, F., & You, J. (2022). Combined effects of nanosized polystyrene and erythromycin on bacterial growth and resistance mutations in Escherichia coli. *Journal of Hazardous Materials*, *422*(August), 126858. doi:10.1016/j.jhazmat.2021.126858

Nizzetto, L., Futter, M., & Langaas, S. (2016). Are agricultural soils dumps for microplastics of urban origin? *Environmental Science & Technology*, *50*(20), 10777–10779. doi:10.1021/acs.est.6b04140 PMID:27682621

NOAA. (2019). *Coral reef ecosystems*. NOAA.

Nobre, C. R., Santana, M. F. M., Maluf, A., Cortez, F. S., Cesar, A., Pereira, C. D. S., & Turra, A. (2015). Assessment of microplastic toxicity to embryonic development of the sea urchin Lytechinus variegatus (Echinodermata: Echinoidea). *Marine Pollution Bulletin*, *92*(1–2), 99–104. doi:10.1016/j.marpolbul.2014.12.050 PMID:25662316

Nomura, T., Tani, S., Yamamoto, M., Nakagawa, T., Toyoda, S., Fujisawa, E., Yasui, A., & Konishi, Y. (2016). Cytotoxicity and colloidal behavior of polystyrene latex nanoparticles toward filamentous fungi in isotonic solutions. *Chemosphere*, *149*, 84–90. doi:10.1016/j.chemosphere.2016.01.091 PMID:26855210

Novotna, K., Cermakova, L., Pivokonska, L., Cajthaml, T., & Pivokonsky, M. (2019). Microplastics in drinking water treatment–Current knowledge and research needs. *The Science of the Total Environment*, *667*, 730–740. doi:10.1016/j.scitotenv.2019.02.431 PMID:30851606

NOWPAP. (2007). *Guidelines for Monitoring Litter on the Beaches and Shorelines of the Northwest Pacific Region*. NOWPAP CEARAC. http://hdl.handle.net/20.500.11822/27232

Nuelle, M. T., Dekiff, J. H., Remy, D., & Fries, E. (2014). A new analytical approach for monitoring microplastics in marine sediments. *Environmental Pollution*, *184*, 161–169. doi:10.1016/j.envpol.2013.07.027 PMID:24051349

O'Brien, S., Okoffo, E. D., Rauert, C., O'Brien, J. W., Ribeiro, F., Burrows, S. D., Toapanta, T., Wang, X., & Thomas, K. V. (2021). Quantification of selected microplastics in Australian urban road dust. *Journal of Hazardous Materials*, *416*(March), 125811. doi:10.1016/j.jhazmat.2021.125811 PMID:33892382

O'Donovan, S., Mestre, N. C., Abel, S., Fonseca, T. G., Carteny, C. C., Cormier, B., Keiter, S. H., & Bebianno, M. J. (2018). Ecotoxicological Effects of Chemical Contaminants Adsorbed to Microplastics in the Clam *Scrobicularia plana*. *Frontiers in Marine Science*, *5*, 143. Advance online publication. doi:10.3389/fmars.2018.00143

O'Donovan, S., Mestre, N. C., Abel, S., Fonseca, T. G., Carteny, C. C., Willems, T., Prinsen, E., Cormier, B., Keiter, S. S., & Bebianno, M. J. (2020). Effects of the UV filter, oxybenzone, adsorbed to microplastics in the clam *Scrobicularia plana*. *The Science of the Total Environment*, *733*, 139102. doi:10.1016/j.scitotenv.2020.139102 PMID:32446057

Ocean Conservancy. (2015). *Stemming the Tide: Land-based strategies for a plastic-free ocean*. McKinsey & Company and Ocean Conservancy. https://oceanconservancy.org/wp-content/uploads/2017/04/full-report-stemming-the.pdf

OECD. (2001). *Extended producer responsibility: A guidance manual for governments*. OECD.

Oehlmann, J., Schulte-Oehlmann, U., Kloas, W., Jagnytsch, O., Lutz, I., Kusk, K. O., Wollenberger, L., Santos, E. M., Paull, G. C., VanLook, K. J. W., & Tyler, C. R. (2009). A critical analysis of the biological impacts of plasticizers on wildlife. *Philosophical Transactions of the Royal Society of London. Series B, Biological Sciences*, *364*(1526), 2047–2062. doi:10.1098/rstb.2008.0242 PMID:19528055

Oelschlägel, M., Zimmerling, J., & Tischler, D. (2018). A review: The Styrene metabolizing cascade of side-chain oxygenation as biotechnological basis to gain various valuable compounds. *Frontiers in Microbiology*, *9*, 9. doi:10.3389/fmicb.2018.00490 PMID:29623070

Ohkita, T., & Lee, S. H. (2006). Thermal degradation and biodegradability of poly (lactic acid)/corn starch biocomposites. *Journal of Applied Polymer Science*, *100*(4), 3009–3017. doi:10.1002/app.23425

Okey, R. W., & Stensel, H. D. (1996). A QSAR based biodegradability model – A QSBR. *Water Research*, *30*(9), 2206–2214. doi:10.1016/0043-1354(96)00098-X

Okshevsky, M., Gautier, E., Farner, J. M., Schreiber, L., & Tufenkji, N. (2020). Biofilm formation by marine bacteria is impacted by concentration and surface functionalization of polystyrene nanoparticles in a species-specific manner. *Environmental Microbiology Reports*, *12*(2), 203–213. doi:10.1111/1758-2229.12824 PMID:31997572

Oliveira, J., Belchior, A., da Silva, V. D., Rotter, A., Petrovski, Ž., Almeida, P. L., Lourenço, N. D., & Gaudêncio, S. P. (2020). Marine Environmental Plastic Pollution: Mitigation by Microorganism Degradation and Recycling Valorization. *Frontiers in Marine Science*, *7*, 1007. doi:10.3389/fmars.2020.567126

Oliveira, M., Ribeiro, A., Hylland, K., & Guilhermino, L. (2013). Single and combined effects of microplastics and pyrene on juveniles (0+ group) of the common goby *Pomatoschistus microps* (*Teleostei, Gobiidae*). *Ecological Indicators*, *34*, 641–647. doi:10.1016/j.ecolind.2013.06.019

Oliveira, P., Barboza, L. G. A., Branco, V., Figueiredo, N., Carvalho, C., & Guilhermino, L. (2018). Effects of microplastics and mercury in the freshwater bivalve *Corbicula fluminea* (Müller, 1774): Filtration rate, biochemical biomarkers, and mercury bioconcentration. *Ecotoxicology and Environmental Safety*, *164*, 155–163. doi:10.1016/j.ecoenv.2018.07.062 PMID:30107325

Orayeva, J. (2020). *New Research on the Possible Effects of Micro-and Nano-plastics on Marine Animals*. IAEA. www.iaea.org/newscenter/news/new-research-on-the-possible-effects-of-micro-and-nano-plastics-on-marine-animals

Oriekhova, O., & Stoll, S. (2018). Heteroaggregation of nanoplastic particles in the presence of inorganic colloids and natural organic matter. *Environmental Science. Nano*, *5*(3), 792–799. doi:10.1039/C7EN01119A

Ory, N. C., Sobral, P., Ferreira, J. L., & Thiel, M. (2017). Amberstripe scad Decapterus muroadsi (Carangidae) fish ingest blue microplastics resembling their copepod prey along the coast of Rapa Nui (Easter Island) in the South Pacific subtropical gyre. *The Science of the Total Environment*, *586*, 430–437. doi:10.1016/j.scitotenv.2017.01.175 PMID:28196756

Pabortsava, K., & Lampitt, R. S. (2020). High concentrations of plastic hidden beneath the surface of the Atlantic Ocean. *Nature Communications*, *11*(1), 4073. doi:10.103841467-020-17932-9 PMID:32811835

Paço, A., Duarte, K., da Costa, J. P., Santos, P. S. M., Pereira, R., Pereira, M. E., Freitas, A. C., Duarte, A. C., & Rocha-Santos, T. A. P. (2017). Biodegradation of polyethylene microplastics by the marine fungus Zalerion maritimum. *The Science of the Total Environment*, *586*, 10–15. doi:10.1016/j.scitotenv.2017.02.017 PMID:28199874

Padervand, M., Lichtfouse, E., Robert, D., & Wang, C. (2020). Removal of microplastics from the environment. A review. *Environmental Chemistry Letters*, *18*(3), 807–828. doi:10.100710311-020-00983-1

Paget, V., Dekali, S., Kortulewski, T., Grall, R., Gamez, C., Blazy, K., Aguerre-Chariol, O., Chevillard, S., Braun, A., Rat, P., & Lacroix, G. (2015). Specific uptake and genotoxicity induced by polystyrene nanobeads with distinct surface chemistry on human lung epithelial cells and macrophages. *PLoS One*, *10*(4), e0123297. doi:10.1371/journal.pone.0123297 PMID:25875304

Palos, R., Gutiérrez, A., Vela, F. J., Olazar, M., Arandes, J. M., & Bilbao, J. (2021). Waste Refinery: The Valorization of Waste Plastics and End-of-Life Tires in Refinery Units. A Review. *Energy & Fuels*, *35*(5), 3529–3557. doi:10.1021/acs.energyfuels.0c03918 PMID:35310012

Palumbo, M. T., & Mingazzini, M. (2011). Toxicity Test With Algae: Evaluation of the Sensitivity Related To the Use of Biomass Versus Growth Rate Endpoint. *16th International MESAEP Symposium on Environmental Pollution.*

Pałyga-Bysiecka, I., Polewczyk, A. M., Polewczyk, M., Kołodziej, E., Mazurek, H., & Pogorzelski, A. (2022). Plastic Bronchitis—A Serious Rare Complication Affecting Children Only after Fontan Procedure? *Journal of Clinical Medicine*, *11*(1), 44. doi:10.3390/jcm11010044 PMID:35011785

Pannetier, P., Fuster, L., Clérandeau, C., Lacroix, C., Gourves, P. Y., Cachot, J., & Morin, B. (2018). Usefulness of RTL-W1 and OLCAB-e3 fish cell lines and multiple endpoint measurements for toxicity evaluation of unknown or complex mixture of chemicals. *Ecotoxicology and Environmental Safety*, *150*, 40–48. doi:10.1016/j.ecoenv.2017.12.027 PMID:29268113

Panseri, S., Martino, P., Cagnardi, P. C., & Tedesco, D. (2018). Feasibility of biodegradable based packaging used for red meat storage during shelflife:a pilot study. *Food Chemistry*, *249*, 22–29. doi:10.1016/j.foodchem.2017.12.067 PMID:29407927

Pan, Z., Guo, H., Chen, H., Wang, S., Sun, X., Zou, Q., Zhang, Y., Lin, H., Cai, S., & Huang, J. (2019). Microplastics in the Northwestern Pacific: Abundance, distribution, and characteristics. *The Science of the Total Environment*, *650*, 1913–1922. doi:10.1016/j.scitotenv.2018.09.244 PMID:30286357

Park, D. H., & Kim, B. S. (2011). Production of poly(3-hydroxybutyrate) and poly(3-hydroxybutyrate-co-4-hydroxybutyrate) by Ralstonia eutropha from soybean oil. *New Biotechnology*, *28*(6), 719–724. doi:10.1016/j.nbt.2011.01.007 PMID:21333767

Parker, L. (2019, June 7). *National Geographic*. Retrieved July 14, 2021, from https://www.nationalgeographic.com/environment/article/plastic-pollution

Park, S. Y., & Kim, C. G. (2019). Biodegradation of micro-polyethylene particles by bacterial colonization of a mixed microbial consortium isolated from a landfill site. *Chemosphere*, *222*, 527–533. doi:10.1016/j.chemosphere.2019.01.159 PMID:30721811

Patagonia. (2021). *Recycled Polyester*. https://eu.patagonia.com/it/en/our-footprint/recycled-polyester.html

Patchaiyappan, A., Dowarah, K., Zaki Ahmed, S., Prabakaran, M., Jayakumar, S., Thirunavukkarasu, C., & Devipriya, S. P. (2021). Prevalence and characteristics of microplastics present in the street dust collected from Chennai metropolitan city, India. *Chemosphere*, *269*, 128757. doi:10.1016/j.chemosphere.2020.128757 PMID:33183789

Patil, S. M., Rane, N. R., Bankole, P. O., Krishnaiah, P., Ahn, Y., Park, Y. K., Yadav, K. K., Amin, M. A., & Jeon, B. H. (2022). An assessment of micro-and nanoplastics in the biosphere: A review of detection, monitoring, and remediation technology. *Chemical Engineering Journal*, *430*, 132913. doi:10.1016/j.cej.2021.132913

Paul, M. B., Stock, V., Cara-Carmona, J., Lisicki, E., Shopova, S., Fessard, V., & Böhmert, L. (2020). Micro-and nano-plastics–current state of knowledge with the focus on oral uptake and toxicity. *Nanoscale Advances*, *2*(10), 4350–4367. doi:10.1039/D0NA00539H

Paul-Pont, I., Lacroix, C., González Fernández, C., Hégaret, H., Lambert, C., Le Goïc, N., Frère, L., Cassone, A.-L., Sussarellu, R., Fabioux, C., Guyomarch, J., Albentosa, M., Huvet, A., & Soudant, P. (2016). Exposure of marine mussels *Mytilus* spp. to polystyrene microplastics: Toxicity and influence on fluoranthene bioaccumulation. *Environmental Pollution*, *216*, 724–737. doi:10.1016/j.envpol.2016.06.039 PMID:27372385

Pauly, J. L., Stegmeier, S. J., Allaart, H. A., Cheney, R. T., Zhang, P. J., Mayer, A. G., & Streck, R. J. (1998). Inhaled cellulosic and plastic fibers found in human lung tissue. *Cancer Epidemiology, Biomarkers & Prevention*, *7*(5), 419–428. PMID:9610792

Paunonen, S. (2013). Strength and barrier enhancement of cellophane and cellulose derivative films: A review. *BioResources*, *8*(2), 3098–3121. doi:10.15376/biores.8.2.3098-3121

Pausch, J., & Kuzyakov, Y. (2018). Carbon input by roots into the soil: Quantification of rhizodeposition from root to ecosystem scale. *Global Change Biology*, *24*(1), 1–12. doi:10.1111/gcb.13850 PMID:28752603

Paustian, K., Andrén, O., Janzen, H. H., Lal, R., Smith, P., Tian, G., Tiessen, H., Noordwijk, M. V., & Woomer, P. L. (1997). Agricultural soils as a sink to mitigate CO_2 emissions. *Soil Use and Management*, *13*(s4), 230–244. doi:10.1111/j.1475-2743.1997.tb00594.x

Pedà, C., Caccamo, L., Fossi, M. C., Gai, F., Andaloro, F., Genovese, L., Perdichizzi, A., Romeo, T., & Maricchiolo, G. (2016). Intestinal alterations in European sea bass *Dicentrarchus labrax* (Linnaeus, 1758) exposed to microplastics: Preliminary results. *Environmental Pollution*, *212*, 251–256. doi:10.1016/j.envpol.2016.01.083 PMID:26851981

Pedersen, A. F., Gopalakrishnan, K., Boegehold, A. G., Peraino, N. J., Westrick, J. A., & Kashian, D. R. (2020). Microplastic ingestion by quagga mussels, Dreissena bugensis, and its effects on physiological processes. *Environmental Pollution*, *260*, 113964. doi:10.1016/j.envpol.2020.113964 PMID:31991349

Peixoto, D., Pinheiro, C., Amorim, J., Oliva-Teles, L., Guilhermino, L., & Vieira, M. N. (2019). Microplastic pollution in commercial salt for human consumption: A review. In *Estuarine* (Vol. 219, pp. 161–168). Coastal and Shelf Science., doi:10.1016/j.ecss.2019.02.018

Peng, B. Y., Su, Y., Chen, Z., Chen, J., Zhou, X., Benbow, M. E., Criddle, C. S., Wu, W.-M., & Zhang, Y. (2019). Biodegradation of Polystyrene by Dark (Tenebrio obscurus) and Yellow (Tenebrio molitor) Mealworms (Coleoptera: Tenebrionidae). *Environmental Science & Technology*, *53*(9), 5256–5265. doi:10.1021/acs.est.8b06963 PMID:30990998

Peng, G., Xu, P., Zhu, B., Bai, M., & Li, D. (2018). Microplastics in freshwater river sediments in Shanghai, China: A case study of risk assessment in mega-cities. *Environmental Pollution, 234*, 448–456. doi:10.1016/j.envpol.2017.11.034 PMID:29207296

Peng, L., Fu, D., Qi, H., Lan, C. Q., Yu, H., & Ge, C. (2020). Micro- and nano-plastics in marine environment: Source, distribution, and threats — A review. *The Science of the Total Environment, 698*, 134254. doi:10.1016/j.scitotenv.2019.134254 PMID:31514025

Peng, X., Chen, M., Chen, S., Dasgupta, S., Xu, H. K., Ta, K., & Bai, S. (2018). Microplastics contaminate the deepest part of the world's ocean. *Geochemical Perspectives Letters, 9*, 1–5. doi:10.7185/geochemlet.1829

Perez-Puyana, V., Felix, M., Romero, A., & Guerrero, A. (2016). Effect of the injection moulding processing conditions on the development of pea protein-based bioplastics. *Journal of Applied Polymer Science, 133*(20), 43306. doi:10.1002/app.43306

Perren, W., Wojtasik, A., & Cai, Q. (2018). Removal of Microbeads from Wastewater Using Electrocoagulation. *ACS Omega, 3*(3), 3357–3364. doi:10.1021/acsomega.7b02037 PMID:31458591

Peters, C. A., & Bratton, S. P. (2016). Urbanization is a major influence on microplastic ingestion by sunfish in the Brazos River Basin, Central Texas, USA. In *Environmental Pollution* (Vol. 210, pp. 380–387). Elsevier Sci Ltd. doi:10.1016/j.envpol.2016.01.018

Petersen, F., & Hubbart, J. A. (2021). The occurrence and transport of microplastics: The state of the science. *The Science of the Total Environment, 758*, 143936. doi:10.1016/j.scitotenv.2020.143936 PMID:33333307

Petroody, S. S. A., Hashemi, S. H., & van Gestel, C. A. M. (2020). Factors affecting microplastic retention and emission by a wastewater treatment plant on the southern coast of Caspian Sea. In *Chemosphere* (Vol. 261). Pergamon-Elsevier Science Ltd. doi:10.1016/j.chemosphere.2020.128179

Phuong, N. N., Poirier, L., Pham, Q. T., Lagarde, F., & Zalouk-Vergnoux, A. (2018). Factors influencing the microplastic contamination of bivalves from the French Atlantic coast: Location, season and/or mode of life? *Marine Pollution Bulletin, 129*(2), 664–674. doi:10.1016/j.marpolbul.2017.10.054 PMID:29106937

Phuong, N. N., Zalouk-Vergnoux, A., Poirier, L., Kamari, A., Châtel, A., Mouneyrac, C., & Lagarde, F. (2016). Is there any consistency between the microplastics found in the field and those used in laboratory experiments? *Environmental Pollution, 211*, 111–123. doi:10.1016/j.envpol.2015.12.035 PMID:26745396

Piarulli, S., & Airoldi, L. (2020). Mussels facilitate the sinking of microplastics to bottom sediments and their subsequent uptake by detritus-feeders. *Environmental Pollution, 266*, 115151. doi:10.1016/j.envpol.2020.115151 PMID:32673992

Piarulli, S., Vanhove, B., Comandini, P., Scapinello, S., Moens, T., Vrielinck, H., Sciutto, G., Prati, S., Mazzeo, R., Booth, A. M., Van Colen, C., & Airoldi, L. (2020). Do different habits affect microplastics contents in organisms? A trait-based analysis on salt marsh species. In *Marine Pollution Bulletin* (Vol. 153). Pergamon-Elsevier Science Ltd. doi:10.1016/j.marpolbul.2020.110983

Picó, Y., & Barceló, D. (2019). Analysis and prevention of microplastics pollution in water: Current perspectives and future directions. *ACS Omega, 4*(4), 6709–6719. doi:10.1021/acsomega.9b00222 PMID:31459797

Piehl, S., Hauk, R., Robbe, E., Richter, B., Kachholz, F., Schilling, J., Lenz, R., Fischer, D., Fischer, F., Labrenz, M., & Schernewski, G. (2021). Combined Approaches to Predict Microplastic Emissions Within an Urbanized Estuary (Warnow, Southwestern Baltic Sea). In Frontiers in Environmental Science (Vol. 9). Frontiers Media SA. doi:10.3389/fenvs.2021.616765

Piehl, S., Leibner, A., Löder, M. G. J., Dris, R., Bogner, C., & Laforsch, C. (2018). Identification and quantification of macro- and microplastics on an agricultural farmland. *Scientific Reports, 8*(1), 1–9. doi:10.1038/s41598-018-36172-y

Pietroiusti, A. (2012). Health implications of engineered nanomaterials. *Nanoscale*, *4*(4), 1231–1247. doi:10.1039/c2nr11688j PMID:22278373

Pinsino, A., Bergami, E., Della Torre, C., Vannuccini, M. L., Addis, P., Secci, M., Dawson, K. A., Matranga, V., & Corsi, I. (2017). Amino-modified polystyrene nanoparticles affect signalling pathways of the sea urchin (*Paracentrotus lividus*) embryos. *Nanotoxicology*, *11*(2), 201–209. doi:10.1080/17435390.2017.1279360 PMID:28091127

Pitt, J. A., Trevisan, R., Massarsky, A., Kozal, J. S., Levin, E. D., & Di Giulio, R. T. (2018). Maternal transfer of nanoplastics to offspring in zebrafish (*Danio rerio*): A case study with nanopolystyrene. *The Science of the Total Environment*, *643*, 324–334. doi:10.1016/j.scitotenv.2018.06.186 PMID:29940444

Pittroff, M., Müller, Y. K., Witzig, C. S., Scheurer, M., Storck, F. R., & Zumbülte, N. (2021). Microplastic analysis in drinking water based on fractionated filtration sampling and Raman microspectroscopy. *Environmental Science and Pollution Research International*, *28*(42), 59439–59451. Advance online publication. doi:10.100711356-021-12467-y PMID:33511538

Pittura, L., Avio, C. G., Giuliani, M. E., d'Errico, G., Keiter, S. H., Cormier, B., Gorbi, S., & Regoli, F. (2018). Microplastics as Vehicles of Environmental PAHs to Marine Organisms: Combined Chemical and Physical Hazards to the Mediterranean Mussels, *Mytilus galloprovincialis. Frontiers in Marine Science*, *5*, 103. Advance online publication. doi:10.3389/fmars.2018.00103

Plastics Europe. (2017). *Plastics – the Facts 2017.* doi:10.1016/j.marpolbul.2013.01.015

Plastics Europe. (2019). *Plastics-the facts.* https://www.plasticseurope.org/application/files/5515/1689/9220/2014plastics the_facts_PubFeb2015.pdf

Plastics Europe. (2020). Plastics – the Facts 2020. In *PlasticEurope*. https://www.plasticseurope.org/en/resources/publications/4312-plastics-facts-2020

PlasticsEurope. (2019). *Plastics - the Facts 2019. An analysis of European plastic production, demand and waste data.* https://plasticseurope.org/wp-content/uploads/2021/10/2019-Plastics-the-facts.pdf

Plummer, R. (2018). *Plastic fantastic: How it changed the world.* https://www.bbc.com/news/business-42646025

Porta, R. (2021). Anthropocene, the plastic age and future perspectives. *FEBS Open Bio*, *11*(4), 948–953. doi:10.1002/2211-5463.13122 PMID:33794071

Porter, D. W., Hubbs, A. F., Mercer, R. R., Wu, N., Wolfarth, M. G., Sriram, K., Leonard, S., Battelli, L., Schwegler-Berry, D., & Friend, S. (2010). Mouse pulmonary dose- and time course-responses induced by exposure to multi-walled carbon nanotubes. *Toxicology*, *269*(2-3), 136–147. doi:10.1016/j.tox.2009.10.017 PMID:19857541

Potts, T., O'Higgins, T., Mee, L., & Pita, C. (2011). Public Perceptions of Europe's Seas: A Policy Brief. Brussels, Belgium: EU FP7 KNOWSEAS Project.

Pranamuda, H., Tokiwa, Y., & Tanaka, H. (1997). Polylactide degradation by an Amycolatopsis sp. *Applied and Environmental Microbiology*, *63*(4), 1637–1640. doi:10.1128/aem.63.4.1637-1640.1997 PMID:16535586

Prata J. C. (2018). Airborne microplastics: Consequences to human health? *Environmental Pollution, 234*, 115–126.

Prata, J., Silva, A., da Costa, J., Mouneyrac, C., Walker, T., Duarte, A., & Rocha-Santos, T. (2019). Solutions and Integrated Strategies for the Control and Mitigation of Plastic and Microplastic Pollution. *Int. J. Environ. Res. Public Health 2019, 2411*(16).

Prata, J. C. (2018). Airborne microplastics: Consequences to human health? *Environmental Pollution, 234*, 115–126. doi:10.1016/j.envpol.2017.11.043 PMID:29172041

Prata, J. C., da Costa, J. P., Duarte, A. C., & Rocha-Santos, T. (2019). Methods for sampling and detection of microplastics in water and sediment: A critical review. *Trends in Analytical Chemistry, 110*, 150–159. doi:10.1016/j.trac.2018.10.029

Prata, J. C., da Costa, J. P., Girão, A. V., Lopes, I., Duarte, A. C., & Rocha-Santos, T. (2019). Identifying a quick and efficient method of removing organic matter without damaging microplastic samples. *The Science of the Total Environment, 686*, 131–139. doi:10.1016/j.scitotenv.2019.05.456 PMID:31176812

Prata, J. C., da Costa, J. P., Lopes, I., Duarte, A. C., & Rocha-Santos, T. (2019). Effects of microplastics on microalgae populations: A critical review. *The Science of the Total Environment, 665*, 400–405. doi:10.1016/j.scitotenv.2019.02.132 PMID:30772570

Prata, J. C., da Costa, J. P., Lopes, I., Duarte, A. C., & Rocha-Santos, T. (2020). Environmental exposure to microplastics: An overview on possible human health effects. *The Science of the Total Environment, 702*, 134455. doi:10.1016/j.scitotenv.2019.134455 PMID:31733547

Prata, J. C., & Lavorante, B. R. B. O. (2017, September). Maria da, M. da C., & Guilhermino, L. (2018). Influence of microplastics on the toxicity of the pharmaceuticals procainamide and doxycycline on the marine microalgae *Tetraselmis chuii. Aquatic Toxicology (Amsterdam, Netherlands), 197*, 143–152. doi:10.1016/j.aquatox.2018.02.015 PMID:29494946

Prata, J. C., Reis, V., da Costa, J. P., Mouneyrac, C., Duarte, A. C., & Rocha-Santos, T. (2021). Contamination issues as a challenge in quality control and quality assurance in microplastics analytics. *Journal of Hazardous Materials, 403*(August), 123660. Advance online publication. doi:10.1016/j.jhazmat.2020.123660 PMID:33264868

Prata, J. C., Reis, V., Matos, J. T. V., da Costa, J. P., Duarte, A. C., & Rocha-Santos, T. (2019c). A new approach for routine quantification of microplastics using Nile Red and automated software (MP-VAT). *The Science of the Total Environment, 690*, 1277–1283. doi:10.1016/j.scitotenv.2019.07.060 PMID:31470490

Praveena, S. M., Shaifuddin, S. N. M., & Akizuki, S. (2018). Exploration of microplastics from personal care and cosmetic products and its estimated emissions to marine environment: An evidence from Malaysia. *Marine Pollution Bulletin, 136*, 135–140. doi:10.1016/j.marpolbul.2018.09.012 PMID:30509794

Privas, E., Leroux, F., & Navard, P. (2013). Preparation and properties of blends composed of lignosulfonated layered double hydroxide/pasticized starch thermoplastics. *Carbohydrate Polymers, 96*(1), 91–100. doi:10.1016/j.carbpol.2013.03.042 PMID:23688458

Provencher, J. F., Covernton, G. A., Moore, R. C., Horn, D. A., Conkle, J. L., & Lusher, A. L. (2020). Proceed with caution: The need to raise the publication bar for microplastics research. *The Science of the Total Environment, 748*, 141426. doi:10.1016/j.scitotenv.2020.141426 PMID:32814297

Puls, J., Wilson, S. A., & Hölter, D. (2011). Degradation of cellulose acetate-based materials: A review. *Journal of Polymers and the Environment, 19*(1), 152–165. doi:10.100710924-010-0258-0

Qiu, R., Song, Y., Zhang, X., Xie, B., & He, D. (2020). Microplastics in Urban Environments: Sources, Pathways, and Distribution. Handbook of Environmental Chemistry, 95, 41–61. doi:10.1007/698_2020_447

Qiu, Q., Tan, Z., Wang, J., Peng, J., Li, M., & Zhan, Z. (2016). Extraction, enumeration and identification methods for monitoring microplastics in the environment. *Estuarine, Coastal and Shelf Science*, *176*, 102–109. doi:10.1016/j.ecss.2016.04.012

Qi, X., Ren, Y., & Wang, X. (2017). New advances in the biodegradation of poly(lactic) acid. *International Biodeterioration & Biodegradation*, *117*, 215–223. doi:10.1016/j.ibiod.2017.01.010

Qi, Y. L., Yang, X. M., Pelaez, A. M., Lwanga, E. H., Beriot, N., Gertsen, H., Garbeva, P., & Geissen, V. (2018). Macro- and micro- plastics in soil-plant system: Effects of plastic mulch film residues on wheat (*Triticum aestivum*) growth. *The Science of the Total Environment*, *645*, 1048–1056. doi:10.1016/j.scitotenv.2018.07.229 PMID:30248830

Qi, Y., Ossowicki, A., Yang, X., Huerta Lwanga, E., Dini-Andreote, F., Geissen, V., & Garbeva, P. (2020). Effects of plastic mulch film residues on wheat rhizosphere and soil properties. *Journal of Hazardous Materials*, *387*, 121711. doi:10.1016/j.jhazmat.2019.121711 PMID:31806445

Qu, X., Su, L., Li, H., Liang, M., & Shi, H. (2018). Assessing the relationship between the abundance and properties of microplastics in water and in mussels. *Science of the Total Environment, 621*(February), 679–686. doi:10.1016/j.scitotenv.2017.11.284

Raddadi, N., & Fava, F. (2019). Biodegradation of oil-based plastics in the environment: Existing knowledge and needs of research and innovation. *The Science of the Total Environment*, *679*, 148–158. doi:10.1016/j.scitotenv.2019.04.419 PMID:31082589

Rafique, A., Irfan, M., Mumtaz, M., & Qadir, A. (2020). Spatial distribution of microplastics in soil with context to human activities: A case study from the urban center. *Environmental Monitoring and Assessment*, *192*(11), 671. Advance online publication. doi:10.100710661-020-08641-3 PMID:33009943

Ragusa, A., Svelato, A., Santacroce, C., Catalano, P., Notarstefano, V., Carnevali, O., Papa, F., Rongioletti, M. C. A., Baiocco, F., Draghi, S., D'Amore, E., Rinaldo, D., Matta, M., & Giorgini, E. (2021). Plasticenta: First evidence of microplastics in human placenta. *Environment International*, *146*, 106274. doi:10.1016/j.envint.2020.106274 PMID:33395930

Rahman, A. U. (2012). *Oxo-Biodegradable Additives for Use in Fossil Fuel Polymer Films and Once-Used Packaging*. Academic Press.

Rai, P. K., Lee, J., Brown, R. J. C., & Kim, K.-H. (2020). Micro-and nanoplastic pollution: Behavior, microbial ecology, and remediation technologies. *Journal of Cleaner Production*, •••, 125240.

Raisuddin, S., Kwok, K. W. H., Leung, K. M. Y., Schlenk, D., & Lee, J. S. (2007). The copepod *Tigriopus*: A promising marine model organism for ecotoxicology and environmental genomics. *Aquatic Toxicology (Amsterdam, Netherlands)*, *83*(3), 161–173. doi:10.1016/j.aquatox.2007.04.005 PMID:17560667

Rajendran, N. N., Puppala, S., Raj, M. S., Angeeleena, B. R., & Venkata Rajam, Ch. (2012). Seaweeds can be a new source for bioplastics. *Journal of Pharmacy Research*, *5*, 1476–1479.

Ramirez, L., Gentile, R. S., Zimmerman, S., & Stoll, S. (2019). Drinking and Lake Geneva Waters. Impact of Water. *Water*.

Rasheed, F. (2011). Production of Sustainable Bioplastic Materials from Wheat Gluten Proteins. The Swedish University of Agricultural Sciences, 4.

Rasmussen, J. W., Martinez, E., Louka, P., & Wingett, D. G. (2010). Zinc oxide nanoparticles for selective destruction of tumor cells and potential for drug delivery applications. *Expert Opinion on Drug Delivery*, *7*(9), 1063–1077. doi:10.1517/17425247.2010.502560 PMID:20716019

Rathi, A., Basu, S., & Barman, S. (2019). Adsorptive removal of fipronil from its aqueous solution by modified zeolite HZSM-5: Equilibrium, kinetic and thermodynamic study. *Journal of Molecular Liquids*, *283*, 867–878. doi:10.1016/j.molliq.2019.02.140

Ratola, N., Ramos, S., Homem, V., Silva, J. A., Jiménez-Guerrero, P., Amigo, J. M., Santos, L., & Alves, A. (2016). Using air, soil and vegetation to assess the environmental behaviour of siloxanes. *Environmental Science and Pollution Research International*, *23*(4), 3273–3284. doi:10.100711356-015-5574-4 PMID:26490903

Razza, F., & Cerutti, A. K. (2017). *Soil Degradable Bioplastics for a Sustainable Modern Agriculture*. Springer. doi:10.1007/978-3-662-54130-2_7

Rech, S., Macaya-Caquilpán, V., Pantoja, J. F., Rivadeneira, M. M., Madariaga, D. J., & Thiel, M. (2014). Rivers as a source of marine litter–a study from the SE Pacific. *Marine Pollution Bulletin*, *82*(1-2), 66–75. doi:10.1016/j.marpolbul.2014.03.019 PMID:24726186

Regulation, E. C. (2008). No. 1272/2008 of the European Parliament and of the Council of 16 December 2008 on classification, labelling and packaging of substances and mixtures, amending and repealing Directives 67/548/EEC and 1999/45/EC, and amending Regulation (EC) No 1907/2006. *Official Journal of the European Union. 2008b L, 353*.

Rehm, R., Zeyer, T., Schmidt, A., & Fiener, P. (2021). Soil erosion as transport pathway of microplastic from agriculture soils to aquatic ecosystems. *The Science of the Total Environment*, *795*, 148774. doi:10.1016/j.scitotenv.2021.148774 PMID:34328923

Rehse, S., Kloas, W., & Zarfl, C. (2016). Short-term exposure with high concentrations of pristine microplastic particles leads to immobilisation of Daphnia magna. *Chemosphere*, *153*, 91–99. doi:10.1016/j.chemosphere.2016.02.133 PMID:27010171

Reichert, J., Arnold, A. L., Hoogenboom, M. O., Schubert, P., & Wilke, T. (2019). Impacts of microplastics on growth and health of hermatypic corals are species-specific. *Environmental Pollution*, *254*, 113074. doi:10.1016/j.envpol.2019.113074 PMID:31473388

Reichert, J., Schellenberg, J., Schubert, P., & Wilke, T. (2018). Responses of reef building corals to microplastic exposure. *Environmental Pollution*, *237*, 955–960. doi:10.1016/j.envpol.2017.11.006 PMID:29146203

Revel, M., Châtel, A., & Mouneyrac, C. (2018). Micro (nano) plastics: A threat to human health? *Current Opinion in Environmental Science & Health*, *1*, 17–23. doi:10.1016/j.coesh.2017.10.003

Revel, M., Lagarde, F., Perrein-Ettajani, H., Bruneau, M., Akcha, F., Sussarellu, R., Rouxel, J., Costil, K., Decottignies, P., Cognie, B., Châtel, A., & Mouneyrac, C. (2019). Tissue-Specific Biomarker Responses in the Blue Mussel *Mytilus* spp. Exposed to a Mixture of Microplastics at Environmentally Relevant Concentrations. *Frontiers in Environmental Science*, *7*, 33. Advance online publication. doi:10.3389/fenvs.2019.00033

Rezaei, M., Riksen, M., Sirjani, E., Sameni, A., & Geissen, V. (2019). Wind erosion as a driver for transport of light density microplastics. *The Science of the Total Environment*, *669*, 273–281. doi:10.1016/j.scitotenv.2019.02.382 PMID:30878934

Rhodes, C. J. (2018). Plastic pollution and potential solutions. *Science Progress*, *101*(3), 207–260. doi:10.3184/003685018X15294876706211 PMID:30025551

Ribeiro, F., Garcia, A. R., Pereira, B. P., Fonseca, M., Mestre, N. C., Fonseca, T. G., Ilharco, L. M., & Bebianno, M. J. (2017). Microplastics effects in *Scrobicularia plana*. *Marine Pollution Bulletin*, *122*(1-2), 379–391. doi:10.1016/j.marpolbul.2017.06.078 PMID:28684108

Ribeiro, F., O'Brien, J. W., Galloway, T., & Thomas, K. V. (2019). Accumulation and fate of nano-and micro-plastics and associated contaminants in organisms. *Trends in Analytical Chemistry*, *111*, 139–147. doi:10.1016/j.trac.2018.12.010

Ricciardi, M., Pironti, C., Motta, O., Miele, Y., Proto, A., & Montano, L. (2021). Microplastics in the Aquatic Environment: Occurrence, Persistence, Analysis, and Human Exposure. *Water (Basel)*, *13*(7), 973. doi:10.3390/w13070973

Richardson, C. R., Burritt, D. J., Allan, B. J. M., & Lamare, M. D. (2021). Microplastic ingestion induces asymmetry and oxidative stress in larvae of the sea urchin *Pseudechinus huttoni*. *Marine Pollution Bulletin*, *168*, 112369. doi:10.1016/j.marpolbul.2021.112369 PMID:33932840

Rico-Martínez, R., Arzate-Cárdenas, M. A., Robles-Vargas, D., Pérez-Legaspi, I. A., Jesús, A.-F., & Santos-Medrano, G. E. (2016). Rotifers as Models in Toxicity Screening of Chemicals and Environmental Samples. In *Invertebrates - Experimental Models in Toxicity Screening* (pp. 57–99). Academic Press.

Riisgård, H. U. (1988). Efficiency of particle retention and filtration rate in 6 species of Northeast American bivalves. Marine ecology progress series. *Oldendorf*, *45*(3), 217–223. doi:10.3354/meps045217

Rillig, M. C. (2012). Microplastic in terrestrial ecosystems and the soil? *Environmental Science & Technology*, *46*(12), 6453–6454. doi:10.1021/es302011r PMID:22676039

Rillig, M. C. (2018). Microplastic disguising as soil carbon storage. *Environmental Science & Technology*, *52*(11), 6079–6080. doi:10.1021/acs.est.8b02338 PMID:29757627

Rillig, M. C. (2020). Plastic and plants. *Nature Sustainability*, *3*(11), 1–2. doi:10.103841893-020-0583-9

Rillig, M. C., & Bonkowski, M. (2018). Microplastic and soil protists: A call for research. *Environmental Pollution*, *241*, 1128–1131. doi:10.1016/j.envpol.2018.04.147 PMID:30029321

Rillig, M. C., Hoffmann, M., Lehmann, A., Liang, Y., Lück, M., & Augustin, J. (2021a). Microplastic fibers affect dynamics and intensity of CO_2 and N_2O fluxes from soil differently. *Microplastics and Nanoplastics*, *1*(1), 3. doi:10.118643591-021-00004-0

Rillig, M. C., & Lehmann, A. (2020). Microplastic in terrestrial ecosystems. *Science*, *368*(6498), 1430–1431. doi:10.1126cience.abb5979 PMID:32587009

Rillig, M. C., Lehmann, A., Machado, A. A. D. S., & Yang, G. (2019a). Microplastic effects on plants. *The New Phytologist*, *223*(3), 1066–1070. doi:10.1111/nph.15794 PMID:30883812

Rillig, M. C., Lehmann, A., Ryo, M., & Bergmann, J. (2019b). Shaping up: Toward considering the shape and form of pollutants. *Environmental Science & Technology*, *53*(14), 7925–7926. doi:10.1021/acs.est.9b03520 PMID:31267727

Rillig, M. C., Leifheit, E., & Lehmann, J. (2021b). Microplastic effects on carbon cycling processes in soils. *PLoS Biology*, *19*(3), e3001130. doi:10.1371/journal.pbio.3001130 PMID:33784293

Rillig, M. C., Ryo, M., Lehmann, A., Aguilar-Trigueros, C. A., Buchert, S., Wulf, A., Iwasaki, A., Roy, J., & Yang, G. (2019c). The role of multiple global change factors in driving soil functions and microbial biodiversity. *Science*, *366*(6467), 886–890. doi:10.1126cience.aay2832 PMID:31727838

Rillig, M. C., Ziersch, L., & Hempel, S. (2017). Microplastic transport in soil by earthworms. *Scientific Reports*, *7*(1), 1362. doi:10.103841598-017-01594-7 PMID:28465618

Rios Mendoza, L. M., & Balcer, M. (2019). Microplastics in freshwater environments: A review of quantification assessment. *Trends in Analytical Chemistry*, *113*, 402–408. doi:10.1016/j.trac.2018.10.020

Rios Mendoza, L. M., Karapanagioti, H., & Álvarez, N. R. (2018). Micro(nanoplastics) in the marine environment: Current knowledge and gaps. *Current Opinion in Environmental Science & Health, 1*, 47–51. doi:10.1016/j.coesh.2017.11.004

Rios, L. M., Moore, C., & Jones, P. R. (2007). Persistent organic pollutants carried by synthetic polymers in the ocean environment. *Marine Pollution Bulletin, 54*(8), 1230–1237. doi:10.1016/j.marpolbul.2007.03.022 PMID:17532349

Rist, S. E., Assidqi, K., Zamani, N. P., Appel, D., Perschke, M., Huhn, M., & Lenz, M. (2016). Suspended micro-sized PVC particles impair the performance and decrease survival in the Asian green mussel *Perna viridis. Marine Pollution Bulletin, 111*(1-2), 213–220. doi:10.1016/j.marpolbul.2016.07.006 PMID:27491368

Rist, S., Baun, A., Almeda, R., & Hartmann, N. B. (2019). Ingestion and effects of micro- and nanoplastics in blue mussel (Mytilus edulis) larvae. *Marine Pollution Bulletin, 140*, 423–430. Advance online publication. doi:10.1016/j.marpolbul.2019.01.069 PMID:30803663

Rist, S., Carney Almroth, B., Hartmann, N. B., & Karlsson, T. M. (2018). A critical perspective on early communications concerning human health aspects of microplastics. *The Science of the Total Environment, 626*, 720–726. doi:10.1016/j.scitotenv.2018.01.092 PMID:29396337

Rivers, M., & Gwinnett, C. (n.d.). *Quantification is more than counting: Actions required to accurately quantify and report isolated marine microplastics.* Elsevier. Retrieved December 17, 2021, from https://www.sciencedirect.com/science/article/pii/S0025326X18308750

Roblin, B., & Aherne, J. (2020). Moss as a biomonitor for the atmospheric deposition of anthropogenic microfibres. *The Science of the Total Environment, 715*, 136973. doi:10.1016/j.scitotenv.2020.136973 PMID:32018105

Rocha, R. J. M., Rodrigues, A. C. M., Campos, D., Cícero, L. H., Costa, A. P. L., Silva, D. A. M., Oliveira, M., Soares, A. M. V. M., & Patrício Silva, A. L. (2020). Do microplastics affect the zoanthid *Zoanthus sociatus? The Science of the Total Environment, 713*, 136659. doi:10.1016/j.scitotenv.2020.136659 PMID:31955109

Rocha-Santos, T., & Duarte, A. C. (2015). A critical overview of the analytical approaches to the occurrence, the fate and the behavior of microplastics in the environment. *Trends in Analytical Chemistry, 65*, 47–53. doi:10.1016/j.trac.2014.10.011

Rochman, C. M. (2015). *The complex mixture, fate and toxicity of chemicals associated with plastic debris in the marine environment.* In M. Bergmann, L. Gutow, & M. Klages (Eds.), *in Marine Anthropogenic Litter* (pp. 117–140). Springer. doi:10.1007/978-3-319-16510-3_5

Rochman, C. M. (2018). Microplastics research - from sink to source. *Science, 360*(6384), 28–29. doi:10.1126cience.aar7734 PMID:29622640

Rochman, C. M., Brookson, C., Bikker, J., Djuric, N., Earn, A., Bucci, K., Athey, S., Huntington, A., McIlwraith, H., Munno, K., De Frond, H., Kolomijeca, A., Erdle, L., Grbic, J., Bayoumi, M., Borrelle, S. B., Wu, T., Santoro, S., Werbowski, L. M., ... Hung, C. (2019). Rethinking microplastics as a diverse contaminant suite. *Environmental Toxicology and Chemistry, 38*(4), 703–711. doi:10.1002/etc.4371 PMID:30909321

Rochman, C. M., Hoh, E., Hentschel, B. T., & Kaye, S. (2013). Long-term field measurement of sorption of organic contaminants to five types of plastic pellets: Implications for plastic marine debris. *Environmental Science & Technology, 47*(3), 1646–1654. doi:10.1021/es303700s PMID:23270427

Rochman, C. M., Hoh, E., Kurobe, T., & Teh, S. J. (2013). Ingested plastic transfers hazardous chemicals to fish and induces hepatic stress. *Scientific Reports, 3*(1), 3263. doi:10.1038rep03263 PMID:24263561

Rochman, C. M., Tahir, A., Williams, S. L., Baxa, D. V., Lam, R., Miller, J. T., Teh, F.-C., Werorilangi, S., & Teh, S. J. (2015). Anthropogenic debris in seafood: Plastic debris and fibers from textiles in fish and bivalves sold for human consumption. *Scientific Reports*, *5*(1), 14340. doi:10.1038rep14340 PMID:26399762

Rodrigues, M. O., Abrantes, N., Gonçalves, F. J. M., Nogueira, H., Marques, J. C., & Gonçalves, A. M. M. (2018). Spatial and temporal distribution of microplastics in water and sediments of a freshwater system (Antuã River, Portugal). *The Science of the Total Environment*, *633*, 1549–1559. doi:10.1016/j.scitotenv.2018.03.233 PMID:29758905

Rogers, K. L., Carreres-Calabuig, J. A., Gorokhova, E., & Posth, N. R. (2020). Micro-by-micro interactions: How microorganisms influence the fate of marine microplastics. *Limnology and Oceanography Letters*, *5*(1), 18–36. doi:10.1002/lol2.10136

Romera-Castillo, C., Pinto, M., Langer, T. M., Álvarez-Salgado, X. A., & Herndl, G. J. (2018). Dissolved organic carbon leaching from plastics stimulates microbial activity in the ocean. *Nature Communications*, *9*(1), 1–7. doi:10.103841467-018-03798-5 PMID:29651045

Ronneberger, D. (1998). Uptake of latex beads as size-model for food of planktonic rotifers. *Hydrobiologia*, *387*(387), 445–449. doi:10.1023/A:1017046711821

Rossiter, D. G. (2021). Are soil phenoforms the new normal? Soil classification and soil mapping in the Anthropocene. *Soil Security*, *5*, 100017. doi:10.1016/j.soisec.2021.100017

Rotini, A., Tornambè, A., Cossi, R., Iamunno, F., Benvenuto, G., Berducci, M. T., Maggi, C., Thaller, M. C., Cicero, A. M., Manfra, L., & Migliore, L. (2017). Salinity-based toxicity of CuO nanoparticles, CuO-bulk and Cu ion to *vibrio anguillarum. Frontiers in Microbiology*, *8*, 2076. doi:10.3389/fmicb.2017.02076 PMID:29118743

Rouillon, C., Bussiere, P. O., Desnoux, E., Collin, S., Vial, C., Therias, S., & Gardette, J. L. (2016). Is carbonyl index a quantitative probe to monitor polypropylene photodegradation? *Polymer Degradation & Stability*, *128*, 200–208. doi:10.1016/j.polymdegradstab.2015.12.011

Rowley, K. H., Cucknell, A.-C., Smith, B. D., Clark, P. F., & Morritt, D. (2020). London's river of plastic: High levels of microplastics in the Thames water column. In *Science of the Total Environment* (Vol. 740). Elsevier. doi:10.1016/j.scitotenv.2020.140018

Rubol, S., Manzoni, S., Bellin, A., & Porporato, A. (2013). Modeling soil moisture and oxygen effects on soil biogeochemical cycles including dissimilatory nitrate reduction to ammonium (DNRA). *Advances in Water Resources*, *62*, 106–124. doi:10.1016/j.advwatres.2013.09.016

Rudin, A., & Choi, P. (2013). *The Elements of Polymer Science & Engineering* (3rd ed.). Academic Press.

Rudyak, V. Y., Efimova, E. A., Guseva, D. V., & Chertovich, A. V. (2018). Thermoset Polymer Matrix Structure and Properties: Coarse-Grained Simulations. *Polymers*, *11*(1), 36. doi:10.3390/polym11010036 PMID:30960020

Ru, J., Huo, Y., & Yang, Y. (2020). Microbial degradation and valorization of plastic wastes. *Frontiers in Microbiology*, *11*, 11. doi:10.3389/fmicb.2020.00442 PMID:32373075

Rummel, C. D., Jahnke, A., Gorokhova, E., Kühnel, D., & Schmitt-Jansen, M. (2017). Impacts of biofilm formation on the fate and potential effects of microplastic in the aquatic environment. *Environmental Science & Technology Letters*, *4*(7), 258–267. doi:10.1021/acs.estlett.7b00164

Ryan, P. G. (1987). The effects of ingested plastic on seabirds: Correlations between plastic load and body condition. *Environmental Pollution*, *46*(2), 119–125. doi:10.1016/0269-7491(87)90197-7 PMID:15092735

Ryan, P. G., Weideman, E. A., Perold, V., Durholtz, D., & Fairweather, T. P. (2020). A trawl survey of seafloor macrolitter on the South African continental shelf. *Marine Pollution Bulletin, 150*, 110741. doi:10.1016/j.marpolbul.2019.110741 PMID:31785848

Ryberg, M. W., Hauschild, M. Z., Wang, F., Averous-Monnery, S., & Laurent, A. (2019). Global environmental losses of plastics across their value chains. *Resources, Conservation and Recycling, 151*, 104459. doi:10.1016/j.resconrec.2019.104459

Sadri, S. S., & Thompson, R. C. (2014). On the quantity and composition of floating plastic debris entering and leaving the Tamar Estuary, Southwest England. *Marine Pollution Bulletin, 81*(1), 55–60. doi:10.1016/j.marpolbul.2014.02.020 PMID:24613232

Sakai, K., Hamada, N., & Watanabe, Y. (1986). Degradation mechanism of poly(vinyl alcohol) by successive reactions of secondary alcohol oxidase and ®-diketone hydrolase from *Pseudomonas* sp. *Agricultural and Biological Chemistry, 50*(4), 989–996. doi:10.1080/00021369.1986.10867494

Sana, S. S., Dogiparthi, L. K., Gangadhar, L., Chakravorty, A., & Abhishek, N. (2020). Effects of microplastics and nanoplastics on marine environment and human health. *Environmental Science and Pollution Research International, 27*(36), 44743–44756. doi:10.100711356-020-10573-x PMID:32876819

Sanchez-Vazquez, S. A., Hailes, H. C., & Evans, J. R. G. (2013). Hydrophobic Polymers from Food Waste: Resources and Synthesis. *Polymer Reviews (Philadelphia, Pa.), 53*(4), 627–694. doi:10.1080/15583724.2013.834933

Sang, B. I., Hori, K., Tanji, Y., & Unno, H. (2002). Fungal contribution to in situ biodegradation of poly(3-hydroxybutyrate-co-3-hydroxyvalerate) film in soil. *Applied Microbiology and Biotechnology, 58*, 241–247. doi:10.100700253-001-0884-5 PMID:11876418

Santana, M. F. M., Moreira, F. T., & Turra, A. (2017). Trophic transference of microplastics under a low exposure scenario: Insights on the likelihood of particle cascading along marine food-webs. *Marine Pollution Bulletin, 121*(1–2), 154–159. doi:10.1016/j.marpolbul.2017.05.061 PMID:28595982

Sarasamma, S., Audira, G., Siregar, P., Malhotra, N., Lai, Y. H., Liang, S. T., Chen, J.-R., Chen, K. H.-C., & Hsiao, C. D. (2020). Nanoplastics cause neurobehavioral impairments, reproductive and oxidative damages, and biomarker responses in zebrafish: Throwing up alarms of wide spread health risk of exposure. *International Journal of Molecular Sciences, 21*(4), 1410. doi:10.3390/ijms21041410 PMID:32093039

Sarıdaş, M. A., Kapur, B., Çeliktopuz, E., Şahiner, Y., & Kargı, S. P. (2021). Land productivity, irrigation water use efficiency and fruit quality under various plastic mulch colors and irrigation regimes of strawberry in the eastern Mediterranean region of Turkey. *Agricultural Water Management, 245*, 106568. doi:10.1016/j.agwat.2020.106568

Sarkar, D. J., Sarkar, S. D., Das, B. K., Manna, R. K., Behera, B. K., & Samanta, S. (2019). Spatial distribution of meso and microplastics in the sediments of river Ganga at eastern India. *The Science of the Total Environment, 694*, 133712. doi:10.1016/j.scitotenv.2019.133712 PMID:31400677

Savinelli, B., Vega Fernández, T., Galasso, N. M., D'Anna, G., Pipitone, C., Prada, F., Zenone, A., Badalamenti, F., & Musco, L. (2020). Microplastics impair the feeding performance of a Mediterranean habitat-forming coral. *Marine Environmental Research, 155*, 104887. doi:10.1016/j.marenvres.2020.104887 PMID:32072989

Savoca, M. S., Tyson, C. W., McGill, M., & Slager, C. J. (2017). Odours from marine plastic debris induce food search behaviours in a forage fish. *Proceedings of the Royal Society B: Biological Sciences, 284*(1860). 10.1098/rspb.2017.1000

Savoca, M. S., McInturf, A. G., & Hazen, E. L. (2021). Plastic ingestion by marine fish is widespread and increasing. *Global Change Biology, 27*(10), 2188–2199. Advance online publication. doi:10.1111/gcb.15533 PMID:33561314

Scanes, E., Wood, H., & Ross, P. (2019). Microplastics detected in haemolymph of the Sydney rock oyster Saccostrea glomerata. *Marine Pollution Bulletin*, *149*, 110537. doi:10.1016/j.marpolbul.2019.110537 PMID:31466014

Scherer, T. M., Fuller, R. C., Lenz, R. W., & Goodwin, S. (1999). Hydrolase activity of an extracellular depolymerase from Aspergillus fumigatus with bacterial and synthetic polyesters. *Polymer Degradation & Stability*, *64*(2), 267–275. doi:10.1016/S0141-3910(98)00201-8

Scheurer, M., & Bigalke, M. (2018). Microplastics in Swiss Floodplain Soils. *Environmental Science & Technology*, *52*(6), 3591–3598. doi:10.1021/acs.est.7b06003 PMID:29446629

Schirinzi, G. F., Pedà, C., Battaglia, P., Laface, F., Galli, M., Baini, M., Consoli, P., Scotti, G., Esposito, V., Faggio, C., Farré, M., Barceló, D., Fossi, M. C., Andaloro, F., & Romeo, T. (2020). A new digestion approach for the extraction of microplastics from gastrointestinal tracts (GITs) of the common dolphinfish (Coryphaena hippurus) from the western Mediterranean Sea. *Journal of Hazardous Materials*, *397*(February), 122794. doi:10.1016/j.jhazmat.2020.122794 PMID:32387826

Schirinzi, G. F., Pérez-Pomeda, I., Sanchís, J., Rossini, C., Farré, M., & Barceló, D. (2017). Cytotoxic effects of commonly used nanomaterials and microplastics on cerebral and epithelial human cells. *Environmental Research*, *159*, 579–587. doi:10.1016/j.envres.2017.08.043 PMID:28898803

Schmidt, C., Krauth, T., & Wagner, S. (2017). Export of Plastic Debris by Rivers into the Sea. *Environmental Science & Technology*, *51*(21), 12246–12253. doi:10.1021/acs.est.7b02368 PMID:29019247

Schnurr, R., Alboiu, V., Chaudhary, M., Corbett, R., Quanz, M., Sankar, K., Srain, H. S., Thavarajah, V., Xanthos, D., & Walker, T. R. (2018). Reducing marine pollution from single-use plastics (SUPs): A review. *Marine Pollution Bulletin*, *137*, 157–171. doi:10.1016/j.marpolbul.2018.10.001 PMID:30503422

Schwabl, Köppel, S., Königshofer, P., Bucsics, T., Trauner, M., Reiberger, T., & Liebmann, B. (2019). Detection of Various Microplastics in Human Stool: A Prospective Case Series. *Annals of Internal Medicine*, *171*(7), 453–457. doi:10.7326/M19-0618 PMID:31476765

Scott, G. (2002). *Degradable Polymers*. Springer. doi:10.1007/978-94-017-1217-0

Seeley, M. E., Song, B., Passie, R., & Hale, R. C. (2020). Microplastics affect sedimentary microbial communities and nitrogen cycling. *Nature Communications*, *11*(1), 2372. doi:10.103841467-020-16235-3 PMID:32398678

Sekino, T., Takahashi, S., & Takamasu, K. (2012). Fundamental study on nanoremoval processing method for microplastic structures using photocatalyzed oxidation. *Key Engineering Materials*, *523*, 610–614. doi:10.4028/www.scientific.net/KEM.523-524.610

Sekudewicz, I., Dabrowska, A. M., & Syczewski, M. D. (2021). Microplastic pollution in surface water and sediments in the urban section of the Vistula River (Poland). In *Science of the Total Environment* (Vol. 762). Elsevier, doi:10.1016/j.scitotenv.2020.143111

Seltenrich, N. (2015). New link in the food chain? Marine plastic pollution and seafood safety. *Environmental Health Perspectives*, *123*(2), A41. doi:10.1289/ehp.123-A34 PMID:25643424

Selvam, S., Jesuraja, K., Venkatramanan, S., Roy, P. D., & Jeyanthi Kumari, V. (2021). Hazardous microplastic characteristics and its role as a vector of heavy metal in groundwater and surface water of coastal south India. *Journal of Hazardous Materials, 402*(August), 123786. doi:10.1016/j.jhazmat.2020.123786

Semmler-Behnke, M., Kreyling, W. G., Lipka, J., Fertsch, S., Wenk, A., Takenaka, S., Schmid, G., & Brandau, W. (2008). Biodistribution of 1.4- and 18-nm gold particles in rats. *Small*, *4*(12), 2108–2111. doi:10.1002mll.200800922 PMID:19031432

Seng, N., Lai, S., Fong, J., Saleh, M. F., Cheng, C., Cheok, Z. Y., & Todd, P. A. (2020). Early evidence of microplastics on seagrass and macroalgae. *Marine and Freshwater Research*, *71*(8), 922–928. doi:10.1071/MF19177

Setälä, O., Fleming-Lehtinen, V., & Lehtiniemi, M. (2014). Ingestion and transfer of microplastics in the planktonic food web. *Environmental Pollution*, *185*, 77–83. doi:10.1016/j.envpol.2013.10.013 PMID:24220023

Setälä, O., Magnusson, K., Lehtiniemi, M., & Norén, F. (2016). Distribution and abundance of surface water microlitter in the Baltic Sea: A comparison of two sampling methods. *Marine Pollution Bulletin*, *110*(1), 177–183. doi:10.1016/j.marpolbul.2016.06.065 PMID:27339742

Shah, A. A., Kato, S., Shintani, N., Kamini, N. R., & Nakajima-Kambe, T. (2014). Microbial degradation of aliphatic and aliphatic-aromatic co-polyesters. *Applied Microbiology and Biotechnology*, *98*(8), 3437–3447. doi:10.100700253-014-5558-1 PMID:24522729

Shang, J., Chai, M., & Zhu, Y. (2003). Solid-phase photocatalytic degradation of polystyrene plastic with TiO2 as photocatalyst. *Journal of Solid State Chemistry*, *174*(1), 104–110. doi:10.1016/S0022-4596(03)00183-X

Sharifinia, M., Bahmanbeigloo, Z. A., Keshavarzifard, M., Khanjani, M. H., & Lyons, B. P. (2020). Microplastic pollution as a grand challenge in marine research: A closer look at their adverse impacts on the immune and reproductive systems. *Ecotoxicology and Environmental Safety*, *204*(July), 111109. doi:10.1016/j.ecoenv.2020.111109 PMID:32798751

Sharma, S., Basu, S., Shetti, N. P., Nadagouda, M. N., & Aminabhavi, T. M. (2021). Microplastics in the environment: Occurrence, perils, and eradication. *Chemical Engineering Journal*, *408*, 127317. doi:10.1016/j.cej.2020.127317 PMID:34017217

Sharma, S., & Chatterjee, S. (2017). Microplastic pollution, a threat to marine ecosystem and human health: A short review. *Environmental Science and Pollution Research International*, *24*(27), 21530–21547. doi:10.100711356-017-9910-8 PMID:28815367

Sharma, S., Kundu, A., Basu, S., Shetti, N. P., & Aminabhavi, T. M. (2020). Sustainable environmental management and related biofuel technologies. *Journal of Environmental Management*, *273*, 111096. doi:10.1016/j.jenvman.2020.111096 PMID:32734892

Sharma, S., Shetti, N. P., Basu, S., Nadagouda, M. N., & Aminabhavi, T. M. (2022). Remediation of per- and polyfluoroalkyls (PFAS) via electrochemical methods. *Chemical Engineering Journal*, *430*, 132895.

Sharpley, R., & Ussi, M. (2014). Tourism and governance in small island developing states (SIDS): The case of Zanzibar. *International Journal of Tourism Research*, *16*(1), 87–96. doi:10.1002/jtr.1904

Shen, M., Zhang, Y., Zhu, Y., Song, B., Zeng, G., Hu, D., Wen, X., & Ren, X. (2019). Recent advances in toxicological research of nanoplastics in the environment: A review. *Environmental Pollution*, *252*, 511–521. doi:10.1016/j.envpol.2019.05.102 PMID:31167159

Shevealy, S., Courtney, K., & Parks, J. (2011). *The Honolulu Strategy: A global framework for prevention and management of marine debris.* United Nations Environment Programme. Retrieved December 13, 2021, from https://marinedebris.noaa.gov/sites/default/files/publications-files/Honolulu_Strategy.pdf

Shi, J., Wu, D., Su, Y., & Xie, B. (2021). Selective enrichment of antibiotic resistance genes and pathogens on polystyrene microplastics in landfill leachate. *The Science of the Total Environment*, *765*, 142775. doi:10.1016/j.scitotenv.2020.142775 PMID:33082042

Shimao, M. (2001). Biodegradation of plastics. *Current Opinion in Biotechnology*, *12*(3), 242–247. doi:10.1016/S0958-1669(00)00206-8 PMID:11404101

Shimao, M., Yamamoto, H., Ninomiya, K., Kato, N., Adachi, O., Ameyama, M., & Sakazawa, C. (1984). Pyrroloquinoline quinone as an essential growth factor for a poly(vinyl alcohol)-degrading symbiont, *Pseudomonas* sp. VM15C. *Agricultural and Biological Chemistry*, *48*(11), 2873–2876. doi:10.1271/bbb1961.48.2873

Shim, W. J., Hong, S. H., & Eo, S. E. (2017). Identification methods in microplastic analysis: A review. *Analytical Methods*, *9*(9), 1384–1391. doi:10.1039/C6AY02558G

Shi, W., Han, Y., Sun, S., Tang, Y., Zhou, W., Du, X., & Liu, G. (2020). Immunotoxicities of microplastics and sertraline, alone and in combination, to a bivalve species: Size-dependent interaction and potential toxication mechanism. *Journal of Hazardous Materials*, *122603*, 122603. Advance online publication. doi:10.1016/j.jhazmat.2020.122603 PMID:32289642

Shoshitaishvili, B. (2021). From Anthropocene to Noosphere: The Great Acceleration. *Earth's Future*, *9*(2).

Shruti, V. C., Pérez-Guevara, F., Roy, P. D., & Kutralam-Muniasamy, G. (2022). Analyzing microplastics with Nile Red: Emerging trends, challenges, and prospects. *Journal of Hazardous Materials*, *423*(August). doi:10.1016/j.jhazmat.2021.127171

Siegfried, M., Koelmans, A. A., Besseling, E., & Kroeze, C. (2017). Export of microplastics from land to sea. A modelling approach. *Water Research*, *127*, 249–257. doi:10.1016/j.watres.2017.10.011 PMID:29059612

Sighicelli, M., Pietrelli, L., Lecce, F., Iannilli, V., Falconieri, M., Coscia, L., Vito, S. D., Nuglio, S., & Zampetti, G. (2018). Microplastic pollution in the surface waters of Italian Subalpine Lakes. *Environmental Pollution*, *236*, 645–651. doi:10.1016/j.envpol.2018.02.008 PMID:29433105

Siipola, V., Pflugmacher, S., Romar, H., Wendling, L., & Koukkari, P. (2020). Low-cost biochar adsorbents for water purification including microplastics removal. *Applied Sciences (Basel, Switzerland)*, *10*(3), 788. doi:10.3390/app10030788

Silva, P. P. G. (2016). *Contaminação e toxicidade de microplásticos em uma área de proteção marinha costeira* [Master's Dissertation]. Escola de Engenharia de São Carlos, University of São Paulo, São Carlos. Retrieved 2021-11-12, from www.teses.usp.br doi:10.11606/D.18.2016.tde-27092016-084059

Silva, A. B., Bastos, A. S., Justino, C. I. L., Duarte, A. C., & Rocha-santos, T. A. P. (2018). Analytica Chimica Acta Microplastics in the environment : Challenges in analytical chemistry -. *RE:view*, *1017*. Advance online publication. doi:10.1016/j.aca.2018.02.043 PMID:29534790

Silva, A. L. P., Prata, J. C., Walker, T. R., Duarte, A. C., Ouyang, W., Barcelò, D., & Rocha-Santos, T. (2021). Increased plastic pollution due to COVID-19 pandemic: Challenges and recommendations. *Chemical Engineering Journal*, *405*, 126683. doi:10.1016/j.cej.2020.126683 PMID:32834764

Silva-Cavalcanti, J. S., Silva, J., França, E. J., Araújo, M., & Gusmão, F. (2017). Microplastics ingestion by a common tropical freshwater fishing resource. *Environmental Pollution*, *221*, 218–226.

Silva, J. A., Tobella, L. M., Becerra, J., Godoy, F., & Matrínez, M. A. (2007). Biosynthesis of poly-β-hydroxyalkanoate by Brevundimonas vesicularis LMG P-23615 and Sphingopyxis macrogoltabida LMG 17324 using acid-hydrolyzed sawdust as carbon source. *Journal of Bioscience and Bioengineering*, *103*(6), 542–546. doi:10.1263/jbb.103.542 PMID:17630126

Simon, M. (2020). *Plastic Rain Is the New Acid Rain.* https://www.wired.com/story/plastic-rain-is-the-new-acid-rain/

Simon, M. (2021). *Plastic Is Falling From the Sky. But Where's It Coming From?* https://www.wired.com/story/plastic-is-falling-from-the-sky/

Singh, B., & Sharma, N. (2008). Mechanistic implications of plastic degradation. In Polymer Degradation and Stability (Vol. 93, Issue 3, pp. 561–584). doi:10.1016/j.polymdegradstab.2007.11.008

Singh, S., Naik, T. S. K., Anil, A. G., Dhiman, J., Kumar, V., Dhanjal, D. S., ... Ramamurthy, P. C. (2021). Micro (nano) plastics in wastewater: A critical review on toxicity risk assessment, behaviour, environmental impact and challenges. *Chemosphere*, 133169. PMID:34890615

Singla, S., Shetti, N. P., Basu, S., Mondal, K., & Aminabhavi, T. M. (2022). Hydrogen production technologies-Membrane based separation, storage and challenges. *Journal of Environmental Management*, *302*, 113963. doi:10.1016/j.jenvman.2021.113963 PMID:34700079

Sjollema, S. B., Redondo-Hasselerharm, P., Leslie, H. A., Kraak, M. H. S., & Vethaak, A. D. (2016). Do plastic particles affect microalgal photosynthesis and growth? *Aquatic Toxicology (Amsterdam, Netherlands)*, *170*, 259–261. doi:10.1016/j.aquatox.2015.12.002 PMID:26675372

Skaf, D. W., Punzi, V. L., Rolle, J. T., & Kleinberg, K. A. (2020). Removal of micron-sized microplastic particles from simulated drinking water via alum coagulation. *Chemical Engineering Journal*, *386*, 123807. doi:10.1016/j.cej.2019.123807

Skjolding, L. M., Ašmonaitė, G., Jølck, R. I., Andresen, T. L., Selck, H., Baun, A., & Sturve, J. (2017). An assessment of the importance of exposure routes to the uptake and internal localisation of fluorescent nanoparticles in zebrafish (*Danio rerio*), using light sheet microscopy. *Nanotoxicology*, *11*(3), 351–359. doi:10.1080/17435390.2017.1306128 PMID:28286999

Slepecky, R. A., & Law, J. H. (1961). Synthesis and degradation of poly-b-hydroxybutyric acid in connection with sporulation of Bacillus megaterium. *Journal of Bacteriology*, *82*, 37–42. doi:10.1128/jb.82.1.37-42.1961 PMID:16561914

Smith, M., Love, D. C., Rochman, C. M., & Neff, R. A. (2018). Microplastics in Seafood and the Implications for Human Health. *Current Environmental Health Reports*, *5*(3), 375–386. doi:10.100740572-018-0206-z PMID:30116998

Smith, S. E., & Read, D. J. (2010). *Mycorrhizal symbiosis*. Academic Press.

Sobhani, Z., Lei, Y., Tang, Y., Wu, L., Zhang, X., Naidu, R., Megharaj, M., & Fang, C. (2020). Microplastics generated when opening plastic packaging. *Scientific Reports*, *10*(1), 1–7. doi:10.103841598-020-61146-4 PMID:32193409

Som, C., Wick, P., Krug, H., & Nowack, B. (2011). Environmental and health effects of nanomaterials in nanotextiles and facade coatings. *Environment International*, *37*(6), 1131–1142. doi:10.1016/j.envint.2011.02.013 PMID:21397331

Song, Y. K., Hong, S. H., Eo, S., Jang, M., Han, G. M., Isobe, A., & Shim, W. J. (2018). Horizontal and vertical distribution of microplastics in Korean coastal waters. *Environmental Science & Technology*, *52*(21), 12188–12197. doi:10.1021/acs.est.8b04032 PMID:30295469

Sonnegaard Poulsen, M., Mose, T., Leth Maroun, L., Mathiesen, L., Ehlert Knudsen, L., & Rytting, E. (2013). Kinetics of silica nanoparticles in the human placenta. *Nanotoxicology*. Advance online publication. doi:10.3109/17435390.2013.812259 PMID:23742169

Sparks, C., Awe, A., & Maneveld, J. (2021). Abundance and characteristics of microplastics in retail mussels from Cape Town, South Africa. *Marine Pollution Bulletin*, *166*(February), 112186. doi:10.1016/j.marpolbul.2021.112186 PMID:33676106

Sridharan, S., Kumar, M., Singh, L., Bolan, N. S., & Saha, M. (2021). Microplastics as an emerging source of particulate air pollution: A critical review. *Journal of Hazardous Materials*, *418*(March), 126245. doi:10.1016/j.jhazmat.2021.126245 PMID:34111744

Staehr, P. A., Sheikh, M., Rashid, R., Ussi, A., Suleiman, M., Kloiber, U., Dahl, K., Tairova, Z., Strand, J., Kuguru, B., & Muhando, C. (2018). Managing human pressures to restore ecosystem health of zanzibar coastal waters. *J. Aquac. Mar. Biol*, *7*(2), 59–70. doi:10.15406/jamb.2018.07.00185

Stanton, T., Johnson, M., Nathanail, P., MacNaughtan, W., & Gomes, R. L. (2019). Freshwater and airborne textile fibre populations are dominated by 'natural', not microplastic, fibres. *The Science of the Total Environment*, *666*, 377–389. doi:10.1016/j.scitotenv.2019.02.278 PMID:30798244

Stapleton, P. (2019). Toxicological considerations of nano-sized plastics. *AIMS Environmental Science*, *6*(5), 367–378. doi:10.3934/environsci.2019.5.367 PMID:31745497

Steer, M., Cole, M., Thompson, R. C., & Lindeque, P. K. (2017). Microplastic ingestion in fish larvae in the western English Channel. *Environmental Pollution*, *226*, 250–259. doi:10.1016/j.envpol.2017.03.062 PMID:28408185

Stock, F., Reifferscheid, G., Brennholt, N., & Kostianaia, E. (2019). *Plastics in the Aquatic Environment-Part II: Stakeholders' Role Against Pollution*. Academic Press.

Stock, F., Kochleus, C., Bänsch-Baltruschat, B., Brennholt, N., & Reifferscheid, G. (2019). Sampling techniques and preparation methods for microplastic analyses in the aquatic environment – A review. *Trends in Analytical Chemistry*, *113*, 84–92. doi:10.1016/j.trac.2019.01.014

Stolte, A., Forster, S., Gerdts, G., & Schubert, H. (2015). Microplastic concentrations in beach sediments along the German Baltic coast. *Marine Pollution Bulletin*, *99*(1–2), 216–229. doi:10.1016/j.marpolbul.2015.07.022 PMID:26198261

Stubbins, A., Law, K. L., Muñoz, S. E., Bianchi, T. S., & Zhu, L. (2021). Plastics in the Earth system. *Science*, *373*(6550), 51–55. doi:10.1126cience.abb0354 PMID:34210876

Stubenrauch, J., & Ekardt, F. (2020). Plastic pollution in soils: Governance approaches to foster soil health and closed nutrient cycles. *Environments*, *7*(5), 38. doi:10.3390/environments7050038

Sturm, M. T., Herbort, A. F., Horn, H., & Schuhen, K. (2020). Comparative study of the influence of linear and branched alkyltrichlorosilanes on the removal efficiency of polyethylene and polypropylene-based microplastic particles from water. *Environmental Science and Pollution Research International*, *27*(10), 10888–10898. doi:10.100711356-020-07712-9 PMID:31953766

Sudhakar, M. P., Magesh, P. D., & Dharani, G. (2020). Studies on the development and characterization of bioplastic film from the red seaweed (Kappaphycus alvarezii). *Environmental Science and Pollution Research International*, *28*(26), 33899–33913. doi:10.100711356-020-10010-z PMID:32935218

Sudhakar, M., Priyadarshini, C., Doble, M., Sriyutha Murthy, P., & Venkatesan, R. (2007). Marine bacteria mediated degradation of nylon 66 and 6. *International Biodeterioration & Biodegradation*, *60*(3), 144–151. doi:10.1016/j.ibiod.2007.02.002

Sugni, M., Mozzi, D., Barbaglio, A., Bonasoro, F., & Candia Carnevali, M. D. (2007). Endocrine disrupting compounds and echinoderms: New ecotoxicological sentinels for the marine ecosystem. *Ecotoxicology (London, England)*, *16*(1), 95–108. doi:10.100710646-006-0119-8 PMID:17253161

Sujathan, S., Kniggendorf, A. K., Kumar, A., Roth, B., Rosenwinkel, K. H., & Nogueira, R. (2017). Heat and Bleach: A Cost-Efficient Method for Extracting Microplastics from Return Activated Sludge. *Archives of Environmental Contamination and Toxicology*, *73*(4), 641–648. doi:10.100700244-017-0415-8 PMID:28550340

Su, L., Nan, B., Craig, N. J., & Pettigrove, V. (2020). Temporal and spatial variations of microplastics in roadside dust from rural and urban Victoria, Australia: Implications for diffuse pollution. *Chemosphere*, *252*, 126567. doi:10.1016/j.chemosphere.2020.126567 PMID:32443265

Sulistyo, E. N., Rahmawati, S., Putri, R. A., Arya, N., & Eryan, Y. A. (2020). Identification of the Existence and Type of Microplastic in Code River Fish, Special Region of Yogyakarta. *EKSAKTA: Journal of Sciences and Data Analysis*, *20*(1), 85–91.

Sundt, P., Schulze, P.-E., & Syversen, F. 2014. *Sources of microplastic- pollution to the marine environment.* Miljødirektoaret/Norwegian Environment Agency. https://d3n8a8pro7vhmx.cloudfront.net/boomerangalliance/pages/507/attachments/original/1481155578/Norway_Sources_of_Microplastic_Pollution.pdf?1481155578

Sun, S., Shi, W., Tang, Y., Han, Y., Du, X., Zhou, W., Hu, Y., Zhou, C., & Liu, G. (2020). Immunotoxicity of petroleum hydrocarbons and microplastics alone or in combination to a bivalve species: Synergic impacts and potential toxication mechanisms. *The Science of the Total Environment*, *138852*. Advance online publication. doi:10.1016/j.scitotenv.2020.138852 PMID:32570313

Sun, X. D., Yuan, X. Z., Jia, Y., Feng, L. J., Zhu, F. P., Dong, S. S., Liu, J., Kong, X., Tian, H., Duan, J. L., Ding, Z., Wang, S. G., & Xing, B. (2020). Differentially charged nanoplastics demonstrate distinct accumulation in Arabidopsis thaliana. *Nature Nanotechnology*, *15*(9), 755–760. doi:10.103841565-020-0707-4 PMID:32572228

Sun, X., Chen, B., Li, Q., Liu, N., Xia, B., Zhu, L., & Qu, K. (2018). Toxicities of polystyrene nano- and microplastics toward marine bacterium *Halomonas alkaliphila. The Science of the Total Environment*, *642*, 1378–1385. doi:10.1016/j.scitotenv.2018.06.141 PMID:30045518

Sun, Y., Xu, W., Gu, Q., Chen, Y., Zhou, Q., Zhang, L., Gu, L., Huang, Y., Lyu, K., & Yang, Z. (2019). Small-sized microplastics negatively affect rotifers: Changes in the key life-history traits and rotifer-*Phaeocystis* population dynamics. *Environmental Science & Technology*, *53*(15), 9241–9251. Advance online publication. doi:10.1021/acs.est.9b02893 PMID:31268695

Sun, Y., Yuan, J., Zhou, T., Zhao, Y., Yu, F., & Ma, J. (2020). Laboratory simulation of microplastics weathering and its adsorption behaviors in an aqueous environment: A systematic review. *Environmental Pollution*, *265*, 114864. doi:10.1016/j.envpol.2020.114864 PMID:32505960

Surak, M. (2018). *Extended producer responsibility.* Encyclopedia Britannica. Retrieved November 17, 2021, from https://www.britannica.com/topic/extended-producer-responsibility

Suresh, S. S., Mohanty, S., & Nayak, S. K. (2017). Composition analysis and characterization of waste polyvinyl chloride (PVC) recovered from data cables. *Waste Management (New York, N.Y.)*, *60*, 100–111. doi:10.1016/j.wasman.2016.08.033 PMID:27594574

Surfers Against Sewage. (2021, July 16). Retrieved from www.sas.org.uk: https://www.sas.org.uk/our-work/plastic-pollution/plastic-pollution-facts-figures/

Suriyamongkol, P., Weselake, R., Narine, S., Moloney, M., & Shah, S. (2007). Biotechnological approaches for the production of polyhydroxyalkanoates in microorganisms and plants – a review. *Biotechnology Advances*, *25*(2), 148–175. doi:10.1016/j.biotechadv.2006.11.007 PMID:17222526

Sushmitha, B. S., Vanitha, K. P., & Rangaswamy, B. E. (2016). Bioplastics - A Review. *International Journal of Modern Trends in Engineering and Research, 3*(4), 411–413.

Sussarellu, R., Suquet, M., Thomas, Y., Lambert, C., Fabioux, C., Pernet, M. E., Le Goïc, N., Quillien, V., Mingant, C., Epelboin, Y., Corporeau, C., Guyomarch, J., Robbens, J., Paul-Pont, I., Soudant, P., & Huvet, A. (2016). Oyster reproduction is affected by exposure to polystyrene microplastics. *Proceedings of the National Academy of Sciences of the United States of America, 113*(9), 2430–2435. doi:10.1073/pnas.1519019113 PMID:26831072

Su, Y., Zhang, Z., Zhu, J., Shi, J., Wei, H., Xie, B., & Shi, H. (2021). Microplastics act as vectors for antibiotic resistance genes in landfill leachate: The enhanced roles of the long-term aging process. In *Environmental Pollution* (Vol. 270). Elsevier Sci Ltd. doi:10.1016/j.envpol.2020.116278

Suzuki, T., Ichihara, Y., Yamada, M., & Tonomura, K. (1973). Some characteristics of *Pseudomonas* O-3 which utilizes polyvinyl alcohol. *Agricultural and Biological Chemistry, 37*(4), 747–756. doi:10.1271/bbb1961.37.747

Syakti, A. D., Jaya, J. V., Rahman, A., Hidayati, N. V., Raza'i, T. S., Idris, F., Trenggono, M., Doumenq, P., & Chou, L. M. (2019). Bleaching and necrosis of staghorn coral (*Acropora formosa*) in laboratory assays: Immediate impact of LDPE microplastics. *Chemosphere, 228*, 528–535. Advance online publication. doi:10.1016/j.chemosphere.2019.04.156 PMID:31051356

Syberg, K., Nielsen, A., Khan, F. R., Banta, G. T., Palmqvist, A., & Jepsen, P. M. (2017). Microplastic potentiates triclosan toxicity to the marine copepod *Acartia tonsa* (Dana). *Journal of Toxicology and Environmental Health - Part A: Current Issues, 80*(23–24), 1369–1371. doi:10.1080/15287394.2017.1385046 PMID:29131715

Ta, A. T., & Babel, S. (2020). Microplastics pollution with heavy metals in the aquaculture zone of the Chao Phraya River Estuary, Thailand. *Marine Pollution Bulletin, 161*, 111747. doi:10.1016/j.marpolbul.2020.111747 PMID:33091841

Tadsuwan, K., & Babel, S. (2021). Microplastic contamination in a conventional wastewater treatment plant in Thailand. In Waste Management & Research (Vol. 39, Issues 5, SI, pp. 754–761). Sage Publications Ltd. doi:10.1177/0734242X20982055

Takata, K., & Hirano, H. (1997). Mechanism of glucose transport across the human and rat placental barrier: A review. *Microscopy Research and Technique, 38*(1-2), 145–152. doi:10.1002/(SICI)1097-0029(19970701/15)38:1/2<145::AID-JEMT15>3.0.CO;2-P PMID:9260845

Tallec, K., Huvet, A., Di Poi, C., González-Fernández, C., Lambert, C., Petton, B., Le Goïc, N., Berchel, M., Soudant, P., & Paul-Pont, I. (2018). Nanoplastics impaired oyster free living stages, gametes and embryos. *Environmental Pollution, 242*(Pt B), 1226–1235.

Tallec, K., Huvet, A., Di Poi, C., González-Fernández, C., Lambert, C., Petton, B., Le Goïc, N., Berchel, M., Soudant, P., & Paul-Pont, I. (2018). Nanoplastics impaired oyster free living stages, gametes and embryos. *Environmental Pollution, 242*, 1226–1235. doi:10.1016/j.envpol.2018.08.020 PMID:30118910

Talsness, C. E., Andrade, A. J. M., Kuriyama, S. N., Taylor, J. A., & vom Saal, F. S. (2009). Components of plastic: Experimental studies in animals and relevance for human health. *Philosophical Transactions of the Royal Society of London. Series B, Biological Sciences, 364*(1526), 2079–2096. doi:10.1098/rstb.2008.0281 PMID:19528057

Talvitie, J., Mikola, A., Koistinen, A., & Setälä, O. (2017). Solutions to microplastic pollution – Removal of microplastics from wastewater effluent with advanced wastewater treatment technologies. *Water Research, 123*, 401–407. doi:10.1016/j.watres.2017.07.005 PMID:28686942

Tamminga, M., Hengstmann, E., & Fischer, E. K. (2018). Microplastic analysis in the South Funen Archipelago, Baltic Sea, implementing manta trawling and bulk sampling. *Marine Pollution Bulletin, 128*, 601–608. doi:10.1016/j.marpolbul.2018.01.066 PMID:29571412

Tang, J., Ni, X., Zhou, Z., Wang, L., & Lin, S. (2018). Acute microplastic exposure raises stress response and suppresses detoxification and immune capacities in the scleractinian coral *Pocillopora damicornis. Environmental Pollution, 243*, 66–74. Advance online publication. doi:10.1016/j.envpol.2018.08.045 PMID:30172125

Tang, N., Liu, X., & Xing, W. (2020). Microplastics in wastewater treatment plants of Wuhan, Central China: Abundance, removal, and potential source in household wastewater. *The Science of the Total Environment, 745*, 141026. doi:10.1016/j.scitotenv.2020.141026 PMID:32726699

Tang, Y., Liu, Y., Chen, Y., Zhang, W., Zhao, J., He, S., Yang, C., Zhang, T., Tang, C., Zhang, C., & Yang, Z. (2021). A review: Research progress on microplastic pollutants in aquatic environments. *The Science of the Total Environment, 766*, 142572. doi:10.1016/j.scitotenv.2020.142572 PMID:33183825

Tang, Y., Rong, J., Guan, X., Zha, S., Shi, W., Han, Y., ... Liu, G. (2019). Immunotoxicity of microplastics and two persistent organic pollutants alone or in combination to a bivalve species. *Environmental Pollution, 113845*. Advance online publication. doi:10.1016/j.envpol.2019.113845 PMID:31883493

Teng, J., Zhao, J., Zhu, X., Shan, E., & Wang, Q. (2021). Oxidative stress biomarkers, physiological responses, and proteomic profiling in oyster (*Crassostrea gigas)* exposed to microplastics with irregular-shaped PE and PET microplastic. *The Science of the Total Environment, 786*, 147425. doi:10.1016/j.scitotenv.2021.147425

Teng, J., Zhao, J., Zhu, X., Shan, E., Zhang, C., Zhang, W., & Wang, Q. (2020). Toxic effects of exposure to microplastics with environmentally relevant shapes and concentrations: Accumulation, energy metabolism and tissue damage in oyster *Crassostrea gigas. Environmental Pollution.* Advance online publication. doi:10.1016/j.envpol.2020.116169 PMID:33302083

Tenorio-Alfonso, A., Sánchez, M. C., & Franco, J. M. (2020). A review of the sustainable approaches in the production of bio-based polyurethanes and their applications in the adhesive field. *Journal of Polymers and the Environment, 28*(3), 749–774. doi:10.100710924-020-01659-1

Ter Halle, A., Jeanneau, L., Martignac, M., Jardé, E., Pedrono, B., Brach, L., & Gigault, J. (2017). Nanoplastic in the North Atlantic Subtropical Gyre. *Environmental Science & Technology, 51*(23), 13689–13697. doi:10.1021/acs.est.7b03667 PMID:29161030

Ter Halle, A., Ladirat, L., Martignac, M., Mingotaud, A. F., Boyron, O., & Perez, E. (2017). To what extent are microplastics from the open ocean weathered? *Environmental Pollution, 227*, 167–174. doi:10.1016/j.envpol.2017.04.051 PMID:28460234

Tetu, S. G., Sarker, I., Schrameyer, V., Pickford, R., Elbourne, L. D. H., Moore, L. R., & Paulsen, I. T. (2019). Plastic leachates impair growth and oxygen production in *Prochlorococcus*, the ocean's most abundant photosynthetic bacteria. *Communications Biology, 2*(1), 184. doi:10.103842003-019-0410-x PMID:31098417

Teuten, E. L., Rowland, S. J., Galloway, T. S., & Thompson, R. C. (2007). Potential for Plastics to Transport Hydrophobic Contaminants. *Environmental Science & Technology, 41*(22), 7759–7764. doi:10.1021/es071737s PMID:18075085

Teuten, E. L., Saquing, J. M., Knappe, D. R. U., Barlaz, M. A., Jonsson, S., Björn, A., Rowland, S. J., Thompson, R. C., Galloway, T. S., Yamashita, R., Ochi, D., Watanuki, Y., Moore, C., Viet, P. H., Tana, T. S., Prudente, M., Boonyatumanond, R., Zakaria, M. P., Akkhavong, K., ... Takada, H. (2009). Transport and release of chemicals from plastics to the environment and to wildlife. *Philosophical Transactions of the Royal Society of London. Series B, Biological Sciences, 364*(1526), 2027–2045. doi:10.1098/rstb.2008.0284 PMID:19528054

The Pew Charitable Trusts & SYSTEMIQ. (2020). *Breaking the Plastic Wave: A Comprehensive Assessment of Pathways Towards Stopping Ocean Plastic Pollution.* https://www.pewtrusts.org/-/media/assets/2020/10/breakingtheplasticwave_mainreport.pdf

Thiagarajan, V., Iswarya, V., P, A. J., Seenivasan, R., Chandrasekaran, N., & Mukherjee, A. (2018, October). Influence of differently functionalized polystyrene microplastics on the toxic effects of P25 TiO2 NPs towards marine algae *Chlorella* sp. *Aquatic Toxicology (Amsterdam, Netherlands)*, *207*, 208–216. doi:10.1016/j.aquatox.2018.12.014 PMID:30638491

Thiele, C. J., Hudson, M. D., & Russell, A. E. (2019). Evaluation of existing methods to extract microplastics from bivalve tissue: Adapted KOH digestion protocol improves filtration at single-digit pore size. *Marine Pollution Bulletin*, *142*(March), 384–393. doi:10.1016/j.marpolbul.2019.03.003 PMID:31232316

Thiele, C. J., Hudson, M. D., Russell, A. E., Saluveer, M., & Sidaoui-Haddad, G. (2021). Microplastics in fish and fishmeal: An emerging environmental challenge? *Scientific Reports*, *11*(1), 1–12. doi:10.103841598-021-81499-8 PMID:33479308

Thiel, M., Hinojosa, I. A., Joschko, T., & Gutow, L. (2011). Spatio-temporal distribution of floating objects in the German Bight (North Sea). *Journal of Sea Research*, *65*(3), 368–379. doi:10.1016/j.seares.2011.03.002

Thomas, M., Jon, B., Craig, S., Edward, R., Ruth, H., John, B., Dick, V. A., Heather, L. A., & Matthew, S. (2020). The world is your oyster: Low-dose, long-term microplastic exposure of juvenile oysters. *Heliyon*, *6*(1), e03103. doi:10.1016/j.heliyon.2019.e03103 PMID:31909270

Thomas, R. T., Nair, V., & Sandhyarani, N. (2013). TiO2 nanoparticle assisted solid phase photocatalytic degradation of polythene film: A mechanistic investigation. *Colloids and Surfaces. A, Physicochemical and Engineering Aspects*, *422*, 1–9. doi:10.1016/j.colsurfa.2013.01.017

Thompson, R.C., Swan, S.H., Moore, C.J., & Vom Saal, F.S. (2009). *Our plastic age.* doi:10.1098/rstb.2009.0054

Thompson, R. C., Olsen, Y., Mitchell, R. P., Davis, A., Rowland, S. J., John, A. W., McGonigle, D., & Russell, A. E. (2004). Lost at sea: Where is all the plastic? *Science*, *304*(5672), 838–838. doi:10.1126cience.1094559 PMID:15131299

Thompson, R. C., Swan, S. H., Moore, C. J., & Vom Saal, F. S. (2009). Our plastic age. Philos. Trans. R. Soc. Lond. Ser. B Biol. *Sci.*, *364*(1526), 1973–1976.

Thompson, R., Moore, C., vom Saal, F., & Swan, S. (2009). Plastics, the environment and human health: Current consensus and future trends. *Philosophical Transactions of the Royal Society of London. Series B, Biological Sciences*, *364*(1526), 2153–2166. doi:10.1098/rstb.2009.0053 PMID:19528062

Thurmund, W. (2010). *Seaweed: A new wave of investment in macroalgae.* Biofuels International.

Thushari, G., & Senevirathna, J. (2020). Plastic pollution in the marine environment. *Heliyon*, *6*(8), e04709. doi:10.1016/j.heliyon.2020.e04709 PMID:32923712

Tibbetts, J. (2015). Managing marine plastic pollution: Policy initiatives to address wayward waste. *Environmental Health Perspectives*, *123*(4), A90–A93. doi:10.1289/ehp.123-A90 PMID:25830293

Tlili, S., Jemai, D., Brinis, S., & Regaya, I. (2020). Microplastics mixture exposure at environmentally relevant conditions induce oxidative stress and neurotoxicity in the wedge clam *Donax trunculus. Chemosphere*, *127344*, 127344. Advance online publication. doi:10.1016/j.chemosphere.2020.127344 PMID:32554011

Tofanelli, M., & Wortman, S. (2020). Benchmarking the agronomic performance of biodegradable mulches against polyethylene mulch film: A meta-analysis. *Agronomy (Basel)*, *2020*(10), 10. doi:10.3390/agronomy10101618

Tokiwa, Y., & Calabia, B. P. (2006). Biodegradability and biodegradation of poly(lactide). *Applied Microbiology, 72*, 244–251. PMID:16823551

Topouzelis, K., Papakonstantinou, A., & Garaba, S. P. (2019). Detection of floating plastics from satellite and unmanned aerial systems (Plastic Litter Project 2018). *International Journal of Applied Earth Observation and Geoinformation, 79*, 175–183. doi:10.1016/j.jag.2019.03.011

Torre, M., Digka, N., Anastasopoulou, A., Tsangaris, C., & Mytilineou, C. (2016). Anthropogenic microfibres pollution in marine biota. A new and simple methodology to minimize airborne contamination. *Marine Pollution Bulletin, 113*(1–2), 55–61. doi:10.1016/j.marpolbul.2016.07.050 PMID:27491365

Torres, F. G., & De-la-Torre, G. E. (2021). Historical microplastic records in marine sediments: Current progress and methodological evaluation. *Regional Studies in Marine Science, 46*, 101868. doi:10.1016/j.rsma.2021.101868

Tosetto, L., Williamson, J. E., & Brown, C. (2017). Trophic transfer of microplastics does not affect fish personality. *Animal Behaviour, 123*, 159–167. doi:10.1016/j.anbehav.2016.10.035

Toussaint, B., Raffael, B., Angers-Loustau, A., Gilliland, D., Kestens, V., Petrillo, M., Rio-Echevarria, I. M., & Van den Eede, G. (2019). Review of micro- and nanoplastic contamination in the food chain. In Food Additives and Contaminants - Part A Chemistry, Analysis, Control, Exposure and Risk Assessment (Vol. 36, Issue 5, pp. 639–673). doi:10.1080/19440049.2019.1583381

Trainic, M., Flores, J. M., Pinkas, I., Pedrotti, M. L., Lombard, F., Bourdin, G., Gorsky, G., Boss, E., Rudich, Y., Vardi, A., & Koren, I. (2020). Airborne microplastic particles detected in the remote marine atmosphere. *Communications Earth & Environment, 1*(1), 1–9. doi:10.103843247-020-00061-y

Tramoy, R., Gasperi, J., Dris, R., Colasse, L., Fisson, C., Sananes, S., Rocher, V., & Tassin, B. (2019). Assessment of the Plastic Inputs From the Seine Basin to the Sea Using Statistical and Field Approaches. *Frontiers in Marine Science, 6*, 151. Advance online publication. doi:10.3389/fmars.2019.00151

Trestrail, C., Walpitagama, M., Miranda, A., Nugegoda, D., & Shimeta, J. (2021). Microplastics alter digestive enzyme activities in the marine bivalve, *Mytilus galloprovincialis. The Science of the Total Environment, 779*, 146418. doi:10.1016/j.scitotenv.2021.146418 PMID:33744572

Trifuoggi, M., Pagano, G., Oral, R., Pavičić-Hamer, D., Burić, P., Kovačić, I., Siciliano, A., Toscanesi, M., Thomas, P. J., Paduano, L., Guida, M., & Lyons, D. M. (2019). Microplastic-induced damage in early embryonal development of sea urchin *Sphaerechinus granularis. Environmental Research, 108815*. Advance online publication. doi:10.1016/j.envres.2019.108815 PMID:31629182

Uheida, A., Mejía, H. G., Abdel-Rehim, M., Hamd, W., & Dutta, J. (2021). Visible light photocatalytic degradation of polypropylene microplastics in a continuous water flow system. *Journal of Hazardous Materials, 406*, 124299. doi:10.1016/j.jhazmat.2020.124299 PMID:33131945

Ummalyma, S. B., Sahoo, D., & Pandey, A. (2020). Microalgal Biorefineries for Industrial Products. In Microalgae Cultivation for Biofuels Production. Academic Press.

UN Environment Programme Report. (2018). *Banning single-use plastic: Lessons and experiences from countries.* UN Environment Programme.

UN. (2015). *The 17 Goals.* https://sdgs.un.org/goals

UNEP & GRID-Arendal. (2016). *Marine Litter Vital Graphics.* UN Environment Programme and GRID-Arendal, Nairobi and Arendal. https://www.unep.org/resources/report/marine-litter-vital-graphics

UNEP. (2014a). *Valuing Plastic: The Business Case for Measuring, Managing and Disclosing Plastic Use in the Consumer Goods Industry*. UN Environment Programme. http://hdl.handle.net/20.500.11822/9238

UNEP. (2014b). *Annex I. UNEA Resolution 1/6 Marine plastic debris and microplastics.* https://wedocs.unep.org/bitstream/handle/20.500.11822/17562/Marine%20Plastic%20Debris%20and%20Microplastic%20Technical%20Report%20Advance%20Copy%20Ann.pdf?%20sequence=2&isAllowed=y

UNEP. (2016a). *Marine Plastic Debris and Microplastics – Global Lessons and Research to Inspire Action and Guide Policy Change*. UN Environment Programme. https://wedocs.unep.org/handle/20.500.11822/7720

UNEP. (2016b). *2/11. Marine plastic litter and microplastics.* https://wedocs.unep.org/bitstream/handle/20.500.11822/11186/K1607228_UNEPEA2_RES11E.pdf?sequence=1&isAllowed=y

UNEP. (2017). *3/7. Marine litter and microplastics.* https://wedocs.unep.org/bitstream/handle/20.500.11822/22773/K1800210%20-%20UNEP-EA-3-RES-7%20-%20Advance.pdf?sequence=15&isAllowed=y

UNEP. (2018a). *Report of the first meeting of the ad hoc open-ended expert group on marine litter and microplastics.* UN Environment Programme. https://papersmart.unon.org/resolution/uploads/k1801471.pdf

UNEP. (2018b). *Africa Waste Management Outlook*. UN Environment Programme. https://wedocs.unep.org/20.500.11822/25514

UNEP. (2018c). *Mapping of global plastics value chain and plastics losses to the environment (with a particular focus on marine environment)*. UN Environment Programme. http://hdl.handle.net/20.500.11822/26745

UNEP. (2019a). *4/6. Marine plastic litter and microplastics.* https://wedocs.unep.org/bitstream/handle/20.500.11822/28471/English.pdf?sequence=3&isAllowed=y

UNEP. (2021). *Drowning In Plastics - Marine Litter and Plastic Waste Vital Graphics*. UN Environment Programme and GRID-Arendal, Nairobi and Arendal. https://wedocs.unep.org/xmlui/bitstream/handle/20.500.11822/36964/VITGRAPH.pdf

UNGC. (2020). *Ocean Stewardship 2030. Ten ambitions and recommendations for growing sustainable ocean business.* New York: UN Global Compact. https://ungc-communications-assets.s3.amazonaws.com/docs/publications/Ocean-Stewardship-2030-Report.pdf

Uruyama, H., Kanamori, T., & Kimura, Y. (2002). Properties and biodegradability of polymer blends of poly(L-lactide) swith different optical purity of the lactate units. *Macromolecular Materials and Engineering*, *287*(2), 116–121. doi:10.1002/1439-2054(20020201)287:2<116::AID-MAME116>3.0.CO;2-Z

Ustabasi, G. S., & Baysal, A. (2020). Bacterial interactions of microplastics extracted from toothpaste under controlled conditions and the influence of seawater. *The Science of the Total Environment*, *703*, 135024. doi:10.1016/j.scitotenv.2019.135024 PMID:31734496

Van Cauwenberghe, L., & Janssen, C. R. (2014). Microplastics in bivalves cultured for human consumption. *Environmental Pollution, 193*, 65–70.

Van Cauwenberghe, L., & Janssen, C. R. (2014). Microplastics in bivalves cultured for human consumption. *Environmental Pollution, 193*, 65–70. doi:10.1016/j.envpol.2014.06.010 PMID:25005888

Van Cauwenberghe, L., Vanreusel, A., Mees, J., & Janssen, C. R. (2013). Microplastic pollution in deep-sea sediments. *Environmental Pollution*, *182*, 495–499. doi:10.1016/j.envpol.2013.08.013 PMID:24035457

Van Colen, C., Vanhove, B., Diem, A., & Moens, T. (2020). Does microplastic ingestion by zooplankton affect predator-prey interactions? An experimental study on larviphagy. *Environmental Pollution*, *256*, 113479. doi:10.1016/j.envpol.2019.113479 PMID:31679869

Van den Berg, P., Huerta-Lwanga, E., Corradini, F., & Geissen, V. (2020). Sewage sludge application as a vehicle for microplastics in eastern Spanish agricultural soils. *Environmental Pollution*, *261*, 114198. doi:10.1016/j.envpol.2020.114198 PMID:32097788

Van Melkebeke, M., Janssen, C., & De Meester, S. (2020). Characteristics and sinking behavior of typical microplastics including the potential effect of biofouling: Implications for remediation. *Environmental Science & Technology*, *54*(14), 8668–8680. doi:10.1021/acs.est.9b07378 PMID:32551546

Van Sebille, E., Gilbert, A., & Spathi, C. (2016). *The ocean plastic pollution challenge: towards solutions in the UK.* Grantham Institute Breifing Paper, 19(19), 3–4. www.imperial.ac.uk/grantham/publications

Van Sebille, E., Aliani, S., Law, K. L., Maximenko, N., Alsina, J. M., Bagaev, A., Bergmann, M., Chapron, B., Chubarenko, I., Cózar, A., Delandmeter, P., Egger, M., Fox-Kemper, B., Garaba, S. P., Goddijn-Murphy, L., Hardesty, B. D., Hoffman, M. J., Isobe, A., Jongedijk, C. E., ... Wichmann, D. (2020). The physical oceanography of the transport of floating marine debris. *Environmental Research Letters*, *15*(2), 023003. doi:10.1088/1748-9326/ab6d7d

Van Sebille, E., England, M. H., & Froyland, G. (2012). Origin, dynamics and evolution of ocean garbage patches from observed surface drifters. *Environmental Research Letters*, *7*(4), 044040. doi:10.1088/1748-9326/7/4/044040

Van Sebille, E., Wilcox, C., Lebreton, L., Maximenko, N., Hardesty, B. D., Van Franeker, J. A., Eriksen, M., Siegel, D., Galgani, F., & Law, K. L. (2015). A global inventory of small floating plastic debris. *Environmental Research Letters*, *10*(12), 124006. doi:10.1088/1748-9326/10/12/124006

van Wijnen, J., Ragas, A. M. J., & Kroeze, C. (2019). Modelling global river export of microplastics to the marine environment: Sources and future trends. *The Science of the Total Environment*, *673*, 392–401. doi:10.1016/j.scitotenv.2019.04.078 PMID:30991329

Vanapalli, K. R., Dubey, B. K., Sarmah, A. K., & Bhattacharya, J. (2021). Assessment of microplastic pollution in the aquatic ecosystems–An indian perspective. *Case Studies in Chemical and Environmental Engineering*, *3*, 100071. doi:10.1016/j.cscee.2020.100071

Varela, J. A., Bexiga, M. G., Åberg, C., Simpson, J. C., & Dawson, K. A. (2012). Quantifying size-dependent interactions between fluorescently labeled polystyrene nanoparticles and mammalian cells. *Journal of Nanobiotechnology*, *10*(1), 39. doi:10.1186/1477-3155-10-39 PMID:23006133

Vazquez, O. A., & Rahman, M. S. (2021). An ecotoxicological approach to microplastics on terrestrial and aquatic organisms: A systematic review in assessment, monitoring and biological impact. *Environmental Toxicology and Pharmacology*, *84*, 103615. doi:10.1016/j.etap.2021.103615 PMID:33607259

Vecchi, S., Bianchi, J., Scalici, M., Fabroni, F., & Tomassetti, P. (2021). Field evidence for microplastic interactions in marine benthic invertebrates. *Scientific Reports*, *11*(1), 1–12. doi:10.103841598-021-00292-9 PMID:34686714

Veerasingam, S., Ranjani, M., Venkatachalapathy, R., Bagaev, A., Mukhanov, V., Litvinyuk, D., Verzhevskaia, L., Guganathan, L., & Vethamony, P. (2020). Microplastics in different environmental compartments in India: Analytical methods, distribution, associated contaminants and research needs. *Trends in Analytical Chemistry*, *133*, 116071. doi:10.1016/j.trac.2020.116071

Veiga, J. M., Fleet, D., Kinsey, S., Nilsson, P., Vlachogianni, T., Werner, S., Galgani, F., Thompson, R. C., Dagevos, J., Gago, J., Sobral, P., & Cronin, R. (2016). *Identifying sources of marine litter.* MSFD GES TG Marine Litter Thematic Report. *JRC Technical Report, EUR, 28309.* Advance online publication. doi:10.2788/018068

Venâncio, C., Ferreira, I., Martins, M. A., Soares, A. M. V. M., Lopes, I., & Oliveira, M. (2019). The effects of nanoplastics on marine plankton: A case study with polymethylmethacrylate. *Ecotoxicology and Environmental Safety, 184,* 109632. doi:10.1016/j.ecoenv.2019.109632 PMID:31514077

Verma, R., Singh, S., Dalai, M. K., Saravanan, M., Agrawal, V. V., & Srivastava, A. K. (2017). Photocatalytic degradation of polypropylene film using TiO2-based nanomaterials under solar irradiation. *Materials & Design, 133,* 10–18. doi:10.1016/j.matdes.2017.07.042

Vethaak, A. D., Lahr, J., Schrap, S. M., Belfroid, A. C., Rijs, G. B., Gerritsen, A., & de Voogt, P. (2005). An integrated assessment of estrogenic contamination and biological effects in the aquatic environment of The Netherlands. *Chemosphere, 59*(4), 511–524. doi:10.1016/j.chemosphere.2004.12.053 PMID:15788174

Vethaak, A., & Leslie, H. (2016). Plastic debris is a human health issue. *Environmental Science & Technology, 50*(13), 6825–6826. doi:10.1021/acs.est.6b02569 PMID:27331860

Vianello, A., Jensen, R. L., Liu, L., & Vollertsen, J. (2019). Simulating human exposure to indoor airborne microplastics using a Breathing Thermal Manikin. *Scientific Reports, 9*(1), 8670. Advance online publication. doi:10.103841598-019-45054-w PMID:31209244

Villalba, M., Pérez, V., Herrera, L., Stepke, C., Maldonado, N., Fredericksen, F., Yáñez, A., & Olavarría, V. H. (2017). Infectious pancreatic necrosis virus infection of fish cell lines: Preliminary analysis of gene expressions related to extracellular matrix remodeling and immunity. *Veterinary Immunology and Immunopathology, 193–194,* 10–17. doi:10.1016/j.vetimm.2017.09.009 PMID:29129223

Vince, J., & Hardesty, B. (2018). Governance solutions to the tragedy of the commons that marine plastics have become. *Frontiers in Marine Science, 5,* 214. doi:10.3389/fmars.2018.00214

Vital, S. A., Cardoso, C., Avio, C., Pittura, L., Regoli, F., & Bebianno, M. J. (2021). Do microplastic contaminated seafood consumption pose a potential risk to human health? *Marine Pollution Bulletin, 171*(April), 112769. doi:10.1016/j.marpolbul.2021.112769 PMID:34358788

Vogt, A., Combadiere, B., Hadam, S., Stieler, K. M., Lademann, J., Schaefer, H., Autran, B., Sterry, W., & Blume-Peytavi, U. (2006). 40 nm, but not 750 or 1,500 nm, nanoparticles enter epidermal CD1a+ cells after transcutaneous application on human skin. *The Journal of Investigative Dermatology, 126*(6), 1316–1322. doi:10.1038j.jid.5700226 PMID:16614727

von Friesen, L. W., Granberg, M. E., Hassellöv, M., Gabrielsen, G. W., & Magnusson, K. (2019). An efficient and gentle enzymatic digestion protocol for the extraction of microplastics from bivalve tissue. *Marine Pollution Bulletin, 142*(March), 129–134. doi:10.1016/j.marpolbul.2019.03.016 PMID:31232285

Von Moos, N., Burkhardt-Holm, P., & Köhler, A. (2012). Uptake and effects of microplastics on cells and tissue of the blue mussel Mytilus edulis L. after an experimental exposure. *Environmental Science & Technology, 46*(20), 11327–11335. doi:10.1021/es302332w PMID:22963286

Vroom, R., Halsband, C., Besseling, E., & Koelmans, A. A. (2016). *Effects of microplastics on zooplankton.* https://library.wur.nl/WebQuery/wurpubs/510036

Vutivoradit, S., & Jakkapattarawong, S. (2018). Stakeholder Participation for sustainable waste management in Phranakorn District, Bangkok. *Proceedings of Academics World 92nd International Conference,* 103-107.

Walker, T., & Xanthos, D. (2018). A call for Canada to move toward zero plastic waste by reducing and recycling single-use plastics. *Resour. Conserv. Recycl.*, 99-100.

Walkinshaw, C., Lindeque, P. K., Thompson, R., Tolhurst, T., & Cole, M. (2020). Microplastics and seafood: Lower trophic organisms at highest risk of contamination. *Ecotoxicology and Environmental Safety*, *190*, 110066. doi:10.1016/j.ecoenv.2019.110066 PMID:31846861

Wallace, R. L., Snell, T. W., Ricci, C., & Nogrady, T. (2006). Rotifera. Biology, Ecology and Systematics. In Guides to the identification of the microinvertebrates of the continental waters of the world. Kenobi Productions and Backhuys Publishers.

Walls, M. (2011). *Deposit–refund systems in practice and theory. Resources for the Future Discussion Paper No. 11–47.* Washington, DC: Resources for the Future.

Walther, A., Yen, N., & Hu, C.-S. (2021). Strategies, actions, and policies by Taiwan's ENGOs, media, and government to reduce plastic use and marine plastic pollution. *Marine Policy*, *126*, 104391. doi:10.1016/j.marpol.2021.104391

Wang, K., Mandal, A., Ayton, E., Hunt, R., Zeller, M.A., & Sharma, S. (2016). Modification of protein rich algal biomass to form bioplastics and odor removal. *Protein Byproduct*, 107-117.

Wang, C., Jiang, L., Liu, R., He, M., Cui, X., & Wang, C. (2021). Comprehensive assessment of factors influencing Nile red staining: Eliciting solutions for efficient microplastics analysis. *Marine Pollution Bulletin*, *171*(July), 112698. doi:10.1016/j.marpolbul.2021.112698 PMID:34245991

Wang, C., Zhao, J., & Xing, B. (2021). Environmental source, fate, and toxicity of microplastics. *Journal of Hazardous Materials*, *407*, 124357. doi:10.1016/j.jhazmat.2020.124357 PMID:33158648

Wang, F., Zhang, M., Sha, W., Wang, Y., Hao, H., Dou, Y., & Li, Y. (2020). Sorption behavior and mechanisms of organic contaminants to nano and microplastics. *Molecules (Basel, Switzerland)*, *25*(8), 1827. doi:10.3390/molecules25081827 PMID:32316227

Wang, J., Li, Y., Lu, L., Zheng, M., Zhang, X., Tian, H., Wang, W., & Ru, S. (2019). Polystyrene microplastics cause tissue damages, sex-specific reproductive disruption, and transgenerational effects in marine medaka (*Oryzias melastigma*). *Environmental Pollution*, *254*, 113024. doi:10.1016/j.envpol.2019.113024 PMID:31454586

Wang, J., Peng, J., Tan, Z., Gao, Y., Zhan, Z., Chen, Q., & Cai, L. (2017). Microplastics in the surface sediments from the Beijiang River littoral zone: Composition, abundance, surface textures and interaction with heavy metals. *Chemosphere*, *171*, 248–258. Advance online publication. doi:10.1016/j.chemosphere.2016.12.074 PMID:28024210

Wang, J., Tan, Z., Peng, J., Qiu, Q., & Li, M. (2016). The behaviors of microplastics in the marine environment. *Marine Environmental Research*, *113*, 7–17. doi:10.1016/j.marenvres.2015.10.014 PMID:26559150

Wang, L., Kaeppler, A., Fischer, D., & Simmchen, J. (2019). Photocatalytic TiO2 micromotors for removal of microplastics and suspended matter. *ACS Applied Materials & Interfaces*, *11*(36), 32937–32944. doi:10.1021/acsami.9b06128 PMID:31429262

Wang, L., Zhang, J., Hou, S., & Sun, H. (2017). A Simple Method for Quantifying Polycarbonate and Polyethylene Terephthalate Microplastics in Environmental Samples by Liquid Chromatography-Tandem Mass Spectrometry. *Environmental Science & Technology Letters*, *4*(12), 530–534. doi:10.1021/acs.estlett.7b00454

Wang, R., Ji, M., Zhai, H., & Liu, Y. (2020). Occurrence of phthalate esters and microplastics in urban secondary effluents, receiving water bodies and reclaimed water treatment processes. *The Science of the Total Environment*, *737*, 140219. doi:10.1016/j.scitotenv.2020.140219 PMID:32783843

Wang, S., Wang, Y., Liang, Y., Cao, W., Sun, C., Ju, P., & Zheng, L. (2020). The interactions between microplastic polyvinyl chloride and marine diatoms: Physiological, morphological, and growth effects. *Ecotoxicology and Environmental Safety*, *203*(July), 111000. doi:10.1016/j.ecoenv.2020.111000 PMID:32736119

Wang, T., Hu, M., Xu, G., Shi, H., Leung, J. Y. S., & Wang, Y. (2021). Microplastic accumulation via trophic transfer: Can a predatory crab counter the adverse effects of microplastics by body defence? *The Science of the Total Environment*, *754*, 142099. doi:10.1016/j.scitotenv.2020.142099 PMID:32911152

Wang, T., Li, B., Zou, X., Wang, Y., Li, Y., Xu, Y., Mao, L., Zhang, C., & Yu, W. (2019). Emission of primary microplastics in mainland China: Invisible but not negligible. *Water Research*, *162*, 214–224. doi:10.1016/j.watres.2019.06.042 PMID:31276985

Wang, W., Ndungu, A. W., Li, Z., & Wang, J. (2017). Microplastics pollution in inland freshwaters of China: A case study in urban surface waters of Wuhan, China. *The Science of the Total Environment*, *575*, 1369–1374. doi:10.1016/j.scitotenv.2016.09.213 PMID:27693147

Wang, W., & Wang, J. (2018). Investigation of microplastics in aquatic environments: An overview of the methods used, from field sampling to laboratory analysis. *Trends in Analytical Chemistry*, *108*, 195–202. doi:10.1016/j.trac.2018.08.026

Wang, W., Yuan, W., Chen, Y., & Wang, J. (2018). Microplastics in surface waters of Dongting Lake and Hong Lake, China. *The Science of the Total Environment*, *633*, 539–545. doi:10.1016/j.scitotenv.2018.03.211 PMID:29579665

Wang, X., Yang, Y. D., Pei, K., Zhou, J., Peixoto, L., Gunina, A., Zeng, Z., Zang, H., Rasmussen, J., & Kuzyakov, Y. (2020). Nitrogen rhizodeposition of legumes and its fate in agroecosystems: Field study and literature review. *Land Degradation & Development*, *32*(1), 410–419. doi:10.1002/ldr.3729

Wang, Y., Yin, J., & Chen, G.-Q. (2014). Polyhydroxyalkanoates, challenges and opportunities. *Current Opinion in Biotechnology*, *30*, 59–65. doi:10.1016/j.copbio.2014.06.001 PMID:24976377

Wang, Z., Zhang, Y., Kang, S., Yang, L., Shi, H., Tripathee, L., & Gao, T. (2021). Research progresses of microplastic pollution in freshwater systems. *The Science of the Total Environment*, *795*, 148888. doi:10.1016/j.scitotenv.2021.148888 PMID:34328911

Wan, Y., Wu, C., Xue, Q., & Hui, X. (2019). Effects of plastic contamination on water evaporation and desiccation cracking in soil. *The Science of the Total Environment*, *654*, 576–582. doi:10.1016/j.scitotenv.2018.11.123 PMID:30447596

Wardrop, P., Shimeta, J., Nugegoda, D., Morrison, P. D., Miranda, A., Tang, M., & Clarke, B. O. (2016). Chemical Pollutants Sorbed to Ingested Microbeads from Personal Care Products Accumulate in Fish. *Environmental Science & Technology*, *50*(7), 4037–4044. doi:10.1021/acs.est.5b06280 PMID:26963589

Waring, R. H., Harris, R. M., & Mitchell, S. C. (2018). Plastic contamination of the food chain: A threat to human health? *Maturitas*, *115*, 64–68. doi:10.1016/j.maturitas.2018.06.010 PMID:30049349

Watts, A. J. R., Urbina, M. A., Corr, S., Lewis, C., & Galloway, T. S. (2015). Ingestion of plastic microfibers by the crab Carcinus maenas and its effect on food consumption and energy balance. *Environmental Science & Technology*, *49*(24), 14597–14604. doi:10.1021/acs.est.5b04026 PMID:26529464

Watts, A. J. R., Urbina, M. A., Goodhead, R., Moger, J., Lewis, C., & Galloway, T. S. (2016). Effect of microplastic on the gills of the shore crab Carcinus maenas. *Environmental Science & Technology*, *50*(10), 5364–5369. doi:10.1021/acs.est.6b01187 PMID:27070459

Webb, S., Gaw, S., Marsden, I. D., & McRae, N. K. (2020). Biomarker responses in New Zealand green-lipped mussels *Perna canaliculus* exposed to microplastics and triclosan. *Ecotoxicology and Environmental Safety*, *201*, 110871. doi:10.1016/j.ecoenv.2020.110871 PMID:32559692

Weber, A., Jeckel, N., Weil, C., Umbach, S., Brennholt, N., Reifferscheid, G., & Wagner, M. (2021). Ingestion and toxicity of polystyrene microplastics in freshwater bivalves. *Environmental Toxicology and Chemistry*, *40*(8), 2247–2260. doi:10.1002/etc.5076 PMID:33928672

Weber, C. J., & Lechthaler, S. (2021). Plastics as a stratigraphic marker in fluvial deposits. *Anthropocene*, *36*, 100314. doi:10.1016/j.ancene.2021.100314

Wegner, A., Besseling, E., Foekema, E. M., Kamermans, P., & Koelmans, A. A. (2012). Effects of nanopolystyrene on the feeding behaviour of the blue mussel (*Mytilus edulis* L.). *Environmental Toxicology and Chemistry*, *31*(11), 2490–2497. doi:10.1002/etc.1984 PMID:22893562

Wei, S., Luo, H., Zou, J., Chen, J., Pan, X., Rousseau, D. P. L., & Li, J. (2020). Characteristics and removal of microplastics in rural domestic wastewater treatment facilities of China. *The Science of the Total Environment*, *739*, 139935. doi:10.1016/j.scitotenv.2020.139935 PMID:32540663

Wei, W., Huang, Q. S., Sun, J., Wang, J.-Y., Wu, S.-L., & Ni, B.-J. (2019). Polyvinyl chloride microplastics affect methane production from the anaerobic digestion of waste activated sludge through leaching toxic bisphenol-A. *Environmental Science & Technology*, *53*(5), 2509–2517. doi:10.1021/acs.est.8b07069 PMID:30758964

Wen, Y., Freeman, B., Ma, Q., Evans, C., Chadwick, D., Zang, H., & Jones, D. (2020). Raising the groundwater table in the non-growing season can reduce greenhouse gas emissions and maintain crop productivity in cultivated fen peats. *Journal of Cleaner Production*, *262*, 121179. doi:10.1016/j.jclepro.2020.121179

Wen, Y., Zang, H., Freeman, B., Musarika, S., Evans, C., Chadwick, D., & Jones, D. (2019). Microbial utilization of low molecular weight organic carbon substrates in cultivated peats in response to warming and soil degradation. *Soil Biology & Biochemistry*, *139*, 107629. doi:10.1016/j.soilbio.2019.107629

WHO. (2019). *Microplastics in drinking-water: World Health Organization*. Geneva: World Health Organization.

Widmer, R., Oswald-Krapf, H., Sinha-Khetriwal, A., Schnellmann, M., & Böni, H. (2005). Global perspectives on the e-waste. *Environmental Impact Assessment Review*, *25*(5), 436–458. doi:10.1016/j.eiar.2005.04.001

Williams, D. F. (1981). Enzymatic hydrolysis of polylactic acid. *Engineering in Medicine*, *10*(1), 5–7. doi:10.1243/EMED_JOUR_1981_010_004_02

Wong, Y.-M., Brigham, C. J., Rha, C. K., Sinskey, A. J., & Sudesh, K. (2012). Biosynthesis and characterization of polyhydroxyalkanoate containing high 3-hydroxyhexanoate monomer fraction from crude palm kernel oil by recombinant Cupriavidus necator. *Bioresource Technology*, *121*, 320–327. doi:10.1016/j.biortech.2012.07.015 PMID:22858502

Worm, B., Lotze, H. K., Jubinville, I., Wilcox, C., & Jambeck, J. (2017). Plastic as a Persistent Marine Pollutant. *Annual Review of Environment and Resources*, *42*(1), 1–26. doi:10.1146/annurev-environ-102016-060700

Wright, S. L., & Kelly, F. J. (2017). Plastic and Human Health: A Micro Issue? *Environmental Science & Technology*, *51*(12), 6634–6647. doi:10.1021/acs.est.7b00423 PMID:28531345

Wright, S. L., Rowe, D., Thompson, R. C., & Galloway, T. S. (2013). Microplastic ingestion decreases energy reserves in marine worms. *Current Biology*, *23*(23), R1031–R1033. doi:10.1016/j.cub.2013.10.068 PMID:24309274

Wu, F., Wang, Y., Leung, J. Y. S., Huang, W., Zeng, J., Tang, Y., Chen, J., Shi, A., Yu, X., Xu, X., Zhang, H., & Cao, L. (2020). Accumulation of microplastics in typical commercial aquatic species: A case study at a productive aquaculture site in China. *The Science of the Total Environment*, *708*, 135432. doi:10.1016/j.scitotenv.2019.135432 PMID:31806295

Wu, Z., Wang, F., Hu, L., Jiang, Y., Wang, X., & Xu, J. (2020). Directional liquefaction of lignocellulose in 1, 4-dioxane–ethanol–formic acid co-solvents. *Journal of Chemical Technology and Biotechnology (Oxford, Oxfordshire)*, *96*(4), 971–979. doi:10.1002/jctb.6606

WWAP (United Nations World Water Assessment Programme). (2017). T*he United Nations World Water Development Report 2017. Wastewater: The Untapped Resource*. UNESCO. https://wedocs.unep.org/20.500.11822/20448

WWF, EMF, & BCG. (2020). *The business case for a UN treaty on plastic pollution*. WWF. https://www.plasticpollutiontreaty.org/UN_treaty_plastic_poll_report.pdf

Xiong, X., Wu, C., Elser, J. J., Mei, Z., & Hao, Y. (2019). Occurrence and fate of microplastic debris in middle and lower reaches of the Yangtze River–from inland to the sea. *The Science of the Total Environment*, *659*, 66–73. doi:10.1016/j.scitotenv.2018.12.313 PMID:30597469

Xue, Y.-H., Sun, Z.-X., Feng, L.-S., Jin, T., Xing, J.-C., & Wen, X.-L. (2020). Algal density affects the influences of polyethylene microplastics on the freshwater rotifer *Brachionus calyciflorus*. *Chemosphere*, *128613*. Advance online publication. doi:10.1016/j.chemosphere.2020.128613 PMID:33131733

Xu, J. L., Thomas, K. V., Luo, Z., & Gowen, A. A. (2019). FTIR and Raman imaging for microplastics analysis: State of the art, challenges and prospects. *Trends in Analytical Chemistry*, *119*, 115629. doi:10.1016/j.trac.2019.115629

Xu, X.-Y., Lee, W. T., Chan, A. K. Y., Lo, H. S., Shin, P. K. S., & Cheung, S. G. (2017). Microplastic ingestion reduces energy intake in the clam *Atactodea striata*. *Marine Pollution Bulletin*, *124*(2), 798–802. doi:10.1016/j.marpolbul.2016.12.027 PMID:28038767

Xu, Y., Chan, F. K. S., He, J., Johnson, M., Gibbins, C., Kay, P., Stanton, T., Xu, Y., Li, G., Feng, M., Paramor, O., Yu, X., & Zhu, Y.-G. (2020). A critical review of microplastic pollution in urban freshwater environments and legislative progress in China: Recommendations and insights. *Critical Reviews in Environmental Science and Technology*, *•••*, 1–44. doi:10.1080/10643389.2020.1801308

Xu, Y., Chan, F. K. S., Johnson, M., Stanton, T., He, J., Jia, T., Wang, J., Wang, Z., Yao, Y., Yang, J., Liu, D., Xu, Y., & Yu, X. (2021). Microplastic pollution in Chinese urban rivers: The influence of urban factors. *Resources, Conservation and Recycling*, *173*, 105686. doi:10.1016/j.resconrec.2021.105686

Xu, Y., Chan, F. K. S., Stanton, T., Johnson, M. F., Kay, P., He, J., Wang, J., Kong, C., Wang, Z., Liu, D., & Xu, Y. (2021). Synthesis of dominant plastic microfibre prevalence and pollution control feasibility in Chinese freshwater environments. *The Science of the Total Environment*, *783*, 146863. doi:10.1016/j.scitotenv.2021.146863 PMID:33872912

Xu, Y., He, Q., Liu, C., & Huangfu, X. (2019). Are Micro- or Nanoplastics Leached from Drinking Water Distribution Systems? *Environmental Science & Technology*, *53*(16), 9339–9340. doi:10.1021/acs.est.9b03673 PMID:31393716

Xu, Y., Lin, L., Xiao, M., Wang, S., Smith, A. T., Sun, L., & Meng, Y. (2018). Synthesis and properties of CO2-based plastics: Environmentally-friendly, energy-saving and biomedical polymeric materials. *Progress in Polymer Science*, *80*, 163–182. doi:10.1016/j.progpolymsci.2018.01.006

Yamashita, K., Yoshioka, Y., Higashisaka, K., Mimura, K., Morishita, Y., Nozaki, M., Yoshida, T., Ogura, T., Nabeshi, H., Nagano, K., Abe, Y., Kamada, H., Monobe, Y., Imazawa, T., Aoshima, H., Shishido, K., Kawai, Y., Mayumi, T., Tsunoda, S., ... Tsutsumi, Y. (2011). Silica and titanium dioxide nanoparticles cause pregnancy complications in mice. *Nature Nanotechnology*, *6*(5), 321–328. doi:10.1038/nnano.2011.41 PMID:21460826

Yang, D., Shi, H., Li, L., Li, J., Jabeen, K., & Kolandhasamy, P. (2015). Microplastic, pollution in table salts from China. *Environmental Science & Technology*, *49*(22), 13622–13627. doi:10.1021/acs.est.5b03163 PMID:26486565

Yang, J. H., Yu, J. G., & Ma, X. F. (2006). A novel plasticizer for the preparation of thermoplastic starch. *Chinese Chemical Letters*, *17*(1), 133–136.

Yang, J., Ching, Y. C., & Chuah, C. H. (2019). Applications of lignocellulosic fibers and lignin in bioplastics: A review. *Polymers*, *11*(5), 1–26. doi:10.3390/polym11050751 PMID:31035331

Yang, L., Li, K., Cui, S., Kang, Y., An, L., & Lei, K. (2019). Removal of microplastics in municipal sewage from China's largest water reclamation plant. *Water Research*, *155*, 175–181. doi:10.1016/j.watres.2019.02.046 PMID:30849731

Yang, L., Zhang, Y., Kang, S., Wang, Z., & Wu, C. (2021). Microplastics in soil: A review on methods, occurrence, sources, and potential risk. *The Science of the Total Environment*, *780*, 146546. doi:10.1016/j.scitotenv.2021.146546 PMID:33770602

Yang, S. S., Wu, W. M., Brandon, A. M., Fan, H. Q., Receveur, J. P., Li, Y., Wang, Z.-Y., Fan, R., McClellan, R. L., Gao, S.-H., Ning, D., Phillips, D. H., Peng, B.-Y., Wang, H., Cai, S.-Y., Li, P., Cai, W.-W., Ding, L.-Y., Yang, J., ... Criddle, C. S. (2018). Ubiquity of polystyrene digestion and biodegradation within yellow mealworms, larvae of Tenebrio molitor Linnaeus (Coleoptera: Tenebrionidae). *Chemosphere*, *212*, 262–271. doi:10.1016/j.chemosphere.2018.08.078 PMID:30145418

Yang, X., Wang, H., Zhang, L., Kong, L., Chen, Y., He, Q., Li, L., Grossart, H. P., & Ju, F. (2021). Marine algae facilitate transfer of microplastics and associated pollutants into food webs. *The Science of the Total Environment*, *787*, 147535. doi:10.1016/j.scitotenv.2021.147535 PMID:33991910

Yang, Y. F., Chen, C. Y., Lu, T. H., & Liao, C. M. (2019). Toxicity-based toxicokinetic/toxicodynamic assessment for bioaccumulation of polystyrene microplastics in mice. *Journal of Hazardous Materials*, *366*, 703–713. doi:10.1016/j.jhazmat.2018.12.048 PMID:30583240

Yang, Y., Yang, J., Wu, W. M., Zhao, J., Song, Y., Gao, L., Yang, R., & Jiang, L. (2015). Biodegradation and mineralization of polystyrene by plastic-eating mealworms. Part 1. Chemical and physical characterization and isotopic tests. *Environmental Science & Technology*, *49*(20), 12080–12086. doi:10.1021/acs.est.5b02661 PMID:26390034

Yano, H., Sugiyama, J., Nakagaito, A. N., Nogi, M., Matsuura, T., Hikita, M., & Handa, K. (2005). Optically transparent composites reinforced with networks of bacterial nanofibers. *Advanced Materials*, *17*(2), 153–155. doi:10.1002/adma.200400597

Yan, W., Hamid, N., Deng, S., Jia, P. P., & Pei, D. S. (2020). Individual and combined toxicogenetic effects of microplastics and heavy metals (Cd, Pb, and Zn) perturb gut microbiota homeostasis and gonadal development in marine medaka (*Oryzias melastigma*). *Journal of Hazardous Materials*, *397*(March), 122795. doi:10.1016/j.jhazmat.2020.122795 PMID:32388101

Yan, Z. J., Zhou, J., Nie, J. W., Yang, Y. D., Zhao, J., Zeng, Z. H., Marshall, M. R., Peixoto, L., & Zang, H. D. (2021). Do cropping system and fertilization rate change water-stable aggregates associated carbon and nitrogen storage? *Environmental Science and Pollution Research International*, *28*(46), 65862–65871. doi:10.100711356-021-15562-2 PMID:34322806

Yan, Z. J., Zhou, J., Yang, L., Gunina, A., Yang, Y. D., Peixoto, L., Zeng, Z. H., Zang, H. D., & Kuzyakov, Y. (2022). Diversified cropping systems benefit soil carbon and nitrogen stocks by increasing aggregate stability: Results of three fractionation methods. *The Science of the Total Environment*, *824*, 153878. doi:10.1016/j.scitotenv.2022.153878 PMID:35167890

Yao, P., Zhou, B., Lu, Y. H., Yin, Y., Zong, Y. Q., Chen, M. Te, & O'Donnell, Z. (2019). A review of microplastics in sediments: Spatial and temporal occurrences, biological effects, and analytic methods. *Quaternary International, 519*(October), 274–281. doi:10.1016/j.quaint.2019.03.028

Yaranal, N. A., Subbiah, S., & Mohanty, K. (2021a). Identification, extraction of microplastics from edible salts and its removal from contaminated seawater. *Environmental Technology and Innovation, 21*, 101253. Advance online publication. doi:10.1016/j.eti.2020.101253

Yaranal, N. A., Subbiah, S., & Mohanty, K. (2021b). Distribution and characterization of microplastics in beach sediments from Karnataka (India) coastal environments. *Marine Pollution Bulletin, 169*, 112550. doi:10.1016/j.marpolbul.2021.112550 PMID:34091249

Yates, M. R., & Barlow, C. Y. (2013). Life Cycle assessment of biodegradable, commercial biopolymers – a critical review. *Resources, Conservation and Recycling, 78*, 54–66. doi:10.1016/j.resconrec.2013.06.010

Yee, M. S. L., Hii, L. W., Looi, C. K., Lim, W. M., Wong, S. F., Kok, Y. Y., Tan, B.-K., Wong, C.-Y., & Leong, C. O. (2021). Impact of microplastics and nanoplastics on human health. *Nanomaterials (Basel, Switzerland), 11*(2), 496. doi:10.3390/nano11020496 PMID:33669327

Ye, S., & Andrady, A. L. (1991). Fouling of floating plastic debris under Biscayne Bay exposure conditions. *Marine Pollution Bulletin, 22*(12), 608–613. doi:10.1016/0025-326X(91)90249-R

Ye, S., Cheng, M., Zeng, G., Tan, X., Wu, H., Liang, J., Shen, M., Song, B., Liu, J., Yang, H., & Zhang, Y. (2020). Insights into catalytic removal and separation of attached metals from natural-aged microplastics by magnetic biochar activating oxidation process. *Water Research, 179*, 115876. doi:10.1016/j.watres.2020.115876 PMID:32387922

Ye, S., Wang, S., Lin, L., Xiao, M., & Meng, Y. (2019). CO2 derived biodegradable polycarbonates: Synthesis, modification and applications. *Advanced Industrial and Engineering Polymer Research, 2*(4), 143–160. doi:10.1016/j.aiepr.2019.09.004

Yin, L., Chen, B., Xia, B., Shi, X., & Qu, K. (2018). Polystyrene microplastics alter the behaviour, energy reserve and nutritional composition of marine jacopever (*Sebastes schlegelii*). *Journal of Hazardous Materials, 360*(August), 97–105. doi:10.1016/j.jhazmat.2018.07.110 PMID:30098534

Yokota, K., Waterfield, H., Hastings, C., Davidson, E., Kwietniewski, E., & Wells, B. (2017). Finding the missing piece of the aquatic plastic pollution puzzle: Interaction between primary producers and microplastics. *Limnology and Oceanography Letters, 2*(4), 91–104. doi:10.1002/lol2.10040

Yong, C. Q. Y., Valiyaveetill, S., & Tang, B. L. (2020). Toxicity of microplastics and nanoplastics in mammalian systems. *International Journal of Environmental Research and Public Health, 17*(5), 1509. doi:10.3390/ijerph17051509 PMID:32111046

Yoshida, S., Hiraga, K., Takehana, T., Taniguchi, I., Yamaji, H., Maeda, Y., Toyohara, K., Miyamoto, K., Kimura, Y., & Oda, K. (2016). A bacterium that degrades and assimilates poly(ethylene terephthalate). *Science, 351*(6278), 1196–1199. doi:10.1126cience.aad6359 PMID:26965627

Yue, W., Yin, C. F., Sun, L., Zhang, J., Xu, Y., & Zhou, N. Y. (2021). Biodegradation of bisphenol-A polycarbonate plastic by Pseudoxanthomonas sp. strain NyZ600. *Journal of Hazardous Materials, 15*.

Yukioka, S., Tanaka, S., Nabetani, Y., Suzuki, Y., Ushijima, T., Fujii, S., Takada, H., Van Tran, Q., & Singh, S. (2020). Occurrence and characteristics of microplastics in surface road dust in Kusatsu (Japan), Da Nang (Vietnam), and Kathmandu (Nepal). *Environmental Pollution, 256*, 113447. doi:10.1016/j.envpol.2019.113447 PMID:31679875

Yu, P., Liu, Z., Wu, D., Chen, M., Lv, W., & Zhao, Y. (2018). Accumulation of polystyrene microplastics in juvenile *Eriocheir sinensis* and oxidative stress effects in the liver. *Aquatic Toxicology (Amsterdam, Netherlands)*, *200*(March), 28–36. doi:10.1016/j.aquatox.2018.04.015 PMID:29709883

Yurtsever, M. (2019). Glitters as a source of primary microplastics: An approach to environmental responsibility and ethics. *Journal of Agricultural & Environmental Ethics*, *32*(3), 459–478. doi:10.100710806-019-09785-0

Yu, S.-P., & Chan, B. K. K. (2020). Intergenerational microplastics impact the intertidal barnacle *Amphibalanus amphitrite* during the planktonic larval and benthic adult stages. *Environmental Pollution*, *115560*. Advance online publication. doi:10.1016/j.envpol.2020.115560 PMID:33254593

Yu, Z., Peldszus, S., & Huck, P. M. (2008). Adsorption characteristics of selected pharmaceuticals and an endocrine disrupting compound-Naproxen, carbamazepine and nonylphenol-on activated carbon. *Water Research*, *42*(12), 2873–2882. doi:10.1016/j.watres.2008.02.020 PMID:18377945

Zang, H., Blagodatskaya, E., Wen, Y., Shi, L., Cheng, F., Chen, H., Zhao, B., Zhang, F., Fan, M., & Kuzyakov, Y. (2020b). Temperature sensitivity of soil organic matter mineralization decreases with long-term N fertilization: Evidence from four Q_{10} estimation approaches. *Land Degradation & Development*, *31*(6), 683–693. doi:10.1002/ldr.3496

Zang, H., Xiao, M., Wang, Y., Ling, N., Wu, J., Ge, T., & Kuzyakov, Y. (2019). Allocation of assimilated carbon in paddies depending on rice age, chase period and N fertilization: Experiment with $^{13}CO_2$ labelling and literature synthesis. *Plant and Soil*, *445*(1-2), 113–123. doi:10.100711104-019-03995-1

Zang, H., Zhou, J., Marshall, M. R., Chadwick, D. R., Wen, Y., & Jones, D. L. (2020a). Microplastics in the agroecosystem: Are they an emerging threat to the plant-soil system? *Soil Biology & Biochemistry*, *148*, 107926. doi:10.1016/j.soilbio.2020.107926

Zarfl, C. (2019). Promising techniques and open challenges for microplastic identification and quantification in environmental matrices. *Analytical and Bioanalytical Chemistry*, *411*(17), 3743–3756. doi:10.100700216-019-01763-9 PMID:30919016

Zbořilova, P., & Pac, J. (2014). *Oxo-Degradable Polyolefinic Material*. Academic Press.

Zbyszewski, M., Corcoran, P. L., & Hockin, A. (2014). Comparison of the distribution and degradation of plastic debris along shorelines of the Great Lakes, North America. *Journal of Great Lakes Research*, *40*(2), 288–299. Advance online publication. doi:10.1016/j.jglr.2014.02.012

Zettler, E. R., Mincer, T. J., & Amaral-Zettler, L. A. (2013). Life in the "plastisphere": Microbial communities on plastic marine debris. *Environmental Science & Technology*, *47*(13), 7137–7146. doi:10.1021/es401288x PMID:23745679

Zhang, S., Liu, X., Hao, X., Wang, J., & Zhang, Y. (2020). Distribution of low-density microplastics in the mollisol farmlands of northeast China. *Science of the Total Environment*, *708*, 135091. doi:10.1016/j.scitotenv.2019.135091

Zhang, Y., Kang, S., Allen, S., Allen, D., Gao, T., & Sillanpää, M. (2020). Atmospheric microplastics: A review on current status and perspectives. Earth-Science Reviews. doi:10.1016/j.earscirev.2020.103118

Zhang, Z., & Chen, Y. (2020). Effects of microplastics on wastewater and sewage sludge treatment and their removal: A review. In Chemical Engineering Journal (Vol. 382). doi:10.1016/j.cej.2019.122955

Zhang, C., Chen, X., Wang, J., & Tan, L. (2017). Toxic effects of microplastic on marine microalgae Skeletonema costatum: Interactions between microplastic and algae. *Environmental Pollution*, *220*, 1282–1288. doi:10.1016/j.envpol.2016.11.005 PMID:27876228

Zhang, C., Wang, C., Cao, G., Wang, D., & Ho, S.-H. (2020). A sustainable solution to plastics pollution: An eco-friendly bioplastic film production from high-salt contained Spirulina sp. residues. *Journal of Hazardous Materials*, *388*, 121773. doi:10.1016/j.jhazmat.2019.121773 PMID:31836373

Zhang, C., Zhou, H., Cui, Y., Wang, C., Li, Y., & Zhang, D. (2019). Microplastics in offshore sediment in the yellow Sea and east China Sea, China. *Environmental Pollution*, *244*, 827–833. doi:10.1016/j.envpol.2018.10.102 PMID:30390456

Zhang, G. S., & Liu, Y. F. (2018). The distribution of microplastics in soil aggregate fractions in southwestern China. *The Science of the Total Environment*, *642*, 12–20. doi:10.1016/j.scitotenv.2018.06.004 PMID:29894871

Zhang, G., & Zhang, F. (2020). Variations in aggregate-associated organic carbon and polyester microfibers resulting from polyester microfibers addition in a clayey soil. *Environmental Pollution*, *258*, 113716. doi:10.1016/j.envpol.2019.113716 PMID:31831225

Zhang, H., Kuo, Y. Y., Gerecke, A. C., & Wang, J. (2012). Co-release of hexabromocyclododecane (HBCD) and nano- and microparticles from thermal cutting of polystyrene foams. *Environmental Science & Technology*, *46*(20), 10990–10996. doi:10.1021/es302559v PMID:23013539

Zhang, H., Obias, V., Gonyer, K., & Dennis, D. (1994). Production of polyhydroxyalkanoates in sucrose-utilizing recombinant Escherichia coli and Klebsiella strains. *Applied and Environmental Microbiology*, *60*(4), 1198–1205. doi:10.1128/aem.60.4.1198-1205.1994 PMID:8017916

Zhang, H., Zhou, Q., Xie, Z., Zhou, Y., Tu, C., Fu, C., Mi, W., Ebinghaus, R., Christie, P., & Luo, Y. (2018). Occurrences of organophosphorus esters and phthalates in the microplastics from the coastal beaches in north China. *The Science of the Total Environment*, *616-617*, 1505–1512. doi:10.1016/j.scitotenv.2017.10.163 PMID:29089130

Zhang, J., Zhang, C., Deng, Y., Wang, R., Ma, E., Wang, J., Bai, J., Wu, J., & Zhou, Y. (2019). Microplastics in the surface water of small-scale estuaries in Shanghai. *Marine Pollution Bulletin*, *149*, 110569. doi:10.1016/j.marpolbul.2019.110569 PMID:31546109

Zhang, K., Xiong, X., Hu, H., Wu, C., Bi, Y., Wu, Y., Zhou, B., Lam, P. K. S., & Liu, J. (2017). Occurrence and Characteristics of Microplastic Pollution in Xiangxi Bay of Three Gorges Reservoir, China. *Environmental Science & Technology*, *51*(7), 3794–3801. doi:10.1021/acs.est.7b00369 PMID:28298079

Zhang, P., Tan, X., Liu, S., Liu, Y., Zeng, G., Ye, S., Yin, Z., Hu, X., & Liu, N. (2019). Catalytic degradation of estrogen by persulfate activated with iron-doped graphitic biochar: Process variables effects and matrix effects. *Chemical Engineering Journal*, *378*, 122141. doi:10.1016/j.cej.2019.122141

Zhang, S., Wang, J., Liu, X., Qu, F., Wang, X., Wang, X., Li, Y., & Sun, Y. (2019). Microplastics in the environment: A review of analytical methods, distribution, and biological effects. *Trends in Analytical Chemistry*, *111*, 62–72. doi:10.1016/j.trac.2018.12.002

Zhang, Y., Chen, Y., Westerhoff, P., Hristovski, K., & Crittenden, J. C. (2008). Stability of commercial metal oxide nanoparticles in water. *Water Research*, *42*(8–9), 2204–2212. doi:10.1016/j.watres.2007.11.036 PMID:18164742

Zhang, Y., Diehl, A., Lewandowski, A., Gopalakrishnan, K., & Baker, T. (2020). Removal efficiency of micro-and nanoplastics (180 nm–125 μm) during drinking water treatment. *The Science of the Total Environment*, *720*, 137383. doi:10.1016/j.scitotenv.2020.137383 PMID:32325555

Zhang, Y., Wang, J., Geng, X., & Jiang, Y. (2021). Does microplastic ingestion dramatically decrease the biomass of protozoa grazers? A case study on the marine ciliate Uronema marinum. *Chemosphere*, *267*, 129308. doi:10.1016/j.chemosphere.2020.129308 PMID:33352364

Zhang, Z., Peng, H., Yang, D., Zhang, J., & Ju, F. (2021). Polyvinyl Chloride Biodegradation Fuels Survival of Invasive Insect Larva and Intestinal Degrading Strain of Klebsiella. *bioRxiv*.

Zhao, S., Zhu, L., & Li, D. (2015). Microplastic in three urban estuaries, China. *Environmental Pollution, 206*, 597–604. doi:10.1016/j.envpol.2015.08.027 PMID:26312741

Zhao, T., Tan, L., Han, X., Wang, X., Zhang, Y., Ma, X., Lin, K., Wang, R., Ni, Z., Wang, J., & Wang, J. (2022). Microplastic-induced apoptosis and metabolism responses in marine Dinoflagellate, *Karenia mikimotoi. The Science of the Total Environment, 804*(238), 150252. doi:10.1016/j.scitotenv.2021.150252 PMID:34798757

Zhao, Y. B., Gao, P. P., & Ni, H. G. (2019). A chemical time bomb: Future risks of microplastics. *Water, Air, and Soil Pollution, 230*(11), 1–5. doi:10.100711270-019-4320-9

Zheng, Y., Li, J., Cao, W., Liu, X., Jiang, F., Ding, J., Yin, X., & Sun, C. (2019). Distribution characteristics of microplastics in the seawater and sediment: A case study in Jiaozhou Bay, China. *The Science of the Total Environment, 674*, 27–35. doi:10.1016/j.scitotenv.2019.04.008 PMID:31003085

Zhou, B., Wang, J., Zhang, H., & Barceló, D. (2019) Microplastics in agricultural soils on the coastal plain of Hangzhou Bay, east China: multiple sources other than plastic mulching film. *Journal of Hazardous Materials, 388*.

Zhou, B., Wang, J., Zhang, H., Shi, H., Fei, Y., Huang, S., Tong, Y., Wen, D., Luo, Y., & Barceló, D. (2020). Microplastics in agricultural soils on the coastal plain of Hangzhou Bay, east China: Multiple sources other than plastic mulching film. *Journal of Hazardous Materials, 388*, 121814. doi:10.1016/j.jhazmat.2019.121814 PMID:31843412

Zhou, J., Gui, H., Banfield, C. C., Wen, Y., Zang, H. D., Dippold, M. A., Charlton, A., & Jones, D. L. (2021a). The microplastisphere: Biodegradable microplastics addition alters soil microbial community structure and function. *Soil Biology & Biochemistry, 156*, 108211. doi:10.1016/j.soilbio.2021.108211

Zhou, J., Wen, Y., Cheng, H., Zang, H., & Jones, D. L. (2022). Simazine degradation in agroecosystems: Will it be affected by the type and amount of microplastic pollution? *Land Degradation & Development, 33*(7), 1128–1136. Advance online publication. doi:10.1002/ldr.4243

Zhou, J., Wen, Y., Marshall, M. R., Zhao, J., Gui, H., Zeng, Z. H., Jones, D. L., & Zang, H. D. (2021b). Microplastics as an emerging threat to plant and soil health in agroecosystems. *The Science of the Total Environment, 787*, 147444. doi:10.1016/j.scitotenv.2021.147444

Zhou, J., Wen, Y., Shi, L. L., Marshall, M. R., Kuzyakov, Y., Blagodatskaya, E., & Zang, H. D. (2021c). Strong priming of soil organic matter induced by frequent input of labile carbon. *Soil Biology & Biochemistry, 152*, 108069. doi:10.1016/j.soilbio.2020.108069

Zhou, J., Zang, H., Loeppmann, S., Gube, M., Kuzyakov, Y., & Pausch, J. (2020). Arbuscular mycorrhiza enhances rhizodeposition and reduces the rhizosphere priming effect on the decomposition of soil organic matter. *Soil Biology & Biochemistry, 140*, 107641. doi:10.1016/j.soilbio.2019.107641

Zhou, Q., Zhang, H., Zhou, Y., Li, Y., Xue, Y., Fu, C., Tu, C., & Luo, Y. (2016). Separation of microplastics from a coastal soil and their surface microscopic features. *Kexue Tongbao. Chinese Science Bulletin, 61*(14), 1604–1611. doi:10.1360/N972015-01098

Zhou, W., Tang, Y., Du, X., Han, Y., Shi, W., Sun, S., Zhang, W., Zheng, H., & Liu, G. (2021). Fine polystyrene microplastics render immune responses more vulnerable to two veterinary antibiotics in a bivalve species. *Marine Pollution Bulletin, 164*, 111995. doi:10.1016/j.marpolbul.2021.111995 PMID:33493858

Zhou, Y., Wang, J., Zou, M., Jia, Z., Zhou, S., & Li, Y. (2020). Microplastics in soils: A review of methods, occurrence, fate, transport, ecological and environmental risks. In *Science of the Total Environment* (Vol. 748, p. 141368). Elsevier. doi:10.1016/j.scitotenv.2020.141368

Zhu, J., & Wang, C. (2020). Recent advances in the analysis methodologies for microplastics in aquatic organisms: Current knowledge and research challenges. *Analytical Methods*, *12*(23), 2944–2957. doi:10.1039/D0AY00143K PMID:32930155

Zhu, J., Yu, X., Zhang, Q., Li, Y., Tan, S., Li, D., Yang, Z., & Wang, J. (2019). Cetaceans and microplastics: First report of microplastic ingestion by a coastal delphinid, Sousa chinensis. *The Science of the Total Environment*, *659*, 649–654. doi:10.1016/j.scitotenv.2018.12.389 PMID:31096394

Zhu, J., Zhang, Q., Li, Y., Tan, S., Kang, Z., Yu, X., Lan, W., Cai, L., Wang, J., & Shi, H. (2019). Microplastic pollution in the Maowei Sea, a typical mariculture bay of China. *The Science of the Total Environment*, *658*, 62–68. doi:10.1016/j.scitotenv.2018.12.192 PMID:30577027

Zhu, X., Zhao, W., Chen, X., Zhao, T., Tan, L., & Wang, J. (2020). Growth inhibition of the microalgae *Skeletonema costatum* under copper nanoparticles with microplastic exposure. *Marine Environmental Research*, *158*(April), 105005. doi:10.1016/j.marenvres.2020.105005 PMID:32501269

Zobkov, M., & Esiukova, E. (2017). Microplastics in Baltic bottom sediments: Quantification procedures and first results. *Marine Pollution Bulletin*, *114*(2), 724–732. doi:10.1016/j.marpolbul.2016.10.060 PMID:27810093

Zumstein, M. T., Schintlmeister, A., Nelson, T. F., Baumgartner, R., Woebken, D., Wagner, M., Kohler, H. P. E., McNeill, K., & Sander, M. (2018). Biodegradation of Synthetic Polymers in Soils: Tracking Carbon into CO_2 and Microbial Biomass. *Science Advances*, *4*(7), eaas9024. doi:10.1126ciadv.aas9024 PMID:30050987

About the Contributors

Sung Hee Joo is a Professor in Post-plastic Specialized Graduate School at the University of Seoul. She has over 20 years of experience in Environmental Engineering and Science. She has expertise in the field of advanced treatment technologies for emerging environmental contaminants, environmental nanotechnology, toxicity assessment of nanomaterials, chemical nanoscience, environmental chemistry, the innovative processes of water/wastewater treatment, the application of membrane technology in wastewater, and the fate and transport of contaminants in the environment. She is a recipient of multiple awards and has published research and review papers in scientific journals and am the author of two books, titled "Applying Nanotechnology for Environmental Sustainability" and "Modern Inorganic Chemistry: Nanotechnology for Environmental Remediation".

* * *

Gilberto Dias de Alkimin (GDA) is biologist with PhD from University of Aveiro (Portugal) in the doctoral program in Biology and Ecology of Global Changes (2020). He works in the area of aquatic ecotoxicology (freshwater and marine environment), histology, histochemistry, ecotoxicological tests, cellular and biochemical analysis. The focus of his studies is metals and pharmaceutical effects in aquatic plants and animals and now he is going through the effects of nano and microplastics. As well as areas related to water treatment (phytoremediation and alternative materials). He has experience in education, with an emphasis on Environmental Education. GDA is also deeply involved in the organization/participation of science communication actions. In the last years, GDA maintained collaborations with other research groups (national and international), giving important contributions about the toxicity of different contaminants, mostly to model organisms.

Sandhya Babel is a full Professor at the Sirindhorn International Institute of Technology (SIIT), Thammasat University, Thailand. Her current research interest includes conversion of waste to energy, recovery of valuable materials from waste, low- cost technologies for wastewater treatment, microplastics, photocatalysis, phytoremediation and adsorption.

Devarati Bagchi (BDS) completed her Bachelor of Dental Surgery from NTR University of Health Sciences, Kakinada, Andhra Pradesh and is currently working as a house surgeon at GITAM Dental College and Hospital, Visakhapatnam, Andhra Pradesh, India. She is a holder of several licensed courses including Medical coding, introductory practices in health informatics and has completed several certified courses related to Clinical Research. Her research interests include pharmacovigilance and Clinical Data Management. She has a niche towards health informatics and is an incoming graduate.

Debasish Banerjee is a senior Technical assistant of Mechanical Engineering Dept. Om Dayal Group of Institutions. Mechanical Engineer and also B.Sc in Physics. Interested areas are Fluid Mechanics, Dynamics of Machine, Mechanical Systems and Material Science.

Soumen Basu, Associate Professor, Thapar Institute of Engineering and Technology, India is currently working in the field of environmental sustainability by advanced functionalized nanomaterials. He is also actively involved in developing chemical sensors and nano-bio sensors. He is actively working on carbon capture and storage (CCS) technology. He completed his Ph.D. from the Indian Institute of Technology, Kharagpur, India and he did his postdoctoral research at the University of Alabama-USA, AIBN-University of Queensland, Australia. He has twelve years of research experience in the field of nanoscience and nanotechnology. He has published more than 130 research articles in reputed international journals.

Maria Bebianno is a full professor at the University of Algarve with great experience in marine contamination and ecotoxicology. She has a PhD in Marine Ecotoxicology At the international level she integrated the Portuguese delegation that negotiated the United Nations Convention on the Law of the Sea and is currently a member of the Group of Experts of the Regular Process for the Evaluation of the State of the Marine Environment including the Socio-Economic Commission of the United Nations. Within the World Ocean Asessment II, Dr Bebianno was a Lead -Members of the chapters "Changes in Liquid and Atmospheric Inputs to the Marine Environment from Land (including through Groundwater), Ships and Offshore Installations", "Changes in inputs and distribution of solid waste in the marine environment (other than dredged material)", Co-Lead-member of the chapters "Changes in inputs to the marine environment of nutrients" and "Changes in Seabed Mining" and co-author of the Summary and of the Approaches to the Assessment Chapters. She was a member of the Portuguese Delegation to the Oslo Convention and Paris Convention (now called OSPAR) on Protecting and Conserving the North-East Atlantic and its Resources and the Barcelona Convention for the Protection of the Marine Environment and the Coastal Region of the Mediterranean, the International Council for the Exploration of the Sea (ICES) and the UNESCO Intergovernmental Oceanographic Commission (IOC). Her research work is developed at the Centre of Marine and Environmental Research (CIMA) of the University of Algarve where she is the coordinator since 2016 and leads the Ecotoxicology and Environmental Chemistry Group.Dr. Maria Bebianno research focused on the effects of organic and inorganic "old" and emerging contaminants (personnel care products, pharmaceuticals, nanomaterials and microplastics) on aquatic organisms from coastal areas to the deep-sea. The team has also enrolled in proteomic research applied to Ecotoxicology. She has been responsible for several research projects funded by the European Union and Portuguese Institutions. She has published more than 221 papers is author of several book chapters and editor of several books and participated in several national and international (EU and others) projects. She has supervised several PhDs some of which co-supervised by colleagues from other EU countries, Brazil and Tunisia, as well as, several Pos-docs some of them from other EU countries. She has developed collaborative research with teams from several universities and research centres of the EU (Spain, France, Ireland, Italy, UK, and Finland) and non-EU countries (Brazil, Cape Verde and China). She is a member of several professional societies (Sociedade de Geografia de Lisboa, Marine Biological

Association of the United Kingdom, SETAC, SECOTOX, SICTA) and presently she was the President from the period (2015-2019) and is since January 2019 chairwomen of the General Assembly of the Portuguese association of Women Scientists-AMONET and is the Portuguese alternate in the European Platform of Women in Science (EPWS). For more details see: https://orcid.org/0000-0003-1492-8566, Scopus Author ID: 7004152715.

Sanchari Biswas (Ph.D) completed her doctorate in Environmental Sciences by specializing in Eco-toxicology from Department of Environmental Studies, GITAM Institute of Science, GITAM (Deemed to be University), Visakhapatnam, Andhra Pradesh, India. She has worked on the effect of heavy metals on birds and ecosystem health. As a part of her post-doctoral work, she currently works as a Research Associate in the conservation biology division at Sálim Ali Centre for Ornithology and Natural History, Anaikatty, Coimbatore. Her research interest includes effects of microplastics and heavy metals on the marine biota and sea-shore birds, toxicological impacts of heavy metals on different environmental matrices. Currently, she is designing a State Action Plan which will aid in conservation of birds across the country.

Gabriela Fernandez is an Adjunct Faculty in the Department of Geography, Principal-Investigator at the Center for Human Dynamics in the Mobile Age, and Graduate Advisor of the Big Data Analytics Master of Science Program at San Diego State University. She received a Ph.D. in Urban Planning, Design, & Policy from the Department of Architecture and Urban Studies at the Politecnico di Milano. Her research interests include urban metabolism ideologies and material flow analysis of metropolitan cities. Identifying urban typologies and socioeconomic indicators in the urban context while promoting public policy, smart cities, UN-SDGs, and vulnerable-populations. She serves as the UNEP delegate of the Major Group for Children & Youth, Marine Litter-&-Micro-Plastics Working-Group. She is Co-Founder & Researcher at the Metabolism of Cities, a NPO with data, tools, & publications related to urban metabolism studies & Director of the Metabolism of Cities Living Lab-at-SDSU working to localize the UN-SDGs in southern-California and Baja California Mexico region.

Debjit Ghosh received his PhD degree in Chemistry from Department of Chemistry, GITAM Institute of Science, GITAM (Deemed to be University), Visakhapatnam, Andhra Pradesh, India. His research interests include Design, synthesis, and investigation of synthetic and natural product-derived medicinal agents; Drug delivery; Isolation and spectroscopic characterization of pure phyto-constituents from herbals; Qualitative and quantitative analysis of phyto-constituents using various chromatographic and spectroscopic techniques; Pharmacological screening and Toxicological assessments both in vitro (cell-based assays) and in vivo (Animal studies).

Nitai C. Giri has completed his M. Sc. in chemistry from IIT Kharagpur, India. He had obtained his Ph.D. in Chemistry from the University of Massachusetts Amherst, USA. He did his postdoctoral research first at the University of Texas at San Antonio and then at Texas A&M University. He is now an assistant professor at the Central Institute of Petrochemical Engineering and Technology, Raipur.

Joanna M. Gonçalves has a BSc in Marine Biology and a MSc in Marine Biology and currently taking a PhD in Marine, Earth and Environmental Science at the Centre for Marine and Environmental Research (CIMA), with specialty in Marine Pollution and Ecotoxicology, at the University of Algarve.

Her research efforts are focused on the biological impacts that environmental concentrations of emerging contaminants, such as nanoplastics, metal nanoparticles and pharmaceuticals, can cause individually and in mixtures, in marine bivalves.

Soumaya Hajji is an Engineer in Geology from National Engineering School in Sfax (ENIS), Tunisia in 2000. She obtained her PhD in Modeling in Hydrogeology in 2015. She obtained her HDR in Environnemntal Hydrogeology and geo-Informatic in 2021. She is a researcher at geochemistry and hydrogeology, modelling and geostatistics at 'Water-Energy-Environment' Research Laboratory (LR3E) in Engineering School Sfax, Tunisia. Her research activities deal with geochemistry, modeling, analysis, optimisation, simulation of groundwater resources, groundwater quality and. She is an Associate Professor in Geology Departement in Faculty of Sciences of Sfax, Tunisia.

Md Saquib Hasnain (PhD) has over 10 years of research experience in the field of drug delivery and pharmaceutical formulation and analyses. Dr. Hasnain is especially proficient in the systematic development and characterization of diverse nanostructured drug delivery systems, controlled release drug delivery systems, bioenhanced drug delivery systems, polymeric composites, nanomaterials and nanocomposites employing Quality by Design approaches. He has contributed to over 60 publications in various high-impact peer-reviewed journals, 100 book chapters, and 20 books. He also serves as the associate editorial board member of the Recent Patent on Drug Delivery & Formulation journal, Academic Editor in Oxidative Medicine and Cellular Longevity journal, as a Review Editor in Drug Metabolism and Transport (specialty section of Frontiers in Pharmacology) and Editorial advisory board member in Materials Science in Energy Technologies. He is also serving as the reviewer of several prestigious journals. Overall, he has earned highly impressive publishing and cited record in Google Scholar (h-index: 29, i10-Index: 86). Hasnain has also participated and presented his research work at over ten conferences in India, and abroad. Prof. Hasnain was also the member of scientific societies of Royal Society of Chemistry, Great Britain, International Association of Environmental and Analytical Chemistry, Switzerland and Swiss Chemical Society, Switzerland.

Erangi Imasha Hewawasam Udullege is a master's graduate in the Engineering and Technology program at Sirindhorn International Institute of Technology (SIIT), Thammasat University, Thailand. Her thesis was on "Microplastics analysis in green mussels in Thailand". She is passionate about research related to emerging environmental contaminants, water treatment, solid waste management, life cycle analysis, and climate change.

Aayushi Kundu is currently working as a Research Scholar in the School of Chemistry and Biochemistry and JRF in TIET-Virginia Tech Center of Excellence in Emerging Materials. She has done her bachelors from Panjab University, Chandigarh, and Masters from Thapar Institute of Engineering and Technology, Patiala. She has worked in the field of photocatalysis and wastewater treatment during her master's thesis. She is currently working in the field of Graphene Quantum dots (GQDs) and Carbon Quantum dots (CQDs) and their sensing applications.

Carol Maione is a natural scientist, currently pursuing her doctoral degree in Industrial Engineering. Her doctoral research is focused on monitoring material flows and pollution cycles across the plastic industry-environment-society nexus, and investigating the role of technology in the transition to a circular economy for plastics. Previous works encompass exploration of plastic pollution in the African seas and related impacts on human communities and marine ecosystems, and quantitative analysis of microplastic accumulations in pelagic biota and their effects on species survival. Research interests include marine pollution, microplastics, earth observation, material flow analysis, ocean and coastal management.

Kaustubha Mohanty is currently Professor at the Department of Chemical Engineering and Head of School of Energy Science & Engineering, Indian Institute of Technology Guwahati. He obtained his PhD in 2006 from IIT Kharagpur and had post-doctoral stints at Ben-Gurion University, Israel and Mc-Master University, Canada. His research interest includes pyrolysis of biomass, biofuels, heterogeneous catalysis, microalgae-based biofuels, membrane-based separations and wastewater treatment process. He is a Fellow of Royal Society of Chemistry, UK, Institute of Engineers, India and Biotech Research Society of India.

Bupe Getrude Mwanza has over 10 years of experience in the Higher Education Sector. She has practical experience in teaching and learning, academic administration, research, and quality assurance in the Higher Education Sector. She has teaching and learning experience in Zambia, Zimbabwe and South Africa. Bupe has a Bachelor of Science in Production Management, Master of Engineering in Manufacturing Systems and Operations Management and PhD in Engineering Management. Bupe's research interests are in, solid waste management, supply-chain management, business systems and system dynamics. She has published in international journals and presented several papers in, countries such as Zambia, Zimbabwe, South Africa, Ghana, Colombia, Singapore, Malaysia, Indonesia, Macao, Thailand, India, Austria and South Korea.

Justine Nathan has a bachelor's degree from the University of the West of England, Bristol (UWE) in Conservation Biology BSc (Hons) . She has a Master Degree on Marine Biology of the University of the Algarve (Portugal). She has worked with impacts of microplastics on fish in Bermuda and is now working with the PlasticSea Project to assess the levels of microplastics in sediment, water and organisms along the coast of Portugal.

Bhanja Prasad Patro is currently working as Director & Head at Central Institute of Petrochemical Engineering & Technology (CIPET) a Government of India Premier Institution. He has 30 years of experience in polymer technology field providing training, consultancy, product & process development, Testing & Quality control of plastics materials & products as per National & International standards,

S. Senthilmurugan is currently a professor at the Department of Chemical Engineering, Indian Institute of Technology Guwahati, India. He obtained his Ph. D from the Indian Institute of Technology Delhi, India in the year 2005. He has eight years of industrial research experience focusing on water and wastewater treatment, industrial process water, sustainable water recycles power, renewable and oil & gas sector. His research interest includes microplastics identification and removal, water management for oil and gas upstream, smart Water grid, Waste to Energy, novel desalination technologies, energy storage, smart microgrids, air purification. He has executed more than 30 research projects and filed 19 patent application (5 granted).

Naveenkumar Ashok Yaranal is a PhD student in the Department of Chemical Engineering, Indian Institute of Technology Guwahati, India. He obtained his M.Tech degree in Chemical Engineering from Manipal Institute of technology, Manipal, India in the year 2016. His research interest includes desalination, membrane technology, wastewater treatment, heterogeneous catalyst, biodiesel and microplastics identification and removal.

Huadong Zang works as an associate professor at China Agricultural University (CAU) since 2019. Before joining CAU, he obtained PhD at the University of Goettingen in 2018 and works as a PostDoc at Bangor University. He has wide experience in agronomy and soil science, and extensive experience in 13C natural abundance techniques and multiple stable/radioactive isotope (13C, 14C, 15N, 18O) labeling approaches. His past research focused on N and C cycles in the plant-soil system, specifically, how N fertilization, temperature, and crop management influence C sequestration, organic matter stabilization, turnover, and priming effects in the agroecosystem. His current research interests in investigating C and nutrients cycling, as well as the plant-plant and plant-microbial-soil interactions in diversified cropping systems and agroecology. In his work he uses a combination of methods including on-station and on-farm experiments, isotopic labeling, zymography, and molecular techniques.

Index

N

O

P

R

S

T

U

V

W

Recommended Reference Books

IGI Global's reference books are available in three unique pricing formats: Print Only, E-Book Only, or Print + E-Book.

Shipping fees may apply.

www.igi-global.com

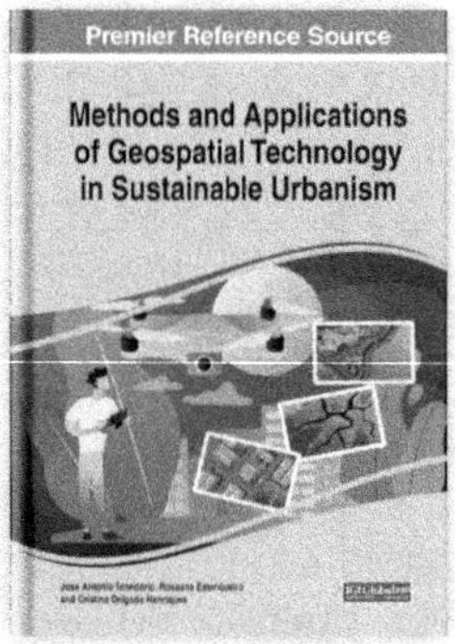

ISBN: 9781799822493
EISBN: 9781799822516
© 2021; 684 pp.
List Price: US$ **195**

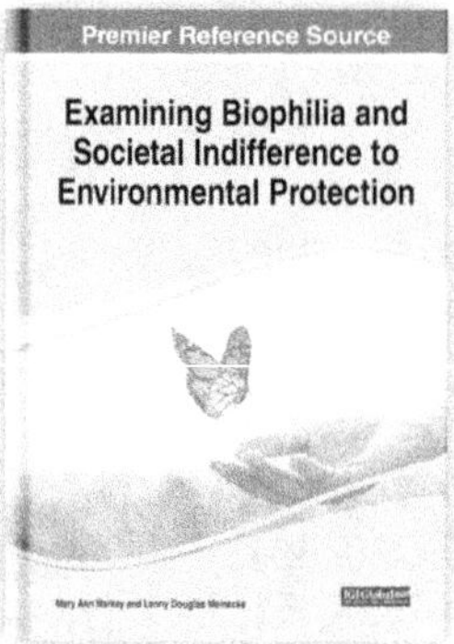

ISBN: 9781799844082
EISBN: 9781799844099
© 2021; 279 pp.
List Price: US$ **195**

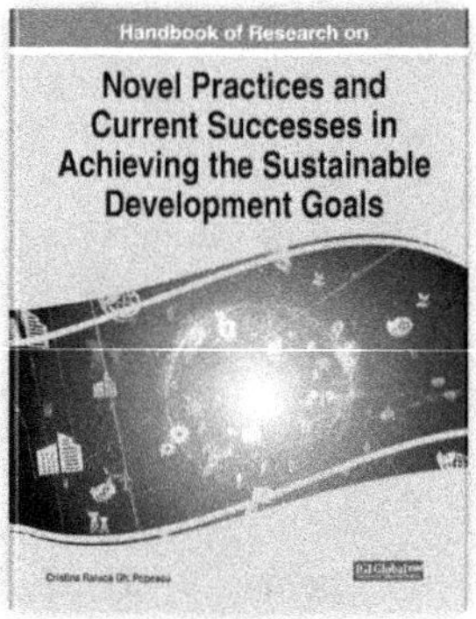

ISBN: 9781799884262
EISBN: 9781799884286
© 2021; 461 pp.
List Price: US$ **295**

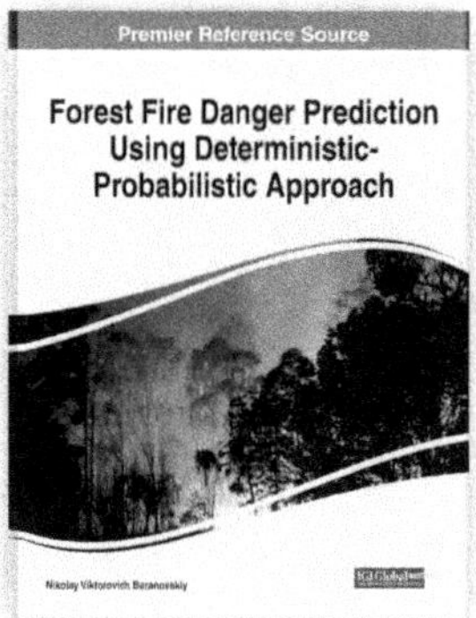

ISBN: 9781799872504
EISBN: 9781799872528
© 2021; 297 pp.
List Price: US$ **195**

ISBN: 9781799875123
EISBN: 9781799875192
© 2021; 416 pp.
List Price: US$ **295**

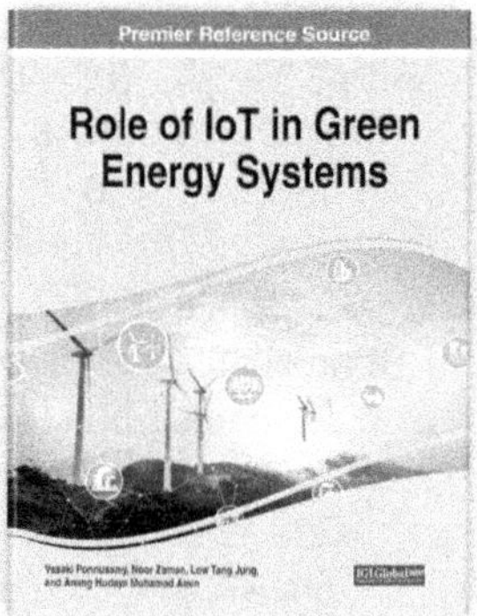

ISBN: 9781799867098
EISBN: 9781799867111
© 2021; 405 pp.
List Price: US$ **195**

Do you want to stay current on the latest research trends, product announcements, news, and special offers?
Join IGI Global's mailing list to receive customized recommendations, exclusive discounts, and more.
Sign up at: **www.igi-global.com/newsletters.**

Publisher of Timely, Peer-Reviewed Inclusive Research Since 1988

IGI Global
PUBLISHER of TIMELY KNOWLEDGE

www.igi-global.com Sign up at www.igi-global.com/newsletters facebook.com/igiglobal twitter.com/igiglobal linkedin.com/igiglobal

www.ingramcontent.com/pod-product-compliance
Lightning Source LLC
LaVergne TN
LVHW060356300926
849162LV00006B/1280
* 9 7 8 1 7 9 9 8 9 7 2 3 1 *